PROGRESS IN BRAIN RESEARCH

VOLUME 56

BRAIN PHOSPHOPROTEINS, CHARACTERIZATION
AND FUNCTION

Recent volumes in PROGRESS IN BRAIN RESEARCH

PROGRESS IN BRAIN RESEARCH

VOLUME 56

# BRAIN PHOSPHOPROTEINS
## Characterization and Function

Proceedings of a Workshop at the State University of Utrecht, September 1981

edited by

Willem Hendrik GISPEN

*Professor of Molecular Neurobiology, Rudolf Magnus Institute for Pharmacology and Institute of Molecular Biology, Padualaan 8, 3508 TB Utrecht (The Netherlands)*

and

Aryeh ROUTTENBERG

*Professor of Psychology and Neurobiology, Cresap Neuroscience Laboratory, 3021 Sheridan Road, Evanston, IL 60201 (U.S.A.)*

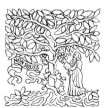

ELSEVIER BIOMEDICAL PRESS
Amsterdam – New York
1982

PUBLISHED BY:
ELSEVIER BIOMEDICAL PRESS
MOLENWERF 1, P.O. BOX 1527
AMSTERDAM, THE NETHERLANDS

SOLE DISTRIBUTORS FOR THE U.S.A. AND CANADA:
ELSEVIER NORTH-HOLLAND INC.
52 VANDERBILT AVENUE
NEW YORK, NY 10017, U.S.A.

**Library of Congress Cataloging in Publication Data**

Main entry under title:

Brain phosphoproteins.

   (Progress in brain research ; v. 56)
   Bibliography: p.
   Includes indexes.
   1. Brain chemistry--Congresses. 2. Phosphoproteins--
Congresses. I. Gispen, Willem Hendrik. II. Routtenberg,
Aryeh. III. Series. [DNLM: 1. Brain chemistry--
Congresses. 2. Nerve tissue proteins--Congresses.
3. Phosphoproteins--Congresses. W1 PR667J v. 56 / WL 300
B8138 1981]
QP376.P7 vol. 56  612'.82s [599.01'88]    82-11501
ISBN 0-444-80412-9 (U.S.)

PRINTED IN BELGIUM

# Preface

This volume contains the contributions of participants in a workshop on "Brain Phosphoproteins: Characterization and Function", which took place at the State University of Utrecht in September 1981.

The impetus for this meeting was based on our belief that the field had reached sufficient maturity to warrant a monograph devoted to this topic. Moreover, the rapid growth of information signalled to us increasing interest in brain phosphoproteins. The time was indeed auspicious, then, to inventory our field and discuss future directions.

The chapters contained in this volume document the progress that has, in fact, been made in the past 3–5 years in the identification, characterization and in some cases purification of several different brain phosphoproteins.

The discussions at the workshop were vigorous and prolonged, leading to a considerable interchange of ideas. The value of having the workshop directed at extended discussion will doubtless provide benefit to the participants' research enterprise.

We wish to acknowledge the encouragement and support provided by Dr. David de Wied. We also wish to thank the participants for their enthusiastic participation at the workshop and their cooperation in the final steps of preparing this volume. We like to thank Drs. Victor Wiegant and Henk Zwiers for taking care of the local organization and Miss Lia Claessens for her outstanding success in running the symposium desk. Finally, the meeting would not have been possible without the support of the Dutch Government, the University of Utrecht and the Dr. Saal van Swanenberg Foundation.

We note with sadness the passing of Malcolm Weller, an early and important contributor to the brain phosphoprotein field. We feel that the contributions in this volume have grown out of his pioneering studies.

The phosphorylation of brain proteins provides an interface between the neurophysiological signalling capacity of the brain and the metabolism of nerve cells. As such it represents a critical step in relating brain function to brain chemistry. The present volume, it is hoped, by summarizing much of the available evidence, will provide a basis for the accelerated development of the functional study of brain phosphoproteins.

*November 1981*                                                      Utrecht, Willem Hendrik Gispen
                                                                      Evanston, Aryeh Routtenberg

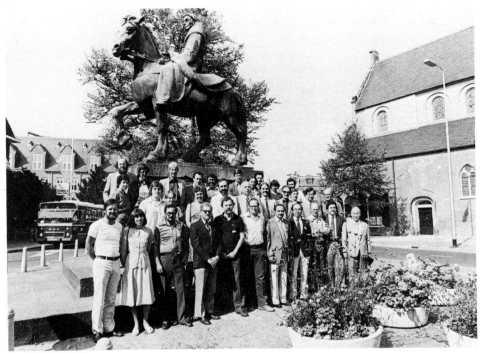

# Participants

Aloyo, V.J.    Div. of Molecular Neurobiology, Institute of Molecular Biology and Rudolf Magnus Institute for Pharmacology, State University of Utrecht, Padualaan 8, 3508 TB Utrecht (The Netherlands)

Bär, P.R.    Institute of Molecular Biology and Rudolf Magnus Institute for Pharmacology, State University of Utrecht, Padualaan 8, 3508 TB Utrecht (The Netherlands)

Baudry, M.    Psychobiology Department, University of California Irvine, Ca 92717 (U.S.A.)

Bowling, Allen    Dept. of Neurology, Yale Medical School, 333 Cedar Street, New Haven, CN 06510 (U.S.A.)

Browning, M.    Dept. of Pharmacology, Yale University, School of Medicine, Cedar Street 333, New Haven, CN 06510 (U.S.A.)

Carlin, Richard K.    Dept. of Cell Biology, The Rockefeller University, New York, NY (U.S.A.)

Cheung, Wai Yiu    Dept. of Biochemistry, St. Jude Children's Research Hospital and the University of Tennessee Center for the Health Sciences, Memphis, TN 38101 (U.S.A.)

Cohen, Rochelle S.    Dept. of Anatomy, University of Illinois at the Medical Center, Chicago, IL 60612 (U.S.A.)

DeLorenzo, Robert J.    Dept. of Neurology, Yale Medical School, 333 Cedar Street, New Haven. CN 06510 (U.S.A.)

Edwards, P.M.    Div. of Molecular Neurobiology, Institute of Molecular Biology, State University of Utrecht, Padualaan 8, 3508 TB Utrecht (The Netherlands)

Ehrlich, Yigal H.    Dept. of Psychiatry, Medical Alumni Building, University of Vermont, College of Medicine, Burlington, VE 05405 (U.S.A.)

Farber, Debora B.    Jules Stein Eye Institute, UCLA School of Medicine, Los Angeles, CA 90024 (U.S.A.)

Frankena, H.    Div. of Molecular Neurobiology, Institute of Molecular Biology, State University of Utrecht, Padualaan 8, 3508 TB Utrecht (The Netherlands)

Garfield, Mark K.    The Neuroscience Unit, Dept. of Psychiatry and Pharmacology, University of Vermont, College of Medicine, Burlington, VE 05405 (U.S.A.)

Gispen, W.H.    Division of Molecular Neurobiology, Institute of Molecular Biology and Rudolf Magnus Institute for Pharmacology, State University of Utrecht, Padualaan 8, 3508 TB Utrecht (The Netherlands)

Goldering, James    Dept. of Neurology, Yale Medical School, 333 Cedar Street, New Haven, CN 06510 (U.S.A.)

Gonzalez, Basilio    Dept. of Neurology, Yale Medical School, 333 Cedar Street, New Haven, CN 06510 (U.S.A.)

Grab, Dennis J.    Dept. of Biochemistry, Ilrad, Nairobi (Kenya)

Graber, Stephen G.    The Neuroscience Research Unit, Dept. of Psychiatry and Biochemistry, University of Vermont, College of Medicine, Burlington, VE 05405 (U.S.A.)

Guy, Paul S.    Dept. of Biochemistry, University of Dundee, Medical Sciences Institute, Dundee, DD1 4HN (Scotland)

Hardie, D. Grahame    Dept. of Biochemistry, University of Dundee, Medical Sciences Institute, Dundee DD1 4HN (Scotland)

Harrison, Janie J.    Cancer Center and Dept. of Molecular Biology, Northwestern University Medical School, 303 East Chicago Avenue, Chicago, IL 60611 (U.S.A.)

Hawkes, Richard    Friedrich Miescher-Institut, P.O. Box 273 CH-4002, Basel (Switzerland)

Heron, Davis    Dept. of Isotope Research, The Weizmann Institute of Science, Rehovot 76100 (Israel)

Hershkowitz, Moshe    Dept. of Isotope Research, The Weizmann Institute of Science, Rehovot 76100 (Israel)

Jacobson, Ronald    Dept. of Neurology, Yale Medical School, 333 Cedar Street New Haven, CN 06510 (U.S.A.)

Jolles, J.    Division of Molecular Neurobiology, Rudolf Magnus Institute for Pharmacology, and Institute of Molecular Biology, State University of Utrecht, Padualaan 8, 3508 TB Utrecht (The Netherlands)

Jungmann, Richard A.    Cancer Center and Dept. of Molecular Biology, Northwestern University Medical School, 303 East Chicago Avenue, Chicago, IL 60611 (U.S.A.)

| | |
|---|---|
| Kaibuchi, Kozo | Dept. of Biochemistry, Kobe University, School of Medicine, Kobe 650 (Japan) |
| Kikkawa, Ushio | Dept. of Biochemistry, Kobe University, School of Medicine, Kobe 650 (Japan) |
| Kleine, Leonard P. | Animal and Cell Physiocology Group, Biological Sciences M54, National Research Council of Canada, Ottawa, Ont. K1A OR6 (Canada) |
| Lee, Seung-Ki | Cancer Center and Dept. of Molecular Biology, Northwestern University Medical School, 303 East Chicago Avenue, Chicago, IL 60611 (U.S.A.) |
| Lenox, Robert M. | The Neuroscience Research Unit, Dept. of Psychiatry, University of Vermont, College of Medicine, Burlington, VE 05405 (U.S.A.) |
| Lopes da Silva, F.H. | Dept. of Animal Physiology, University of Amsterdam, Kruislaan 320, 1098 SM Amsterdam (The Netherlands) |
| Lynch, G. | Psychobiology Department, University of California, Irvine, CA 92717 (U.S.A.) |
| Mahler, Henry R. | Dept. of Chemistry and the Molecular, Cellular and Developmental Biology Program, Indiana University, Bloomington. IN 47405 (U.S.A.) |
| Matsubara, Tsukasa | Dept. of Biochemistry, Kobe University School of Medicine, Kobe 650 (Japan) |
| Matus, Andrew | Friedrich Miescher-Institut, P.O. Box 273, CH-4002, Basel (Switzerland) |
| Miles, Michael F. | Cancer Center and Dept. of Molecular Biology, Northwestern University Medical School, 303 East Chicago Avenue, Chicago, IL 60611 (U.S.A.) |
| Milkowski, Deborah | Cancer Center and Dept. of Molecular Biology, Northwestern Univ. Medical School, 303 East Chicago Avenue, Chicago, IL 60611 (U.S.A.) |
| Minakuchi, Ryoji | Dept. of Biochemistry, Kobe University School of Medicine Kobe 650 (Japan) |
| Naito, Shigetaka | Mental Health Research Institute and the Department of Psychiatry and Pharmacology, The University of Michigan, Ann Arbor, MI 48109 (U.S.A.) |
| Ng, Meelian | Friedrich Miescher-Institut, P.O. Box 273, CH-4002, Basel (Switzerland) |
| Niday, E. | Friedrich Miescher-Institut, P.O. Box 273, CH-4002 Basel (Switzerland) |
| Nishizuka, Yasutomi | Dept. of Biochemistry, Kobe University School of Medicine, Kobe 650 (Japan) |
| Oestreicher, A.B. | Division of Molecular Neurobiology, Rudolf Magnus Institute for Pharmacology and Institute of Molecular Biology, State university of Utrecht, Padualaan 8, 3508 TB Utrecht (The Netherlands) |
| Petrali, Elena H. | Dept. of Physiology, College of Medicine, University of Saskatchewan, Saskatoon, S7N OWO (Canada) |
| Ratner, Nancy | Dept. of Chemistry and the Molecular, Cellular and Development Biology Program, Indiana University. Bloomington, IN 47405 (U.S.A.) |
| Roberts, Sidney | Dept. Biol. Chemistry, School of Medicine and Brain Research Institute, University of California Center for the Health Sciences Los Angeles, CA 90024 (U.S.A.) |
| Rodnight, Richard | Dept. of Biochemistry, Institute of Psychiatry De Crespigny Park, London SE5 8AF (England) |
| Routtenberg, Aryeh, | Cresap Neuroscience Laboratory, 2021 Sheridan Road, Northwestern University, Evanston, IL 60201 (U.S.A.) |
| Samuel, David | Dept. of Isotope Research, The Weizmann Institute of Science, Rehovot, 76100 (Israel) |
| Sano, Kimihiko | Dept. of Biochemistry, Kobe University, School of Medicine Kobe 650 (Japan) |
| Schlichter, Doris J. | Dept. of Biochemistry, University of Tennessee Knoxville, TN 37916 (U.S.A.) |
| Schotman, P. | Div. of Molecular Neurobiology, Institute of Molecular Biology, State University of Utrecht, Padualaan 8, 3508 TB Utrecht (The Netherlands) |
| Schrama, L.H. | Div. of Molecular Neurobiology, Institute of Molecular Biology, State University of Utrecht, Padualaan 8, 3508 TB Utrecht (The Netherlands) |
| Schweppe, John S. | Cancer Center and Dept. of Molecular Biology, Northwestern University Medical School, 303 East Chicago Avenue, Chicago IL 60611 (U.S.A.) |
| Shinitzky, Meir | Dept. Of Membrane Research, The Weizmann Institute of Science, Rehovot 76100 (Israel) |
| Siekevitz, Philip | Dept. of Cell Biology, The Rockefeller University, New York, NY (U.S.A.) |
| Sörensen, Roger G. | Dept. of Chemistry, Texas Christian University, Fort Worth, TX 76129 (U.S.A.) |
| Sulakhe, Prakash V. | Dept. of Physiology, College of Medicine, University of Saskatchewan, Saskatoon S7N OWO (Canada) |
| Takai, Yoshimi | Dept. of Biochemistry, Kobe University School of Medicine, Kobe 650 (Japan) |
| Thomas, G. | Friedrich Miescher Institut, P.O. Box 273, CH 4002 Basel (Switzerland) |
| Tielen, A.M. | Institute for Medical Physics, MFI-TNO, Da Costakade 45, 2861 PN Utrecht (The Netherlands) |
| Ueda, Tetsufumi | Mental Health Research Institue and the Department of Psychiatry and Pharmacology, The University of Michigan, Ann Arbor, MI 48109 (U.S.A.) |

Whittemore, Scott R.    The Neuroscience Research Unit, Dept. of Psychiatry and Physiology-Biophysics, University of Vermont, College of Medicine, Burlington, VE 05405 (U.S.A.)

Wiegant, V.M.    Rudolf Magnus Institute for Pharmacology, State University of Utrecht, Vondellaan 6, 3521 GD Utrecht (The Netherlands)

Yu, Binzu    Dept. of Biochemistry, Kobe University, School of Medicine, Kobe 650 (Japan)

Zwiers, H.    Div. of Molecular Neurobiology, Institute of Molecular Biology and Rudolf Magnus Institute for Pharmacology State University of Utrecht, Padualaan 8, 3508 TB Utrecht (The Netherlands)

# Contents

# Aspects of Protein Phosphorylation in the Nervous System with Particular Reference to Synaptic Transmission

RICHARD RODNIGHT

*Department of Biochemistry, Institute of Psychiatry,*
*De Crespigny Park, London SE5 8AF U.K.*

## INTRODUCTION

Few fields of biochemistry have seen such explosive progress in recent years as the one we are concerned with in this book. Some 15 years ago the phosphorylation of hydroxyamino acids in proteins was thought to be a relatively uncommon biochemical event, involving only a few acceptor proteins and catalysed by one or two protein kinase enzymes. Now we recognize several families of protein kinases dependent on a variety of co-factors, as well as kinases which on present evidence do not require an activating factor. Even more impressive is the very wide range of polypeptides now known to accept phosphate from ATP as a result of kinase action, a range that includes at least 25 enzymes and several structural proteins (Weller, 1979; Krebs and Beavo, 1979; Cohen, 1980). In the nervous system the great importance of this ubiquitous process of cellular control is demonstrated by numerous observations showing that structures derived from mammalian synapses are probably the richest and most diversified known source of protein phosphorylating systems (defined as complexes of protein kinase, acceptor protein and protein phosphatase). For recent reviews on various aspects of protein phosphorylation in neural tissue see Williams and Rodnight (1977), Greengard (1978), Kometiani et al. (1978), Routtenberg (1979), Rodnight (1979, 1980 a,b, 1981), Dunkley (1981) and Rodnight et al. (1982).

In parallel with the discovery of the great diversity of phosphoproteins in mammalian cells, and particularly in cells of neural origin, has come a revolution in techniques for detecting and characterizing the polypeptide chains of proteins on a micro scale. I refer to the development of powerful two-dimensional electrophoretic methods for the analysis of cellular proteins. At a recent EMBO workshop the possibility was seriously discussed of eventually making by this technique a complete catalogue of all animal cell proteins (Clark, 1981). The formidable nature of such a task is indicated by the fact that two-dimensional studies have already shown that membrance structures from *E. coli* possess in excess of 600 distinct polypeptides. In mammalian tissues the number is believed to be of the order of 10 000 in given cell type, of which many are presumably located in the plasma membrane. Such knowledge is of great significance for students of the nervous system, where the limiting cell membrane is a key structure for functional processes. As to how many neuronal membrane polypeptides are normally phosphorylated, clearly we have little idea at present, but the number must greatly exceed the 20 or so major phosphate acceptors described in the literature; a conservative guess would suggest several hundred. Moreover, many of these minor phosphoproteins may be characteristic of specific neuronal cell types and therefore only appear as minor in heterogeneous membrane preparations made from whole tissue.

The reason why synaptic structures have evolved such a complex array of protein phosphorylating systems is presumably related to a great complexity in the molecular events concerned with neuronal communication. In fact, as has been pointed out elsewhere (Greengard, 1978; Neary et al., 1981) the post-translational modification of membrane-located proteins in synapses represents an attractive molecular mechanism for the modulation of both short- and long-term aspects of synaptic transmission. This general statement seems particularly true of protein phosphorylation, since this is a readily reversible process that occurs rapidly with a high degree of specificity, and can reasonably be assumed to lead to conformational change and therefore to modulation of membrane functions with the potential for signal amplification; moreover through the control of protein dephosphorylation reversibility can conceivably be delayed and thus lead to long-lasting modifications in membrane properties.

In the present Chapter I shall give a broad overview of certain aspects of the subject, based mainly on recent work from my own laboratory, but also filling in on certain facets that are not covered in other chapters.

## SUBCELLULAR STUDIES

It is logical to start with these aspects since only at the subcellular level is the full potential of the tissue's phosphorylating systems displayed. The general approach of incubating subcellular fractions of brain tissue with $[\gamma-^{32}P]$ATP and observing the transfer of phosphate to protein as a result of endogenous protein kinase activity is well known and widely used. However, strictly speaking this approach does not directly measure protein kinase activity: tissue fractions invariably contain protein phosphatase activity, and the observed incorporation is therefore compounded of the net transfer of phosphate to vacant sites and the turnover of previously phosphorylated sites. Since dephosphorylation is rate-limiting in turnover (Weller and Rodnight, 1971) the speed and magnitude of $^{32}P$ incorporated into a polypeptide depends upon the extent to which it has been dephosphorylated during tissue fractionation, as well as on the activity state of its associated phosphatase. A further complication is the very rapid breakdown of ATP in the reaction mixture catalysed by ATPase activity which may result in the hydrolysis of the major part of the donor within seconds of initiating the reaction (Wiegant et al., 1978). Clearly these considerations limit the extent to which data from this approach can be interpreted in terms of the kinetics of protein kinase action. In theory the most meaningful results should be obtained from reaction conditions using very short (e.g. <1 sec) incubation times and a high ratio of ATP to tissue protein. In practice most workers compromise and use low ATP concentrations (<20 $\mu$M) in order to maintain an acceptable specific radioactivity and incubation times of 15–60 sec.

Apart from these methodological considerations concerning the labelling reaction, there are several cogent reasons for questioning the physiological significance of endogenous protein phosphorylation in membrane fragments that require discussion.

(1) *All synaptic membrane preparations are contaminated to some extent with non-synaptic structures*

The question of the purity of membrane preparations putatively derived from synapses is a vexed one, but there is nevertheless compelling evidence to suggest that with few exceptions the main phosphate acceptors in typical preparations are located in fragments of synaptic plasma membranes. Some of this evidence is mentioned later and for a more detailed discussion see Sörensen et al. (1981) and Rodnight et al. (1982).

*(2) Cell disruption may lead to association of kinases and phosphatases with unphysiological protein substrates*

Matus et al. (1980) have drawn attention to this problem with evidence that certain cytoplasmic proteins tend to stick to the postsynaptic densities after cell disruption. It has also been investigated in another tissue (Brunner et al., 1978). However, artifactual associations of kinases with unphysiological substrates during preparative procedures are likely to be reversed by exposure of the membrane fragments to solutions of high ionic strength, and as will be mentioned later, the majority of protein phosphorylating systems are not affected by such treatment.

*(3) Protein dephosphorylation and proteolysis may occur during preparation*

It must be assumed that extensive protein dephosphorylation of membrane proteins occurs during subcellular fractionation and it is unfortunate that no satisfactory inhibitor of this process is available that does not also seriously interfere with fractionation procedures. Proteolysis during preparation is a serious risk and has hardly been considered, except by Burke and DeLorenzo (1981) with respect to cytosolic phosphorylating systems.

*(4) Redistribution of regulatory factors may occur during preparation*

The possibility of a redistribution of regulatory subunits of cyclic AMP-dependent protein kinases occurring during preparation needs to be considered seriously, although evidence from the erythrocyte membrane suggests that the regulatory subunit of the membrane kinase is more tightly bound than the catalytic subunit (Rubin et al., 1972).

*(5) ATP has access to the external membrane surface during incubation*

Current evidence from experiments with intact synaptosomes supports the conclusion that virtually all of the cyclic AMP (cAMP)-dependent phosphorylating activity is located intra-terminally, indicating no support for the existence of ecto-kinases dependent on cyclic AMP (Weller, 1977; Sörensen et al., 1981; Rodnight et al., 1982; see also below). However, most of the $Ca^{2+}$-calmodulin-dependent activity appears to be non-occluded in synaptosomal preparations and must therefore be located either in the postsynaptic densities (for which there is considerable evidence) or on the external surface of the terminal membrane. The fact that ATP is released from synaptic terminals (Potter and White, 1980), either as a purinergic transmitter, or along with other transmitters, indicates that the concept of ecto-kinase activity may have functional implications. There are several reports of ecto-kinase acitivity occurring in other tissues (e.g. Kang et al., 1978).

*(6) Vesicle formation from membrane fragments may limit access of ATP to sites of enzyme action*

Electron microscopy of typical preparations suggests that vesiculation of the membrane fragments does indeed occur (Jones and Matus, 1974; Rodnight, 1981). Probably this results in some restriction of the access of ATP to all sites since it is well known that detergents (e.g. Triton X-100) increase the activity of many phosphorylating systems, particularly those dependent on cAMP. However, detergents do not uncover activity towards substrates not seen under normal conditions, although not all the cAMP-dependent systems are equally affected. For example in our experience, 0.5% Triton X-100 trebles the cAMP-stimulated activity towards an acceptor identified as an autophosphorylated regulatory subunit of a cAMP-dependent protein kinase (mol. wt. 52 000 — see Table II) while only having a minimal effect on the activity of other cAMP-dependent systems. Moreover the $Ca^{2+}$-activated systems are either unaffected or inhibited by detergents. Thus for most purposes little is gained by including detergents in the reaction mixture.

It can be seen therefore that considerable caution is needed in interpreting the results of endogenous protein phosphorylation reactions. However, the approach is clearly an essential complement to studies of cell containing tissues in vitro and to in vivo studies, and so we need to consider, on another level, some further questions that need answers before physiologically meaningful conclusions may be drawn. These are listed in Table I. I will return to consider the limited progress that has been made on these problems from my point of view after describing our own results, but it should be pointed out that several authors in this book deal in depth with special aspects of these questions.

TABLE I

SOME QUESTIONS RAISED BY THE PHENOMENON OF INTRINSIC
PROTEIN PHOSPHORYLATION IN SYNAPTOSOMAL MEMBRANES

1. Topography within membrane structure: are the acceptor polypeptides and/or their associated enzymes integral or peripheral? How fluid is the enzyme substrate interaction?

2. Sub-synaptic location of acceptors: are they present in the terminal membrane and/or the postsynaptic membrane or the postsynaptic densities?

3. How many distinct types of kinase are involved? What is the status of kinase activity independent of cAMP or $Ca^{2+}$-calmodulin?

4. What is the specificity, if any, to neuronal systems utilizing different neurotransmitters?

*Methods*

*Tissue preparation*

A modification of the method of Jones and Matus (1974), omitting $Ca^{2+}$ from the sucrose solutions, was used to prepare membrane fragments from rat (adult Wistar, both sexes) tissue. In view of its heterogenous character and following Dunkley (1981) I prefer to refer to this preparation as one of "synaptosomal membrane fragments" rather than the usual "synaptic plasma membrane fragments". The whole of the forebrain was taken, excluding the central structures (thalamus, septum and mid brain); the preparation is therefore predominantly derived from cerebral cortex tissue, but includes the hippocampus and part of the striatum. Animals were killed by decapitation; tissue was dissected within 1 min and homogenized within 5 min of death. After dilution and spinning out, membrane fragments from the gradient received an additional centrifugal wash with 4 mM imidazole HCl (pH 7.0) to decrease contamination with endogenous $Ca^{2+}$. For further details see Holmes and Rodnight (1981). Preparations were stored at $-20°C$ in 50% (v/v) glycerol in 2 mM imidazole HCl (pH 7.0) at a protein concentration of 5 mg/ml. Present evidence, gathered from 3 years experience, indicates that these storage conditions maintain full phosphorylating activity, including sensitivity to cAMP, $Ca^{2+}$ and calmodulin, for periods of at least 12 months. However, I accept that it should not be concluded that glycerol-stored membrane fragments necessarily possess identical properties to fresh unfrozen material.

*Phosphorylation reactions*

For studying cAMP-dependent reactions the following medium (final volume 80 $\mu$l) was used: 30 mM Tris–HCl (pH 7.4 at 37°C), 1 mM $MgSO_4$, 0.25 mM EGTA, 20 $\mu$M [$\gamma$-

$^{32}$P]ATP, 100 $\mu$g of membrane protein, with or without 50 $\mu$M cAMP. For Ca$^{2+}$-dependent reactions the same medium was used, but with 0.5 mM CaCl$_2$ and 4 $\mu$g of calmodulin substituted for cAMP. The ratio of ATP (nmole) to protein (mg) was therefore 16. Incubation time was 10 sec and the reactions were always started by the rapid injection of the membrane preparation into the rapidly agitated preincubated reaction mixture at 37°C. Termination was achieved by the rapid injection of the usual SDS–mercaptoethanol "stopping solution" (see Holmes and Rodnight, 1981). After solubilisation the samples were not boiled; electrophoresis was normally done the following day after storage at 5°C. These are the standard conditions referred to in the figure legends; variations are indicated in the text.

*Gel electrophoresis*

A discontinuous polyacrylamide slab gel procedure was used essentially as described earlier (Holmes and Rodnight, 1981). The length of the resolving gel was 13.5 cm. Because single concentration gels of 10% acrylamide or higher were unsuitable for resolving the high molecular weight acceptors and because gels of concentration <10% invariably led to 'bunching' of the polypeptides in the range 45 K–55 K (K = 10$^3$), several attempts were made, within the 13.5 cm dimension, to develop a gradient system capable of separating the whole range of the main phosphate acceptors in the preparations. The nearest approach to this aim was obtained with exponential gradient gels of 6–17% acrylamide, but resolution in the range 45 K–55 K dalton was still inconsistent (for a reasonably successful separation using this system see Fig. 11). For most work therefore single concentration gels of 5% or 7% acrylamide were used for the higher molecular weight polypeptides (>100 K) and 10% gels for the remainder. The latter were excellent for resolving the range 40 K–80 K, but failed to resolve the high and very low (<20 K) molecular weight components.

Apparent molecular weights were derived from relative mobilities determined in gels of 6 different acrylamide concentrations. The following proteins were used as standards: apoferritin (450 K), myosin (200 K), phosphorylase *b* (197 K), bovine serum albumin (68 K), ovalbumin (45 K) and in some cases the "30" band (27.5 K) of the rat heart preparation of Giometti et al. (1980). (This preparation was also used as a source of myosin). Ferguson plots were constructed and used to calculate free mobilities of all standards and acceptors (Gower and Rodnight, 1982). Of the standards only apoferritin gave a deviant free mobility; values for phosphorylated polypeptides are given in Table I, where it can be seen that the high molecular weight acceptors (>250 K but with the exception of O$_{3b}$cAMP) and one other ($\gamma_5$) possess free mobilities that are clearly lower than the others. This means that molecular weight estimates for these acceptors are particularly approximate and in the case of O$_1$, O$_2$ and O$_{3a}$ only minimal estimates can be quoted. The present estimates, however, may reasonably be considered more realistic than those quoted formerly by our group (Rodnight, 1980a,b, 1981; Holmes and Rodnight 1981), and which are given in Table II for comparison.

*Calmodulin* was prepared by the method of Walsh and Stevens (1978), omitting the final DEAE cellulose column. The product yielded a single band on electrophoresis.

### General characteristics of protein phosphorylating systems in synaptosomal membranes

Under this heading I refer primarily to the pattern of phosphorylated acceptors in our standard preparation of predominantly cerebral cortex tissue from the rat, as revealed by our methods. It is important to emphasize this point, because in some respects our results differ from those of other laboratories (e.g. Ehrlich et al., 1977a; Walter et al., 1978; De Blas et al.,

6

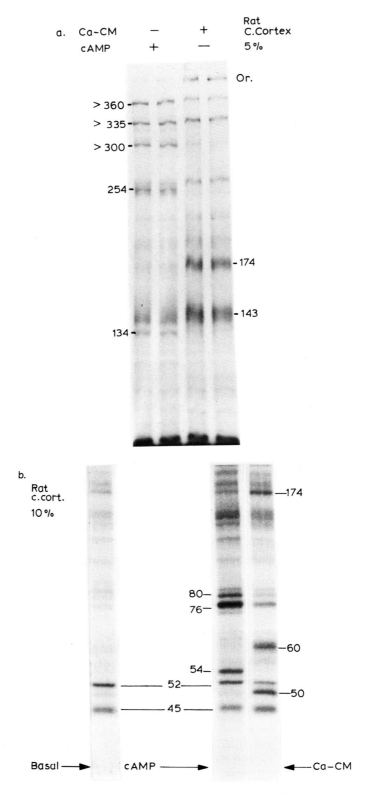

Fig. 1. Typical radioautographs of gels prepared from membrane fragments made from adult rat cerebral cortex labelled under standard conditions. Molecular weights are $\times 10^{-3}$. (a) High molecular acceptors separated on a 5% gel (basal phosphorylation not shown); (b) lower molecular weight acceptors separated on a 10% gel. In both cases 20 $\mu$M [$\gamma$-$^{32}$P]ATP of specific radioactivity around 1000 cpm/pmole was used.

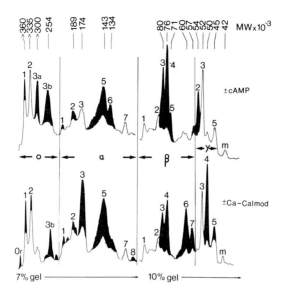

Fig. 2. Composite densitometric scans (expanded × 3) of radioautographs of gels prepared from membrane fragments from adult rat cerebral cortex and labelled under standard conditions. In this experiment a 6–17 % exponential gradient gel was used to separate the high molecular weight acceptors. The ATP concentration was 20 $\mu$M for both cAMP and Ca²⁺-calmodulin systems. The black areas indicate stimulation by activating factors and were derived by superimposing scans from membrane fragments labelled under basal conditions and run in parallel.

1979; Routtenberg, 1979). Undoubtedly the main factors contributing to these differences are variations in procedure, but it is also becoming clear that phosphorylation patterns are not necessarily constant between different brain regions and between species.

Representative radioautographs and densitometric scans are illustrated in Figs. 1 and 2, and Table II summarizes the main characteristics of the typical pattern. It must be recognized that two-dimensional analysis may eventually show that many of these phosphorylated bands are complex. The designation follows previous practice (Rodnight, 1979) and will be used in this text except for $\beta_3$ and $\beta_4$, now generally known through Greengard's extensive work (Greengard, 1978) as proteins Ia and Ib (or collectively as protein I), and $\gamma_5$, which I will refer to as B-50, the term coined by the Utrecht group (Zwiers et al., 1980).

Considering first the relatively high molecular weight acceptors (O and $\alpha$ regions) phosphorylated by cAMP-dependent kinase activity, only $O_{3a}$ has been tentatively identified. It appears to correspond exactly to a polypeptide described in bovine and rat preparations of brain by Lohmann et al. (1980) and identified by these authors as a microtubular-associated protein (MAP$_2$). In our electrophoresis system it also co-migrates with MAP$_2$ (H. Gower, unpublished observations), occurs at a high level in the cytosol and perhaps most significantly is readily extracted from membrane preparations by exposure to high salt solutions, both before and after labelling. It seems likely therefore that this acceptor is only peripherally associated with membranes and its presence there may be considered an artifact of subcellular fractionation. By contrast two other major acceptors in this region, $O_{3b}$ (cAMP) and $\alpha_5$, together with their associated kinases are not significantly extracted by salt and may therefore represent tightly bound proteins, integral to the membrane structure. At present there are no clues as to their identity, but it is of interest to note that $\alpha_5$ is absent from preparations made from cerebellum (Fig. 3). It corresponds on the Coomassie Blue stained gels to a minor polypeptide, that always

## TABLE II

### PROTEIN ACCEPTORS FOR ENDOGENOUS KINASE ACTIVITY IN SYNAPTOSOMAL MEMBRANES

| Designation | Present estimate of mol. wt. $(\times 10^{-3})$[a] | Previous estimate of mol. wt. $(\times 10^{-3})$[b] | Free mobility in polyacrylamide[c] | Activating factor for phosphorylation | Percentage remaining after high salt wash[d] | Occurrence in cerebellar membrane fragments[e] | Comments |
|---|---|---|---|---|---|---|---|
| Ca-orig | >400 | Not determined | — | $Ca^{2+}$, calmod. | Uncertain | Uncertain | Scarcely enters 5% gel (see Fig. 1a) |
| $O_1$ | >360 | 209 | 165 | cAMP, $Ca^{2+}$, calmod. | 40–60 | + | Kinase has low sensitivity to cAMP |
| $O_2$ | >335 | 204 | 206 | $Ca^{2+}$, calmod. | 70 | +++ | — |
| $O_{3a}$ | >300 | 198 | 217 | cAMP only | >15 | Absent | Identified in bovine brain as microtubular associated protein ($MAP_2$) |
| $O_{3b}$ (cAMP) | 254 | 195 | 253 | cAMP | >80 | +++ | These two acceptors run together on 8% gels but separate on gels of lower and higher concentrations; this behaviour reflects the low free mobility of the $Ca^{2+}$-stimulated system |
| $O_{3b}$ ($Ca^{2+}$) | ~254 | 195 | 225 | $Ca^{2+}$, calmod. | >80 | +++ | |
| $\alpha_1$ | 214 | Not determined | 238 | cAMP, $Ca^{2+}$, calmod. | 30–60 | Absent | Quantitatively minor |
| $\alpha_2$ | 189 | Not determined | 238 | cAMP | >80 | Absent | Poorly separated from $\alpha_3$ |
| $\alpha_3$ | 174 | 162 | 237 | $Ca^{2+}$, calmod. | >80 | Absent | Kinase appears to have an unusually high affinity for ATP for a $Ca^{2+}$-dependent system (see Fig. 6) |
| $\alpha_5$ | 143 | 138 | 249 | cAMP, $Ca^{2+}$, calmod. | >80 | Absent | Always seen as a broad diffuse peak. Phosphorylation more sensitive to $Ca^{2+}$ than cAMP |
| $\alpha_6$ | 139 | Not determined | 254 | cAMP | Uncertain | +++ | Poorly separated as a shoulder on $\alpha_5$ (except in cerebellum — see Fig. 3) |
| $\beta_2$ | 82 | Not determined | ? | None known | 30–60 | +++ | |
| $\beta_3$ | 80 | 86 | 247 | cAMP, $Ca^{2+}$, calmod. | 30–60 | ++ | Proteins 1a and 1b of Greengard's laboratory[9] |
| $\beta_4$ | 76 | 79 | 249 | cAMP | <25 | ++ | Derived from cytosol |
| $\beta_5$ | 74 | Not determined | 248 | $Ca^{2+}$, calmod. | >80 | ++ | ?DPH-L[h] and 62 K acceptor of Grab et al.[i] |
| $\beta_6$ | 60 | 68 | 250 | $Ca^{2+}$, calmod. | >80 | +++ | Equal to $\beta_6$ in cerebellum and colliculus; 50% of $\beta_6$ in cerebral cortex |
| $\beta_7$ | 57 | 62 | 248 | | | | |
| $\gamma_2$ | 54 | 59 | 249 | cAMP | 30–60 | ++ | Regulatory subunit of cAMP protein kinase[j]; ? F(p50)[k] |
| $\gamma_3$ | 52 | 54 | 250 | Not known | <25 | ++ | The most prominent acceptor phosphorylated in basal conditions. Kinase has a high affinity for ATP |

| | | | | | | | |
|---|---|---|---|---|---|---|---|
| $\gamma_4$ | 50 | 50 | 245 | Ca$^{2+}$, calmod. | >80 | Trace | ? DPH-M[h] and 51 K acceptor of Grab et al.[i] According to these authors the major postsynaptic density protein |
| $\gamma_5$ | ~45 | 47 | 232 | Ca$^{2+}$ only | Uncertain | + + | B-50[l]. Main phosphorylation by 'C' kinase[m], but seems also to act as acceptor for Ca$^{2+}$-calmodulin kinase. Anomalous free mobility |
| 'M' | 42 | 40 | 248 | ?Ca$^{2+}$, calmod. | – | – | $\alpha$ Subunit of pyruvate dehydrogenase[n]; contaminant of mitochondrial origin |

[a] Gower and Rodnight (1982). Values are the means of values determined on a series of gel concentrations ranging from 5 % to 14 % acrylamide, using a wide range of standards. Values for O$_1$, O$_2$ and O$_{3a}$ are minimal estimates, (a) because no satisfactory standard of molecular weight higher than 300 000 is available, and (b) because these acceptors exhibit anomalous free mobilities.

[b] From Holmes and Rodnight (1981); see also Rodnight (1980a).

[c] Determined from Ferguson plots (see Neville, 1971). Log mobilities, determined on a series of gel concentrations, were plotted against gel concentration and the straight line extrapolated to zero. For convenience the values quoted are 100[log (100 x relative mobility)] at 0 % acrylamide.

[d] Both unlabelled and labelled membrane fragments were washed with 250 mM NaCl and peak heights compared with untreated fragments (= 100). Where losses occurred they were comparable in both situations, indicating acceptor rather than (or as well as) kinase was being removed. These results are preliminary, but were quite consistent for values >80 % and <25 %.

[e] A comparison between membrane fragments made from cerebral cortex and from cerebellum is shown in Fig. 3. Tissue from the colliculi resembles cerebellar tissue.

[f] Lohmann et al. (1980).

[g] Ueda and Greengard (1977); Greengard (1978).

[h] DeLorenzo, (1981).

[i] Grab et al. (1981).

[j] Walter et al. (1978).

[k] DeBlas et al. (1979).

[l] Zwiers et al. (1980).

[m] Aloyo, Zwiers and Gispen, this volume.

[n] Browning et al. (1981).

10

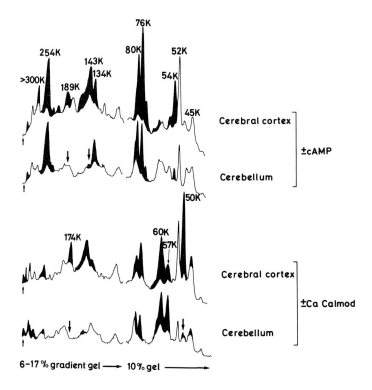

Fig. 3. Composite densitometric scans (expanded × 3) of radioautographs prepared from membrane fragments made from rat cerebral cortex and cerebellar tissue, and labelled under standard conditions. See Fig. 2 for further details.

runs as a broad diffuse band and is therefore reminiscent of band 3, the anion transporting glycoprotein (mol. wt. ∼ 100 K) of erythrocyte membranes (Rothstein et al., 1976).

With respect to acceptors in the $\gamma$ region phosphorylated by cAMP-dependent kinase activity, a major difference between these results and those of Malher's group is the presence in this region in our work of only one major acceptor ($\gamma_2$), instead of the three observed by these workers and designated by them D(p66), E(p54) and F(p50) (De Blas et al., 1979; Sörensen et al., 1981). We suspect that of these F(p50) corresponds to our $\gamma_2$ (54 K), but would appear to co-migrate in their system with our basally phosphorylated $\gamma_3$ (52 K). It is also possible that in our work the protein kinase that phosphorylates $\gamma_3$ is the catalytic subunit of a cAMP-dependent enzyme that for some reason loses its regulatory subunit during subcellular fractionation, but I think this unlikely on present evidence. E(p54) may correspond to a minor acceptor which in our work was originally designated $\gamma_1$ (see Rodnight, 1979) and later ignored as it was only seen inconsistently; it is however just evident in Figs. 2 and 11. D(p66) may correspond to an acceptor phosphorylated in a cAMP-dependent reaction that is regularly observed by us in preparations from caudate nucleus (see Fig. 11), but has never been seen in cerebral cortex tissue. The same difference between cortical and striatal tissue is seen particularly well in bovine (ox) brain (Fig. 4). However, Lohmann et al. (1980) observe in preparations of bovine cerebral cortex three cAMP-dependent acceptor systems (mol. wt. 52 K, 54 K and 58 K) which roughly correspond to those described by De Blas et al. (1979) in the rat. Two of these (52 K and 58 K) bound the photoaffinity label, 8-N$_3$-[$^{32}$P]cAMP, and were therefore identified as the autophosphorylated regulatory subunits of type II cAMP-dependent protein

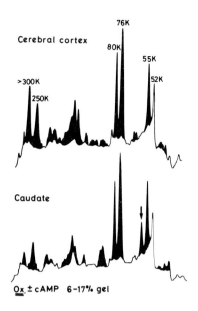

Fig. 4. Densitometric scans (expanded × 3) of radioautographs of a 6–17% gradient gel prepared from membrane fragments made from bovine (ox) cerebral cortex and caudate tissue, and labelled under standard conditions with and without cAMP (see Fig. 2 for further details). The extra acceptor in the caudate phosphorylated in a cAMP-dependent reaction is indicated by an arrow.

kinase; they probably correspond to the 55 K peak in Fig. 4 (in bovine brain preparations $\gamma_2$ migrates slightly slower than in rat material) and to the extra peak we observe only in striatal tissue. In one respect, however, I agree with Lohmann et al. (1980) in that they also do not find our striatum-specific acceptor (D(p66) of De Blas et al., 1979) in cerebral cortex preparations from the rat. Clearly more work is required to sort out the regional patterns of cAMP-dependent systems.

Turning to the $Ca^{2+}$-dependent systems, three categories can be discerned: (a) acceptors phosphorylated apparently by both $Ca^{2+}$-calmodulin-dependent and cAMP kinases ($O_1$, $\alpha_1$, $\alpha_5$ and protein I); (b) acceptors only phosphorylated by $Ca^{2+}$-calmodulin kinase activity ($O_2$, $O_{3b}$-$Ca^{2+}$, $\alpha_3$, $\beta_6$, $\beta_7$ and $\gamma_4$); and (c) one acceptor (B-50) that is maximally phosphorylated in the presence of $Ca^{2+}$ without the inclusion of calmodulin. With respect to category (a) only in the case of protein I has it been shown conclusively (Huttner et al., 1981; Kennedy and Greengard, 1981) that the two kinase activities transfer phosphate to different sites on the same polypeptide chain. In category (b) systems $\alpha_3$ and $\gamma_4$ are of particular interest. They are both absent from membrane fragments made from cerebellar tissue (Fig. 3) and ontogenetic studies (Holmes and Rodnight, 1981) have shown that in the rat they only appear in the cortex after the onset of synaptogenesis, i.e. around Day 12. The absence in the cerebellum of an acceptor corresponding to $\gamma_4$ was also noted by Grab et al. (1981), who consider that in the cerebral cortex it corresponds to the major postsynaptic density protein. Since there are major differences in structure and calmodulin content between postsynaptic densities isolated from the cerebral cortex and cerebellum (Carlin et al., 1980), the absence of $\gamma_4$ in the cerebellum may reflect a special function for this acceptor in the cerebral cortex. Two other acceptors observed by Grab et al. (1981) in cerebral cortical postsynaptic densities, and assigned molecular weights of 62 K and 58 K, appear to correspond to our $\beta_6$ and $\beta_7$. However, both these

12

acceptors occur in the cerebellum where $\beta_7$ is always distinctly elevated compared to cortical tissue (Fig. 3), and their development in the rat is gradual from birth onwards (Holmes and Rodnight, 1981). Grab et al. (1981) tentatively suggest their 62 K acceptor ($\beta_6$) may be a subunit of a cyclic nucleotide phosphodiesterase.

The remaining $Ca^{2+}$-dependent system, the B-50 acceptor and its kinase, are considered in detail by Aloyo et al. (this volume). I will also return in the present chapter to discuss briefly our views on its cellular location.

In all of the work described above the ATP concentration for the $Ca^{2+}$-dependent reactions was 20 $\mu$M, a concentration which approximates to the $K_m$ for the cAMP-dependent protein kinases. Under these conditions endogenous $Ca^{2+}$ and calmodulin present in the membrane preparations make an appreciable contribution to the basal phosphorylation. Later work, however, has shown that this ATP concentration is suboptimal for the $Ca^{2+}$-dependent systems, the enzymes of which possess a lower affinity for ATP. This difference in affinity for the two main types of protein kinase activity in synaptic membranes appears to account for early observations showing that the pattern of protein phosporylation varies with ATP concentration, even at very short (2 sec) incubation times (Fig. 5). A more detailed analysis was therefore undertaken in which the response of both cAMP and $Ca^{2+}$-calmodulin-dependent systems to a range of concentrations of ATP (of constant specific radioactivity), during 2 sec incubation times was examined. The data are too crude for rigorous kinetic analysis since even using these short incubation times some non-specific ATP hydrolysis occurs. Nevertheless by plotting peak heights for the main acceptors against log ATP concentration a clear indication of

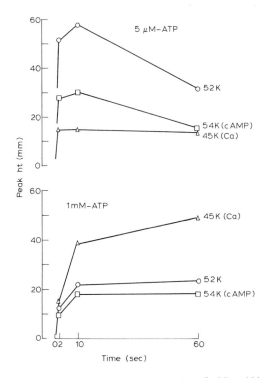

Fig. 5. Time course of the phosphorylation of three acceptors by a low (5 $\mu$M) and high (1 mM) concentration of ATP. In this experiment the specific radioactivity of the ATP varied by a factor of 10 between the two concentrations. The 1 mM ATP samples were there fore exposed to X-ray paper for a longer period.

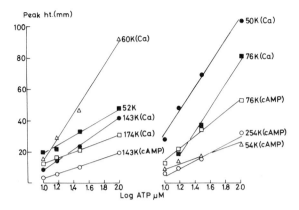

Fig. 6. The effect of ATP concentration on the relative phosphorylation of different acceptors. Membrane fragments (rat, cerebral cortex) were labelled in quadruplicate for 2 sec with 10 $\mu$M, 15 $\mu$M, 30 $\mu$M and 100 $\mu$M [$\gamma$-$^{32}$P]ATP of constant specific radioactivity (400 cpm/pmole). In other respects labelling conditions were standard for both the cAMP and Ca$^{2+}$-calmodulin series. The labelled fragments were fractionated on 7% and 10% gels and a series of radioautographs prepared and scanned. Peak heights were measured and plotted against log ATP concentration. Each point is the mean of 4–8 observations.

a difference of affinity was obtained (Fig. 6). The difference in slope is particularly striking for the Ca$^{2+}$-dependent phosphorylation of protein Ib (76 K), $\beta_6$ (60 K) and $\gamma_4$ (50 K); interestingly the reaction phosphorylating $\alpha_3$ (174 K) appears to possess an affinity similar to that of the cAMP-dependent systems. The practical consequence of this finding is that when studying Ca$^{2+}$-dependent reactions the use of a relatively high ATP concentration of relatively low specific radioactivity (e.g. 100 $\mu$M, 250 cpm/pmole) results in a strikingly lower level of basal phosphorylation and therefore a more pronounced stimulation by Ca$^{2+}$ and calmodulin (Rodnight et al., 1982).

## Sensitivity to cations

### Sodium ions

In several respects the cAMP- and Ca$^{2+}$-calmodulin-dependent kinase activities are distinguished by their response to cations other than Ca$^{2+}$. Of particular interest is the inhibition of the cAMP-dependent systems by Na$^+$ which contrasts with the relative insensitivity of Ca$^{2+}$-dependent systems to this cation (Fig. 7). This inhibitory effect of Na$^+$ is not given by K$^+$, which at 25 mM concentration causes <15% inhibition of the cAMP-dependent phosphorylation of protein Ia, and Ib and $\gamma_2$ (54 K). The Na$^+$ effect is therefore unlikely to be a non-specific physiochemical action on membrane structure. In fact concentrations of Na$^+$ as low as 1 mM produced a reproducible inhibition ( $\sim$ 20%) of $^{32}$P incorporation into protein I. It has yet to be established whether the inhibition is due to a direct action on the protein kinase rather than on a protein phosphatase, but it does not appear to be related to activation of the Na$^+$,K$^+$-ATPase and consequent reduction in the ATP pool available for phosphorylation (R. Rodnight, unpublished observations). On present evidence, therefore, it appears possible that the cAMP-dependent phosphorylation of membrane protein is sensitive to the physiological fluctuations in internal Na$^+$ concentration which accompany depolarization. Finally a practical consequence of this observation is that in assaying endogenous cAMP-dependent protein kinase activity the use of Na$^+$ as a counter ion for amine buffers such as HEPES should be avoided.

14

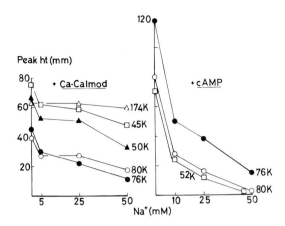

Fig. 7. The effect of $Na^+$ on phosphorylation of several acceptors in fragments prepared from rat cerebral cortex. Standard labelling conditions were used with 20 $\mu M$ ATP as donor.

*Magnesium ions*

$Mg^{2+}$ concentrations in excess of that required to saturate the ATP as Mg-ATP have complex and interesting actions. At ATP concentrations below 100 $\mu M$ more than 95 % of the ATP is in the form of Mg-ATP at 1 mM $Mg^{2+}$ concentration. Nevertheless higher $Mg^{2+}$ concentrations stimulate before inhibiting endogenous kinase activity, and in several different patterns. In our experience the cAMP-dependent systems are all stimulated by $Mg^{2+}$ concentrations up to 5 mM, but are then progressively inhibited, although the difference between 5 and 10 mM is not very great (H. Gower and R. Rodnight, unpublished observations). However, the basal phosphorylation follows a similar activation–inhibition pattern and therefore the degree of stimulation given by cAMP is largely unaffected. In our view therefore there is little justification for using a higher $Mg^{2+}$ concentration than 1 mM for studying the cAMP-dependent systems, especially since the in vivo intracellular concentration of free $Mg^{2+}$ is considered to be about 1 mM (Wolff et al., 1977).

In the case of the $Ca^{2+}$-dependent activity, two patterns emerge. With proteins Ia and Ib, and also the B-50 system, $Mg^{2+}$ stimulated phosphorylation in concentrations up to 5–10 mM and then progressively inhibited the activity. In contrast the phosphorylation of all the other $Ca^{2+}$-calmodulin-dependent systems was not inhibited by $Mg^{2+}$ concentrations greater than 10 mM, even as high as 50 mM; representative examples of the two patterns are given in Fig. 8. It is of interest to note that the acceptors whose phosphorylation is inhibited by high concentrations of $Mg^{2+}$ are believed to be located presynaptically, while the others, in particular $\alpha_3$ and $\gamma_4$, probably have a postsynaptic location.

*Calcium ions*

$Ca^{2+}$ is generally inhibitory for the cAMP-dependent systems, as shown by the stimulation of these systems given by EGTA due to chelation of endogenous $Ca^{2+}$. The effect of a wide range of $Ca^{2+}$ concentrations in the presence of excess calmodulin on $Ca^{2+}$-dependent activity towards several acceptors is shown in Fig. 9. Sensitivity to 'available' $Ca^{2+}$ (free $Ca^{2+}$ plus calmodulin-bound $Ca^{2+}$) was remarkably steep in the range pCa 7 to pCa 6 with half maximal stimulation being obtained with a concentration of about 200 nM. This value lies well within the range of physiological fluctuations of free internal $Ca^{2+}$ (Llinas et al., 1976) and compares well with the concentration of free $Ca^{2+}$ required to activate other calmodulin-dependent

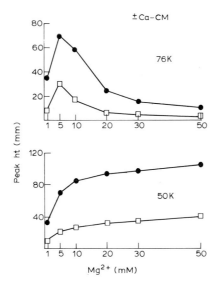

Fig. 8. The effect of Mg²⁺ on the phosphorylation of protein Ib and $\gamma_4$ (50 K) in fragments prepared from rat cerebral cortex. Standard labelling conditions were used with 20 μM ATP as donor. EDTA (0.2 mM) was added to the upper buffer during electrophoresis to correct for the distortion which occurred when samples containing high Mg²⁺ concentrations were applied. □, basal; ●, with Ca²⁺.

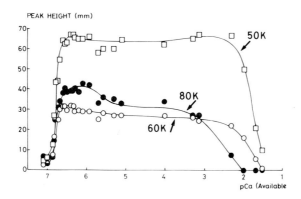

Fig. 9. The effect of Ca²⁺ on the phosphorylation of several acceptors in fragments prepared from rat cerebral cortex. Standard labelling conditions were used with 100 μM ATP as donor. The available Ca²⁺ is defined as the sum of free [Ca²⁺] and the [Ca²⁺] bound to calmodulin. This was calculated by a computer programme (Perrin and Sayce, 1967) incorporating 10 stability constants (see Rodnight et al., 1982 for more detail).

enzymes such as the erythrocyte Ca²⁺ ATPase (Downes and Michell, 1981). The concentration at which Ca²⁺ inhibits phosphorylation varies between systems, but in general inhibition occurs above 1 mM.

### Location of phosphate acceptors

In view of the extensive studies on this aspect of the subject carried out by Mahler's group (De Blas et al., 1979; Sörensen et al., 1981; Mahler et al., this volume) and by Greengard's laboratory with respect to protein I (Ueda et al., 1979; Bloom et al., 1979) I will confine my remarks to a few topics. In general it can now be safely concluded, as already noted, that the major part of the cAMP-dependent phosphorylating activity is located within the presynaptic terminal (Weller, 1977, Sorensen et al., 1981). Certainly in our experience this applies to protein I, $\gamma_2$ and $O_{3b}$ cAMP. By contrast experiments using intact synaptosomes exposed to ATP indicate that the $Ca^{2+}$-calmodulin-dependent systems transferring to $\alpha_3$, $\alpha_5$, $\beta_6$, $\beta_7$ and $\gamma_4$ (but not protein I) are located outside the terminal, probably in the postsynaptic densities (Rodnight et al., 1982).

Another approach is illustrated in Fig. 10 which provides a useful summary of the heterogeneity of synaptosomal membrane preparations. A lysed $P_2$ fraction was subjected to centrifugal density gradient fractionation. The experiment shows that the two main membrane fractions are enriched in all systems, that the crude vesicle fraction is unique in containing only protein Ia, Ib and a little $\gamma_3$ and that the crude mitochondrial fraction contains two prominent phosphorylated acceptors of low molecular weight. The great enrichment of protein I in vesicles was first shown by Ueda et al. (1979) and confirmed by immunocytochemistry by Bloom et al. (1979). Although it is not evident from this experiment (since the vesicle fraction was contaminated with myelin) the concentration of protein I in highly purified vesicles is at least 20 times higher than in the membrane fraction (Ueda et al., 1979). It remains an open question as to whether the occurence of protein I in membrane fractions reflects artifactual contamination with vesicles or the occurrence of vesicular proteins in the membrane as a result of 'exocytotic fusion'.

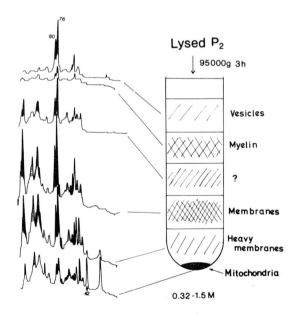

Fig. 10. Densitometric scans prepared from radioautographs of gels prepared from gradient particulate fractions made from rat cerebral cortex. $P_2$ fraction (Jones and Matus, 1974) was lysed and centrifuged as indicated on a continuous sucrose gradient. Fractions were collected, treated by the same procedure as used for routine membrane preparations and labelled under standard conditions with and without cAMP or $Ca^{2+}$-calmodulin with 20 $\mu$M ATP. Labelled membranes were fractionated on 10% gels and the radioautographs scanned. The black areas represent stimulation by cAMP and the hatched areas stimulation by $Ca^{2+}$-calmodulin (acceptors phosphorylated by both systems are black).

The two low molecular weight acceptors in the mitochondrial fraction are in fact typical of purified mitochondria and have been identified as the $\alpha$ subunit of pyruvate dehydrogenase (42 K) and a subunit of succinyl CoA synthetase (Morgan and Routtenberg, 1980; Browning et al., 1981; Steiner and Smith, 1981). A possible role for the phosphorylation of pyruvate dehydrogenase in the phenomenon of long-term potentiation is considered by Browning et al. (this volume).

The remaining acceptor whose location I wish to discuss is that of the B-50 kinase system, extensively investigated by the Utrecht group (Zwiers et al. and Aloyo et al., this volume). Probably more is known about the biochemical function of this phosphorylation system than of any of the other systems in synaptic membranes. The phosphorylation of the B-50 acceptor is regulated by ACTH (Zwiers et al., 1979) and there is strong evidence that it constitutes a catalytic or regulatory factor concerned in the phosphorylation of diphosphoinositide to triphosphoinositide, (Jolles et al., 1980). Determination of its cellular location may therefore provide important clues as to the sites of action of ACTH in the nervous system and of physiological roles of the polyphosphoinositides. Immunocytochemical studies of its location in the cerebellum (Oestreicher et al., 1981) suggest that the B-50 system is confined to the synapse rich molecular layer and Sörensen et al. (1981) (see also Mahler et al., this volume) consider it to be located in presynaptic terminals. Certainly our experience with intact synaptosomes confirms that the B-50 system is occluded, but two other facts complicate the picture. First, ontogenetic studies (Holmes and Rodnight, 1981) have shown that the level of the B-50 acceptor in the rat brain is exceptionally high in the first 10 days of life, i.e. before the onset of synaptogenesis. Secondly, mild lesions of the striatum induced by a low dose (5 nmoles) of kainic acid, but still sufficient to result in major losses of all the neuronally located phosphorylating systems, does not result in any loss of the B-50 acceptor (Fig. 11). Higher doses of kainate, such as those used by Sieghart et al. (1978, 1980) do cause some dimunition

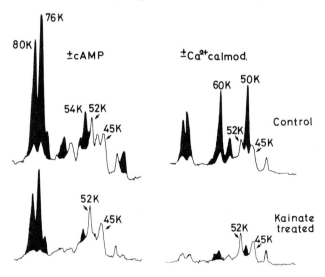

Fig. 11. Densitometric scans (expanded × 3) of radioautographs of gels from synaptosomal membrane fragments made from rat caudate nucleus tissue pretreated in vivo with kainic acid. The dose of kainate was 5 nmoles stereotaxically injected into the striatum; survival time was 5 days. For further details of presentation see Fig. 2. Standard labelling conditions were used with 20 $\mu$M ATP as donor for the cAMP-dependent systems and 100 $\mu$M ATP for the $Ca^{2+}$-calmodulin-dependent systems. This experiment is also an example of a reasonably satisfactory separation of all the main acceptors on a single exponential gradient gel of 6–17% acrylamide.

in the level of B-50 phosphorylation, but proportionally the loss is very little compared with the virtual destruction of all other systems except $\gamma_3$. One possible interpretation of this experiment is that the B-50 system is confined to synaptic terminals with perikarya located outside the striatum, e.g. those of the nigro-striatal dopaminergic tract or the corticostriatal glutamatergic tracts.

*Discussion*

Partial answers are now available to the questions posed in Table I. One acceptor ($O_{3a}$ or MAP$_2$) is clearly a peripheral protein, although it is not known whether this association is artifactual and arises solely as a consequence of cell disruption. It is not known whether MAP$_2$ carries its own kinase to the membrane or is phosphorylated by a membrane-bound enzyme. It is of interest to note that Matus et al. (1981) have shown that MAPs are preferentially associated with dendritic microtubules. Several other acceptors and their kinases may turn out to be integral to the synaptic membrane or to be tightly bound to synaptic densities: this applies to both components of $O_{3b}$ and to $\alpha_2$, $\alpha_3$, $\alpha_5$, $\beta_6$, $\beta_7$ and $\gamma_4$. For the rest the nature of their association with the membrane or densities remains uncertain. The interesting question of the influence of membrane fluidity on substrate enzyme interactions is discussed by Hershkowitz et al. later in this volume.

Of the tightly bound phosphorylating systems only $O_{3b}$ cAMP, $\alpha_5$ (cAMP phosphorylation only) and possibly $\gamma_2$ appear to be located in presynaptic terminals (R. Rodnight, unpublished observations). The others, which are all phosphorylated in $Ca^{2+}$-calmodulin-dependent reactions are almost certainly located in non-terminal areas of the synapse, which in the case of $\beta_6$, and $\gamma_4$ appear on present evidence to be the postsynaptic densities (Grab et al., 1981). The subsynaptic location of phosphate acceptors is discussed further by Mahler et al. (this volume) and by Cohen et al. (this volume).

With regard to the diversity of membrane-bound protein kinases, four types are discernable: a cAMP-dependent kinase, shown by Walter et al. (1979) in the rat to be the type II enzyme; one or more $Ca^{2+}$-calmodulin-dependent enzymes; the phospholipid requiring 'C' enzyme (Nishizuka et al., 1979; this volume) which appears to be responsible for the phosphorylation of the B-50 acceptor (Aloyo et al., this volume); and the kinase phosphorylating $\gamma_3$ (52 K) for which no activating factor has been found. No doubt further research will reveal a more complex picture; in particular I suspect that heterogeneity will be found in the $Ca^{2+}$-dependent kinases. However, a calmodulin-dependent kinase with a broad specificity has been described (Waisman et al., 1978). It is also worth noting that only in a few cases have the amino acid sites of phosphorylation in synaptic membranes been identified; in this respect recent work demonstrating in non-neural systems the existence of protein kinases which transfer phosphate specifically to the hydroxyl groups of tyrosine residues merits attention. Finally, it is necessary to note here that my group have been quite unable to confirm, using both post-mortem tissue and fresh biopsy tissue, a report by Boehme et al. (1978) claiming the presence of cGMP-dependent protein kinase activity in membrane fragments prepared from human cerebral cortex (L. Martinez-Millan and R. Rodnight, unpublished observations).

With regard to specificity to neuronal cell systems characterized by different neurotransmitters, some intriguing pointers are available which strongly suggest that some acceptors may be neurone-specific. The striking difference in the cerebellar pattern (Fig. 3) supports this conclusion, as does recent work by Dolphin and Greengard (1981a) which suggests that in the cerebellum protein I is highly enriched in granule cells. Further studies using specific lesioning techniques may help to develop this important aspect of the subject.

## STUDIES IN VITRO IN INTACT TISSUE OR
## SYNAPTOSOMES

The early observations of our group on the protein phosphorylation response in cerebral cortex slices, first discovered by P.J. Heald in 1957, have been outlined on several occasions (Rodnight, 1977; 1980b; Williams and Rodnight, 1977). In summary brief depolarization of respiring $^{32}$P-labelled cerebral cortex slices by the application of electrical pulses results in an increased incorporation of phosphate into vacant protein-bound serine hydroxyl groups. The response is tetrodotoxin sensitive and mediated via a $\beta$-noradrenergic receptor which is most probably (although this has never been proved) linked to adenylate cyclase. The $^{32}$P incorporated as a result of depolarization or exposure to noradrenaline proved to be extremely rapidly dephosphorylated on disruption of the tissue and so far this lability has prevented the isolation and characterization of the acceptor protein(s). Briefly, although dephosphorylation can be effectively inhibited by $Ca^{2+}$ or $Zn^{2+}$ (Rodnight, 1977) these heavy metal cations render subfractionation of the tissue impossible. Fixation of the whole tissue slice with the usual 'stopping reagent' (SDS–mercaptoethanol) followed by unidimensional electrophoresis results in enormously high background labelling and uninterpretable patterns; two-dimensional analysis of such complex polypeptide mixtures are obviously desirable.

The problem of post-experimental dephosphorylation of $^{32}$P-labelled intact tissues and unacceptable background labelling has led other workers to develop a different approach, often referred to as the "back phosphorylation" assay. A important example of this approach, due to Greengard's group, was applied to a study of the phosphorylation state of protein I in rat cerebral cortex slices (Forn and Greengard, 1978). No attempt was made to isotopically label the tissue during incubation, and at the termination of the experiment the tissue was fixed by homogenizing it in 5 mM zinc acetate to arrest phosphatase action; after centrifuging protein I was extracted from the particulate fraction with 2 M citric acid and phosphorylated under standard conditions with exogenous partially purified cAMP-dependent protein kinase and $[\gamma$-$^{32}$P]ATP as donor. The amount of label incorporated under these conditions was shown to be inversely proportional to the original state of phosphorylation of protein I in the tissue slice, with a high level of incorporation reflecting a low phosphorylation state and vice versa. Forn and Greengard concluded that in slices incubated without the addition of pharmacological agents protein I was present almost entirely in the dephosphorylated form. Incubation of the tissue with cAMP (or its analogues), with phosphodiesterase inhibitors or depolarization of the tissue with high $K^+$ or vertradine all resulted in an increase in the phosphorylation state of protein I; in the case of the depolarizing agents the response of protein I was $Ca^{2+}$-dependent.

Attemps in this work to demonstrate an effect of a variety of putative neurotransmitters on the phosphorylation state of protein I yielded uniformly negative results, suggesting either that the depolarization response was not receptor mediated but perhaps related to the mechanism of transmitter release, or that the neuronal circuitory is too complex in the cerebral cortex for a response to be demonstrable through a single class of receptor. However, in later work from this group it proved possible to demonstrate a receptor-mediated increase in the phosphorylation state of protein I in the superior cervical ganglion (Nestler and Greengard, 1980) and in slices of the facial motor nucleus of the rat (Dolphin and Greengard, 1981b). In the facial nucleus some 2% of the synaptic terminals are serotoninergic where they represent a facilitatory input from the raphe magnus. Exposure of slices of this tissue to serotonin increased the phosphorylation state of protein I by 30% in a response that was partially blocked by the serotonin antagonist mianserin. For several reasons the authors conclude that this response is mediated via presynaptic receptors and may be involved in the mechanism of the facilitation of synaptic transmission controlled by this serotoninergic pathway.

The application of the ''back phosphorylation'' approach to the assay of protein I is really a special case, since this particular acceptor is readily extracted from the tissue by mild acid treatment and may then be rephosphorylated by adding back the specific kinase. This procedure is clearly inapplicable when screening for possible changes in the phosphorylation state of a range of phosphate acceptors in intact tissues resulting from pharmacological or electrophysiological treatment. The alternative approach has been simply to prepare membrane fractions from incubated tissue by the usual techniques and then measure endogenous protein phosphorylation, a procedure known as the "post hoc" assay (e.g. Ehrlich et al., 1977b; Browning et al., 1979; Bär et al., 1980). Several applications of the "post hoc" assay are described later in this volume (Routtenberg; Lopes da Silva et al.; Browning et al.) and I will confine my remarks here to general points. It is clear that changes in the amount of phosphate incorporated into an acceptor induced by a treatment of the intact tissue are interpretable either in terms of an altered phosphorylation state or, less likely, in terms of a stable modification in the activity state of the appropriate protein kinase. It should be noted, however, that the *absence* of differences in apparent phosphorylation state between control and treated tissue using this approach cannot be interpreted at all, since post-incubation dephosphorylation may have eliminated these differences. Even if the response in the intact tissue results in a lower phosphorylation state for a particular acceptor, an increase in the incorporation in the "post hoc" assay will only be detectable if the corresponding acceptor in the control tissue has not been dephosphorylated during cellular fractionation. In view of these considerations it is perhaps surprising that meaningful results have been obtained with this approach by several investigators. The most developed research concerns the increase in the phosphorylation state of the $\alpha$ subunit of pyruvate dehydrogenase induced specifically in hippocampal slices by conditions of electrical stimulation resulting in long-term potentiation (Browning et al., 1979, this volume). It is possible, however, that in this case the "post hoc" assay approach is only applicable because pyruvate dehydrogenase phosphatase is loosely coupled with its substrate and subject to rigorous control (Denton and Halestrap, 1979).

The technical problems encountered in labelling brain slices with $[^{32}P]PO_4^{3-}$ have proved less serious in studies of incubated synaptosomes. These structures therefore constitute an excellent model system for investigating roles for protein phosphorylation in presynaptic processes. Krueger et al. (1977) found that exposure of prelabelled synaptosomes to depolarizing agents such as high $K^+$ and veratridine, as well as to the calcium ionophore A23187, stimulated the incorporation of $^{32}P$ into protein I by a $Ca^{2+}$-dependent mechanism. The phosphoprotein response to depolarization was rapid, reaching a maximum within 10 sec in a time course that matched the uptake of $^{45}Ca$ by the synaptosomes. This result has been confirmed in my laboratory using electrical field stimulation as a depolarizing stimulus (D. De Souza and R. Rodnight, unpublished observations). However, Krueger et al. were unable to detect any effect of a range of putative neurotransmitters on protein I phosphorylation in synaptosomes, a finding which suggests that the phosphorylation state of this acceptor is regulated by voltage-dependent $Ca^{2+}$ channels independently of receptor activation. Later work by this group (Huttner and Greengard, 1979) using tryptic digests of protein I demonstrated that the sites phosphorylated as a result of exposing synaptosomes to depolarizing agents corresponded to the sites phosphorylated by ATP in lysed synaptosomes by the $Ca^{2+}$-calmodulin-dependent kinase activity.

A similar approach was used by Michaelson and Avissar (1979) in a study of $^{32}P$-labelled cholinergic synaptosomes from *Torpedo*. The use of a purely cholinergic tissue enabled transmitter release provoked by high $K^+$ or A23187 to be reliably measured concomitantly with a phosphorylation response. The latter consisted of an increased incorporation into an acceptor of 100 000 dalton mediated by a $Ca^{2+}$-dependent mechanism. The time courses of acetylcholine release and phosphorylation of the 100 K acceptor were impressively similar, but as the authors recognize such co-incidence does not necessarily demonstrate a causal relationship.

## IN VIVO PHOSPHORYLATION STUDIES

As Routtenberg (1979) has pointed out the relationship of phosphorylation reactions observed in vitro (both at the subcellular and intact tissue level) to the in vivo situation is crucial if we are to understand roles of protein phosphorylation in CNS functioning. Two recent studies have approached the problem by injecting $[^{32}P]PO_4^{3-}$ intracerebrally and subsequently isolating the tissue and fractionating the labelled proteins by electrophoresis (Berman et al., 1980; Mitrius et al., 1981). Both studies demonstrated the feasibility of demonstrating the in vivo labelling of specific phosphoproteins. Berman et al. (1980) noted, not surprisingly, that the electrophoretic pattern of phosphorylated polypeptides derived from tissue labelled with $[^{32}P]PO_4^{3-}$ injected intraventricularly in vivo, was different from that in membranes labelled with $[\gamma^{-32}P]ATP$ in vitro. The extent to which post-mortem dephosphorylation rather than in vivo control mechanisms contributed to this difference is not known. Mitrius et al. (1981) injected $[^{32}P]PO_4^{3-}$ sterotaxically into the striatum and hippocampus and attempted to overcome the dephosphorylation problem by fixing the tissue, either by immersing the animal in liquid nitrogen or by focussed microwave irradiation. In some experiments radioactivity was injected into conscious unrestrained animals via chronic implants. It is difficult to judge how effective the fixation procedures were since results were essentially similar whether the animals were killed by decapitation, microwave fixation or immersion in liquid nitrogen. However, some similarities between the in vivo and in vitro labelling patterns were observed, although it is difficult to interpret these since in most cases only whole tissue was analysed in the in vivo experiments. In conclusion these are pioneer experiments of great potential and when the techniques are refined significant progress may be anticipated.

## ENVOI

In the past it would have been appropriate to conclude a review of this nature with some discussion of the functional implications of the subject. It is fast becoming clear, however, that protein phosphorylation is such a universal control mechanism in cellular processes embracing numerous macromolecules, that although its involvement in all aspects of synaptic transmission may be anticipated, it is proving difficult to obtain firm evidence for causal relationships. In the mammalian CNS investigations of presynaptic mechanisms are most likely to yield progress with the present techniques available. Thus study of phosphorylation reactions in isolated vesicles and in intact synaptosomes strongly suggest that protein I and possibly other polypeptides phosphorylated by $Ca^{2+}$-calmodulin-dependent reactions (DeLorenzo, 1981, this volume), are involved in some aspect of transmitter storage or release. However, on kinetic grounds alone it seems unlikely that a protein phosphorylation event is at the centre of the final release mechanism, whether this is envisaged as occurring by exocytosis or some other process. Another presynaptic mechanism which, by analogy with the sarcoplasmic reticulum (Demaille, 1981), may be modulated by the phosphorylation of membrane protein is the active transport of $Ca^{2+}$ out of the terminal by the $Ca^{2+}$-ATPase, an enzyme whose activity is regulated in synaptic membranes by calmodulin (Sobue et al., 1979). With regard to the involvement of protein phosphorylation in postsynaptic events in the mammalian CNS progress has been disappointing, mainly because of difficulties in observing molecular events in the postsynaptic membrane in intact tissues and to isolating postsynaptic membranes at the subcellular level. Once the latter is unequivocably achieved under non-denaturing conditions and it is possible to recognize the characteristic postsynaptic membrane phosphate acceptors, interpretation of experiments in the intact tissue will become feasible. It seems likely, however, that in the immediate future more progress will be made in these aspects by investigating simpler neuronal systems, such as occur in the molluscs (for two recent examples see Castelluci et al., 1980; Kaczmarek et al., 1980).

## ACKNOWLEDGEMENT

I wish to thank the Medical Research Council of the U.K. for support.

### REFERENCES

Bär, P.R., Schotman, P., Gispen, W.H., Tielen, A.M. and Lopes da Silva, F.H. (1980) Changes in synaptic membrane phosphorylation after tetanic stimulation in the dendate area of the rat hippocampal slice. *Brain Res.*, 198: 478–484.

Berman, R.F., Hullihan, J.P., Kinnier, W.J. and Wilson, J.E. (1980) Phosphorylation of synaptic membranes. *J. Neurochem.*, 34: 431–437.

Bloom, F.E., Ueda, T., Battenberg, E. and Greengard, P. (1979) Immunocytochemical localization in synapses, of protein I, an endogenous substrate for protein kinases in mammalian brain. *Proc. nat. Acad. Sci (Wash.)*, 76: 5982–5986.

Boehme, D.H., Kosecki, R. and Marks, N. (1978) Protein phosphorylation in human synaptosomal membranes: evidence for the presence of substrates for cyclic nucleotide guanosine 3'-5'-monophosphate dependent protein kinases. *Brain Res. Bull.*, 3: 697–700.

Browning, M., Dunwiddie, T., Bennett, W., Gispen, W. and Lynch, G. (1979) Synaptic phosphoproteins: specific changes after repetitive stimulation of the hippocampal slice. *Science*, 203: 60–62.

Browning, M., Bennett, W.F., Kelly, P. and Lynch, G. (1981) The 40000 phosphoprotein influenced by high frequency synaptic stimulation is the alpha-subunit of pyruvate dehydrogenase. *Brain Res.*, 218: 255–266.

Brunner, G., Bauer, H.C., Sater, D. and Speth, V. (1978) Artefacts produced during plasma membrane isolation. I. Cell disruption causes alteration in the structure of the plasma membranes of thymocytes. *Biochim. biophys. Acta*, 507: 419–424.

Burke, B.E. and DeLorenzo, R. (1981) $Ca^{2+}$- and calmodulin-stimulated endogenous phosphorylation of neurotubulin. *Proc. nat. Acad. Sci. (Wash.)*, 78: 991–995.

Carlin, R.K., Grab, D.J. and Siekevitz, P. (1980) Isolation and characterization of postsynaptic densities from various brain regions: enrichment of different types of postsynaptic densities. *J. Cell Biol.*, 86: 831–843.

Castellucci, V.F., Kandel, E.R., Schwartz, J.H., Wilson, F.D., Nairn, A.C. and Greengard, P. (1980) Intracellular injection of the catalytic subunit of cyclic AMP-dependent protein kinase stimulates facilitation of transmitter release underlying behavioural sensitization in Aplysia. *Proc. natl. Acad. Sci. (Wash.)*, 77: 7492–7496.

Clark, B.F.C. (1981) Towards a total human protein map. *Nature (Lond.)*, 292: 491–492.

Cohen, P. (Ed.) (1980) *Recently Discovered Systems of Enzyme Regulation by Reversible Phosphorylation*, Elsevier/North-Holland, Amsterdam.

De Blas, A.L., Wang, Y.-J., Sorensen, R. and Mahler, H.R. (1979) Protein phosphorylation in synaptic membranes regulated by adenosine 3':5'-monophosphate: regional and subcellular distribution of the substrates. *J. Neurochem.*, 33: 647–659.

DeLorenzo, R.J. (1981) Calcium, calmodulin and synaptic function: modulation of neurotransmitter release, nerve terminal protein phosphorylation, and synaptic vesicle morphology by calcium and calmodulin. In *Regulatory Mechanisms of Synaptic Transmission*, R. Tapia and C.W. Cotman (Eds.), Plenum Press, New York, pp. 205–239.

Demaille, J.G. (1981) Cyclic AMP and $Ca^{2+}$-dependent protein kinases and their concerted effects on $Ca^{2+}$ fluxes. *Biochem. Soc. Trans.*, 9: 380–381.

Denton, R.M. and Halestrap, A.P. (1979) Regulation of pyruvate metabolism in mammalian tissues. *Essays Biochem.*, 15: 37–77.

Dolphin, A.C. and Greengard, P. (1981a) Presence of protein I, a phosphoprotein associated with synaptic vesicles, in cerebellar granule cells. *J. Neurochem.*, 36: 1627–1631.

Dolphin, A.C. and Greengard, P. (1981b) Serotonin stimulates phosphorylation of protein I in the facial motor nucleus of rat brain. *Nature (Lond.)*, 289: 76–79.

Downes, P. and Michell, R.H. (1981) Human erythrocyte membranes exhibit a cooperative calmodulin-dependent $Ca^{2+}$-ATPase of high calcium sensitivity. *Nature (Lond.)*, 290: 270–271.

Dunkley, P.R. (1981) Phosphorylation of synaptosomal membrane proteins and evaluation of nerve cell function. In *New Approaches to Nerve and Muscle Disorders. Basic and Applied Contributions*, A.D. Kidman, J.K. Tomkins and R.A. Westerman (Eds.), Excerpta Medica, Amsterdam, pp. 38–51.

Ehrlich, Y.H., Davis, L.G., Gilfoil, T. and Brunngraber, E.G. (1977a) Distribution of endogenously phosphorylated proteins in subcellular fractions of rat cerebral cortex. *Neurochem. Res.*, 2: 533–548.

Ehrlich, Y.H., Rabjohns, R.R. and Routtenberg, A. (1977b) Experiential input alters the phosphorylation of specific proteins in brain membranes. *Pharmacol. biochem. Behav.*, 6: 169–174.

Forn, J. and Greengard, P. (1978) Depolarizing agents and cyclic nucleotides regulate the phosphorylation of specific neuronal proteins in rat cerebral cortex slices. *Proc. nat. Acad. Sci. (Wash.)*, 75: 5195–5199.

Giometti, C.M., Anderson, N.G., Tollaksen, S.L., Edwards, J.J. and Anderson, N.L. (1980) Analytical techniques for cell fractions. XXVII. Use of heart proteins as reference standards in two-dimensional electrophoresis. *Analyt. Biochem.*, 102: 47–58.

Gower, H., and Rodnight, R. (1982) Intrinsic protein phosphorylation in synaptic plasma membrane fragments from the rat. General characteristics and migration behaviour on polyacrylamide gels of the main phosphate acceptors. *Biochim. biophys. Acta*, in press.

Grab, D.J., Carlin, R.K. and Siekevitz, P. (1981) Function of calmodulin in postsynaptic densities. II Presence of a calmodulin-activatable protein kinase activity. *J. Cell Biol.*, 89: 440–448.

Greengard, P. (1978) *Cyclic Nucleotide Phosphorylated Proteins and Neuronal Function*, Raven Press, New York.

Holmes, H. and Rodnight, R. (1981) Ontogeny of membrane-bound protein phosphorylating systems in the rat. *Develop. Neurosci.*, 4: 79–88.

Huttner, W.B. and Greengard, P. (1979) Multiple phosphorylation sites in protein I and their differential regulation by cyclic AMP and calcium. *Proc. nat. Acad. Sci. (Wash.)*, 76: 5402–5406.

Huttner, W.B., DeGennaro, L.J. and Greengard, P. (1981) Differential phosphorylation of multiple sites in purified protein I by cyclic AMP-dependent and calcium-dependent protein kinases. *J. biol. Chem.*, 256: 1482–1491.

Jolles, J., Zwiers, H., van Dougen, J.J., Schotman, P., Wirtz, K.W.A. and Gispen, W.H. (1980) Modulation of brain phosphoinositide metabolism by ACTH-sensitive protein phosphorylation. *Nature (Lond.)*, 286: 623–626.

Jones, D.H. and Matus, A.I. (1974) Isolation of synaptic plasma membrane from brain by combined isolation sedimentation density gradient centrifugation. *Biochim. biophys. Acta*, 356: 276–287.

Kaczmarek, L.K., Jennings, K.R., Strumwasser, F., Nairn, A.C., Walter, U., Wilson, F.D. and Greengard, P. (1980) Microinjection of catalytic subunit of cyclic AMP-dependent protein kinase enhances calcium action potentials of bag cell neurons in cell culture. *Proc. nat. Acad. Sci (Wash.)*, 77: 7487–7491.

Kang, E.S., Gates, R.E. and Farmer, D.M. (1978) Localisation of the catalytic subunit of a cyclic AMP-dependent protein kinase(s) and acceptor proteins on the external surface of the fat cell membrane. *Biochem. biophys. Res. Commun.*, 83: 1561–1569.

Kennedy, M.B. and Greengard, P. (1981) Two calcium/calmodulin dependent protein kinases which are highly concentrated in brain phosphorylate protein I at distinct sites. *Proc. nat. Acad. Sci. (Wash.)*, 78: 1293–1297.

Kometiani, P., Kometiani, Z. and Mikeladze, D. (1978) 3′,5′-AMP dependent protein kinase and membrane ATPases of the nerve cell. *Progr. Neurobiol.*, 11: 223–247.

Krebs, E.G. and Beavo, J.A. (1979) Phosphorylation and dephosphorylation of enzymes. *Ann.Rev.Biochem.*, 49: 923–959.

Krueger, B.K., Forn, J. and Greengard, P. (1977) Depolarization-induced phosphorylation of specific proteins, mediated by calcium ion influx, in rat brain synaptosomes. *J. biol, Chem.*, 252: 2764–2773.

Llinas, R., Steinberg, I.Z. and Walton, K. (1976) Presynaptic calcium currents and their relation to synaptic transmission: Voltage clamp study in squid giant axon and theoretical model for calcium gate. *Proc. nat. Acad. Sci. (Wash.)*, 73: 2918–2922.

Lohmann, S.M., Walter, U. and Greengard, P. (1980) Identification of endogenous substrate proteins for cAMP-dependent protein kinase in bovine brain. *J. biol. Chem.*, 225: 9985–9992.

Matus, A., Pehling, G., Ackermann, M. and Maeder, J. (1980) Brain postsynaptic densities: their relationship to glial and neuronal filaments. *J. Cell Biol.*, 87: 346–359.

24

Matus, A., Bernhardt, R. and Hugh-Jones, T. (1981) High molecular weight microtubule-associated proteins are preferentially associated with dendritic microtubules in brain. *Proc. nat. Acad. Sci. (Wash.)*, 78: 3010–3014.

Michaelson, D.M. and Avissar, S. (1979) $Ca^{2+}$-dependent protein phosphorylation of purely cholinergic Torpedo synaptosomes. *J. biol. Chem.*, 245: 12542–12546.

Mitrius, J.C., Morgan, D.G. and Routtenberg, A. (1981) In vivo phosphorylation following [$^{32}$P]orthophosphate injection into neostriatum or hippocampus: selective and rapid labelling of electrophoretically separated brain proteins. *Brain Res.*, 212: 67–81.

Morgan, D.G. and Routtenberg, A. (1980) Evidence that a 41000 dalton brain phosphoprotein is pyruvate dehydrogenase. *Biochem. biophys. Res. Commun.*, 95: 569–576.

Neary, J.T., Crow, T. and Alkon, D.L. (1981) Change in a specific phosphoprotein band following associative learning in Hermissenda. *Nature (Lond.)* 293: 658–660.

Nestler, E.J. and Greengard, P. (1980) Dopamine and depolarizing agents regulate the state of phosphorylation of protein I in the mammalian superior cervical sympathetic ganglion. *Proc. nat. Acad. Sci. (Wash.)*, 77: 7479–7483.

Neville, Jr., D.M. (1971) Molecular weight determination of protein-dodecyl sulphate complexes by gel electrophoresis in a discontinuous buffer system. *J. biol. Chem.*, 246: 6328–6334.

Nishizuka, Y., Takai, Y., Hashimoto, E., Kishimoto, A., Kuroda, Y., Sakai, K. and Yamamura, H. (1979) Regulatory and functional compartment of three multifunctional protein kinase systems. *Mol. cell. Biochem.*, 23: 153–165.

Oestreicher, A.B., Zwiers, H., Schotman, P. and Gispen, W.H. (1981) Immunohistochemical localisation of a phosphoprotein (B-50) isolated from rat brain synaptic plasma membranes. *Brain Res. Bull.*, 6: 145–153.

Perrin, D.D. and Sayce, I.G. (1967) Computer calculation of equilibrium concentrations in mixtures of metal ions and complexing species. *Talanta*, 14: 883–842.

Potter, P. and White, T.D. (1980) Release of adenosine triphosphate from synaptosomes from different regions of rat brain. *Neuroscience*, 5: 1351–1356.

Rodnight, R. (1977) Phosphorylation of membrane proteins in the brain. In *Mechanisms Regulation and Special Functions of Protein Synthesis in the Brain*, S. Roberts, A. Lajtha and W.H. Gispen (Eds.), Elsevier/North-Holland, Amsterdam, pp. 255–266.

Rodnight, R. (1979) Cyclic nucleotides as second messengers in synaptic transmission. *Int. Rev. Biochem.*, 26: 1–80.

Rodnight, R. (1980a) Cyclic nucleotides, calcium ions and protein phosphorylation in synaptic transmission. In *Synaptic Constituents in Health and Disease*, M. Brzin, D. Sket and H. Bachelard (Eds.), Pergamon Press, Llubljana–Oxford, pp. 81–96.

Rodnight, R. (1980b) Molecular aspects of the actions of cyclic nucleotides at synapses. *Neurochem. int.*, 2: 113–122.

Rodnight, R. (1981) Molecular aspects of brain function. In *Investigations of Brain Function*, A.W. Wilkinson (Ed.), Plenum Press, New York, pp. 197–215.

Rodnight, R., Gower, H., Martinez-Millan, L. and De Souza, D. (1982) Features of the calcium ion and calmodulin dependent protein kinase activity in fragments of synaptosomal membranes from the rat. In *Molecular Aspects of Nervous Stimulation, Transmission and Learning and Memory*, J.A. Rodriguez and R. Caputto (Eds.), Raven Press, New York, in press.

Rothstein, A., Cabantchik, Z.I. and Krauf, P. (1976) Mechanism of ion transport in red blood cells: roles of membrane proteins. *Fed. Proc.*, 35: 3–10.

Routtenberg, A. (1979) Anatomical localization of phosphoprotein and glycoprotein substrates of memory *Prog. Neurobiol.*, 12: 85–113.

Rubin, C.S. Erlichman, J. and Rosen, O.M. (1972) Cyclic adenosine 3′,5′-monophosphate-dependent protein kinase of human erythrocyte membranes. *J. biol. Chem.*, 247: 6135–6139.

Sieghart, W., Forn, J., Schwartz, R., Coyle, J.T. and Greengard, P. (1978) Neuronal localisation of specific brain phosphoproteins. *Brain Res.*, 156: 345–350.

Sieghart, W., Schulman, H. and Greengard, P. (1980) Neuronal localization of $Ca^{2+}$-dependent protein phosphorylation in brain. *J. Neurochem.*, 34; 548–553.

Sobue, K., Ichida, S., Yoshida, H., Yamazaki, R. and Kakuichi, S. (1979) Occurrence of a $Ca^{2+}$- and modulator protein-activatable ATPase in the synaptic plasma membranes of brain. *FEBS Lett.*, 99: 199–202.

Sörensen, R.G., Kleine, L.P. and Mahler, H.R. (1981) Presynaptic localisation of phosphoprotein B-50. *Brain Res. Bull.*, 7: 57–61.

Steiner, A.W. and Smith, R.A. (1981) Endogenous protein phosphorylation in rat brain motochondria: occurrence of a novel ATP-dependent form of the autophosphorylated enzyme succinyl CoA synthetase. *J. Neurochem.*, 37: 582–593.

Ueda, T. and Greengard, P. (1977) Adenosine 3′:5′-monophosphate regulated phosphoprotein system of neuronal membranes. I. Solubilisation purification and some properties of an endogenous phosphoprotein. *J. biol. Chem.*, 252: 5155–5163.

Ueda, T., Greengard, P., Berzins, K., Cohen, R.J., Blomberg, F., Grab, D.J. and Siekevitz, P. (1979) Subcellular distribution in cerebral cortex of two proteins phosphorylated by a cyclic AMP-dependent protein kinase. *J. Cell Biol.*, 83: 308–319.

Waisman, D.M., Singh, T.J. and Wang, J.H. (1978) The modulator-dependent protein kinase. A multifunctional protein kinase activatable by the calcium-dependent modulator protein of the cyclic nucleotide system. *J. biol. Chem.*, 253: 3387–3390.

Walsh, M. and Stevens, F.C. (1978) Preparation characteristics and properties of a novel triple-modified derivative of the $Ca^{2+}$-dependent protein modulator. *Canad. J. Biochem.*, 56: 420–429.

Walter, U., Kanof, P., Schulman, H. and Greengard, P. (1978) Adenosine 3′,5′-monophosphate receptor proteins in mammalian brain. *J. biol. Chem.*, 253: 6275–6280.

Walter, U., Lohmann, S.M. Sieghart, W. and Greengard, P. (1979) Identification of the cyclic AMP-dependent protein kinase responsible for the endogenous phosphorylation of substrate proteins in synaptic membrane fraction from rat brain. *J. biol. Chem.*, 254: 12235–12239.

Weller, M. (1977) Evidence for the presynaptic location of adenylate cyclase and cyclic AMP-stimulated protein kinase which is bound to synpatic membranes. *Biochim. biophys. Acta*, 469: 350–354.

Weller, M. (1979) *Protein Phosphorylation*, Prior Ltd., London.

Weller, M. and Rodnight, R. (1971) Turnover of protein bound phosphorylserine in membrane preparations of ox brain catalysed by intrinsic kinase and phosphatase activity. *Biochem. J.*, 124: 393–406.

Wiegant, V.M. Zwiers, H., Schotman, P. and Gispen, W.H. (1978) Endogenous phosphorylation of rat brain synaptosomal plasma membranes in vitro: some methodological aspects. *Neurochem. Res.*, 3: 443–453.

Williams, M. and Rodnight, R. (1977) Protein phosphorylation in nervous tissue: possible involvement in nervous tissue function and relationship to cyclic nucleotide metabolism. *Progr. Neurol.*, 8: 183–250.

Wolff, D.J., Poivier, P.G., Brostrom, C.O. and Brostrom, M.A. (1977) Divalent cation binding properties of bovine brain $Ca^{2+}$-dependent regulator protein. *J. Biol. Chem.*, 252: 4108–4117.

Zwiers, H., Tonnaer, J., Wiegant, V.M., Schotman, P. and Gispen, W.H. (1979) ACTH-sensitive protein kinase from rat brain membranes. *J. Neurochem.*, 33: 247–256.

Zwiers, H., Schotman, P. and Gispen, W.H. (1980) Purification and some characteristics of an ACTH-sensitive protein kinase and its substrate protein in rat brain membranes. *J. Neurochem*, 34: 1689–1699.

# Identification and Topography
# of Synaptic Phosphoproteins

HENRY R. MAHLER *, LEONARD P. KLEINE **, NANCY RATNER and ROGER G. SORENSEN ***

*Department of Chemistry and the Molecular,
Cellular and Developmental Biology Program,
Indiana University, Bloomington, IN 47405, U.S.A.*

## INTRODUCTION

Like other groups, many of them represented at this symposium, we have been interested in phosphorylation–dephosphorylation reactions of proteins at the synapse as a possible basis for the modification through use of neuronal contacts. Several mutually non-exclusive suppositions can be advanced as to how these or other covalent alterations of synaptic membrane proteins might thus affect neuronal plasticity (Fig. 1) (e.g. Greengard, 1976, 1978; Nathanson, 1977; Williams and Rodnight, 1977; Mahler et al., 1977; Gispen, 1979; Ehrlich, 1979; Carlin et al., 1980; Schoffeniels and Dandrifosse, 1980; Hanbauer et al., 1980; Burgoyne, 1981; Rodnight, this volume). (i) Ion channels or their gates may be responsive to phosphorylation. (ii) Synaptic strength, or the density of synaptic contacts, might depend on the state of phosphorylation, and in this manner provide another means of affecting the efficacy of synaptic transmission directly. (iii) The state of phosphorylation of one or more proteins may affect functionality, catalytic or regulatory potency of membrane constituents, and thus alter their capacity to release, bind or otherwise interact with relevant neuroactive ligands such as transmitters, hormones, pharmacological agents, etc. Alternatively the ability of integral membrane proteins to interact with peripheral and/or cytoskeletal proteins may be influenced by the state of phosphorylation of one or more components of this system and thereby control membrane properties and binding of ligands to membrane receptors. (iv) The state of phosphorylation of certain membrane constituents may provide signals or addresses for the recognition, attachment and eventual integration of soluble macromolecules by the membrane

* Recipient of Research Career Award K06 05060 from the Institute of General Medical Sciences. Research supported by Research Grant NS 08309 from the National Institute of Neurological and Communicative Disorders and Stroke.

** Present address: Dr. Leonard P. Kleine, Animal and Cell Physiology Group, Biological Sciences M54, National Research Council of Canada, Ottawa, Ont. K1A0R6, Canada.

*** Present address: Mr. Roger G. Sorensen, Department of Chemistry, Texas Christian University, Fort Worth, TX 76129, U.S.A.

*Abbreviations:* CaM, calmodulin; DTT, dithiothreitol; EGTA, ethyleneglycol bis($\beta$-aminoethylether)-*N,N,N', N'*-tetraacetic acid; HEPES, 4-(2-hydroxyethyl)-1-piperazine-ethane-sulfonic acid; IBMX, isobutyl-methylxanthine; $M_{app}$, apparent molecular weight; PDH, pyruvate dehydrogenase ($\alpha_2\beta_2$); $\alpha$-PDH, $\alpha$ subunit of PDH; SDS, sodium dodecyl sulfate; PSD, postsynaptic density; PSM–PSD, preparation containing a majority of PSDs attached to postsynaptic membranes; SM, synaptic membranes; TEMED, *N,N,N',N'*-tetramethylethylenediamine.

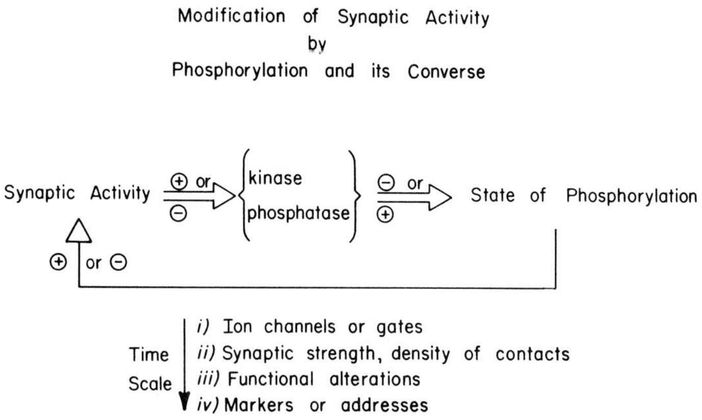

28

Modification of Synaptic Activity
by
Phosphorylation and its Converse

Fig. 1. Modification of synaptic activity by phosphorylation and its converse.

resulting in its long-lasting modification. Since the activities of the enzymes responsible for phosphorylation (protein kinases) and dephosphorylation (protein phosphatases) may themselves be responsive to some concomitant of neuronal activity, either directly or indirectly, in a stimulatory or inhibitory fashion (see this Symposium), one can envisage the phosphorylation–dephosphorylation cycle as occupying a crucial position in a variety of positive or negative feedback loops.

To convert some of these suppositions from vague generalities to the level of testable hypotheses requires the prior establishment of a minimal set of clearly defined experimental objectives. Among them, most investigators would probably agree, is the definition of the potential for modification of synaptic proteins of known structure, function and localization within the junctional complex. Some notable progress toward these objectives has already been achieved by Greengard and his collaborators. They have demonstrated that an entity, with an as yet ill-defined function, called protein I (or more recently "Synapsin") is specifically confined to synapses of the central and peripheral nervous system (DeCamilli et al., 1979; Bloom et al., 1979; Goelz et al., 1981). In the former it is localized both postsynaptically (in the postsynaptic density) (Ueda et al., 1979; Grab et al., 1981) and presynaptically (principally in synaptic vesicles) (Ueda et al., 1979; Bloom et al. 1979; DeCamilli et al., 1979; Sieghart et al., 1980). It is susceptible to phosphorylation at two sets of sites: the first in a reaction requiring either cAMP or $Ca^{2+}$ and the second in one dependent on $Ca^{2+}$ plus calmodulin (CaM) (Huttner and Greengard, 1979; Kennedy and Greengard, 1981; Huttner et al., 1981). In this contribution we provide evidence for the definite identification, requirements for phosphorylation, and localization of three additional proteins present in purified synaptic membrane preparations: $\alpha$-PDH, the $\alpha$ subunit of pyruvate dehydrogenase (Reed, 1974; Krebs and Beavo, 1979); $R_{II}^{\beta}$, the brain-specific regulatory subunit of the cAMP-dependent protein kinase (Krebs and Beavo, 1979; Kelly and Cotman, 1978; Walter et al., 1979; Rubin et al., 1979; Lohmann et al., 1980), and B-50, a brain-specific protein (Oestreicher et al., 1981), originally identified in and isolated from light brain membranes by Zwiers, Gispen and their collaborators, the phosphorylation of which is inhibited by ACTH (Zwiers et al., 1976, 1978, 1979, 1980).

METHODS AND MATERIALS

*Phosphorylation of SM*

The SM preparations used were prepared by the method of Jones and Matus (1974) as modified by Salvaterra and Matthews (1980) using 30–40-day-old Sprague–Dawley rats. SM (100 $\mu$g protein unless otherwise indicated) were phosphorylated for 10 sec at 37° C essentially as described by DeBlas et al. (1979), in 50 $\mu$l of a buffer containing 50 mM HEPES (pH 7.6), 1 mM DTT, 0.5 mM EGTA, 6 mM MgCl$_2$, 1.0 mM theophylline or IBMX and 5 or 25 $\mu$M [$\gamma$-$^{32}$P]ATP (10–40 Ci/mmole, New England Nuclear, Boston, MA). Reaction was started with ATP and stopped with dissociation buffer (DeBlas et al., 1979). Protein kinase activity was assayed by spotting reaction mixtures on phosphocelluose paper (Witt and Roskoski, 1975) and its products determined by the gel techniques described below, subsequent to exposure to dissociation buffer and boiling for 5 min (DeBlas et al., 1979). The final concentrations of modulators, when added, were cAMP (10 $\mu$M), CaCl$_2$ (0.5 or 5 $\mu$M$_T$) and CaM (0.54 $\mu$g, 0.6 $\mu$M).

*Phosphorylation of α-PDH*

Pure PDH from beef heart in both its unphosphorylated and phosphorylated forms were the generous gifts of Prof. Lester J. Reed of the University of Texas, Austin. For phosphorylation (L.J. Reed, personal communication) 1.65 mg of crystalline PDH tetramer ($\alpha_2\beta_2$) were incubated overnight on ice in 0.7 ml of a buffer containing 0.02 M K phosphate (pH 7.0), 1.0 mM MgCl$_2$, 0.1 mM EDTA and 0.5 mM DTT with 3 % by weight of transacetylase–kinase subcomplex and [$\gamma$-$^{32}$P]ATP. Unreacted labeled ATP was removed by passage through a column of Sephadex G-25 and the labeled sample was shown to contain 3.1 nmoles of $^{32}$P per nmole ($\sim$ 154 $\mu$g) of tetrameric PDH.

*One-dimensional gel electrophoresis*

A modification of the gel system described by Laemmli (1970) was used: 10 % acrylamide, 0.1 % bisacrylamide running gels, 9.5 cm long (0.375 M Tris pH 8.8, 0.1 % SDS, 0.1 % ammonium persulfate and 0.05 % TEMED) polymerized for a minimum of 4 h. Stacking gels contained 4 % acrylamide, 0.04 % bisacrylamide, 0.125 M Tris pH 6.8, 0.1 % SDS, 0.1 % ammonium persulfate and 0.1 % TEMED (polymerized for 1 h). Running buffer contained 0.025 M Tris, 0.19 M glycine, and 0.1 % SDS; final pH = 8.4. Electrophoresis was performed at 30 mA per slab (approx. 3.5 h). Gels were stained in 40 % MeOH, 10 % acetic acid, 0.04 % Coomassie Brilliant Blue for 4 h, destained overnight in 10 % MeOH, 10 % acetic acid, 0.004 % Coomassie Brilliant Blue and further destained in 10 % acetic acid. Apparent molecular weights ($M_{app}$) were determined by parallel electrophoresis of molecular weight standards obtained from Bio-Rad [myosin ($200 \times 10^3$), $\beta$-galactosidase ($116.5 \times 10^3$), phosphorylase B ($94 \times 10^3$), BSA ($68 \times 10^3$), ovalbumin ($43 \times 10^3$), carbonic anhydrase ($30 \times 10^3$), soybean trypsin inhibitor ($21 \times 10^3$)]. Internal standards were provided by certain abundant membrane proteins ($M_{app}$ in parentheses), namely $\alpha$-tubulin ($57 \times 10^3$), $\beta$-tubulin ($55 \times 10^3$), and actin ($45 \times 10^3$). For autoradiography dried gels were exposed to Kodak SB-5 medical X-ray film at $-20°$ C.

*Two-dimensional analysis*

Two-dimensional (isoelectric focusing and electrophoretic) analysis on polyacrylamide gels was carried out essentially as described by O'Farrell (1975), using the SDS solubilization and sample preparation methods of Ames and Nikaido (1976), except that the final concentration of SDS in the solubilization mixture was 2 %. A 2 : 2 : 1 ratio of 4–6 : 6–8 : 3.5–10 ampholines was used the isoelectric focusing gels, and the second dimension SDS–polyacrylamide gel system was as described above.

### Fingerprint analysis by partial proteolysis

Enzymatic digestions with *Staphylococcus aureus* V8 protease or papain in a 4 % acrylamide spacer gel and separation on 15 % acrylamide gels were performed as described by Cleveland et al. (1977). Samples were excised from dried gels, incubated in stacking buffer for 30 min, placed in sample wells of a second SDS–polyacrylamide slab gel and overlayed with protease in the amounts described in the figures. Electrophoresis was started at 4 mA/slab for 10 h and completed at 25 mA/slab. Proteolysis occurred in situ during the stacking phase.

### Purified proteins

Regulatory subunits of cAMP-dependent protein kinase from brain of types I and II, referred to as $R_I^\beta$ and $R_{II}^\beta$, respectively, were isolated as described by Rubin et al. (1979); purified B-50 was obtained according to Zwiers et al. (1980) and compared to authentic samples kindly provided by Dr. Zwiers. CaM was prepared from bovine brain as described by Watterson et al. (1980).

### Materials

Papain, cAMP, theophylline and IBMX were obtained from Sigma Chemical Co., St. Louis, MO; ultrapure urea from Schwarz/Mann, Orangeburg, NY; protease from *S. aureus* V8 from Miles Laboratories, Elkhart, IN, and all reagents for electrophoresis and electrofocusing from Bio-Rad, Richmond, CA.

## RESULTS AND DISCUSSION

### Identification of proteins phosphorylated in synaptic membranes

### Phosphorylation systems and substrates

When purified synaptic membranes (SM) from rat cerebral cortex or other brain regions are exposed to short pulses of $[\gamma\text{-}^{32}P]ATP$, and the products of the reactions catalyzed by the endogenous protein kinases separated and analyzed on one-dimensional polyacrylamide gels, more than 25 (groups of) products can be identified (DeBlas et al., 1979; Ng and Matus, 1979a,b; Matus et al., 1980a; Mahler and Sorensen, 1980; Mahler et al., 1981). For the present purposes we have elected to concentrate on a group of prominent products within a range of apparent molecular weights ($M_{app}$) in our standard system * between 40 and 60 × 10³, and examined the effect of four potential cofactors or modulators on their phosphorylation. These are: (a) $Mg^{2+}$ (6 mM) alone; (b) same plus cAMP (10 $\mu$M); (c) $Mg^{2+}$ plus $Ca^{2+}$ at a relatively low concentration (0.5 mM corresponding to $[Ca]_{free} = 5\ \mu$M); (d) same as (c) in the presence of CaM (0.54 $\mu$g) and (e) no $Mg^{2+}$ but high $Ca^{2+}$ (5 mM, corresponding to $[Ca]_{free} = \geqslant 4$ mM). Activity (e) may correspond to that described by Takai et al. (1979) and by

---

\* In this report we employ the following nomenclature for polypeptides: P*N* refers to a protein with an apparent molecular weight in our standard system (Methods and Materials) equal to *N* × 10³, i.e. P43 is a polypeptide with $M_{app} = 43 \times 10^3$. Phosphoproteins are referred to as P*N*p and if their positive effectors are known they are indiscated in parentheses, e.g. P45p (cAMP).

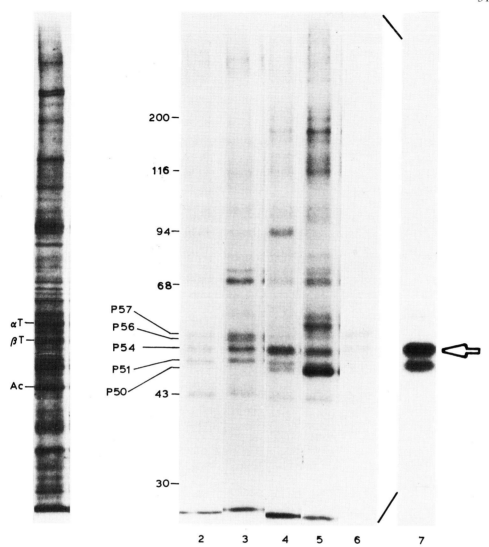

Fig. 2. Comparison of phosphoprotein substrates and the effect of different modulators. Autoradiograph of samples of phosphorylated SM separated on one-dimensional SDS slab gels (see Methods and Materials). The apparent $M_R \times 10^{-3}$ of phosphoproteins relative to standards [myosin (200), $\beta$-D-galactosidase (116.5), phosphorylase $b$ (94), bovine serum albumin (68), ovalbumin (43) and carbonic anhydrase (30)] is shown on the left. The various lanes were loaded with different proteins, as follows: (1) SM (25 $\mu$g), stained with Coomassie Blue: the bands identified (by 2D and fingerprinting techniques) as $\alpha$-tubulin, $\beta$-tubulin and actin are shown; (2) SM (25 $\mu$g), background phosphorylation; (3) SM (25 $\mu$g), plus 10 $\mu$M cAMP; (4) SM (25 $\mu$g), plus 0.5 mM $Ca_T^{2+}$; (5) SM (25 $\mu$g), as (4) plus 3 $\mu$M CaM; (6) SM (25 $\mu$g), with 5.0 mM $Ca_T^{2+}$ in the absence of $Mg^{2+}$ (7) B-50 preparation (2 $\mu$g) with B-50 itself indicated by an arrow.

Wrenn et al. (1980). The results of a typical set of experiments are shown in Fig. 2. They are qualitatively unaffected by increases in ATP concentration from our standard 5 to 25 $\mu$M and/or length of exposure to it from 10 to 60 sec and may be summarized as follows. (i) Addition of cAMP stimulates the phosphorylation of four proteins P57, P56, P54 and P51 in the range of interest, as well as that of a prominent doublet P75-P80 probably corresponding to protein I (see below). (ii) Addition of low concentrations of $Ca^{2+}$ results in the phosphorylation of proteins P54 and P50 (as well as other sets at P95 and P180). (iii) Supplementation of this system with external CaM [for a recent symposium on CaM function including phosphorylation see Watterson and Vincenzi (1980); see also Schulman and Greengard (1978); De Lorenzo (1980); Grab et al. (1981)] results in a pronounced stimulation of the phosphorylation of P50 and the appearance of a doublet at P58 plus P59 — as well as of phosphorylation of the protein I doublet at P75 plus P80 — and of sets of polypeptides at P120-P150 and P170-P210. (iv) The presence of $Ca^{2+}$ in high concentrations results in the phosphorylation of three substrates P51, P54 and P57. (v) Phosphorylation of a polypeptide P44 prominent in the base line ($Mg^{2+}$) system appears to be inhibited by the addition of $Ca^{2+}$, even at low concentrations. Subsequent studies, some of them described below, have resulted in the firm identification of several of these entities as summarized in Table I. In addition, by analogy with published studies, P75-P80p(cAMP) and P75-P80p(Ca/CaM) are virtually certain to correspond to protein I (see Introduction, DeBlas et al., 1979; Carlin et al., 1890; Grab et al., 1981; Ueda, this volume), and we have some evidence that P51p(cAMP) is identical to $R_I^\beta$, the type I regulatory subunit of cAMP-dependent protein kinase from brain (Krebs and Beavo, 1979; Kelly et al., 1979; Rubin et al., 1979; Geahlen et al., 1981).

TABLE I

IDENTIFICATION OF SYNAPTIC PHOSPHOPROTEINS

| Species | pI | Identity | Method of analysis used * | | | |
|---------|-----|----------|---|---|---|---|
| | | | A | B | C | D |
| P44p | 7.6 | $\alpha$-PDH | + | + | + | |
| P54p(Ca) | 4.6 | B-50** | + | + | + | |
| P54p(cAMP) | 5.1 | $R_{II}^\beta$ | + | + | + | + |
| P56p(cAMP) | 6.9 | | | | + | |
| P57p(cAMP) | 5.2 | $R_{II}^\beta$ | + | + | + | + |

\* Comparison with authentic pure proteins by A, comigration in 1D gels; B, comigration in 2D gels; C, fingerprints of partial digest; D, methods A, B, C applied to protein covalently modified by photoaffinity labeling with 8-azido cAMP.
\*\* Confirmed by ACTH inhibition.

*P44 is $\alpha$-PDH*

Studies in two different laboratories had suggested that a hippocampal phosphoprotein, subject to modulation by behavioral or electrophysiological manipulations, was identical with $\alpha$-PDH, the $\alpha$ subunit of pyruvate dehydrogenase, a mitochondrial enzyme (Morgan and Routtenberg, 1980; Routtenberg and Benson, 1980; Browning et al., 1980a,b, 1981). We have extended and confirmed this identification for the synaptic phosphoprotein P44p. Some of the evidence for this assertion is presented in Fig. 3A. Here the $M_{app}$ of this protein (lane 4) equals $43\,500 \pm 500$, established by comparison either with external protein standards (lane 1), or the prominent SM protein at $M_{app} = 45\,000$ (lane 2), previously identified by us as actin by 2D (Fig. 4) and fingerprint techniques. It comigrates exactly with authentic $\alpha$-PDH, as demonstrated in Fig. 3 either with a protein stain (lane 3) or after $^{32}P$ labeling by its specific kinase (lane 7) or by a crude preparation isolated from SM (lane 5). The identification has been

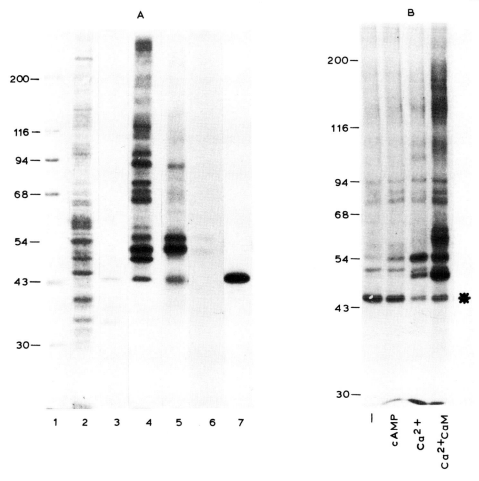

Fig. 3. $\alpha$-PDH is a prominent phosphoprotein in SM preparations. A: Lanes 1–3: proteins stained with Coomassie Brilliant Blue. Lane 1, standard proteins and their $M_R$ (see Fig. 2); lane 2, SM; lane 3, purified $\alpha$-PDH. Lanes 4–7: radioautographs. Lane 4, phosphorylated SM; Lane 5, purified PDH phosphorylated with a crude kinase preparation extracted from SM; lane 6, as in lane 5, without PDH; lane 7, $\alpha$-PDH phosphorylated by PDH kinase. B: radioautographs of SM phosphorylated under the conditions defined in Fig. 2 and Methods. The asterisk marks the position of the band defined In A.

substantiated further by 2D techniques (Fig. 4 below) where spot 5, corresponding to P44p comigrates with $\alpha$-PDH, and comparison of fingerprints of the two phosphoproteins (not shown) using partial digestion with the protease from *Staphylococcus aureus* V8 and with papain. The decrease of the extent of phosphorylation of $\alpha$-PDH by added $Ca^{2+}$ seen in lanes 3 and 4 of Fig. 3B is quite real and reproducible and had been observed by us in earlier studies (Mahler and Sorensen, 1980; Sorensen et al., 1981; also see Fig. 2). It is probably due to the known activation of PDH phosphatase by this ion (Reed, 1974; Sugden et al., 1978; Teague et al., 1979) and is also observed with interterminal mitochondria in intact synaptosomes rendered permeable by 0.1 % saponin (Sorensen et al., 1981). These observations suggest that there exist close coupling between the concentration of intraterminal $Ca^{2+}$ and the activity of PDH and through it mitochondrial respiration, energy generation (Browning et al., 1981) and

34

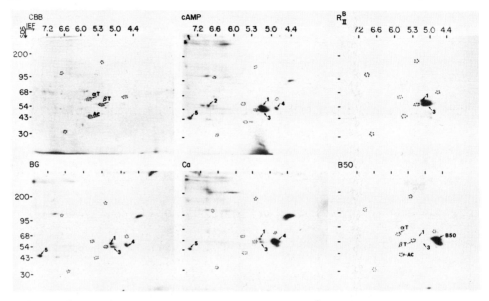

Fig. 4. Two-dimensional analysis of SM phosphoproteins. The $M_{app} \times 10^{-3}$ is indicated on the side. The pH gradient is denoted on the top. CBB (top left), Coomassie Blue stained gel obtained after two-dimensional separation of SM (100 $\mu$g). The circled proteins are used as reference points for all autoradiographs. $\alpha$T, $\alpha$-tubulin; $\beta$T, $\beta$-tubulin; Ac, actin. Other panels are autoradiographs: BG, SM (100 $\mu$g) phosphorylated in buffer alone (background phosphorylation); cAMP, SM phosphorylated in the presence of 10 $\mu$M cAMP; Ca, SM phosphorylated in the presence of 0.5 mM $Ca_T^{2+}$; $R_{II}^B$ and B50, phosphorylated purified proteins (see Methods), 10 and 20 $\mu$g respectively were used for the analysis.

all processes dependent thereon. They emphasize the key role of the potential regulation of and by PDH in intracellular (Reed, 1974; Leiter et al., 1978; Krebs and Beavo, 1979; Seals et al., 1979; Seals and Czech, 1981; McDonald et al., 1981) and synaptic (Morgan and Routtenberg, 1980; Browning et al., 1980a,b; Routtenberg, this volume; Browning, this volume) regulatory events.

*Resolution of P54p: P54p(cAMP) is $R_{II}^B$ and P54p(Ca) is B-50*

Extensive data similar to those presented in Fig. 2 indicated that phosphorylation of a polypeptide with a $M_{app} = 54\,000$ (mobility just below $\beta$-tubulin) appeared to be stimulated either by cAMP or by $Ca^{2+}$ plus CaM. Was this due to phosphorylation of a single protein substrate by two separate systems, analogous to what had already been demonstrated for protein I? Examination of the phosphoprotein product on 2D gels (Fig. 4) showed that it consisted of two discrete components that appeared to be identical with $R_{II}^B$ [P54p(cAMP)] and B-50 [P54p(Ca)] respectively. Further corroboration came from experiments using (a) fingerprinting by partial proteolysis; (b) binding of the radioactive photoaffinity analog 8-N$_3$-[$^{32}$P]cAMP for the identification of cAMP receptors (identical with regulatory subunits of protein kinase — Krebs and Beavo, 1979) followed by their analysis by means of 1D, 2D and fingerprinting techniques; (c) inhibition of the phosphorylation reaction by ACTH or ACTH$_{1-24}$, but not ACTH$_{1-10}$ (Zwiers et al., 1976, 1978, 1979, 1980). Experiments of type (a) disclosed that P54p(cAMP) (Spot 3, Fig. 4) and P57p(cAMP) (spot 1, Fig. 4) both produced identical fingerprints, which were indistinguishable from those generated by purified, phosphorylated $R_{II}^B$ either before or after its resolution into its two phosphoprotein components (Fig.

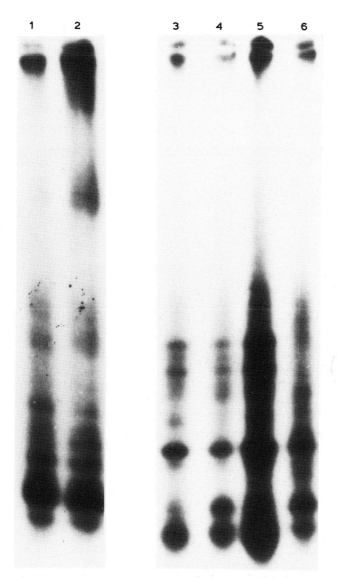

Fig. 5. Comparison of cAMP-binding proteins by fingerprint analysis. Autoradiograph of the peptide maps generated by various preparations, previously covalently labeled with 8-$N_3$-[$^{32}$P]cAMP (see Methods), cut from 1D gels and subjected to digestion with 0.3 $\mu$g *S. aureus* protease per lane for 10 h. (1) SM-P50(cAMP); (2) $R_I^B$-P50(cAMP); (3) SM-P54(cAMP); (4) SM-P57(cAMP); (5) $R_{II}^B$-P54(cAMP); (6) $R_{II}^B$-P57(cAMP).

4, top right). However, this set of fingerprints was completely different from that generated by a second set constituted by P54p(Ca) (spot 4, Fig. 4). Experiments of type (b) showed that both SM and isolated $R_{II}^B$ contained two major cAMP receptor species at P54 and P57. They all generated identical fingerprint patterns (Fig. 5) and corresponded respectively to the completely dephosphorylated and fully phosphorylated form of the same regulatory subunit. This conclusion is based on studies using experimentally dephosphorylated (by potato acid phosphatase — see Geahlen et al., 1981) and rephosphorylated (by endogenous or exogenous kinase) proteins. Furthermore there was substantial comigration on 2D gels between cAMP receptor P54 with P54p(cAMP) and cAMP receptor P57 with P57p(cAMP). Finally, experiments of type (c) clearly demonstrated that formation of P54p(Ca), but not of P54p(cAMP), was inhibited by ACTH and its active analogs.

## *Disposition of synaptic phosphoproteins*

Under this heading we describe experiments designed to answer a number of related questions, namely: (1) Can we assign the proteins just described to discrete entities of the synapse such as its pre- or postsynaptic membrane or its specializations, such as presynaptic mitochondria or postsynaptic densities (PSD)? (2) Can we refine the assignment of membrane proteins to include their topology, i.e. assign them to the internal or external surface of their respective membrane, and can we obtain any evidence for a transmembrane orientation for some of them? And finally, (3) can we begin to accumulate evidence concerning the horizontal (in plane) arrangements of these and other membrane proteins and the possible relevance of such topographical factors and constraints on phosphorylation and other membrane functions?

### *Localization of phosphoproteins*

We have recently published the results of some experiments dealing with this problem (Sorensen et al., 1981). The approaches used in these and more current studies, as well as the results obtained, are summarized in Tables II and III, respectively. Membrane composition has been monitored by both morphological and enzymatic markers: presence or absence of PSDs or the characteristic PSD protein (see below) for postsynaptic components, cristate organelles or their fragments and succinate dehydrogenase for mitochondria. The inferences to be discussed rest on both positive and negative evidence: as shown in Table III absence of a particular protein in fractions enriched in presynaptic membranes is correlated with its presence in ones enriched in postsynaptic membranes, and the converse. Enrichment of a component in fractions known to be contaminated by mitochondria correlates well with its disappearance from fractions known to contain few or no mitochondria. Two phosphoproteins

TABLE II

PREPARATIONS USED FOR ESTABLISHING DISTRIBUTION
OF SYNAPTIC PHOSPHOPROTEIN

| Preparation * | Fractions examined | Membranes present of affected |
|---|---|---|
| PSM–PSD | 0.32/1.0 M sucrose interface | Largely presynaptic |
| | 1.50/2.0 M sucrose interface | Postsynaptic w. PSD attached; (intraterminal) Mt |
| PSD | PSDs from gradient | PSD, some PSM–PSD |
| Synaptosomes | Intact synaptosomes | PSM–PSD plus external surface of presynaptic membrane |
| | Permeabilized synaptosomes (Saponin-treated) | Dto plus internal surface of presynaptic; intraterminal Mt |
| IOV | Inside-out presynaptic membrane vesicles (ghosts) | Presynaptic; no Mt contamination |
| 5-step gradient | Lysed synaptosomal membranes 5 disc. steps plus pellet | Membranes increasing in density, PSM–PSD and Mt content |

* For methods of preparation see Sorensen et al. (1981), except for PSD, see Carlin et al. (1980).

TABLE III

DISTRIBUTION OF PHOSPHOPROTEINS IN SM FRACTIONS

| Phosphoprotein | Preparation * | PSM–PSD | | PSD | Synaptosomes | | IOV | | Gradient | | |
|---|---|---|---|---|---|---|---|---|---|---|---|
| Subfraction | | 0.32/1.0 | 1.5/2.0 | | Intact | Perm[b] ** | Baseline | +Ca$^{2+}$ | 0.32/0.6 | 0.6/0.8 | 0.95/1.0 |
| P44p | α-PDH | – | + | – | ± | + | – | – | – | – | + |
| P50p(Ca/CaM) | | ± | + | + | + | + | – | + | – | ± | + |
| P54p(Ca) | B-50 | + | – | – | – | + | ± | + | + | + | – |
| P54p(cAMP) | | ± | – | + | – | + | + | – | – | + | – |
| Protein Ip(Ca/CaM) | R$_{II}^{B}$ | ± | – | + | – | + | + | ± | – | – | + |
| Protein Ip(cAMP) | | + | – | ± | – | + | + | ± | ± | + | – |

* For methods of preparation see Table II.

** Permeabilized.

38

exhibit unambiguous localization patterns: (i) P44p ($\alpha$-PDH) is present wherever mitochondria are found, and this is true of both intraterminal and cell body mitochondria. This
inference is consistent with the known localization of pyruvate dehydrogenase in the mitochondrial matrix (Reed, 1974; Leiter et al., 1978). (ii) P54p(Ca) (B-50) is localized presynaptically and appears to be present in membranes of low buoyant density. This assignment is
consistent with the original demonstration of the presence of this protein on and its isolation
from light synaptic membranes (Zwiers et al., 1978, 1979, 1980). It also agrees with its
postulated function in modifying the presynaptic membrane (Jolles et al., 1980). The possibility that some of this protein is located postsynaptically but has been lost in the course of
preparation of the postsynaptic fractions is considered highly unlikely for two reasons: it is
absent from the SPM–PSD fraction, which is obtained under rather mild conditions, as well as

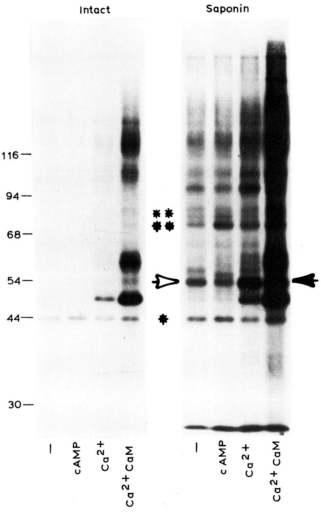

Fig. 6. Phosphorylation patterns of intact and permeabilized (saponin-treated) synaptosomes (Hajos, 1975; McGraw
et al., 1980). Phosphoproteins are identified as follows: P43p ($\alpha$-PDH, single asterisk; P54p(Ca) or B-50, empty
arrow; P54p(cAMP) or $R_{II}^{B}$, solid arrow; protein I doublet, double asterisks. Reprinted from Brain Res. Bull., with
permission.

from intact synaptosomes in which other postsynaptic proteins with similar requirements for phosphorylation are clearly evident (Fig. 6). The remainder of the phosphoproteins are present in fractions enriched in either presynaptic and postsynaptic membranes and their attachments, but exhibit a complementary pattern. Those phosphorylated by kinase(s) activated by cAMP appear to be concentrated in the presynaptic, and those affected by the $Ca^{2+}$-CaM-dependent kinase(s) in the postsynaptic membrane compartment (Ueda et al., 1979; Carlin et al., 1980). This is brought out most clearly by a comparison of the two relatively pure preparations represented by the presynaptic inverted membrane vesicles (IOV) and the PSD, shown here in Figs. 7A and B, respectively. The IOV exhibit pronounced phosphorylation of all SM substrates affected by the cAMP-dependent kinase, while detection of the relatively weakly phosphorylated substrates by the $Ca^{2+}$-CaM kinase in these metal ion-depleted membranes, isolated in the presence of EDTA, becomes evident only on increasing the $Ca^{2+}$ concentration. Incidentally, this concentration of $Ca^{2+}$ completely suppresses the cAMP-dependent phosphorylation of Protein I. In contrast, in the PSD the $Ca^{2+}$-CaM reaction appears to be preponderant, with two principal products P50p and P61p (Carlin et al., 1980; Grab et al., 1981). This is also the pattern observed with our PSM–PSD preparation isolated without the use of detergent. However, unlike the latter, the PSDs obtained by the use of Triton X-100 retain substantial cAMP-dependent phosphorylation of appropriate substrates. In part this difference is due to the retention of an active cAMP-dependent kinase, but even more significant is an activation of both sets of kinase reactions by exposure to the detergent, enhancing the mutual accessibility of the enzyme and its substrates. We shall return to this effect in due course.

*Topology of phosphoproteins*

The reactions observed with permeabilized synaptosomes and inverted presynaptic membranes suggest that the great majority of all phosphorylatable sites on the proteins of the presynaptic membrane are located on its interior (synaptoplasmic) aspect. Alternatively, or in addition, they may be due to the insertion of the responsible kinases at this location. If, as has been suggested, synaptic transmitter storage vesicles account for a high proportion of both the cAMP-dependent (Ueda et al., 1979; Bloom et al., 1979) and Ca/CaM-dependent phosphorylation systems (de Lorenzo, 1980), and if transmitter release depends on exocytosis coincident with fusion of vesicle and presynaptic membranes (see Llinas and Heuser, 1977, for review), then the various phosphoproteins should be found on the *inside* of the synaptic vesicles. This prediction implies that they should be inaccessible to surface probes in *intact* vesicles (Mahler et al., 1977) and become accessible only upon their lysis or fusion with the presynaptic membrane and is subject to experimental verification.

*Transmembrane location of presynaptic phosphoproteins*

Even though the actual phosphorylation of these proteins takes place on the interior aspect of the membrane, there remains the interesting possibility that some of them may penetrate the bilayer and protrude beyond the exterior aspect into the junctional space. This model can be tested by examining the effect of a prior exposure of intact synaptosomes to trypsin (e.g. Smith and Loh, 1979) on their subsequent phosphorylation. In such experiments a negative outcome cannot be interpreted, but positive results lead to interesting inferences *provided* appropriate controls can be devised to show that the trypsin treatment by itself has not affected the integrity and permeability of the synaptosome. A set of such experiments is shown in Fig. 8. That the synaptosomes remain intact after exposure to trypsin is clearly seen by the increase in phosphorylation of all substrates (except P44) after saponin treatment. The phosphorylation of

40

P44 does not increase after permeabilization of synaptosomes indicating that most of this substrate is contributed by contaminating mitochondria. There is no decrease in the phosphorylation of any of the substrates after exposure of intact synaptosomes to trypsin with the possible exception of P50, P58 and P59 ($Ca^{2+}$-CaM). An internal control to demonstrate that the trypsin was active is seen by the decrease in $Ca^{2+}$ and $Ca^{2+}$-CaM substrates in the intact trypsin-treated synaptosomes relative to the intact synaptosomes not exposed to trypsin. This kinase activity in the intact synaptosomes is presumably due to lysed synaptosomes or contaminating membranes. Therefore, the cAMP-dependent substrates would seem to be localized on the interior aspect of the membranes as are the $Ca^{2+}$- and $Ca^{2+}$-CaM-dependent substrates with the exception of P50, P58 and P59 ($Ca^{2+}$-CaM) which may be transmembrane.

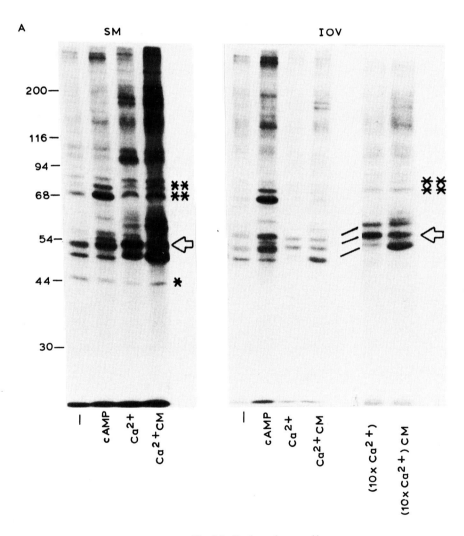

Fig. 7A. For legend see p. 41.

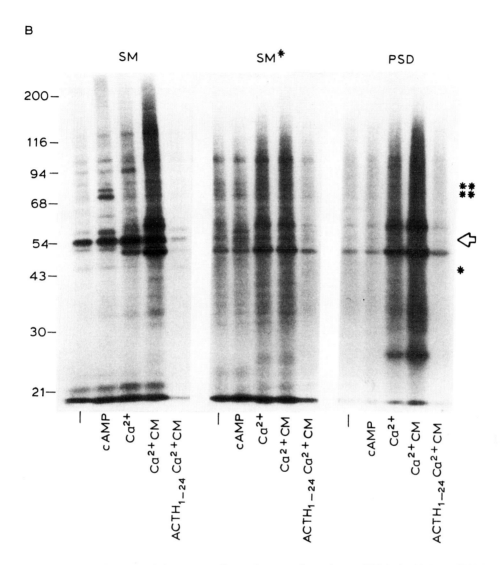

Fig. 7. Comparison of phosphorylation patterns of inverted presynaptic membranes (IOV) in A with those of PSD in B. For part A, 100 μg of SM or IOV (Gill et al., 1981) were phosphorylated under standard conditions and 30 μg of protein per lane analyzed. IOV were also phosphorylated in the presence of 5 mM $Ca_T^{2+}$ (indicated as "$10 \times Ca^{2+}$"). For part B, PSD, SM and SM treated with Triton X-100 to be loaded on the gradients (SM*), were prepared as described in Methods; for all three fractions 50 μg of protein were phosphorylated and for analysis we used 23 μg (SM), 4 μg (SM*) and 2.7 μg (PSD) per lane.

*Topography of synaptic phosphoproteins: Removal of in plane constraints*

While studying the phosphorylation of subsynaptic fractions such as PSM–PSD and especially of PSD isolated by the use of detergents (Cohen et al., 1977; Carlin et al., 1980) we were surprised that their rate of reaction appeared greatly increased over that characteristic of SM. Analysis of the effect disclosed that it could be resolved into at least four components: (i) an enrichment of some of the substrates and, perhaps their kinase, in these postsynaptic fractions (Grab et al., 1981); (ii) an activation by aging (i.e. length of exposure at 0–4° C during isolation); (iii) an increase as the protein concentration was decreased relative to the constant ATP concentration in the standard phosphorylation system; and (iv) an activation due to exposure to detergent. Of them, effect (iv) is particularly striking and is clearly indicated by the results shown in Fig. 7B, where we have taken care to eliminate effects (ii) and (iii) by equalizing both the extent of preexposure and the amount of protein in the reaction mixture. Since we had to decrease the amount of protein analyzed in the gel by factors of 5.8 and 8.5 for SM * (i.e. the detergent-treated membrane), and PSD respectively, it is evident that treatment with detergent is itself responsible for a significant increase in activity. This conclusion is corroborated by a direct determination of protein kinase activity as shown in Table IV. It is not unreasonable to interpret this activation — which is not restricted to Triton X-100 but is also produced by low concentrations of a number of different nonionic detergents (DeBlas, unpublished observation) — in terms of the removal of lateral, in plane, constraints that have prevented free accessibility of the kinases to acceptor sites on the substrates.

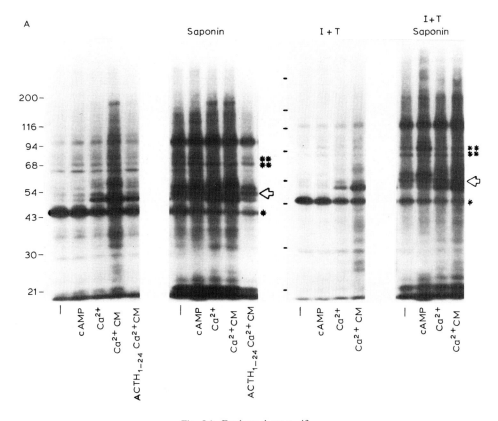

Fig. 8A. For legend see p. 43.

43

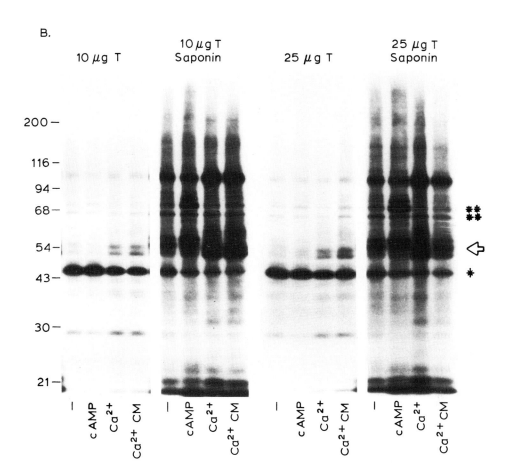

Fig. 8. Effect of trypsin on synaptosome phosphorylation. Synaptosomes (5 mg/ml) were exposed to soybean trypsin inhibitor (I) + trypsin (T) (10 or 25 μg/ml), singly or in combination, incubated at 30° C for 30 min (Smith and Loh, 1979) and the reaction stopped by the addition of inhibitor, if not already present. Aliquots of synaptosomes from each treatment were permeabilized with saponin (0.2 mg/ml). All samples were phosphorylated (see Fig. 2 for conditions) and analyzed on SDS gels. A: Untreated (no T) (48 μg protein/lane) and control (I + T) (40 μg protein/lane) synaptosomes, intact and permeabilized (saponin). B: Trypsin-treated synaptosomes (40 μg protein/lane), intact and permeabilized.

TABLE IV

PROTEIN KINASE ACTIVITIES OF SM AND ITS SUBFRACTIONS

Effect of exposure to 0.5% Triton X-100.

| Fractions | Modulators | | | |
|-----------|-----|------|------|------|
| | – | cAMP | $Ca^{2+}$ | $Ca^{2+}$,CaM |
| SM | 19.7 | 32.5 (12.8) | 42.5 (22.8) | 61.6 (41.9) |
| SM* | 219.8 | 261.7 (41.9) | 344.0 (124.2) | 531.7 (311.9) |
| PSD | 43.6 | 47.1 (3.5) | 151.7 (108.1) | 307.4 (263.8) |

Protein kinase activity in pmoles phosphate bound $mg^{-1}$ $10\ sec^{-1}$. Numbers in parentheses are corrected for baseline activity.

### Nature of phosphoproteins in the PSD

The high rate and extent of the phosphorylation reactions in PSDs makes it possible to subject a contentious question to a critical examination, namely the problem of the possible modification by this reaction of the major constituent proteins of the structure. These, most investigators now agree, are composed of (a) a novel protein specific to the PSD (PSD protein) with a mobility on SDS gels between $\beta$-tubulin and actin, (b) $\alpha$- and $\beta$-tubulin, and (c) actin (e.g. Banker et al., 1974; Wang and Mahler, 1976; Mahler et al. 1977; Kelly and Cotman, 1978; Matus et al., 1980a,b; Carlin et al., 1980). We have determined their relative concentration in SM, PSM–PSD and PSD preparations. Some typical results are shown in Table V. We have also subjected them to phosphorylation and analyzed the results both on 1D (Sorensen et al., 1981) (Fig. 7B) and 2D gels (Fig. 9). The results shown there clearly indicate that while *all* these structural proteins — including tubulin (see also Burke and De Lorenzo, 1981) — are subject to a low level of phosphorylation, the *major* protein responsible for phosphorylation by the Ca/CaM-dependent system is provided by P50 (PSD protein). The question now arises whether the apparent absence of phosphorylation of these structural proteins in unmodified membranes (Fig. 7B, SM vs. SM*) is of potential functional or regulatory significance.

TABLE V

ENRICHMENT OF FILAMENTOUS PROTEINS IN POSTSYNAPTIC MEMBRANES

Fraction of total (% ± S.E.M.).

| | Actin (P45) | α-Tubulin (P57) | β-Tubulin (P55) | PSD protein (P48) |
|---|---|---|---|---|
| SPM ($n = 5$) | 5.4±0.5 | 5.9±0.1 | 5.5±0.3 | 3.9±0.2 |
| PSM–PSD ($n = 5$) | 4.1±0.1 | 5.4±0.4 | 5.7±0.5 | 7.4±0.3 |
| PSD ($n = 4$) | 2.9±0.2 | 6.2±0.5 | 5.7±0.9 | 11.6±1.2 |

$n$, number of experiments.

Apparent molecular weights are based on mobilities in SDS-polyacrylamide gels as described in Methods.

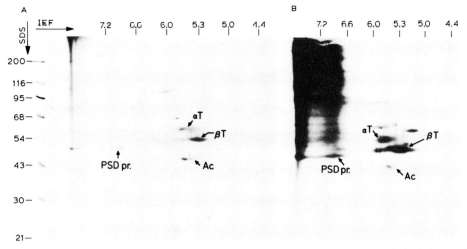

Fig. 9. Two-dimensional analysis of PSD phosphoproteins. A: Coomassie Blue stained gel obtained after two-dimensional separations of PSD (100 μg). B: autoradiograph of PSD (100 μg) phosphorylated in the presence of $Ca^{2+}$ and CaM. αT, α-tubulin; βT, β-tubulin; Ac, actin; PSD pr., the major PSD protein.

## SUMMARY AND CONCLUSIONS

Purified preparations of synaptic plasma membranes contain more than 25 polypeptides susceptible to phosphorylation by resident kinases that are dependent on a variety of activators such as cAMP, $Ca^{2+}$ at low (Ca < 5 μM) concentration enhanced by CaM and $Ca^{2+}$ at high (mM) concentration. Among the more prominent phosphoproteins are ones with $M_{app} = 44 \times 10^3$ and two different proteins with $M_{app} = 54 \times 10^3$, one formed in a $Ca^{2+}$- and another in a cAMP-requiring reaction, that can be separated on 2D gels. The $44 \times 10^3$ protein has been identified as the α subunit of pyruvate dehydrogenase and is localized in both cell body and intraterminal mitochondria. The protein phosphorylated in the presence of $Ca^{2+}$ is identical with phosphoprotein B-50 and appears to exhibit a localization confined to the interior surface of presynaptic membranes. The protein phosphorylated in the cAMP-dependent reaction has been identified as the regulatory, brain-specific, type II subunit of cAMP-dependent protein kinase and is located on pre- as well as postsynaptic membranes. Treatment of synaptic and postsynaptic membranes with low concentrations of nonionic detergents appears to facilitate interaction of membrane-bound kinases with potential substrates, resulting in an extensive phosphorylation of many membrane proteins, some of them protected from this modification in intact membranes.

## ACKNOWLEDGEMENTS

We are greatly indebted to Prof. Lester J. Reed of the University of Texas, Austin for providing us with purified pyruvate dehydrogenase and its subunits, including the phosphorylated α subunit formed with its authentic kinase, and for valuable advice. We also enjoyed our continued collaboration with Prof. W.H. Gispen and Dr. H. Zwiers of the State University of Utrecht, The Netherlands, with the resulting transatlantic exchanges of information, material and personnel.

46

REFERENCES

Ames, G.F.-L. and Nikaido, K. (1976) Two-dimensional gel electrophoresis of membrane proteins. *Biochemistry*, 15: 616–623.

Banker, G., Churchill, L. and Cotman, C.W. (1974) Proteins of the postsynaptic density. *J. Cell Biol.*, 63: 456–465.

Bloom, F.E., Ueda, T., Battenberg, E. and Greengard, P. (1979) Immunocytochemical localization, in synapses, of protein I, an endogenous substrate for protein kinases in mammalian brain. *Proc. nat. Acad. Sci. (Wash.)*, 76: 5982–5986.

Browning, M., Baudry, M., Bennett, W., Kelly, P. and Lynch, G. (1980a) Evidence that high frequency stimulation influences the phosphorylation of pyruvate dehydrogenase and that the activity of this enzyme is linked to mitochondrial calcium sequestration. *Soc. Neurosci.*, 6: 197 (Abstr. 71.2).

Browning, M., Bennett, M. and Lynch, G. (1980b) Phosphorylase kinase phosphorylates a brain protein which is influenced by repetitive synaptic activation. *Nature (London)*, 278: 273–275.

Browning, M., Baudry, M., Bennett, W.F. and Lynch, G. (1981) Phosphorylation-mediated changes in pyruvate dehydrogenase activity influence pyruvate-supported calcium accumulation by brain mitochondria. *J. Neurochem.*, 36: 1932–1940.

Burgoyne, R.D. (1981) A possible role of synaptic membrane protein phosphorylation in the regulation of muscarinic acetylcholine receptors. *FEBS Lett.*, 122: 288–292.

Burke, B.E. and de Lorenzo, R.J. (1981) $Ca^{2+}$- and calmodulin-stimulated endogenous phosphorylation of neurotubulin. *Proc. nat. Acad. Sci. (Wash.)*, 78: 991–995.

Carlin, R.K., Grab, D.J., Cohen, R.S. and Siekevitz, P. (1980) Isolation and characterization of postsynaptic densities from various brain regions: Enrichment of different types of postsynaptic densities. *J. Cell Biol.*, 86: 831–843.

Cleveland, D.W., Fischer, S.G., Kirschner, M.W. and Laemmli, U.K. (1977) Peptide mapping by limited proteolysis in sodium dodecyl sulfate and analysis by gel electrophoresis. *J. biol. Chem.*, 252: 1102–1106.

Cohen, R.S., Blomberg, F., Berzins, K. and Siekevitz, P. (1977) The structure of postsynaptic densities isolated from dog cerebral cortex. I. Overall morphology and protein composition. *J. Cell Biol.*, 74: 181–203.

DeBlas, A.L., Wang, Y.-J., Sorensen, R. and Mahler, H.R. (1979) Protein phosphorylation in synaptic membranes regulated by adenosine 3':5'-monophosphate: Regional and subcellular distribution of the endogenous substrates. *J. Neurochem.*, 33: 647–658.

DeCamilli, P., Ueda, T., Bloom, F.E., Battenberg, E. and Greengard, P. (1979) Widespread distribution of protein I in the central and peripheral nervous system. *Proc. nat. Acad. Sci. (Wash.)*, 76: 5977–5981.

De Lorenzo, R.J. (1980) Role of calmodulin in neurotransmitter release and synaptic function. *Ann. N.Y. Acad. Sci.*, 356: 92–109.

Ehrlich, Y.H. (1979) Phosphoproteins as specifiers for mediators and modulators in neuronal function. In: Modulators, Mediators and Specifiers in Brain Function. *Adv. exp. Med. Biol.*, 116: 75–101.

Geahlen, R.L., Allen, S.M. and Krebs, E.G. (1981) Effect of phosphorylation on the regulatory subunit of the type I cAMP-dependent protein kinase. *J. biol. Chem.*, 256: 4536–4540.

Gill, D.L., Grollman, E.F. and Kohn, L.D. (1981) Calcium transport mechanisms in membrane vesicles from guinea pig brain synaptosomes. *J. biol. Chem.*, 256: 184–192.

Gispen, W.H. (1979) On the neurochemical mechanism of action of ACTH in adaptive capabilities of the nervous system. *Progr. Brain Res.*, 54: 193–206.

Goelz, S.E., Nestler, E.J., Chehrazi, B. and Greengard, P. (1981) Distribution of protein I in mammalian brain as determined by a detergent-based radioimmunoassay. *Proc. nat. Acad. Sci. (Wash.)*, 78: 2130–2134.

Grab, D.J., Carlin, R.K. and Siekevitz, P. (1981) Function of calmodulin in postsynaptic densities. II. Presence of a calmodulin-activatable protein kinase activity. *J. Cell Biol.*, 89: 440–448.

Greengard, P. (1976) Possible role for cyclic nucleotides and phosphorylated membrane proteins in postsynaptic actions of neurotransmitters. *Nature (Lond.)*, 260: 101–108.

Greengard, P. (1978) Phosphorylated proteins as physiological effectors. *Science*, 199: 146–152.

Hajos, F. (1975) An improved method for the preparation of synaptosomal fractions in high purity. *Brain Res.*, 93: 485–489.

Hanbauer, I., Pradhan, S. and Yang, H.-Y.T. (1980) Role of calmodulin in dopaminergic transmission. *Ann. N.Y. Acad. Sci.*, 356: 292–303.

Huttner, W.B. and Greengard, P. (1979) Multiple phosphorylation sites in protein I and their differential regulation by cyclic AMP and calcium. *Proc. nat. Acad. Sci. (Wash.)*, 76: 5402–5406.

Huttner, W.B., De Gennaro, L.J. and Greengard, P. (1981) Differential phosphorylation of multiple sites in purified protein I by cyclic AMP-dependent and calcium-dependent protein kinases. *J. biol. Chem.*, 256: 1482–1488.

Jolles, J., Zwiers, H., van Dongen, C.J., Schotman, P., Wirtz, K.W.A. and Gispen, W.H. (1980) Modulation of brain polyphosphoinositide metabolism by ACTH-sensitive protein phosphorylation. *Nature (Lond.)*, 286: 623–625.

Jones, D.H. and Matus, A.I. (1974) Isolation of synaptic plasma membrane from brain by combined flotation–sedimentation density gradient centrifugation. *Biochim. biophys. Acta*, 356: 276–287.

Kelly, P.T. and Cotman, C.W. (1978) Synaptic proteins. Characterization of tubulin and actin and identification of a distinct postsynaptic density polypeptide. *J. Cell Biol.*, 79: 173–183.

Kelly, P.T., Cotman, C.W. and Largen, M. (1979) Cyclic AMP-stimulated protein kinases at brain synaptic junction. *J. biol. Chem.*, 254: 1564–1575.

Kennedy, M.B. and Greengard, P. (1981) Two calcium/calmodulin-dependent protein kinases, which are highly concentrated in brain, phosphorylate protein I at distinct sites. *Proc. nat. Acad. Sci. (Wash.)*, 78: 1293–1297.

Krebs, E.G. and Beavo, J.A. (1979) Phosphorylation–dephosphorylation of enzymes. *Ann. Rev. Biochem.*, 48: 923–959.

Laemmli, U.K. (1970) Cleavage of structural proteins during the assembly of the head of bacteriophage T4. *Nature (Lond.)*, 227: 680–685.

Leiter, A.B., Weinberg, M., Isohashi, F., Utter, M.F. and Linn, T. (1978) Relationship between phosphorylation and activity of pyruvate dehydrogenase in rat liver mitochondria and the absence of such a relationship for pyruvate carboxylase. *J. biol. Chem.*, 253: 2716–2723.

Llinas, R.R. and Heuser, J.E. (Eds.) (1977) *Depolarization-release Coupling Systems in Neurons*. MIT Press, Boston, MA.

Lohmann, S.M., Walter, U. and Greengard, P. (1980) Identification of endogenous substrate proteins for cAMP-dependent protein kinase in bovine brain. *J. biol. Chem.*, 255: 9985–9992.

Mahler, H.R. and Sorensen, R. (1980) Modulation by $Ca^{2+}$ calmodulin of synaptic protein phosphorylation. *Trans. Am. Soc. Neurochem.*, 11: 237 (Abstr. 336).

Mahler, H.R., Wang, Y.-J., DeBlas, A. and Crawford, G. (1977) Topography of membrane proteins at vertebrate synapses. In *Mechanisms, Regulation and Special Function of Protein Synthesis in the Brain*, S. Roberts, A. Lajtha and W.H. Gispen (Eds.), Elsevier/North-Holland Biomedical Press, Amsterdam, pp. 205–220.

Mahler, H.R., Kleine, L.P. and Sorensen, R.G. (1981) Topography of synaptic phosphoproteins. *Trans. Am. Soc. Neurochem.*, 12: 213 (Abstr. 287).

Matus, A.I., Ng, M.L. and Mazat, J.-P. (1980a) Protein phosphorylation in synaptic membranes: Problems of interpretation. In *Protein Phosphorylation and Bio-Regulation*, G. Thomas, E.J. Podesta and J. Gordon (Eds.), S. Karger, Basel, pp. 25–35.

Matus, A., Pehling, G., Ackermann, M. and Maeder, J. (1980b) Brain postsynaptic densities: Their relationship to glial and neuronal filaments. *J. Cell Biol.*, 87: 346–359.

McDonald, J.M., Pershadsingh, H.A., Kiechle, F.L. and Jarett, L. (1981) Parallel stimulation in adipocytes of the plasma membrane $Ca^{2+}$-transport/$(Ca^{2+} + Mg^{2+})$-ATPase system and mitochondrial pyruvate dehydrogenase. A supernatant factor derived from isolated plasma membranes. *Biochem. biophys. Res. Commun.*, 100: 857–864.

McGraw, C.F., Somlyo, A.V. and Blaustein, M.P. (1980) Localization of calcium in presynaptic nerve terminals. An ultrastructural and electron microprobe analysis. *J. Cell Biol.*, 85: 228–241.

Morgan, D.G. and Routtenberg, A. (1980) Evidence that a 41,000 dalton brain phosphoprotein is pyruvate dehydrogenase. *Biochem. biophys. Res. Commun*, 95: 569–576.

Nathanson, J.A. (1977) Cyclic nucleotides and nervous system function. *Physiol. Rev.*, 57: 157–256.

Ng, M. and Matus, A. (1979a) Protein phosphorylation in isolated plasma membranes and postsynaptic junctional structures from brain synapses. *Neurosci. Res.*, 4: 169–180.

Ng, M. and Matus, A. (1979b) Long duration phosphorylation of synaptic membrane proteins. *Neuroscience*, 4: 1265–1274.

Oestreicher, A.B., Zwiers, H., Schotman, P. and Gispen, W.H. (1981) Immunohistochemical localization of a phosphoprotein (B-50) isolated from rat brain synaptosomal plasma membranes. *Brain Res. Bull.*, 116: 145–153.

O'Farrell, P. (1975) High-resolution two-dimensional electrophoresis of proteins. *J. biol. Chem.*, 250: 4007–4021.

Reed, L.J. (1974) Multienzyme complexes. *Acc. chem. Res.*, 7: 40–46.

Routtenberg, A. and Benson, G.E. (1980) In vitro phosphorylation of a 41,000-MW protein band is selectively increased 24 hr after footshock or learning. *Behav. neural Biol.*, 29: 168–175.

Rubin, C.S., Rangel-Aldao, R., Sarkar, D., Erlichman, J. and Fleischer, N. (1979) Characterization and comparison of membrane-associated and cytosolic cAMP-dependent protein kinase. Physiocochemical and immunological studies on bovine cerebral cortex protein kinases. *J. biol. Chem.*, 254: 3797–3805.

Salvaterra, P.M. and Matthews, D.A. (1980) Isolation of rat brain subcellular fraction enriched in putative neurotransmitter receptors and synaptic junctions. *Neurochem. Res.*, 5: 181–195.

48

Schoffeniels, E. and Dandrifosse, G. (1980) Protein phosphorylation and sodium conductance ın nerve membrane. *Proc. nat. Acad. Sci. (Wash.)*, 77: 812–816.

Schulman, H. and Greengard, P. (1978) $Ca^{2+}$-dependent protein phosphorylation system in membranes from various tissues, and its activation by 'calcium-dependent regulator''. *Proc. nat. Acad. Sci. (Wash.)*, 75: 5432–5436.

Seals, J.R. and Czech, M.P. (1981) Characterization of a pyruvate dehydrogenase activator released by adipocyte plasma membranes in response to insulin. *J. biol. Chem.*, 256: 2894–2899.

Seals, J.R., McDonald, J.M. and Jarett, L. (1979) Insulin effect on protein phosphorylation of plasma membranes and mitochondria in a subcellular system from rat adipocytes. II. Characterization of insulin-sensitive phosphoproteins and conditions for observations of the insulin effect. *J. biol. Chem.*, 254: 6998–7001.

Sieghart, W., Schulman, H. and Greengard, P. (1980) Neuronal localization of $Ca^{2+}$-dependent protein phosphorylation in brain. *J. Neurochem.*, 34: 548–553.

Smith, A.P. and Loh, H.H. (1979) Architecture of the nerve ending membrane. *Life Sci.*, 24: 1–20.

Sorensen, R.G., Kleine, L.P. and Mahler, H.R. (1981) Presynaptic localization of phosphoprotein B-50. *Brain Res. Bull.*, 7: 57–61.

Sugden, P.H., Hutson, N.J., Kerbey, A.L. and Randle, P.H. (1978) Phosphorylation of additional sites on pyruvate dehydrogenase inhibits its reactivation by pyruvate dehydrogenase phosphate phosphatase. *Biochem. J.,* 146: 433–435.

Takai, Y., Kishimoto, A., Iwasa, Y., Kawahara, Y., Mori, T., and Nishizuka, Y. (1979) Calcium-dependent activation of a multifunctional protein kinase by membrane phospholipids. *J. biol. Chem.*, 254: 2693–3695.

Teague, W.M., Pettit, F.H., Yeaman, S.J. and Reed, L.J. (1979) Function of phosphorylation sites on pyruvate dehydrogenase. *Biochem. biophys. Res. Commun.*, 87: 244–252.

Ueda, T., Greengard, P., Berzins, K., Cohen, R.S., Blomberg, F., Grab, D.J. and Siekevitz, P. (1979) Subcellular distribution in cerebral cortex of two proteins phosphorylated by a cAMP-dependant protein kinase. *J. Cell Biol.*, 83: 308–319.

Walter, U., Lohmann, S.M., Sieghart, W. and Greengard, P. (1979) Identification of the cyclic AMP-dependent protein kinase responsible for endogenous phosphorylation of substrate proteins in synaptic membrane fraction from rat brain. *J. biol. Chem.*, 254: 12235–12239.

Wang, Y.-J. and Mahler, H.R. (1976) Topography of the synaptosomal plasma membrane. *J. Cell Biol.*, 71: 639–658.

Watterson, D.M. and Vincenzi, F.F. (Eds.) (1980) *Calmodulin and Cell Functions. Ann. N.Y. Acad. Sci.*, Vol. 356.

Watterson, D.M., Sharief, F. and Vanaman, T.C. (1980) The complete amino acid sequence of the $Ca^{2+}$-dependent modulator protein (calmodulin) of bovine brain. *J. biol. Chem.*, 255: 962–975.

Williams, M. and Rodnight, R. (1977) Protein phosphorylation in nervous tissue: Possible involvement in nervous tissue function and relationship to cyclic nucleotide metabolism. *Progr. Neurobiol.*, 8: 183–250.

Witt, J.J. and Roskoski, Jr., R. (1975) Rapid protein kinase assay using phosphocellulose-paper absorption. *Analyt. Biochem.*, 66: 253–258.

Wrenn, R.W., Katoh, N., Wise, B.C. and Kuo, J.F. (1980) Stimulation by phosphatidylserine and calmodulin of calcium-dependent phosphorylation of endogenous proteins from cerebral cortex. *J. biol. Chem.*, 255: 12042–12046.

Zwiers, H., Veldhuis, D.H., Schotman, P. and Gispen, W.H. (1976) ACTH, cyclic nucleotides, and brain protein phosphorylation in vitro. *Neurochem. Res.*, 1: 669–677.

Zwiers, H., Wiegant, V.M., Schotman, P. and Gispen, W.H. (1978) ACTH-induced inhibition of endogenous rat brain protein phosphorylation in vitro: Structure activity. *Neurochem. Res.*, 3: 455–463.

Zwiers, H. Tonnaer J., Wiegant, V.M., Schotman, P. and Gispen, W.H. (1979) ACTH-sensitive protein kinase from rat brain membranes. *J. Neurochem.*, 33: 247–256.

Zwiers, H., Schotman, P. and Gispen, W.H. (1980) Purification and some characteristics of an ACTH-sensitive protein kinase and its substrate protein in rat brain membranes. *J. Neurochem.*, 34: 1689–1699.

# Phosphoproteins in Postsynaptic Densities

ROCHELLE S. COHEN[1], RICHARD K. CARLIN[2],
DENNIS J. GRAB[3] and PHILIP SIEKEVITZ[2]

[1] *Department of Anatomy, University of Illinois at the Medical Center, Chicago, IL 60612 ;* [2] *Department of Cell Biology, The Rockefeller University, New York, NY, U.S.A. ; and* [3] *Department of Biochemistry, ILRAD, Nairobi, Kenya*

## INTRODUCTION

The postsynaptic density (PSD) is a dense submembranous filamentous array located behind and in intimate contact with the postsynaptic membrane (Akert et al., 1969) (Fig. 1). PSDs have been isolated from synaptosomal plasma membranes and synaptosomes using various detergents (see review by Siekevitz, 1981). Cotman et al. (1974) used N-lauroyl sarcosinate, Matus and Walters (1975) used deoxycholate and Cohen et al. (1977) used Triton X-100. It has been shown by Matus and Taff-Jones (1978) that the Triton X-100-derived PSD is more similar to the PSD in situ than that isolated using N-lauroyl sarcosinate or deoxycholate.. Using Triton

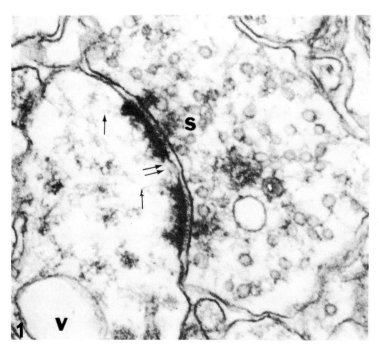

Fig. 1. Electron micrograph of synapse from canine cerebral cortex cut normal to the plane of the junction. s, synaptic vesicles; v, vacuole in the postsynaptic cell. Double arrows indicate hole in PSD; single arrows indicate postsynaptic cell filamentous material seen to be attached to the central mass of the PSD. × 75 000.

50

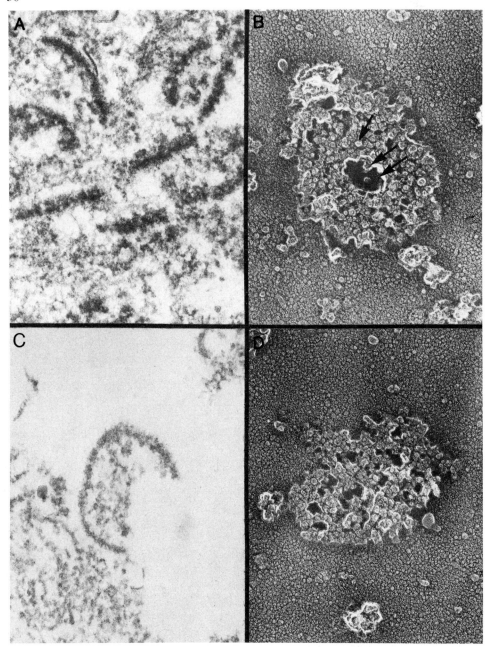

Fig. 2. Electron microscope images of PSDs isolated from cerebral cortex and from cerebellum. A: Thin section, showing cross-sectional view of PSD preparation from cerebral cortex. × 100 500. B: Replica preparation, with rotary shadowing of PSDs from cerebral cortex. × 118 000. C: Thin section, showing cross-sectional view of PSD preparation from cerebellum. × 100 500. D: Replica preparation, with rotary shadowing of PSDs from cerebellum. × 118 000. Double arrows point to the large central hole in B, while single arrows point to 20–30 nm particulate bodies.

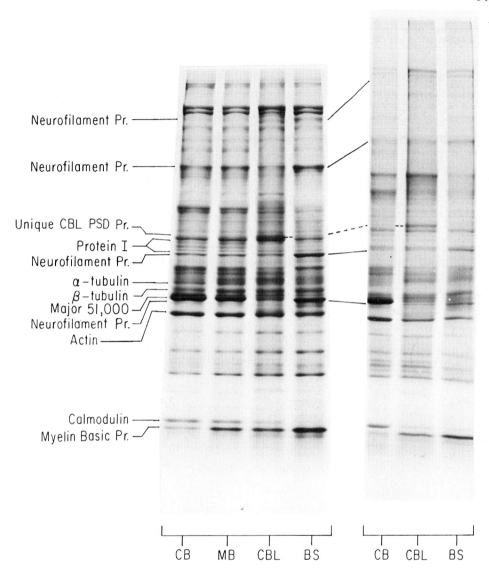

Neurofilament Pr.

Neurofilament Pr.

Unique CBL PSD Pr.
Protein I
Neurofilament Pr.
α–tubulin
β–tubulin
Major 51,000
Neurofilament Pr.
Actin

Calmodulin
Myelin Basic Pr.

CB   MB   CBL   BS      CB  CBL  BS

Fig. 3. SDS PAGE profile of proteins of PSDs from different brain parts. Equal amounts (100 μg protein) from each preparation were run on the gels. The markers on the left indicate the positions of known proteins in the PSD preparation (cf. text); of these only the myelin basic protein and the intermediate filament proteins are believed to be contaminants. The two photographs represent two different isolations, with the solid lines between them showing the positions of the intermediate filament bands and with the dotted line indicating the position of a protein unique to the cerebellar PSD preparation. The two brain stem profiles indicate the high variability of intermediate filament content. The cerebellum PSD preparation shows a reduced content of the 51 000 dalton protein and calmodulin, while the brain stem preparation almost completely lacks the bands corresponding to these two proteins. The profiles of the cerebral cortex and midbrain PSD preparations are similar. CB, cerebrum; MB, midbrain; CBL, cerebellum; BS, brain stem.

X-100 we have isolated a PSD fraction from cerebral cortex, midbrain and cerebellum (Cohen et al., 1977; Carlin et al., 1980a) (Fig. 2). In the cerebral cortex and midbrain (Cohen et al., 1977; Carlin et al., 1980a) the isolated PSD resembles that of the density seen in situ, particularly with respect to its thickness ($\sim$ 57 nm) (Fig. 2A) being similar to the postsynaptic density seen in the type I synapse of Gray (1959) or the asymmetric synapse of Colonnier (1968). A striking morphological feature of the cerebral cortex and midbrain PSD is a large central perforation (Cohen and Siekevitz, 1978; Peters and Kaiserman-Abramof, 1969; Carlin et al., 1980a) (Figs. 1 and 2B); they are also composed of aggregates 20–30 nm in diameter (Fig. 2B). PSDs isolated from the cerebellum (Carlin et al., 1980a), however, are thinner ($\sim$ 33 nm) (Fig. 2C), lack the larger perforation (Fig. 2D), but have a lattice structure and lack the 20–30 nm aggregates (Fig. 2C, D) being more like the PSD seen in the Type II synapse of Gray (1959) or the symmetric synapse of Colonnier (1968) (Carlin et al., 1980a).

Canine cerebral cortex and midbrain PSDs have identical protein patterns with SDS–polyacrylamide gel electrophoresis (SDS PAGE) (Carlin et al., 1980a) and contain about 10 major and at least 20 minor proteins (Fig. 3). No membranes are seen by electron microscopy and the phospholipid content is 1% or less (Cohen et al., 1977). No nucleic acid was found either so that the structure is composed almost exclusively of protein (Cohen et al., 1977). Enzymatic marker studies and radioactive mixing experiments reveal 0.1–6% contamination of the PSD fraction by mitochondrial, synaptic vesicle, plasma membrane and myelin membrane proteins (Cohen et al., 1977). Myelin basic protein (Cohen et al., 1977) and intermediate filament protein (Carlin et al., 1980a) have been identified as contaminants. There are no $Mg^{2+}$- or $Ca^{2+}$-ATPase (Cohen et al., 1977) nor adenylate cyclase (Grab et al., 1979) activities present in the fraction. A cAMP-dependent protein kinase (Ueda et al., 1979) and the two substrates for this kinase, proteins Ia and Ib are present. The presence of actin has been identified by amino acid analysis (Blomberg et al., 1977), immunology (Blomberg et al., 1977) and by gel mobility (Matus and Taff-Jones, 1978). Kelly and Cotman (1978) have identified forms of actin in their N-lauroyl sarcosinate-derived preparation. There are indications that tubulin may be present (Blomberg et al., 1977), although the amount may be questionable (Carlin and Siekevitz, in press).

Calmodulin has been identified (Grab et al., 1979) in these PSDs by the following criteria: (1) the 18 000 dalton protein from the PSD fraction is similar to both purified canine and porcine brain calmodulin in stimulating a partially purified cyclic nucleotide phosphodiesterase in a calcium-dependent manner (Grab et al., 1981a); (2) all three proteins comigrate as a single band on SDS–polyacrylamide gels; (3) the amino acid composition of the 18 000 dalton protein is similar to that of whole brain calmodulin and contains $\varepsilon$-N-trimethyllysine; (4) the protein from the PSD and canine brain and porcine brain calmodulin all exhibit an enhanced migration rate on polyacrylamide gels in the presence of calcium, but not of magnesium (Fig. 4), indicating strong calcium binding. Also, purified calmodulin from porcine brain, canine brain, and PSDs could be reconstituted in the presence of calcium, but not of magnesium, into a PSD rendered deficient in calmodulin by treatment with EGTA. Wood et al. (1980) and Lin et al. (1980) have confirmed the biochemical localization of calmodulin in PSDs in situ using immunohistochemical methods.

Furthermore, in studying the functions of calmodulin in cerebral cortex PSDs, the presence of the following proteins was confirmed: a calmodulin-activatable cyclic nucleotide phosphodiesterase (Grab et al., 1980, 1981a), a calmodulin-activatable protein kinase (Grab et al., 1980, 1981b), and calmodulin-binding proteins including primarily the major 51 000 dalton protein and secondarily, the regions at 60 000, 140 000, 230 000 dalton and lesser amounts of a number of other proteins (Grab et al., 1980; Carlin et al., 1980a; Carlin et al., 1981). The

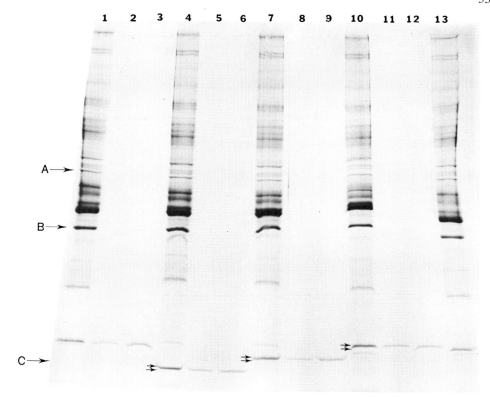

Fig. 4. Effect of different divalent cations on migration on SDS PAGE of the 18 000 mol. wt. postsynaptic density protein and purified canine and porcine brain calmodulin. SDS PAGE was performed as described in the text except that EDTA was omitted from the upper reservoir buffer. The samples contained 1 mM EDTA, pH 7.8, and either 10 mM $CaCl_2$, $MnCl_2$, or $MgCl_2$. After a few minutes incubation on ice, the samples (88 $\mu$g postsynaptic density or 5 $\mu$g calmodulin) were prepared for SDS PAGE. The single arrows on the left indicate the positions on the gel of (A) bovine serum albumin, (B) ovalbumin, and (C) sperm whale myoglobin; the double arrows indicate the position of the 18 000 mol. wt. proteins under the different conditions. (1) postsynaptic density alone; (2) canine brain calmodulin alone; (3) porcine brain calmodulin alone; (4) postsynaptic density + $CaCl_2$; (5) canine brain calmodulin + $CaCl_2$; (6) porcine brain + $CaCl_2$; (7) postsynaptic density + $MnCl_2$; (8) canine brain calmodulin + $MnCl_2$; (9) porcine brain calmodulin + $MnCl_2$; (10) postsynaptic density + $MgCl_2$; (11) canine brain calmodulin + $MgCl_2$; (12) porcine brain calmodulin + $MgCl_2$; (13) postsynaptic density alone.

role that these proteins may play in PSD function will be discussed in greater detail below.

In addition, the protein composition of PSDs isolated from canine cerebellum was examined with SDS PAGE and this will also be discussed below.

## SUBCELLULAR DISTRIBUTION OF PHOSPHOPROTEINS

Because of our interest in the possible role that the PSD plays in synaptic function and because of the increasing evidence that many of the effects of cAMP in nervous tissue are mediated through changes in the state of phosphorylation of specific proteins, particularly in synaptic membranes (Dunkely et al., 1976; Routtenberg and Ehrlich, 1975; Ueda and Greengard, 1977; Ueda et al., 1973), we studied (Ueda et al., 1979) the subcellular distribution of phosphoproteins in canine cerebral cortex, specifically two substrate proteins, proteins

Ia and Ib, collectively referred to as protein I, which are specific to neuronal membranes (Ueda and Greengard, 1977). Protein I serves as a substrate for cAMP-dependent protein kinase present in synaptic membranes and is phosphorylated in intact synaptosomes in response to veratridine-induced or potassium-induced influx of $Ca^{2+}$ ions (Kreuger et al., 1977). This protein has been purified from calf cerebral cortex to apparent homogeneity and has been partially characterized (Ueda and Greengard, 1977). In collaboration with T. Ueda and P. Greengard, we have studied the subcellular localization of proteins Ia and Ib using biochemical methods including subcellular fractionation of canine cerebral cortex and SDS–polyacrylamide gel electrophoresis (Ueda et al., 1979).

TABLE I

SPECIFIC AMOUNTS OF PROTEINS Ia AND Ib IN VARIOUS
SUBCELLULAR FRACTIONS FROM DOG CEREBRAL CORTEX

| Fraction | Protein Ia | Protein Ib |
|---|---|---|
| | pmole/mg protein | |
| Homogenate | 6.2 | 5.1 |
| Synaptosomal | 9.6 | 13.7 |
| Synaptosomal supernate | not detected | not detected |
| Crude synaptic membrane (after lysis) | 6.6 | 9.9 |
| Intrasynaptosomal mitochondria | 5.4 | 8.1 |
| Lower synaptic membrane (with PSD) | 16.1 | 23.4 |
| Postsynaptic density | 23.2 | 35.6 |
| Crude synaptic vesicle | 27.8 | 39.1 |
| Synaptic vesicle fraction 1 | 98.8 | 162.1 |
| Synaptic vesicle fraction 2 | 46.0 | 83.5 |
| Synaptic vesicle fraction 3 | 19.9 | 27.6 |
| Synaptic vesicle fraction 4 | 14.0 | 19.2 |

The table shows that of the subcellular fractions, obtained by methods described by Ueda et al. (1979), the synaptic vesicle fractions had the highest concentrations of proteins Ia and Ib, followed in declining order by the postsynaptic density fraction and by the synaptic membrane fraction.

The specific amounts of proteins Ia and Ib in subcellular fractions are shown in Table I and the electron micrographs of some of the corresponding fractions are seen in Fig. 5. Proteins Ia and Ib were most highly enriched in synaptic vesicle fractions and also present in the PSD and synaptic membrane fractions in significant amounts. Immunocytochemical studies of the localization of protein I by Bloom et al. (1979) have verified these findings.

Fig. 6 shows SDS–polyacrylamide gels and their corresponding autoradiograms of the phosphorylation of proteins Ia and Ib in PSD and crude synaptic vesicle fractions and the extraction of these proteins from these fractions with EGTA. When these two fractions were incubated with radioactive ATP, many of the proteins in each fraction were phosphorylated. However, only the phosphorylation of the 73 000 and 68 000 dalton protein was increased by the addition of cAMP. This is seen in slots 5 and 6 for these two proteins in the PSD fraction, and slots 7 and 8 for the crude synaptic vesicle fraction. Occasionally, the phosphorylation of the 26 000 and 60 000 dalton proteins was also increased by the addition of cAMP (Ueda et al., 1979).

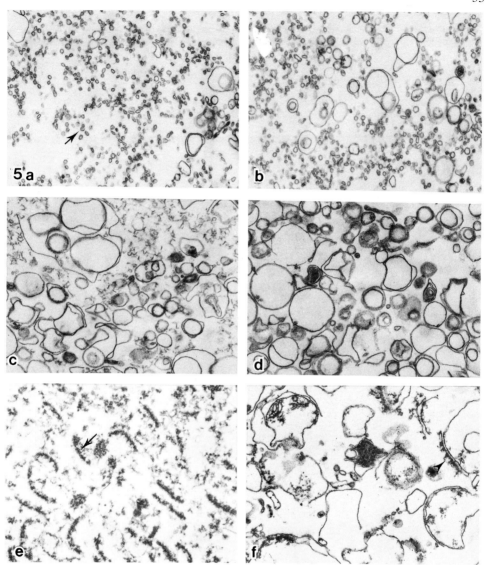

Fig. 5. Electron micrographs of various subcellular fractions. a–d: Various synaptic vesicle fractions taken from the sucrose density gradient as described in Ueda et al. (1979) × 23 750. a: The 0.4 M sucrose band contains predominantly synaptic vesicles of 40–50 nm diameter (arrow) with occasional larger vesicular membranes of varying dimensions. This layer corresponds to the fraction (synaptic vesicle fraction 1) with the highest specific amounts of proteins Ia and Ib. b: The 0.6 M sucrose band, in which the number of large vesicular membranes increases. c: The 0.8 M sucrose band; synaptic vesicles are rarely seen, but the band contains many large membrane vesicles and some unidentified membranous fragments. d: The pellet, which is almost completely devoid of synaptic vesicles. Large membrane vesicles predominate. e: Postsynaptic density fraction. Single arrow indicates PSDs with attached subsynaptic web material. This fraction is high in its specific content of proteins Ia and Ib. × 23 750. f: Synaptic membrane fraction. This fractions contains synaptosomal plasma membranes, some with recognizable synapses, as indicated by the arrow. This fraction has a high specific content of proteins Ia and Ib, although not so high as that of the synaptic vesicle and PSD fractions. × 19 000.

56

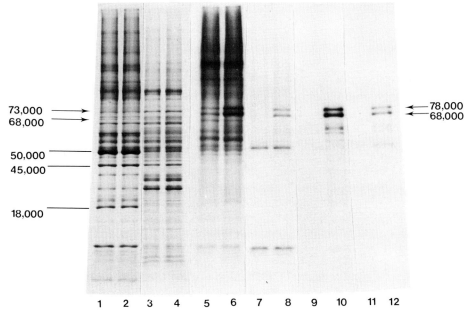

Fig. 6. Phosphorylation of proteins in the postsynaptic density and crude synaptic vesicle fractions. The fractions were isolated, and incubated, as described in Ueda et al. (1979), with partially purified protein kinase added to all the fractions and cAMP added as indicated below. The samples were treated with SDS and electrophoresed as described in Ueda et al. (1979). The Coomassie-Blue-stained protein profiles are shown in slots 1 and 2 for 60 μg of the postsynaptic density fraction and in slots 3 and 4 for 60 μg of the crude synaptic vesicle fraction. Slots 5 and 6 show the autoradiograms of the same postsynaptic density fraction and slots 7 and 8 show the autoradiograms of the same crude synaptic vesicle fraction. The gels shown in slots 1, 3, 5 and 7 are fractions incubated in the absence of cAMP, while slots 2, 4, 6 and 8 are of fractions incubated in the presence of 10 M cAMP. Replicate samples of the postsynaptic density and crude synaptic fractions were incubated in the presence of both protein kinase and cAMP, and were then treated with either 0.32 M sucrose–1 mM $NaHCO_3$ (solution B) or 100 mM EGTA. The treated samples were centrifuged and the pellets and supernates were prepared for gel electrophoresis. Slot 9 shows the autoradiogram of the postsynaptic density supernate after treatment with solution B, and slot 10 shows it after treatment with EGTA in solution B; slot 11 shows the autoradiogram of the crude synaptic vesicle supernate after treatment with solution B, and slot 12 shows it after treatment with EGTA in solution B. Not shown in the figure are the pelleted residues after the extraction treatments. These indicated that proteins Ia and Ib were still in the postsynaptic density and vesicle residue after solution B treatment but were absent from these residues after treatment with EGTA in solution B. The arrows indicate the positions of proteins Ia and Ib.

Proteins Ia and Ib in the PSD fraction are similar, if not identical, to proteins Ia and Ib in the crude synaptic vesicle fraction. Firstly, in addition to serving as substrates for cAMP-dependent kinase, the 73 000 and 68 000 dalton proteins in the two fractions gave identical gel mobilities (Fig. 6) and moved in the same way in the same gel system as proteins Ia and Ib (not shown), prepared as described earlier (Ueda and Greengard, 1977). These proteins had apparent molecular weights of 86 000 and 80 000 dalton, in the Laemmli gel system used earlier and because of its probable elongated shape it would show different mobilities in different gel systems (Ueda et al., 1979).

Secondly, proteins Ia and Ib from the PSD and crude synaptic vesicle fractions showed similar extractability by EGTA. This is seen in Fig. 6 in which the phosphorylated PSD and crude synaptic vesicle fractions were incubated in either sucrose/$NaHCO_3$, pH 8.1, alone, or sucrose/$NaHCO_3$ supplemented with 100 mM EGTA, then sedimented and the resulting supernates and pellets analyzed by SDS–gel electrophoresis. Fig. 6 shows that EGTA extracted the phosphorylated 73 000 and 68 000 dalton proteins from the PSD fraction (slot 10) and also from the crude synaptic vesicle fraction (slot 12). Treatment with 0.32 M sucrose and 1 mM NaHCO₃, pH 8.1, extracted these two proteins only in small amounts from the PSD fraction (slot 9) and from the crude synaptic vesicle fraction (slot 11). It has previously been observed (Blomberg et al., 1977), using SDS PAGE, that treatment of PSD fraction with EGTA extracted all of two minor Coomassie-Blue-stained 73 000 and 68 000 dalton proteins.

Thirdly, when both the 73 000 and 68 000 dalton proteins were extracted by NH₄Cl from the PSD and synaptic vesicle fractions, phosphorylated and then subjected to limited proteolysis by *Staphylococcus aureus* protease in the presence of 0.1% SDS, similar, if not identical, digestion patterns were obtained (not shown). Therefore, based on the aforementioned evidence, it appears that proteins Ia and Ib in the PSD and crude synaptic vesicle fraction are the same proteins (Ueda et al., 1979).

In addition, the PSD fraction has been found to contain cAMP-dependent protein Ia and Ib kinase activity (Ueda et al., 1979). In the phosphorlyation experiments described above, an

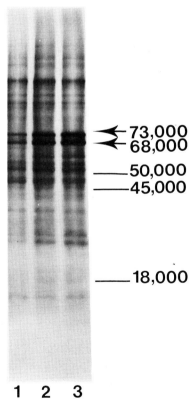

Fig. 7. Autoradiogram indicating the presence of a cAMP-dependent protein kinase in postsynaptic densities. The composition of the reaction mixture, containing 60 μg of PSD protein is as described in Ueda et al. (1979), but with the addition of cAMP and protein kinase only where noted. The reactions were stopped by the addition of TCA to a final concentration of 30% (w/v), and the precipitated proteins were subjected to SDS–gel electrophoresis and autoradiography. PSDs were incubated as follows: slot 1, without cAMP or protein kinase; slot 2, with 10 μM cAMP, but without protein kinase; slot 3, with 10 μM cAMP plus 8 units of protein kinase. The arrows indicate the positions of proteins Ia and Ib.

exogenous protein kinase was added to the reaction mixtures. Proteins Ia and Ib could still be phosphorylated in a cAMP-dependent manner upon omission of the exogenous protein kinase (Fig. 7, slots 1 and 2). Furthermore, addition of cAMP alone to the PSD fraction was sufficient to elicit optimal phosphorylation of proteins Ia and Ib; the addition of exogenous purified protein kinase did not cause a further increase in phosphorylation (Fig. 7, compare slots 2 and 3). These results imply that the PSD has an intrinsic cAMP-dependent protein kinase.

Evidence in support of the presence of a cAMP-dependent protein kinase in the PSD was obtained using the photo-affinity analogue 8-$N_3$-[$^{32}$P]cAMP which quantitatively labels the type I and type II cAMP-dependent protein kinases, both in cytosol and in membrane fractions of mammalian tissue (Walter and Greengard, 1978; Walter et al., 1978). Purified PSD fractions incorporated 0.22 pmole of 8-$N_3$-[$^{32}$P]cAMP into the type I cAMP-dependent protein kinase and 0.37 pmole into the type II cAMP-dependent protein kinase per mg of PSD protein (U. Walter and P. Greengard, unpublished observations). It has also been found (Kelly et al., 1979; Weller and Morgan, 1976) that cAMP-dependent protein kinase activity is present in a Triton X-100 insoluble synaptic junction complex fraction.

Phosphorylation experiments (Ueda et al., 1979) with crude synaptic vesicle preparations showed that addition of cAMP alone also caused phosphorylation of proteins Ia and Ib; however, the results were variable when purified synaptic vesicle preparations were used and therefore, no conclusion can be made regarding the association of a cAMP-dependent kinase with synaptic vesicles.

Because protein I is present in synaptic vesicles and PSDs it may play both presynaptic and postsynaptic physiological roles in nerve cells (Ueda et al., 1979).

## ROLE OF CALMODULIN IN RELATION TO PHOSPHOPROTEINS IN THE PSD

### *Cyclic nucleotide phosphodiesterase activation*

Because of the presence of calmodulin in the PSD (Grab et al., 1979) and because one of the functions of calmodulin in whole brain is to activate a specific nucleotide phosphodiesterase (Cheung, 1970; Filburn et al., 1978; Kakiuchi and Yamazaki, 1970; Klee et al., 1979; Vanaman et al., 1976), the presence of a calmodulin-activatable cyclic nucleotide phosphodiesterase was investigated in a Triton X-100-derived PSD fraction from canine cerebral cortex (Grab et al., 1981a). Previous studies have shown the localization of cyclic nucleotide phosphodiesterase at neuronal postsynaptic thickenings using histochemical techniques (Florendo et al., 1971) and this was confirmed by others (see Daly, 1977). Ariano and Appleman (1979) have shown histochemically the presence of a calmodulin-activatable cyclic nucleotide phosphodiesterase activity at postsynaptic sites in rat brain. Therien and Mushynski (1979) found a cAMP-phosphodiesterase activity associated with the synaptic membrane fraction. Cotman et al. (1974) also noted a cAMP-phosphodiesterase activity in a Sarkosyl-derived PSD preparation from rat brain.

The PSD fraction from canine cerebral cortex contains an endogenous cyclic nucleotide phosphodiesterase activity that is dependent on $Mn^{2+}$ and/or $Mg^{2+}$ but not on $Ca^{2+}$ (Grab et al., 1980; Grab et al., 1981a). This particular activity was not decreased upon removal of the calmodulin from the PSD nor was it increased when calmodulin was added back to a PSD preparation made deficient in calmodulin. The enzymatic activity, however, could be extracted by sonication of the PSDs and S-300 Sephacryl column chromatography of this soluble

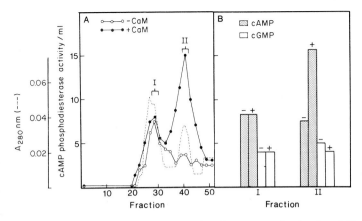

Fig. 8. S-300 Sephacryl column chromatography of the sonicated supernatant fraction from PSDs isolated from cerebral cortex. A: Elution profile of cyclic nucleotide phosphodiesterase activity in the absence or presence of 1 mM $Ca^{2+}$ + 1.5 $\mu$g bovine calmodulin. B: Column fractions I and II noted in A were pooled as indicated by the brackets in A, and were incubated in either 2 mM cAMP or 2 mM cGMP both in the absence or presence of $Ca^{2+}$ and bovine calmodulin as described in A. Activity is expressed as nmole inorganic phosphate produced/30 min at 30°C.

fraction revealed two peaks of activity: fraction I (excluded peak) and fraction II (215 000 dalton).

The fraction I activity preferred cAMP over cGMP and was not activated by calmodulin (Fig. 8). The fraction II activity had an approximately 4-fold lower $K_m$ for cGMP over cAMP and was activatable by calmodulin (Fig. 8). A crude whole brain calmodulin-dependent cyclic nucleotide phosphodiesterase activity eluted on the Sephacryl column in the same position as peak II so that it seems that fraction II from the PSD contains a calmodulin-activatable cyclic nucleotide phosphodiesterase activity, and that this activity resides in a complex similar to that obtained from the entire cerebral cortex (Grab et al., 1980, 1981a).

So, it can be stated that while a portion of the solubilized cyclic nucleotide phosphodiesterase activity is calmodulin-activatable, this activation is concealed in intact PSDs and in the sonicated, solubilized fraction before gel filtration (Grab et al., 1980, 1981a). One explanation for this is the presence of the heat-labile calmodulin-inhibitor protein (Wang and Desai, 1977; Klee and Krinks, 1978) which is found in the PSD as detected by immunohistochemical methods (Wood et al., 1980). However, addition of excess calmodulin, which should have overcome this inhibition, did not, while it did increase a protein kinase activity in the PSD (Grab et al., 1980, 1981a). A second possibility is that the phosphodiesterase in the PSD is inhibited by myelin basic protein, a contaminant in the PSDs (Cohen et al., 1977) and which has been implicated in the inhibition of the activation of whole brain phosphodiesterase by calmodulin (Grand and Perry, 1979). However, treatment of the intact PSD fraction, the sonicated extract, or fraction I with antibody to myelin basic protein had a variable effect; in some cases a stimulation was observed, while in other cases no stimulation was observed (Grab et al., 1980, 1981a). Also when fraction I was coincubated with a partially purified calmodulin-dependent cyclic nucleotide phosphodiesterase from canine cerebral cortex, the results were additive in both the absence and presence of exogenous calmodulin, indicating that fraction I did not contain an unbound inhibitor (Grab et al., 1980, 1981a). Another possibility is that the lack of activation of the PSD phosphodiesterase is caused by small amounts of Triton X-100 adsorbed onto the PSD, since recently Sharma (1981) has noted that 15 $\mu$M Triton

60

X-100 caused a 50% inhibition of the calmodulin activatability of a soluble phosphodiesterase preparation.

It is therefore assumed that there are two forms of cyclic nucleotide phosphodiesterase, one activatable by calmodulin and one not, and that the former activity is seen when the two activities are separated into fractions I and II (Grab et al., 1980, 1981a).

It is therefore possible that the calmodulin present in the PSD modulates the activity of the cyclic nucleotide phosphodiesterase in the PSD during changing neurophysiological states. Such changes could result in increased susceptibility of the enzyme to calmodulin activation. The consequent decrease in localized cyclic nucleotide concentration could affect the cyclic nucleotide-dependent protein kinase found to be present in the PSD (Berzins et al., 1978; Ueda et al., 1979; Grab et al., 1980, 1981a).

*Protein kinase activation*

The presence of calmodulin-activatable cyclic nucleotide phosphodiesterase in the PSD (Grab et al., 1980, 1981a) prompted an investigation of a calmodulin-activatable protein kinase activity in the Triton X-100-derived PSD fraction from canine cerebral cortex (Grab et al., 1981b). The involvement of calmodulin in stimulating the $Ca^{2+}$-dependent phosphorylation of two proteins, 51 000 and 62 000 dalton, in lysed synaptosomes and in crude synaptosomal plasma membrane fraction was shown by Schulman and Greengard (1978a, b). Evidence recently presented by Grab et al. (1980, 1981b) localizes the calmodulin-activatable protein kinase activity to the PSD.

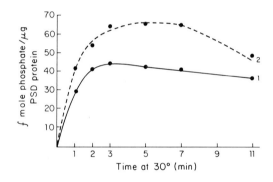

Fig. 9. Incorporation of $^{32}PO_4$ into total PSD protein. Fresh PSDs (80 $\mu$g) were incubated for various times at 30°C with [$\gamma$-$^{32}$P]ATP and the reaction was stopped with 5 ml ice-cold 5% TCA–1% pyrophosphate as described in the text. The samples were then transferred onto paper discs and prepared for scintillation counting. The data are expressed as femtomoles phosphate incorporation per microgram total PSD protein. (1) PSDs incubated in the presence of 10 mM $Mg^{2+}$ alone; (2) PSDs incubated as in (1) except that 0.5 mM $Ca^{2+}$ and 4 $\mu$g chick brain calmodulin were also present.

This was demonstrated firstly by incubation of a PSD fraction with labeled ATP and $Mg^{2+}$ for various times in the absence and presence of $Ca^{2+}$ and calmodulin. Fig. 9 shows that incorporation of $^{32}PO_4$ into total PSD protein in the presence of $Mg^{2+}$ reached a maximal level after 3 min. of incubation at 30°C. The addition of $Ca^{2+}$ and calmodulin, however, resulted in a 30% increase over the $Mg^{2+}$ control (Grab et al., 1981b). It should be noted that the PSD preparation contains little or no $Ca^{2+}$- or $Mg^{2+}$-ATPase activity (Cohen et al., 1977).

To determine which of the proteins were phosphorylated, the PSD fraction after incubation was subjected to SDS PAGE. As seen in Figs. 10 and 16 addition of $Ca^{2+}$ to the PSD fraction

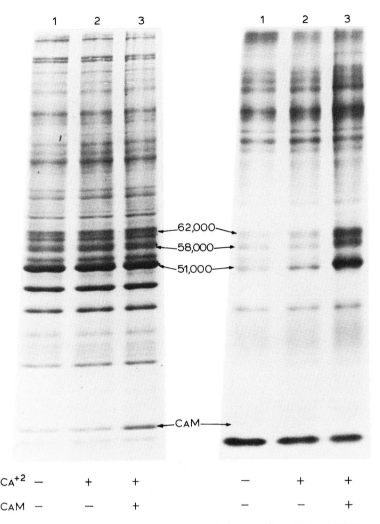

Fig. 10. SDS PAGE of phosphorylated PSD proteins. The incubation conditions (3 min at 30°C) as well as SDS PAGE and autoradiography were performed as described by Grab et al. (1981b). The Coomassie-Blue-stained gels, 120 μg PSD protein, are shown in A, while the autoradiograms of the stained gels are shown in B. The arrows indicate the relative molecular masses of select regions on the gel. The absence or presence of either 0.5 mM Ca²⁺ and/or 4 μg canine brain calmodulin is shown at the bottom of the figure. The phosphorylated band below the calmodulin in B is the contaminating myelin basic protein.

resulted in a slight increase in phosphorylation of the protein(s) in the major 51 000 dalton region (Fig. 10, slot 2). In the presence of both Ca²⁺ and exogenous calmodulin there was a marked increase in the phosphorylation of two major regions in the PSD fraction at 51 000 and 62 000 daltons (Fig. 10, slot 3; Fig. 16, slot 5). There was also an occasional increase in a 58 000 dalton band. Fig. 11, however, shows the average increases in phosphorylation of the PSD proteins on SDS PAGE for 6–8 experiments. The data therefore indicate that the PSD contains an endogenous calmodulin-activatable protein kinase as well as its substrate proteins; the activity is probably on the surface of the PSD, as it responds to added calmodulin (Grab et al., 1981b).

## EFFECT OF CALMODULIN ON THE PHOSPHORYLATION OF PSD PROTEINS ON SDS-PAGE

| $M_R$ REGION | PHOSPHATE INCORPORATED* | | |
|---|---|---|---|
| | −CALMODULIN | +CALMODULIN | % INCREASE |
| 230,000 | 1.3 | 1.5 | 15 |
| 180,000 | 2.4 | 3.1 | 29 |
| 150,000 | 2.8 | 3.4 | 21 |
| 105,000 | 1.9 | 2.2 | 16 |
| 100,000 | 1.1 | 1.3 | 18 |
| 70,000 | 1.2 | 1.6 | 33 |
| 62,000 | 1.0 | 2.1 | 110 |
| 58,000 | 1.6 | 1.7 | 6 |
| 51,000 | 1.0 | 2.8 | 180 |
| 45,000 | 0.3 | 0.3 | 0 |

\* FEMTOMOLE/UG TOTAL PSD PROTEIN

Fig. 11. Effect of $Ca^{2+}$ and calmodulin on the phosphorylation of PSD proteins. Separate PSD preparations (100 $\mu$g protein) from 6–8 different canine cerebral cortices were incubated with [$\gamma$-$^{32}$P] ATP for 3 min both in the presence or absence of 0.5 mM $Ca^{2+}$ and 4 $\mu$g canine brain calmodulin. Various protein regions were cut out of the wet gels and counted in 10 ml double distilled $H_2O$. The data are expressed as the mean (ISE) incorporation of phosphate into an individual protein region per total PSD protein incubated (fmole/$\mu$g). When cAMP was used in place of $Ca^{2+}$ and calmodulin, the final concentration was 10 $\mu$M.

While the above experiments involve the addition of exogenous calmodulin, similar results can be obtained with mild sonication of the PSD preparation for 10–15 sec in water or low ionic strength buffer or by freezing the preparation at −80°C followed by thawing in water or low ionic strength buffer; a marked increase in phosphorylation in the 51 000 and 62 000 dalton regions can be seen by the addition of $Ca^{2+}$ alone (Fig. 12A, compare slot 3, freeze-thawed and calcium alone with Fig. 12B, slot 6, freeze-thawed incubated in the presence of [$^{32}$P]ATP, $Ca^{2+}$ and canine brain calmodulin). Furthermore, there is a comparatively small increase in the phosphorylation of proteins Ia and Ib as seen in Fig. 12A when a comparison is made between slot 1, which shows PSDs incubated in the presence of $Mg^{2+}$ alone, and slot 3, which shows PSDs incubated with the addition of $Ca^{2+}$. This demonstrates two kinase systems in the PSD

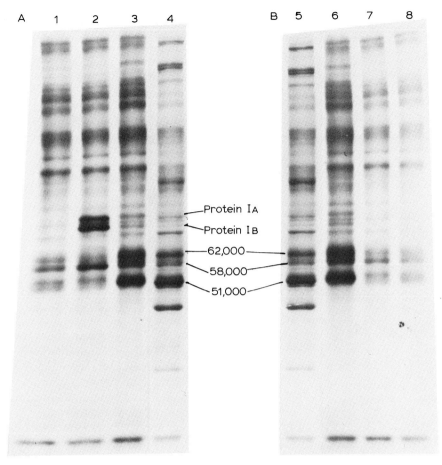

Fig. 12. Effects of freeze-thawing, EGTA, and chlorpromazine on the calmodulin-activatable protein kinase activity in the PSD. PSDs were homogenized and frozen in double-distilled H$_2$O in a dry ice–methanol bath and stored overnight at $-80°$C. The samples were then thawed under warm running tap water and immediately put on ice before use. The PSDs were then incubated with [$\gamma$-$^{32}$P]ATP as described by Grab et al. (1981b). Slot 4 shows the Coomassie-Blue-stained gel of this freeze-thawed PSD preparation (75 $\mu$g protein). The autoradiograms of the freeze-thawed PSDs incubated under varying conditions are shown in slots 1–3. (1) PSDs incubated in the presence of 10 mM Mg$^{2+}$ alone. (2). 10 $\mu$M cyclic AMP. (3) Same as (1) but with the addition of 0.5 mM Ca$^{2+}$. B shows the effects of both EGTA and chlorpromazine on calmodulin-dependent protein kinase activity in the PSD. Slot 5 again shows the Coomassie-Blue-stained gel of the freeze-thawed PSD preparation (75 $\mu$g). Slots 6–8 show the autoradiograms of the freeze-thawed PSD in the presence of [$\gamma$-$^{32}$P]ATP and Ca$^{2+}$ and 3 $\mu$g canine brain calmodulin with the following additions: (6) no additions, (7) 1 mM EGTA, and (8) 1 mM chlorpromazine.

which are different in both activation and substrate requirements and as will be discussed below, in the nature of the two kinases (Grab et al., 1981b).

The results of other experiments demonstrating the ability of Ca$^{2+}$ and calmodulin to activate the PSD kinase activity are seen in Fig. 12B. Freeze-thawed PSDs that were used in the experiment depicted in Fig. 12A were incubated with labeled ATP in the presence of Mg$^{2+}$, Ca$^{2+}$ and calmodulin. As can be seen in slot 7 of the autoradiogram in Fig. 12B, Ca$^{2+}$ chelation with EGTA, which also removes calmodulin from PSD (Grab et al., 1979), inhibits the calmodulin-stimulated phosphorylation to the Mg$^{2+}$ control level (see slot 1, Fig. 12A). Similarly, addition of 1 mM chlorpromazine (slot 8), an antipsychotic agent known to bind

64

calmodulin in the presence of Ca²⁺ (Levin and Weiss, 1978), also inhibited the phosphorylation to the control level (Grab et al., 1981b).

In order to show that the increased phosphorylation was dependent on calmodulin, a calmodulin-deficient PSD preparation was prepared as described previously (Grab et al., 1979), sonicated, and incubated with labeled ATP, Mg²⁺, and Ca²⁺ (Grab et al., 1981b). If the kinase was dependent upon the Ca²⁺ alone, the activity would have been exposed by the sonication. However, a Ca²⁺ stimulation of protein kinase activity was not able to be induced unless exogenous calmodulin was added back to the system. Fig. 13 shows that proteins whose phosphorylation was increased in this reconstituted system were similar to those seen when either exogenous calmodulin is added to a fresh, unchanged PSD preparation (Fig. 10), or when Ca²⁺ is added to a freeze-thawed or sonicated PSD preparation (Fig. 12). The calmodulin-activatable protein kinase activity in the reconstituted system reached saturation levels, and the final level of total phosphate incorporated was similar to that found for the native PSD preparation when incubated with calmodulin (compare Fig. 13B to Fig. 9). It is noteworthy

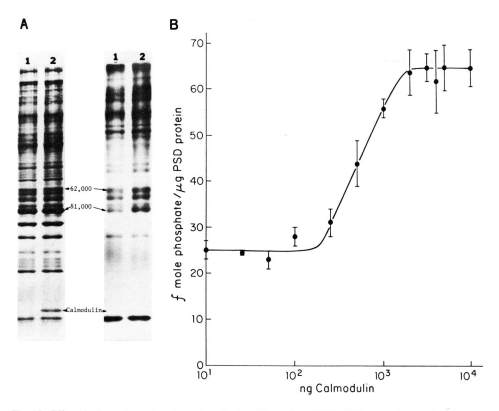

Fig. 13. Effect of calmodulin on phosphorylation of calmodulin-deficient PSDs. PSDs made deficient in calmodulin (Grab et al., 1979) were incubated in the standard phosphorylation reaction mixture, as described in Grab et al. (1981b). In A, 100 μg calmodulin-deficient PSDs were sonicated and then incubated in the presence of 0.5 mM Ca²⁺ alone (slot 1) or with the addition of 4 μg canine brain calmodulin (slot 2). The Coomassie-Blue-stained gels are shown on the left and the corresponding autoradiograms are shown on the right. In B, 25 μg of the calmodulin-deficient PSDs were incubated in the presence of Ca²⁺ and increasing amounts (10¹–10⁴ ng) of canine brain calmodulin. The reaction was stopped with 5% TCA–1% pyrophosphate and the samples counted for radioactivity as described in Grab et al. (1981b). The data are expressed as femtomoles phosphate incorporated per microgram total PSD protein and the curve represents the mean (± S.E.) of triplicate determinations.

that the calmodulin which was added back into the PSD is probably reconstituted into its proper place in the structure, as it is capable of activating the calmodulin-activatable protein kinase system present there.

It has also been found (Grab et al., 1981b) that the calmodulin-activatable protein kinase phosphorylates domains in the 51 000 dalton PSD protein which are different from those phosphorylated by the general kinase activity, rather than increasing the activity of the same domains. PSDs were phosphorylated in the absence or presence of calmodulin and subjected to SDS PAGE. The 51 000 dalton protein was digested with papain and the phosphorylated fragments analyzed by autoradiography. Quantitatively, 3.3 times more phosphate incorporation occurred in the presence of $Ca^{2+}$ plus calmodulin than in the $Mg^{2+}$-incubated control. Qualitatively, papain proteolysis of the 51 000 dalton protein phosphorylated in the presence of $Mg^{2+}$ alone yielded three discernable radioactive peptide fragments with molecular weights of 14 800 (1), 12 300 (2) and 10 950 (3) (Fig. 14). Approximately 50% of the phosphate incorporated into the entire 51 000 dalton protein occurred in the 12 300 dalton peptide fragment, while 25 and 10% of the total phosphate was incorporated into the 10 950 and 14 800 dalton fragments, respectively. On the other hand, the overall autoradiographic pattern

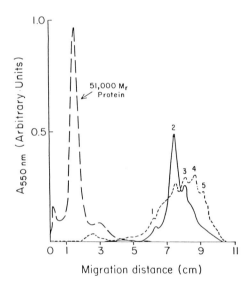

Fig. 14. A scan of the autoradiogram after limited proteolysis by papain of the phosphorylated 51 000 dalton PSD protein. A PSD fraction (100 $\mu$g) was phosphorylated in the absence or presence of $Ca^{2+}$ as described by Grab et al. (1981b). After electrophoresis, the gel was briefly stained and destained, and the portion of the gel containing the major 51 000 dalton protein band, which was easily separated from the marker 51 000 dalton intermediate brain filament protein, was cut out and soaked in 54 mM Tris–sulfate (pH 6.1) for 1 h. In this experiment 3.3 times more $^{32}PO_4$ was incorporated into the 51 000 dalton protein in the presence of $Ca^{2+}$ plus calmodulin than in the $Mg^{2+}$-incubated control (3 fmoles vs. 0.7 fmole/$\mu$g total PSD protein respectively). After soaking in buffer the protein band was subjected to a second SDS gel electrophoresis (15% separating gel with a 3% stacking gel) in the absence or presence of 1 $\mu$g papain according to the method of Cleveland et al. (1977), except that the Neville buffer system (1971) was used. After drying, the gel was subjected to autoradiography and the exposure time normalized so that the intensities of the 51 000 dalton regions in both the $Mg^{2+}$ and $Ca^{2+}$/calmodulin samples were identical. Scanning of the autoradiograms was performed at 550 nm using the Zeiss Spektraphotometer PM6. The figure is a composite of the scan of three slots, the untreated 51 000 dalton protein, and the two papain-treated samples. The phosphorylated band seen above the 51 000 dalton protein region is probably an aggregated form of the 51 000 dalton protein that failed to enter the separating gel. The estimated molecular weights of the phospho-peptide peaks 1–5, as compared to standards run at the same time are: (1) 14 800; (2) 12 300; (3) 10 950; (4) 9 350; (5) 8 150.

of proteolysis products of the 51 000 dalton protein after calmodulin-activatable phosphorylation was significantly different; in this case there were two additional radioactive peptide fragments at 9350 (4) and 8150 (5) dalton (Fig. 14). Phosphate incorporation into the smaller molecular weight peptides 2–5 were similar being 20–25% of the total incorporated phosphate. So it appears that not only is there an overall increase in the amount of phosphate incorporated into the 51 000 dalton protein catalyzed by the PSD calmodulin-activatable protein kinase, but the kinase acts to phosphorylate sites in the protein different from those acted upon by the more general kinase activity(s) present in the PSD. It is thought that there is only one major phosphorylated protein in this region (Carlin et al., 1981). However, it is possible that two populations of the 51 000 dalton protein exist in the cerebral cortex PSD, one phosphorylated by the $Mg^{2+}$ protein kinase, and the other by the calmodulin-activatable protein kinase which binds calmodulin (Carlin et al., 1981).

Because the calmodulin-activatable protein kinase in the PSD can phosphorylate the protein substrates for the endogenous cAMP-dependent protein kinase, proteins Ia and Ib, although not as intensely as it does the 51 000 and 62 000 dalton regions, experiments were performed to elucidate the interrelationships between these two endogenous protein kinase systems in the PSD (Grab et al., 1981b). A fresh PSD preparation was phosphorylated in the presence of $Mg^{2+}$ and with cAMP or calmodulin alone or in combination, together with the specific inhibitor of the catalytic subunit of cAMP-dependent protein kinases (Ashby and Walsh, 1972) or with the calmodulin inhibitor chlorpromazine (Levin and Weiss, 1978). Table II shows the results of these experiments (Grab et al., 1981b). When PSDs were incubated in either the presence of cAMP or calmodulin, the phosphorylation of protein I (Ia and Ib) increased to a

TABLE II

EFFECT OF THE INHIBITOR OF THE cAMP-DEPENDENT PROTEIN
KINASE ON THE CALMODULIN-ACTIVATABLE PROTEIN KINASE
IN THE PSD

| Additions * | Increase relative to the control | | |
|---|---|---|---|
| | Protein I | 62 000 Mr protein | 51 000 Mr protein |
| cAMP | 1.6 | 0 | 0 |
| Calmodulin | 1.2 | 4.0 | 5.1 |
| cAMP + calmodulin | 2.7 | 4.0 | 5.3 |
| + 40 μg inhibitor | 1.7 | 4.0 | 5.5 |
| + 80 μg inhibitor | 1.7 | 4.5 | 5.3 |
| + 120 μg inhibitor | 1.5 | 4.2 | 5.0 |
| + 120 μg inhibitor + chlorpromazine | 0 | 0 | 0 |
| cAMP + chlorpromazine | 1.4 | 0.4 | 0.1 |
| cAMP + 120 μg inhibitor | 0.1 | 0 | 0.1 |
| Calmodulin + chlorpromazine | 0.4 | 0 | 0 |
| Calmodulin + 120 μg inhibitor | 1.3 | 4.2 | 5.1 |

* The concentrations of added components are as follows: 10 μM cyclic AMP, 1 mM chlorpromazine, and 3 μg bovine brain calmodulin plus 0.5 mM $CaCl_2$.
Fresh PSDs (50 μg) were phosphorylated in the presence of 50 mM PIPES (pH 7.0), 10 mM $MgCl_2$, 1 mM isobutylmethylxanthine, 0.2 mM EGTA, and 5 μM [γ-$^{32}$P]ATP for 3 min at 30°C under the conditions given below. SDS PAGE was performed as described by Grab et al. (1981). After drying, the gel was subjected to autoradiography and the regions corresponding to protein I (Ia + Ib), the 62 000 dalton protein, and the major 51 000 dalton PSD protein, were scanned at 550 nm in a Gilford model 240 spectrophotometer (Gilford Instrument Laboratories, Inc., Oberlin, OH). The data are expressed as the increase in peak intensity relative to the $Mg^{2+}$ incubated control.

similar degree, 160% or 129%, respectively. When cAMP and calmodulin were incubated together, the phosphorylation of protein I increased in an almost additive way (270%). On the other hand, in regard to the 51 000 and 62 000 dalton bands, while calmodulin caused a large increase in phosphate incorporation, cAMP had no significant effect on the phosphorylation of these two regions. Also, the cAMP-dependent protein kinase inhibitor almost completely blocked the activation of protein I phosphorylation by cAMP, but had no effect on preventing the calmodulin-induced phosphorylation of the 51 000 and 62 000 dalton proteins. When calmodulin was added to the incubation media with cAMP, the inhibitor protein was only able to reduce the total additive activation of protein I phosphorylation from 270 to 150%, while having no effect on the phosphorylation of the 51 000 and 62 000 dalton proteins. In PSDs incubated with calmodulin plus chlorpromazine, the phosphorylation of the 51 000 and 62 000 dalton bands was completely blocked, while protein I phosphorylation was inhibited about 67%. Chlorpromazine had little effect on the cAMP-induced phosphorylation of protein I. Incubation with both the inhibitor of cAMP-dependent protein kinase and chlorpromazine blocked the activation of protein I, the 51 000 and 62 000 dalton bands. The calmodulin-activatable protein kinase may phosphorylate protein I at a site different from the cAMP-dependent protein kinase in the PSD, as suggested by Huttner and Greengard (1979) and Kreuger et al. (1977) working with synaptosomes. The cAMP protein kinase, however, does not interact with the substrates for the calmodulin-activatable protein kinase system. It may be that the calmodulin system is a more general one, preferring the 51 000 and 62 000 dalton proteins because of some strict geometry inherent in the PSD structure, rather than a strict substrate specificity (Grab et al., 1981b).

It should be noted that while in earlier reports (Schulman and Greengard, 1978a, b) added calmodulin stimulated the phosphorylation of the 51 000 and 62 000 dalton proteins in lysed synaptosomes and in crude synaptic membrane fractions, this phenomenon is probably due to the presence of the PSD in both of these fractions. It has been found that there was a 2-fold increase by calmodulin in the phosphorylation of these two protein regions in the PSD using a synaptic membrane fraction, indicating that the proteins phosphorylated in the synaptic membrane fraction are probably PSD in origin. In support of this Ng and Matus (1979) also found that the specific activity of general phosphoprotein labeling is about 2-fold higher in the PSD than in the synaptic membrane preparation from which it was derived (Grab et al., 1981b).

*Calmodulin-binding proteins in the postsynaptic density*

The relatively large amount of calmodulin in the PSD as well as the presence of calmodulin-activitable cyclic nucleotide phosphodiesterase and calmodulin-activatable protein kinase, suggested that this protein plays an important role in the regulation of synaptic transmission. Consequently, the interaction of PSD calmodulin with other PSD proteins was examined by binding calmodulin, radioiodinated by the lactoperoxidase method, to SDS–polyacrylamide gels (Carlin et al., 1980b, 1981). The results of such an experiment are shown in Fig. 15. Slot 1 shows the Coomassie Blue staining of the PSD. Slot 2 shows the autoradiogram of the gel after treatment with radioiodinated calmodulin; radioiodinated calmodulin is found to primarily bind the major 51 000 dalton protein of the PSD, with intermediate binding to the proteins at the 60 000, 140 000, 230 000 and in the experiment shown, to the 165 000 dalton regions, and with lesser binding to the proteins at lower molecular weights. The radioiodinated calmodulin binding is specific as indicated by various controls. The binding activity is removed by addition of either EGTA (slot 3), EDTA (slot 4), or chlorpromazine (slot 5), or by preincuba-

68

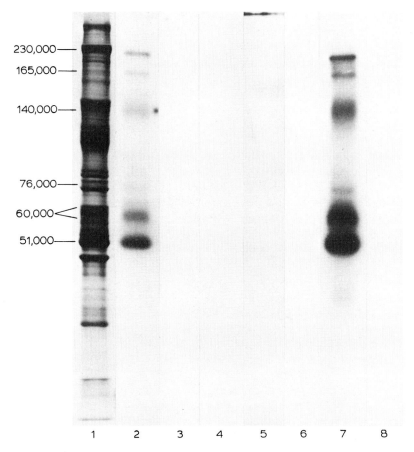

Fig. 15. Binding of radioiodinated calmodulin to proteins from cerebral cortex PDSs separated on SDS–polyacrylamide gels. The method of binding is described by Carlin et al. (1981) with 175 $\mu$g PSD proteins being used in all slots.
The molecular weights of the major calmodulin-binding proteins are shown on the left. Slot 1 shows the Coomassie
Blue staining of the PSD preparation. Slot 2 shows the autoradiograph of the gel after treatment with radioiodinated
calmodulin. Slots 3–8 show autoradiography of the requisite controls. The binding of calmodulin was performed in the
presence of: slot 3, 2 mM EGTA; slot 4, 0.1 mM EDTA; slot 5, 1 mM chlorpromazine. Slot 6 shows the effect of
preincubation with 1 mg unlabeled calmodulin for 2 h, while slot 7 shows the effect of preincubation with 5 mg BSA
for 2 h. Slot 8: the gel was washed with 1 mM EGTA for 12 h after binding of radioiodinated calmodulin and then the
autoradiograph was made. Autoradiographs were exposed at − 90°C for 6 h using a Dupont Cronex Lightning-Plus 4H
enhancing screen.

tion of the gel with unlabeled calmodulin (slot 6). If the gel is first labeled, washing the gel
subsequently with EGTA removes all binding (slot 8). Addition of randomly chosen protein,
BSA, enhanced the binding of calmodulin to the gel (compare slots 2 and 7). Further support of
the specificity of the interaction of the lactoperoxidase-iodinated calmodulin with PSD
proteins comes from an experiment where calmodulin was also iodinated by the chloramine-T
method, which inactivates calmodulin. Gels having either PSD proteins or histone were both
incubated with either calmodulin labeled by the lactoperoxidase method or with calmodulin
labeled by the chloramine-T method. Both these preparations were capable of binding to
histones; however, only the lactoperoxidase-iodinated calmodulin bound to PSD proteins,

indicating that the interaction of lactoperoxidase is specific and not caused by simple ionic interactions.

The 51 000 dalton protein, which is the major substrate for the calmodulin-activatable protein kinase (Grab. et al., 1981b) is also the protein that binds calmodulin most effectively (Carlin et al., 1981). Purified calcineurin, the heat-labile binding protein (Wang and Desai, 1977; Klee and Krinks, 1978) and a purified cAMP phosphodiesterase comigrated with two bands in the 60 000 dalton region of the PSD. Also the radioiodinated calmodulin was found to bind calcineurin previously run on an SDS gel (Grab et al., 1980; Carlin et al., 1980b, 1981).

## PROTEIN PHOSPHORYLATION IN PSDs FROM VARIOUS BRAIN REGIONS

In order to gain insight into the possible role played by the PSD in synaptic function, we isolated PSDs, using Triton X-100, from various general brain regions, to observe any differences that might exist among them. PSDs were isolated from cerebral cortex, midbrain and cerebellum and were compared by electron microscope morphology as described above and by protein composition and protein phosphorylation (Carlin et al., 1980a).

In comparison with the protein composition of cerebral cortex and midbrain PSDs, as described above, cerebellar PSDs lacked the 51 000 dalton protein, contained 2 times less calmodulin and contained a unique protein at 73 000 dalton (Carlin et al., 1980a) (Fig. 3).

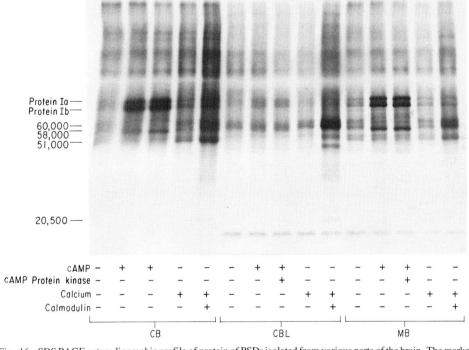

Fig. 16. SDS PAGE autoradiographic profile of protein of PSDs isolated from various parts of the brain. The markers on the left indicate the positions of those proteins whose phosphorylation was increased the most by the additions given on the bottom. The incubation conditions are given in Carlin et al. (1980a). The band that is uniformly phosphorylated under all conditions in all samples near the bottom of the gel (17 000 dalton) is the myelin basic protein. CB, cerebrum; CBL, cerebellum, MB, midbrain.

The results of phosphorylation by ATP of PSD proteins from different brain parts in the absence or presence of cAMP and of calcium and calmodulin are shown in the autoradiogram in Fig. 16. In PSDs from cerebral cortex, cerebellum and midbrain, addition of cAMP to the phosphorylation mixture resulted in increased phosphorylation of three proteins: protein Ia (73 000 dalton) and protein Ib (68 000 dalton) as described above, and a minor protein at 57 000 dalton. The phosphorylation of proteins Ia and Ib occurred in all cases whether or not a purified protein kinase was added, indicating that a cAMP-dependent protein kinase, fully accessible to the substrate protein and to cAMP, is located in the PSD in these preparations. The amounts of protein I in the cerebral cortex and midbrain seem to be identical (Fig. 16), as noted by the increased phosphorylation of these proteins; on the other hand, cerebellum PSDs contained much less of proteins Ia and Ib as noted by their decreased phosphorylations. However, immunocytochemical results of Bloom et al. (1979) gave larger amounts of protein I in various areas of the cerebellum than in the cerebral cortex. The discrepancy between the results may be explained by the observation that in both methods (Bloom et al., 1979; Ueda et al., 1979) the amount of protein I in the PSD is much smaller than in the synaptic vesicles, and the smaller amounts of protein I in cerebellar PSDs as compared to those isolated from cerebral cortex may be masked by the much higher amounts in the synaptic vesicles in both cases. Reddington and Mehl (1979) compared cAMP-dependent phosphorylation from different brain parts and found that synaptic membrane preparations from cerebrum, midbrain and cerebellum all had the same amounts of proteins believed to be identical to proteins Ia and Ib. DeBlas et al. (1979), however, using a total particulate fraction from various brain areas, found two phosphorylated proteins, believed to be analogous to proteins Ia and Ib, in higher amounts in the cerebrum than in the cerebellum.

Ca$^{2+}$ plus calmodulin stimulated the phosphorylation of the 51 000 and 62 000 dalton bands in the cerebral cortex (Carlin et al., 1980b; Grab et al., 1980, 1981) and midbrain (Carlin et al., 1980b), while cerebellar PSDs (Carlin et al., 1980b) showed a decreased phosphorylation of the 51 000 dalton protein (Fig. 16), as expected from the marked decrease in amount of this protein in these PSDs (Fig. 3). The increase in the phosphorylation of the 62 000 dalton band approximated those of cerebral cortex PSDs (Fig. 16). The major protein phosphorylated in the cerebellum PSDs was one at 58 000 dalton (Fig. 16), with a protein at approximately 48 000 dalton being uniquely phosphorylated in these PSDs (Fig. 16). As can be seen from Fig. 16, calcium stimulation was not fully activated unless exogenous calmodulin was also added. If the PSD is frozen or sonicated first, the calcium-stimulated phosphorylation is increased and occasionally equals that with added calcium plus calmodulin (Grab et al., 1980, 1981), suggesting that the calmodulin is not directly accessible to the protein kinase but is within close proximity (Carlin et al., 1980a).

Based on the afore-mentioned ultrastructural data (Carlin et al., 1981), we assume that the cerebral cortex and midbrain PSD fraction represents an enrichment of type I synapses in these fractions and that the cerebellum PSD fraction represents an enrichment of type II synapses in these fractions. By comparing the protein composition and phosphorylation patterns of PSDs derived from these various brain areas we proposed a mechanism of PSD function in type I and type II synapses (Carlin et al., 1980a). Firstly, the major difference in protein composition between cerebral cortex and midbrain PSDs is in the amount of major 51 000 dalton protein and calmodulin (Carlin et al., 1980a). There is very little 51 000 dalton protein in the cerebellum-derived PSDs, so that the 51 000 dalton protein may be unique to asymmetric type I synapses irregardless of the transmitter involved (Carlin et al., 1980a). This is in agreement with the work of Rostas et al. (1979), based on the high amounts of this protein in synaptic junctional complexes isolated from various cerebral cortex and midbrain regions thought to have asymmetric synapses. Another difference is that cerebellum-derived PSDs have 50% less calmodulin than those derived from cerebral cortex (Fig. 3) (Carlin et al., 1980a). This is in agreement with the work of Sobue et al. (1979) where the concentration of calmodulin in membrane preparations from cerebral cortex and cerebellum were determined. Perhaps the higher concentration of calmodulin in cerebral cortex-derived synapses suggests that calmodulin may play an important role in these synapses; detectable amounts of calmodulin in cerebellum-derived PSDs, however, may still suggest a role for calmodulin in these types of synapses (Carlin et al., 1980a).

Furthermore, in the presence of $Ca^{2+}$ and calmodulin, cerebral cortex-derived PSDs exhibit increased phosphorylation of the major 51 000 and 62 000 dalton proteins (Carlin et al., 1980a). Since protein phosphorylation has been proposed to be important in synaptic function (Greengard, 1978), the exclusive presence of the major 51 000 dalton band in cerebral cortex and midbrain PSDs may imply that phosphorylation of this protein is involved in the modulation of postsynaptic potentials in type I synapses (Carlin et al., 1980a). Furthermore, the predominance of the increased phosphorylation, upon addition of $Ca^{2+}$ and calmodulin, of the 58 000 dalton protein in cerebellum may implicate its possible involvement in the modulation of postsynaptic potentials in type II synapses (Carlin et al., 1980a). The phosphorylation of the 62 000 dalton protein cannot be entirely designated to type II synapses since this protein is present in both types of PSD. Whether this protein is involved in the function of both types of PSD or is present in the cerebral cortex PSD fraction because of the presence of PSDs from type II synapses in that fraction in small amounts has not yet been determined.

While cAMP-dependent phosphorylation of cerebral cortex, midbrain and cerebellum PSDs produces a similar pattern, with the major phosphorylated bands being proteins Ia and Ib (Ueda et al., 1979) and the minor phosphorylated band (57 000 daltons) possibly representing autophosphorylation of the regulatory subunit of the cAMP-dependent protein kinase (Uno et al., 1976), cerebral cortex-derived PSDs have much greater phosphorylation of proteins Ia and Ib upon addition of cAMP than do cerebellum PSDs. Therefore, the cAMP-dependent phosphorylations may be involved in the function of type I synapses and not that of the type II synapses. As previously mentioned, however, in the cerebral cortex, protein I is more highly enriched in the synaptic vesicles than in PSDs, so that is also has a presynaptic role (Ueda et al., 1979).

## ROLE OF CALMODULIN AND
## PHOSPHOPROTEINS IN PSD FUNCTION

PSDs isolated from cerebral cortex and midbrain represent an enrichment of PSDs derived from asymmetric or Gray type I synapses and those isolated from cerebellum represent an enrichment of PSDs from symmetric or Gray type II synapses (Carlin et al., 1980a). It is not known why this enrichment occurs during subcellular fractionation, as both types of synapses occur in both brain areas (Carlin et al., 1980a). The general classification of synapses into types I and II (Gray, 1959) or asymmetric and symmetric synapses (Colonnier, 1968) has prompted Eccles (1964) to propose that type I synapses mediate excitation responses and type II synapses mediate inhibitory responses. Based on work reviewed by Eccles (1964) and by Walberg (1968), the hypothesis that was postulated was that in the hippocampus a correlation existed between type I structure and known excitatory synapses and between type II structure and known inhibitory synapses, although in the cerebellum the evidence is more ambiguous. Work in support of this proposal came from Landis et al. (1974), on olfactory bulb synapses, and by Landis and Reese (1974), on cerebellar cortex synapses, who correlated known excitatory and inhibitory properties of certain synapses in these regions and the prevalence of either type I or type II differentiations there.

These assumptions together with the work previously reported from this laboratory (Carlin et al., 1980a) had led us to postulate that the enriched population of thick PSDs from the cerebral cortex and midbrain are derived from type I excitatory synapses and that the enriched population of thinner PSDs from cerebellum arise from type II inhibitory synapses (Carlin et al., 1980a). Thus, the differences in protein composition and also protein phosphorylation may be of functional significance and these are summarized in Table III (Carlin et al., 1980a). Firstly, there is a much larger amount of the 51 000 dalton protein, of calmodulin, and of the

TABLE III

SUMMARY OF POSTULATED CHARACTERISTICS OF PSDs FROM
TYPE I AND TYPE II SYNAPSES

| Characteristics | Type I | Type II |
|---|---|---|
| Function | Excitatory | Inhibitory |
| Morphology | Thick disk, with large perforation in center; presence of aggregates | Thin disk, lattice-like structure with no large central perforation; little or no aggregates |
| Enrichment of proteins | Major 51 000 $M_r$, protein I, calmodulin | 74 000 $M_r$ |
| Enrichment of calmodulin-dependent phosphorylation | 51 000 $M_r$ | 58 000 $M_r$<br>48 000 $M_r$ |
| Enrichment of cAMP-dependent phosphorylation | Proteins Ia and Ib | – |

substrate proteins Ia and Ib for the cAMP-activatable protein kinase in PSDs from cerebral cortex and midbrain over that in the PSDs from the cerebellum, suggesting that these proteins may be involved in excitatory modulation of the transmission signal which occurs at these synapses. Although each population from each of the two sources is a mixture of different kinds of synapses specific for different neurotransmitters and we do not know whether a given PSD has both cAMP-activatable and calmodulin-activatable systems, the involvement of cAMP in modulating excitatory acetylcholine responses intitiated by dopamine has been reported by Libet (1979).

Secondly, results regarding the phosphorylation of some of the proteins of the PSD, provides additional support for this hypothesis. Cerebral cortex PSDs have increased phosphorylation of the major 51 000 and 62 000 dalton proteins in the presence of calcium and calmodulin, while cerebellum PSDs have a greatly reduced phosphorylation under these conditions in the 51 000 dalton region (Carlin et al., 1980a; Grab et al., 1981b). Since Greengard (1978) has proposed that protein phosphorylation is important in synaptic function, the uniqueness of the 51 000 dalton protein in cerebral cortex and midbrain PSDs may suggest that phosphorylation of this protein is involved in the modulation of postsynaptic potentials in type I synapses (Carlin et al., 1980a). Similarly, increased phosphorylation of the 58 000 dalton band in the cerebellum upon addition of $Ca^{2+}$ and calmodulin may implicate its involvement in the generation of postsynaptic potentials in type II synapses (Carlin et al., 1980a).

Thirdly, evidence exists implicating the involvement of calmodulin in the excitation process at the synapse. Calmodulin is found in large amounts (5–10% total PSD protein) in PSDs derived from cerebral cortex and midbrain and is reduced by 50% of this in cerebellum PSDs. Furthermore, calmodulin- and cAMP-activatable protein kinase activities as well as the major 51 000 dalton protein which is phosphorylated by the calmodulin-activatable protein kinase, are enriched in PSDs isolated from cerebral cortex as compared to PSD isolated from the cerebellum. Therefore, the calmodulin and cAMP protein kinase systems together may play a significant role in the excitation response. Also, calmodulin activates a cAMP phosphodiesterase in these PSDs (Grab et al., 1980, 1981a). The interrelationships between cAMP and calmodulin at the PSD may be twofold; cAMP levels may be directly altered by $Ca^{2+}$ activation of the calmodulin-activatable phosphodiesterase present, consequently altering the effects of cAMP-dependent protein kinase in the PSD or the endogenous calmodulin-activatable protein kinase may phosphorylate the catalytic subunit of the calmodulin-activatable phosphodiesterase and in this way control the system (Grab et al., 1981b).

Calmodulin may be involved in excitatory responses by mediating the effects of calcium (Carlin et al., 1981). For example, chlorpromazine, a drug that binds and inactivates calmodulin (Levin and Weiss, 1978), reduced miniature endplate potential amplitutes at the neuromuscular junction (Argov and Yaari, 1979). $Mn^{2+}$, a divalent cation which can partially bind calmodulin (Grab et al., 1979), partially inactivated the excitatory postsynaptic potential in cat spinal cord (Krnjevic et al., 1979). Thus, the larger amounts found in cerebral cortex and midbrain PSDs together with the presence of the 51 000 dalton protein in these PSDs suggest the binding of these two proteins to each other is somehow involved in the modulation and possible generation of postsynaptic excitatory responses (Carlin et al., 1980a, 1981; Grab et al., 1980). This may be mediated by (a) modulation of the action of the protein directly by calmodulin and (b) modulation of the action of the protein by the calcium-calmodulin-dependent phosphorylation (Grab et al., 1981b). In this regard, phosphorylation of the 51 000 dalton protein by the calcium–calmodulin–dependent protein kinase did not release bound calmodulin from the PSDs as shown on SDS PAGE, implying that calmodulin could be bound to the phosphorylated protein (Carlin et al., 1981).

## ACKNOWLEDGEMENTS

We gratefully acknowledge Gudrun Pettersson for typing of this manuscript.

The work on which this report was based was supported in part by the following granting agencies: PHS-NS 15889 to R.S. Cohen; NIH Postdoctoral Fellowship 5-F32-NS06005 to R. Carlin; NIH Postdoctoral Fellowship I-F32-NS05693 to D. Grab; NIH grant PHS-NS 12726 to P. Siekevitz.

### REFERENCES

Akert, K., Moore, H., Pfenninger, K. and Sandri, C. (1969) Contributions of new impregnation methods and freeze-etching to the problems of synaptic fine structure. *Progr. Brain Res.*, 31: 223–240.

Argov, Z. and Yaari, Y. (1979) The action of chlorpromazine at an isolated cholinergic synapse. *Brain Res.*, 164: 227–236.

Ariano, M.A. and Appleman, M.M. (1979) Biochemical characterization of postsynaptically localized cyclic nucleotide phosphodiesterase. *Brain Res.*, 177: 301–309.

74

Ashby, C.D. and Walsh, D.A. (1972) Characterization of the interaction of a protein inhibitor with adenosine 3′,5′-monophosphate-dependent protein kinases. *J. biol. Chem.*, 247: 6637–6642.

Berzins, K., Cohen, R.S., Blomberg, F., Siekevitz, P., Ueda, T. and Greengard, P. (1978) Specific occurrence in the postsynaptic density (PSD) and synaptic vesicles (SV) of two proteins phosphorylated by a cAMP-dependent protein kinase. *J. Cell Biol.*, 79 (2, Pt. 2): 96a (Abstr.).

Blomberg, F., Cohen, R.S. and Siekevitz, P. (1977) Structure of postsynaptic densities isolated from dog cerebral cortex. II. Characterization and arrangement of some of the major proteins within the structure. *J. Cell Biol.*, 74: 204–225.

Bloom, F.E., Ueda, T., Battenberg, E. and Greengard, P. (1979) Immunocytochemical localization, in synapses, of protein I, an endogenous substrate for protein kinases in mammalian brain. *Proc. nat. Acad. Sci. (Wash.)*, 76: 5982–5986.

Carlin, R.K. and Siekevitz, P., *J. Neurochem.*, in press.

Carlin, R.K., Grab, D.J., Cohen, R.S. and Siekevitz, P. (1980a) Isolation and characterization of postsynaptic densities from various brain regions. Enrichment of different types of postsynaptic densities. *J. Cell Biol.*, 86: 831–843.

Carlin, R.K., Grab, D.J. and Siekevitz, P. (1980b) The binding of radioiodinated calmodulin to proteins on denaturing gels. *Ann. N.Y. Acad. Sci.*, 356: 73–74.

Carlin, R.K., Grab, D.J. and Siekevitz, P. (1981) Function of calmodulin in postsynaptic densities. III. Calmodulin-binding proteins of the postsynaptic density. *J. Cell Biol.*, 89: 449–455.

Cheung, W.Y. (1970) Cyclic 3′,5′-nucleotide phosphodiesterase. *Biochem. biophys. Res. Commun.*, 38: 533–538.

Cleveland, D.W., Fisher, S.G., Kirschner, M.W. and Laemmli, V.I. (1977) Peptide mapping by limited proteolysis in sodium dodecyl sulfate and analysis by gel electrophoresis. *J. biol. Chem.*, 252: 1102–1106.

Cohen, R.S. and Siekevitz, P. (1978) The form of the postsynaptic density: A serial section study. *J. Cell Biol.*, 78: 36–46.

Cohen, R.S., Blomberg, F., Berzins, K. and Siekevitz, P. (1977) Structure of postsynaptic densities isolated from dog cerebral cortex. I. Overall morphology and protein composition. *J. Cell Biol.*, 74: 181–203.

Colonnier, M. (1968) Synaptic patterns of different cell types in the different laminae of the cat visual cortex. An electron microscope study. *Brain Res.*, 9: 268–287.

Cotman, C.W., Banker, G., Churchill, L. and Taylor, D. (1974) Isolation of postsynaptic densities from rat brain. *J. Cell Biol.*, 63: 441–445.

Daly, J.W. (1977) The formation, degradation, and function of cyclic nucleotides in the nervous system. *Int. Rev. Neurobiol.*, 20: 105–168.

DeBlas, A.L., Wang, Y.-J., Sorensen, R. and Mahler, H.P. (1979) Protein phosphorylation in synaptic membranes regulated by adenosine 3′,5′-monophosphate: Regional and subcellular distribution of the endogenous substrates. *J. Neurochem.*, 33: 647–659.

Dunkley, P.R., Holmes, H. and Rodnight, R. (1976) Phosphorylation of synaptic-membrane proteins from ox cerebral cortex in vitro. *Biochem. J.*, 157: 661–666.

Eccles, J.C. (1964) *The Physiology of Synapses*. Springer Verlag, New York.

Filburn, C.R., Colpo, F. and Sacktor, B. (1978) Regulation of cyclic nucleotide phosphodiesterases of cerebral cortex by $Ca^{2+}$ and cyclic GMP. *J. Neurochem.*, 30: 337–346.

Florendo, N.T., Barnett, R.J. and Greengard, P. (1971) Cyclic 3′,5′-nucleotide phosphodiesterase: cytochemical localization in cerebral cortex. *Science*, 173: 745–747.

Grab, D.J., Berzins, K., Cohen, R.S. and Siekevitz, P. (1979) Presence of calmodulin in postsynaptic densities isolated from canine cerebral cortex. *J. biol. Chem.*, 254: 8690–8696.

Grab, D.J., Carlin, R.K. and Siekevitz, P. (1980) The presence and functions of calmodulin in the postsynaptic density. *Ann. N.Y. Acad. Sci.*, 356: 55–72.

Grab, D.J., Carlin, R.K. and Siekevitz, P. (1981a) Function of calmodulin in postsynaptic densities. I. Presence of a calmodulin-activatable cyclic nucleotide phosphodiesterase activity. *J. Cell Biol.*, 89: 433–439.

Grab, D.J., Carlin, R.K. and Siekevitz, P. (1981b) Function of calmodulin in postsynaptic densities. II. Presence of calmodulin-activatable protein kinase activity. *J. Cell Biol.*, 89: 440–448.

Grand, R.J. and Perry, S.V. (1979) Calmodulin-binding proteins from brain and other tissues. *Biochem. J.*, 183: 285–295.

Gray, E.G. (1959) Axosomatic and axo-dendritic synapses of the cerebral cortex: an electron microscope study. *J. Anat.*, 93: 420–433.

Greengard, P. (1978) *Cyclic Nucleotides, Phosphorylated Proteins, and Neuronal Functions*. Raven Press, New York.

Huttner, W.B. and Greengard, P. (1979) Multiple phosphorylation sites in protein I and their differential regulation by cyclic AMP and calcium. *Proc. nat. Acad. Sci. (Wash.)*, 76: 5402–5406.

Kakiuchi, S. and Yamazaki, R. (1970) Calcium-dependent phosphodiesterase activity and the activating factor (PAF) from brain. III. Studies on cyclic 3',5'-nucleotide phosphodiesterase. *Biochem. biophys. Res. Commun.,* 41: 1104–1110.

Kelly, P.T. and Cotman, C.W. (1978) Synaptic proteins: Characterization of tubulin and actin and identification of a distinct postsynaptic density protein. *J. Cell Biol.,* 79: 173–183.

Kelly, P.T., Cotman, C.W. and Largen, M. (1979) Cyclic AMP-stimulated protein kinases at brain synaptic junctions. *J. biol. Chem.,* 254: 1564–1575.

Klee, C.B. and Krinks, M.H. (1978) Purification of cyclic 3',5'-nucleotide phosphodiesterase inhibitory protein by affinity chromatography on activator protein coupled to Sepharose. *Biochemistry,* 17: 120–126.

Klee, C.B., Crouch, T.H. and Krinks, M.H. (1979) Subunit structure and catalytic properties of bovine brain Ca$^{2+}$-dependent cyclic nucleotide phosphodiesterase. *Biochemistry,* 18: 722–729.

Kreuger, B.K., Forn, J. and Greengard, P. (1977) Depolarization induced phosphorylation of specific proteins, mediated by calcium ion influx, in rat brain synaptosomes. *J. biol. Chem.,* 252: 2764–2773.

Krnjevic, K., Lamour, Y., MacDonald, J.F. and Nistri, A. (1979) Depression of monosynaptic excitatory postsynaptic potentials by Mn$^{2+}$ and Co$^{2+}$ in cat spinal cord. *Neuroscience,* 4: 1331–1339.

Landis, D.M.D. and Reese, T.S. (1974) Differences in membrane structure between excitatory and inhibitory synapses in cerebellar cortex. *J. comp. Neurol.,* 155: 93–126.

Landis, D.M.D., Reese, T.S. and Raviola, E. (1974) Differences in membrane structure between excitatory and inhibitory components of the reciprocal synapse in the olfactory bulb. *J. comp. Neurol.,* 155: 67–92.

Levin, R.M. and Weiss, B. (1978) Specificity of the binding to trifluoperazine to the calcium-dependent activator of phosphodiesterase and to a series of other calcium-binding proteins. *Biochim. biophys. Acta,* 540: 197–204.

Libet, B. (1979) Which postsynaptic action of dopamine is mediated by cAMP? *Life Sci.,* 24: 1043–1058.

Lin, C., Dedman, J.R., Brinkley, B.R. and Means, A.R. (1980) Localization of calmodulin in rat cerebellum by immunoelectron microscopy. *J. Cell Biol.,* 85: 473–480.

Matus, A.I. and Taff-Jones, D.H. (1978) Morphological and molecular composition of isolated postsynaptic junctional structures. *Proc. R. Soc. Lond. B, Biol. Sci.,* 203: 135–151.

Matus, A.I. and Walters, B.B. (1975) Ultrastructure of the synaptic junctional lattice isolated from mammalian brain, *J. Neurocytol.,* 4: 369–375.

Neville, Jr., D.M. (1971) Molecular weight determination of protein-dodecyl sulfate complexes by gel electrophoresis in a discontinuous buffer system. *J. biol. Chem.,* 246: 6328–6334.

Ng, M. and Matus, A. (1979) Long duration phosphorylation of synaptic membrane proteins. *Neuroscience,* 4: 1265–1274.

Peters, A. and Kaiserman-Abramof, I.R. (1969) The small pyramidal neuron of the rat cerebral cortex. The synapses from dendritic spines. *Z. Zellforsch. mikrosk. Anat.,* 100: 487–506.

Reddington, M. and Mehl, E. (1979) Synaptic membrane proteins as substrates for cAMP-stimulated protein phosphorylation in various regions of rat brain. *Biochim. biophys. Acta,* 555: 230–238.

Rostas, J.A.P., Kelly, P.T., Pesin, R.H. and Cotman, C.W. (1979) Protein and glycoprotein composition of synaptic junctions prepared from descrete synaptic regions and different species. *Brain Res.,* 168: 161–167.

Routtenberg, A. and Ehrlich, Y.H. (1975) Endogenous phosphorylation of four cerebral cortical membrane proteins: Role of cyclic nucleotide, cAMP and divalent cations. *Brain Res.,* 92: 415–430.

Schulman, H. and Greengard, P. (1978a) Stimulation of brain membrane phosphorylation by calcium and an endogenous heat-stable protein. *Nature (Lond.),* 271: 478–479.

Schulman, H. and Greengard, P. (1978b) Ca$^{2+}$-dependent protein phosphorylation system in membranes from various tissues, and its activation by calcium-dependent regulator. *Proc. nat. Acad. Sci. (Wash.),* 75: 5432–5436.

Sharma, R.K. (1981) Inhibition of cyclic nucleotide phosphodiesterase by calmodulin and Triton X-100 complex. *Fed. Proc.,* 40: 1739.

Siekevitz, P. (1981) Isolation of post-synaptic densities from cerebral cortex. In *Research Methods in Neurochemistry,* Vol. 3, N. Marks and R. Rodnight (Eds.), Plenum Press, New York, pp. 75–89.

Sobue, K., Muramoto, Y., Yamazaki, R. and Kakiuchi, S. (1979) Distribution in rat tissue of modulator-binding protein of particulate nature. *FEBS Lett.,* 105: 105–109.

Therien, H. and Mushynski, W.E. (1979) Characterization of the cyclic 3',5'-nucleotide phosphodiesterase activity associated with synaptosomal plasma membranes and synaptic junctions. *Biochim. biophys. Acta,* 585: 201–209.

Ueda, T. and Greengard, P. (1977) Adenosine 3',5'-monophosphate-regulated phosphoprotein system of neuronal membranes. I. Solubilization, purification and some properties of an endogenous phosphoprotein. *J. biol. Chem.,* 252: 5155–5163.

Ueda, T., Maeno, H. and Greengard, P. (1973) Regulation of endogenous phosphorylation of specific proteins in synaptic membrane fractions from rat brain by adenosine 3',5'-monophosphate. *J. biol. Chem.,* 248: 8295–8305.

76

Ueda, T., Greengard, P., Berzins, K., Cohen, R.S., Blomberg, F., Grab, D.J. and Siekevitz, P. (1979) Subcellular distribution in cerebral cortex of two proteins phosphorylated by a cAMP-dependent protein kinase. *J. Cell Biol.*, 83: 308–319.

Uno, I., Ueda, T. and Greengard, P. (1976) Adenosine 3′,5′-monophosphate regulated phosphorylation system of neuronal membranes. II. Solubilization, purification, and some properties of an endogenous 3′,5′-monophosphate-dependent protein kinase. *J. biol. Chem.*, 252: 5164–5174.

Vanaman, T.C., Sharief, F., Awramik, L., Mendel, P.A. and Watterson, D.M. (1976) Chemical and biological properties of the ubiquitous troponin-C like protein from non-muscle tissues, a multifunctional $Ca^{2+}$-dependent regulator protein. In *Contractile Systems in Non-Muscle Tissues*, S.V. Perry, A. Margreth, R.S. Adelstein (Eds.), Elsevier/North-Holland, New York, pp. 165–176.

Walberg, F. (1968) Morphological correlates of postsynaptic inhibitory processes. In *Structure and Function of Inhibitory Neuronal Mechanisms*, C. von Euler, S. Skoglund and V. Soderberg, (Eds.), Pergamon Press, New York, pp. 7–13.

Walter, U. and Greengard, P. (1978) Quantitative labeling of the regulatory subunit of type II cAMP-dependent protein kinase from bovine heart by a photoaffinity analog. *J. cyclic Nucl. Res.*, 4: 437–444.

Walter, U., Kanof, P., Schulman, H. and Greengard, P. (1978) Adenosine 3′,5′-monophosphate receptor proteins in mammalian brain. *J. biol. Chem.*, 253: 6275–6280.

Wang, J.H. and Desai, R. (1977) Modulator binding protein, bovine brain protein exhibiting calcium-dependent assocation with the protein modulator of cyclic nucleotide phosphodiesterase. *J. biol. Chem.*, 252: 4175–4184.

Weller, M. and Morgan, E.G. (1976) Localization in the synaptic junction of the cyclic AMP-stimulated intrinsic protein kinase activity of synaptosomal plasma membranes. *Biochim. biophys. Acta*, 433: 223–228.

Wood, J.G., Wallace, R.W., Whitaker, J.N. and Cheung, W.Y. (1980) Immunocytochemical localization of calmodulin and a heat-labile calmodulin-binding ganglia from mice brain. *J. Cell Biol.*, 84: 66–76.

# Immunocytochemical Localization
# of Identified Proteins in Brain
# by Monoclonal Antibodies

RICHARD HAWKES, MEELIAN NG, EVELYN NIDAY and ANDREW MATUS

*Friedrich Miescher-Institut, P.O.Box 273, CH 4002, Basel, Switzerland*

## INTRODUCTION

As the contributions to this symposium illustrate, most of what is known about brain phosphoproteins is based upon biochemical studies of subcellular fractions. Much of the interest in these molecules arises because they are concentrated in brain subcellular fractions enriched in synaptosomal plasma membranes (SPM) (Weller and Rodnight, 1971; Johnson et al., 1971). This apparent relationship between phosphoproteins and membranes of the synaptic surface led to the proposal that the turnover of phosphate bound to these molecules plays some role in the physiological events of synaptic transmission (Greengard, 1976; Williams and Rodnight, 1977).

However, several recent lines of evidence have emphasized the difficulties of identifying these phosphoproteins with particular aspects of synaptic physiology. We investigated the turnover rate of protein-bound phosphate in SPM fractions with the objective of determining the time course of effects associated with the different phosphopeptides which can be resolved by gel electrophoresis (Ng and Matus, 1979b). This study revealed several apparently anomalous aspects of the phosphorylation process, among which the irreversibility of much of the phosphorylation induced in vitro was the most striking. Problems of this kind led us to question the origin of the phosphoproteins and associated enzymes which occur in these subcellular fractions (Matus et al., 1980). What, for example, is the cellular origin of the kinase and phosphatase activities present in SPM preparations? Are they truly endogenous to the synapse or have they merely been adventitiously co-isolated during subcellular fractionation?

These interpretational problems are made more difficult by considering the purity of the subcellular fractions which are called "synaptosomal plasma membrane preparations". Like all subcellular fractions they are not truly pure, they are enriched relative to other subcellular isolates from the same tissue (Neville, 1975). Indeed all workers agree that SPM fractions from brain contain somewhere between 80 and 90% synaptic membranes as judged by a combination of morphological assessment and content of marker enzymes (reviewed by Matus, 1978). The major contaminants arise from mitochondria and myelin. Thus some 20% of even the best SPM preparation is of non-synaptic origin.

This situation has recently been shown to be even worse for the postsynaptic density. PSDs have proved to be avid binding sites for exogenous proteins, including myelin basic protein (Cohen et al., 1977) and both neuronal and glial filament proteins (Matus et al., 1980). Since the phosphoproteins and their associated enzymes which are present in the SPM fraction are severalfold more concentrated in PSDs (Ng and Matus, 1979a; Ueda et al., 1979; Kelly et al.

1979) this gives us an additional reason to question the provenance of the phosphorylation phenomena associated with these fractions.

The case for being conservative in ascribing phosphorylation effects seen in SPM fractions to the synaptic plasma membranes themselves is further indicated by practical examples. One is the phosphopeptide complex known as protein I (Ueda and Greengard, 1977; Ueda, this volume). Immunocytochemistry has recently revealed that synaptic vesicles are the primary and probably the only site of these proteins in nervous tissue (De Camili et al., 1979; Greengard, 1981). The other is the 40 000 mol. wt. protein whose phosphorylation is depressed during post-tetanic potentiation in the hippocampus (Browning et al., 1979). Subsequent work has demonstrated that rather than being associated with the synaptic membranes, as its physiological correlates might first suggest, it is in fact a component of the mitochondrial enzyme pyruvate dehydrogenase (Morgan and Routtenberg, 1980; Browning et al., this volume). These phenomena are nonetheless interesting even though not situated in the synaptic plasma membranes, but their very existence demonstrates that biochemical studies of brain subcellular fractions are insufficient to lead to a valid conclusion about the cellular site of a particular phosphorylation event (or any other kind of biochemical phenomenon for that matter).

Immunochemical methods offer a solution to some of these difficulties. Immunocytochemical staining has proved a useful way of determining the location within the brain of proteins including phosphate acceptors such as protein I and molecules such as calmodulin which are involved in modulating protein phosphorylation (Wood et al., 1980). Recently introduced immunochemical methods have made it possible to determine accurately which polypeptides an antibody reacts with (Towbin et al., 1979). The combination of this technique with immunocytochemical staining of brain sections has proved a good means of determining the cellular affiliation of proteins within the brain as well as a sensitive means of detecting exogenous contaminants of brain subcellular fractions (Matus et al., 1980). In this paper we describe a range of monoclonal antibodies (*mabs*) raised against the SPM fraction. Their properties illustrate both the range of non-synaptic material which can be expected in such preparations and also demonstrate the value of lymphocyte cloning technology for producing immunological probes for genuinely synaptic proteins.

## MATERIAL AND METHODS

The methods for subcellular fractionation (Matus et al., 1980), gel electrophoresis (Laemmli, 1970) and immunochemical staining of gel blots (Towbin et al., 1979; Matus et al., 1980) have all been described before.

Our method for monoclonal antibody production from lymphocyte hybridomas is essentially that of Galfré et al. (1977). In the experiments described in detail below, a panel of BALB/c mice were immunized twice intraperitoneally with 3–5 mg of SPM proteins. A month after the second injection the mice were again boosted and those two animals with the highest anti-SPM serum titers were chosen for hybridoma production. $10^8$ spleen cells were fused by polyethylene glycol 1500 to $10^7$ cells of the HGPRT-deficient myeloma line X63Ag8.653 and cultured in selective medium (Littlefield, 1964) in $500 \times 1.0$ ml culture wells over a feeder layer of $10^6$ spleen cells per well. The cultures were maintained at $37°$ C in a 95 % air/5 % $CO_2$ atmosphere. The culture medium was replaced every 3 days. Hybridoma colonies appeared in about 2/3 of the wells and the culture supernatants were tested for anti-SPM antibodies after 2–3 weeks (Hawkes et al., 1982c).

To screen for anti-SPM antibodies we use a solid phase immunoassay — the dot immuno-binding assay (Hawkes et al., 1982a). Approximately 0.5 $\mu$l aliquots of a 1.0 mg/ml sus-pension of SPM in saline are "dotted" onto small squares of cellulose nitrate filter and allowed to dry, thereby becoming tightly bound. The dots are then incubated for 30 min in 10% normal horse serum in TBS (50 mM Tris–HCl buffer pH 7.4, 200 mM NaCl) to block residual protein-binding sites on the filter. Testing for anti-SPM antibodies involves a series of three incubations. Firstly, the dot is incubated overnight in the hybridoma supernatant, then for 3 h in 0.1% horseradish peroxidase-conjugated rabbit anti-mouse Ig, and finally for 5–10 min in 0.06% 4-chloro-1-naphthol, 0.01% hydrogen peroxide in TBS. The filter is washed for 15 min in TBS between incubations. Those hybridoma media containing anti-SPM antibodies turn the dot blue.

Immunocytochemical studies were made on 40 $\mu$m vibrotome sections of rat cerebellum from animals fixed by cardiac perfusion with 4% formaldehyde, 0.2% glutaraldehyde in 0.1 M phosphate buffer pH 7.4. Sections were stained by an indirect immunoperoxidase procedure as described previously (Matus et al., 1979) except that 4-chloro-1-naphthol was used as substrate.

## RESULTS

Our *mabs* were raised against synaptosomal plasma membranes from rat cerebellum with the express aim of identifying polypeptides characteristic of specific organelles, cell types and tissue regions in the brain. We use the cerebellum for the same reasons that attracted other workers in the past: simple cytoarchitecture, readily distinguishable cell types and, in the rat, mainly postnatal histogenesis. Hybridoma clones secreting anti-SPM antibodies were first identified by the dot immunobinding assay (Hawkes et al., 1982a). The individual *mabs* were then further screened to identify polypeptide antigens and to determine the antigen distribution within the cerebellar cortex. We identify polypeptide antigens by protein blotting (Towbin et al., 1979). In this technique, the proteins of SPM are separated by gel electrophoresis in polyacrylamide and are then transferred laterally onto cellulose nitrate paper where they form a faithful replica of the original gel. The protein blot may then be stained by an indirect immunoperoxidase procedure to identify those polypeptides recognized by a particular *mab*. The distribution of the antigens within the cerebellar cortex is determined by the immunope-roxidase staining of rat cerebellar sections.

The fusion we discuss in this review produced 176 independent anti-SPM antibody-se-creting primary hybridoma lines (Hawkes et al., 1982c). These fall into four general classes: (i) those which react both with brain sections and protein blots; (ii) those positive histo-chemically but not on protein blots; (iii) those positive only on protein blots; and (iv) those which, while they still react on dots, are negative both on protein blots and brain sections.

There are several plausible explanations for this spectrum of behavior. The positive results which all our *mabs* give in the dot immunobinding assay against SPM which had not been treated with fixative or detergent may reflect the reaction of the antibody with the antigen in its native conformation in the membrane. In favor of this interpretation, we have shown that a range of enzymes all retain their activities through a dot assay. We cannot assume that all anti-SPM *mabs* automatically recognize the native antigen conformation — it is inherent in our selection procedure that only those which are positive in the dot assay are studied further. The failure of individual *mabs* to react on a protein blot could arise either by the loss of antigenicity following detergent denaturation or because the antigen is a molecule to which the gel

80

electrophoresis and blotting technique is unsuited. Likewise, negative results in the immuno-peroxidase staining of tissue sections could involve either a problem of antibody access to the antigen or the loss of antigenicity through tissue fixation. Whatever the reason in any specific case, it is evident that if the full potential of an immunization and lymphocyte fusion of this type is to be realized, then a range of different assay methods must be employed.

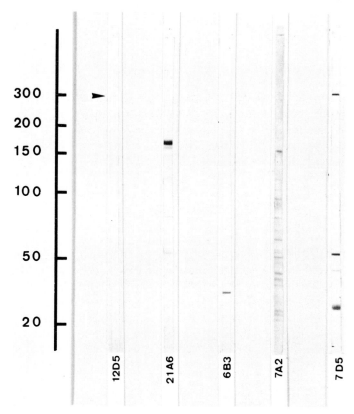

Fig. 1. Immunoblots prepared from SDS-gels in which the polypeptides of a brain SPM fraction had been separated, electrophoretically transferred to cellulose nitrate sheet and then stained with 177 different monoclonal antibodies of which 5 are shown. They are identified by code letters at the base of each column. A scale indicating calculated molecular weight ($\times 10^{-3}$) appears at the left. The single faint polypeptide band detected by 12D5 is indicated by an arrowhead.

Fig. 1 shows a series of 2 mm wide strips, all cut from a single slab gel protein blot, in which the proteins of cerebellar SPM have been separated. Each strip has been stained with a different *mab*. Some of these stain only one polypeptide band (e.g. 6B3), others stain more than one (e.g. 7D5) and a few stain a large number of bands (e.g. 7A2). Even in those cases where a large number of bands are recognized, we can usually be sure that the antibody is monoclonal because the same pattern of bands is stained by antibodies from several independent primary hypridoma lines and because the pattern is maintained through limiting dilution cloning.

Multiple stained bands on an protein blot can arise in any of a number of different ways. It might be that the determinant recognized is "trivial", for example a short amino acid primary sequence found frequently and at random on many proteins or a common post-translational modification which might be widespread among polypeptides. The determinant might be associated with a protein family. A single antigen-bearing polypeptide in vivo may degrade during isolation to yield a spectrum of antigenic degradation products. The antibody may be of low specificity and extensively cross-react between antigenic species. Whatever the case, Fig. 1 emphasizes that by using *mabs* we are studying the characteristics of a determinant rather than a molecule. It also serves to emphasize the value of explicitly identifying the antigen(s) recognized by a *mab*.

A second consistent feature of the *mab* staining of protein blots, also exemplified in Fig. 1, is that the staining intensity of different bands varies between very strong (e.g. 21A6) and very faint (e.g. 12D5). We can account for this in three ways: low antibody titer or affinity; poor preservation of antigenicity during protein blotting; and low absolute amounts of the antigen. Typically, for example in the case of 12D5, it does not seem that antibody titer or affinity is important because the same weak staining is seen with antibody from different primary hybridoma lines (which would not be expected to have the same affinities), the staining is unaffected by a 10-fold change in antibody concentration, and the staining of tissue sections is

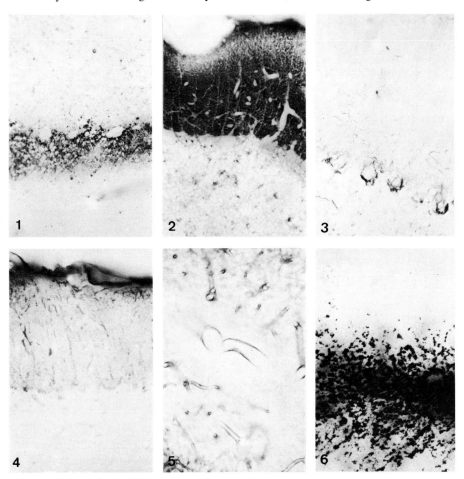

Fig. 2. A set of six sections of rat cerebellar cortec stained with different monoclonal antibodies by an immunoperoxidase procedure. (1) 12D5; (2) 21A6; (3) 6B3; (4) 7A2; (5) 7D5; (6) 17B3. Each can be compared to the appropriate polypeptide staining patterns shown in Fig. 1 except 17B3 which does not stain any bands on gel blots of SPM.

strong. We suspect that the absolute amount of determinant present on the blot is the limiting factor in most cases.

The monoclonal antibodies from this one fusion reacted with a variety of cellular structures in immunocytochemical tests. The staining patterns obtained in cerebellar cortex with six of the *mabs* are shown in Fig. 2. These included various components of neurons, glial cells and, in one case, some component associated with the lining of blood vessels (frame 5, Fig. 2). Below, we discuss two of these *mabs* in greater detail.

*MIT-23: a neuron-specific polypeptide whose expression correlates with terminal neuronal differentiation*

A number of our independent primary hybridoma lines produce antibodies which react with a single polypeptide band of molecular weight 23 000 on SDS-gel blots (Fig. 3a). Immuno-peroxidase staining of adult rat cerebellum with these *mabs* gives strong labeling of the cell bodies, dendrites and axon hillocks of the Purkinje cells (Fig. 3b) with less strong staining in the remainder of the cerebellar cortex and no staining in the white matter. Staining in the granular layer is associated both with granule and Golgi II cells and in the molecular layer, in amongst the strongly stained Purkinje cell dendrites, are staining profiles of both basket and stellate neurons. Although there is general staining of cerebellar neurons, the glial cells, by contrast, are unstained. When the neuronal staining is examined at higher magnifications it resolves into numerous discrete deposits rather than being uniformly distributed (Fig. 3b).

A similar punctate staining pattern also occurs in neurons in cerebellar primary cultures and in neuroblastoma in culture. When viewed in the electron microscope, the antibody staining is seen to be associated with neuronal mitochondria. We have therefore called this protein MIT-23 (Hawkes et al., 1982b). It is necessary to be cautious about this ultrastructural assignment because it has been shown that peroxidase staining of mitochondria can occur as an artifact of formaldehyde fixation (Wood et al., 1980). We feel that it is not an artifact in the case of MIT-23 because punctate deposits are also seen in cells fixed with acetone and because tests on various unfixed subcellular fractions of rat brain show MIT-23 to be enriched along with the mitochondria.

Although in the adult MIT-23 is a prominent feature of most, if not all, neurons of the cerebellar cortex, its distribution in the neonate is strikingly restricted. From birth to 10 days of age, MIT-23 is confined exclusively to the growing Purkinje cells (Fig. 3c). In older animals, the expression of MIT-23 correlates with the onset of terminal differentiation of the neurons. Thus there is no staining of the external granular layer which contains the granule cell neuroblasts and granule cell staining is only seen once the postmitotic cells have migrated into the internal granular layer. According to this interpretation, the Purkinje cells are stained at birth because these neurons are already postmitotic. The adult staining pattern is qualitatively established by about day 20 when the other types of neuroblasts in the cerebellar cortex cease dividing. These results suggest that MIT-23 can be used to pinpoint neurons at the onset of terminal differentiation.

*12D5: a monoclonal antibody which specifically recognizes components of the granular layer*

MIT-23 is an example of a polypeptide antigen which is probably found in all neurons. The antigen recognized by *mab* 12D5 is representative of a further level of specificity, a determinant restricted, within the cerebellar cortex, to the granular layer. 12D5 reacts on protein blots with a single polypeptide band of apparent molecular weight 270 000 (Fig. 1). In immunoperoxidase-stained sections of the cerebellar cortex (Fig. 2, frame 1) only the granular layer is strongly stained with merely a sparse scattering of stain deposits in the molecular layer.

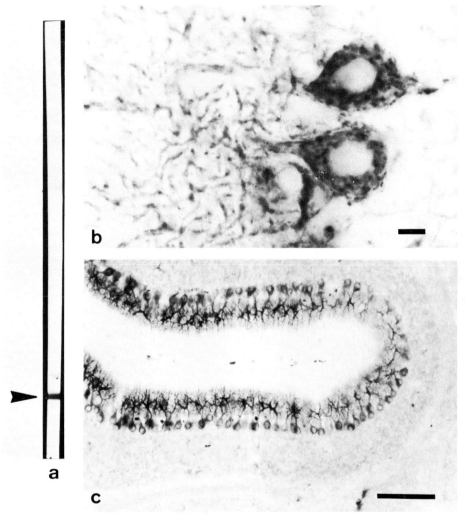

Fig. 3. Results obtained with monclonal antibody against antigen MIT-23. a: Staining of a gel blot (as in Fig. 1) showing the single 23 000 mol. wt. polypeptide which the antibody reacts with. b: Immunoperoxidase staining of rat cerebellar cortex showing reaction product associated with granules in the cell bodies and dendrites of Purkinje neurons. Calibration bar = 10 μm. c: Anti-MIT-23 stained section of cerebellar cortex from a 10-day-old rat. The staining is limited to postmitotic Purkinje cells. Calibration bar = 100 μm.

Whereas anti-MIT-23 stains Purkinje cells especially strongly, 12D5 does not stain them at all. The strong staining in the granular layer is associated with the synaptic glomeruli which occur in between the islands of granule cell bodies. This is suggestive of a specific reaction with some extremely localized tissue element such as mossy fiber axon terminals or specialized glial structure associated with them. Ultrastructural studies are underway to resolve this question.

## DISCUSSION

Because of the combined possibilities of identifying specific polypeptide antigens by protein blotting and of determining their distribution by immunohistochemistry, antibodies are widely recognized as the reagents of choice for determining the cytological localization of specific proteins in the brain. Unfortunately, conventional antibodies suffer from two important drawbacks. Firstly, in order to obtain a monospecific antiserum it is first necessary to have a pure antigen, an ideal it is difficult to approach with many of the more interesting proteins in the nervous system. Secondly, even when a pure protein is available, there are still likely to be multiple antigenic determinants, antibody affinities and so forth, making it impossible to be certain that the immunocytological and immunochemical results reflect the behavior of the self-same antibody.

These problems were solved by the invention of *mabs* which have the pre-eminent virtue that each lymphocyte hybridoma clone produces a unique antibody whose antigenic specificity can be unequivocally defined, so the culture medium from each clonal hybrid line contains antibody of only one specificity which must alone be responsible for all antibody-mediated effects. There is another advantage of *mabs* which is of even greater immediate value. The cloning procedures allow single antibody specificities to be recovered from an animal immunized with a complex mixture of antigens. Therefore, we can immunize a mouse with a crude subcellular fraction and realistically expect to recover antibodies of high biochemical and cytological specificities.

The opportunity presented by monoclonal antibody technology has been exploited by a number of laboratories interested in neuroimmunology. Previous studies of the mammalian brain have reported *mabs* which distinguish central from peripheral neurons (Cohen and Selvendran, 1981; Vulliamy et al., 1981), and various glial subclasses one from another (Bartlett et al., 1981; Lagenauer et al., 1980). Other *mabs* bind differentially to various cell types and regions of the retina (Barnstable, 1980; Trisler et al., 1981). In these studies, however, the particular antigen(s) responsible for the various staining patterns have not been identified. Neither has a study so far been reported in which *mabs* have been used specifically as reagents for surveying the kinds of antigens associated with synaptosomal plasma membrane-enriched brain subcellular fractions. As the results reported here indicate, use and characterization of anti-SPM *mabs* support and extend previous evidence (Cohen et al., 1977; Matus et al., 1980) pointing to the significant contamination of SPM fractions by proteins originating outside the synaptic plasma membranes. Among the antigens detected in SPM fractions by our *mabs* are a large number directed against glial antigens (e.g. 7A2, Fig. 2, frame 4), some directed against mitochondria (e.g. MIT-23), some apparently against components of neuronal internediate filaments (e.g. 6B3), some against myelin components (e.g. 17B3) and even one directed against components of the lining of blood vessels (7D5). There seems little point in arguing the virtues of one or other method of preparing SPM fractions in considering the implications of these contaminants — they have been found in SPM produced by different fractionation schedules to those we employ, and in the morphologically more pure PSD fraction the level of contaminants is even higher (Cohen et al., 1977; Matus et al., 1980).

What these findings suggest is that functional studies of brain subcellular fractions, which in the present context means the characterization of phosphoproteins and their associated enzymes, should be performed together with alternative techniques for identifying the endogenous sites at which the active molecules are found. The use of monoclonal antibodies for identifying particular polypeptides and determining their cytological affiliation in whole tissue, provides an appropriate approach to this problem.

ACKNOWLEDGEMENTS

We thank M. Ackermann and G. Pehling for technical assistance.

REFERENCES

Barnstable, C.J. (1980) Monoclonal antibodies which recognize different cell types in the rat retina. *Nature (Lond.)*, 286: 231–235.

Bartlett, P.F., Noble, M.D., Pruss, R.M., Raff, M.C., Rattray, S. and Williams, C.A. (1981) Rat neural antigen 2 (RAN-2): a cell surface antigen on astrocytes, ependymal cells, Müller cells and lepto-meninges defined by a monoclonal antibody. *Brain Res.*, 204: 339–351.

Browning, M., Dunwiddie, T., Bennet, W., Gispen, W. and Lynch, G. (1979) Synaptic phosphoproteins: specific changes after repetitive stimulation of the hippocampal slice. *Science*, 203: 60–62.

Cohen, J. and Selvendran, Y. (1981) A neuronal cell surface antigen is found in the CNS but not in peripheral neurones. *Nature (Lond.)*, 291: 421–423.

Cohen, R.S., Blomberg, F., Berzins, K. and Siekevitz, P. (1977) The structure of postsynaptic densities isolated from dog cerebral cortex. I. Overall morphology and protein composition. *J. Cell Biol.*, 74: 181–203.

De Camilli, P., Ueda, T., Bloom, F.E., Battenberg, E. and Greengard, P. (1979) Widespread distribution of protein I in the central and peripheral nervous systems. *Proc. nat. Acad. Sci. (Wash.)*, 76: 5977–5981.

Galfré, G., Howe, S., Milstein, C., Butcher, G.W. and Howard, J.C. (1977) Antibodies to major histocompatibility antigens produced by hybrid cell lines. *Nature (Lond.)*, 266: 550–552.

Greengard, P. (1976) Possible role for cyclic nucleotide phosphorylated membrane proteins in postsynaptic actions of neurotransmitters. *Nature (Lond.)*, 260: 101–108.

Greengard, P. (1981) In *The Harvey Lectures*, Academic Press, New York, in press.

Hawkes, R., Niday, E. and Gordon, J. (1982a) A dot immunobinding assay for monoclonal and other antibodies. *Anal. Biochem.*, 119: 142–147.

Hawkes, R., Niday, E. and Matus, A. (1982b) MIT-23: a mitochondrial marker for terminal neuronal differentiation defined by a monoclonal antibody. *Cell*, 28: 253–258.

Hawkes, R., Niday, E. and Matus, A. (1982c) Monoclonal antibodies identify novel neural antigens. *Proc. nat. Acad. Sci. (Wash.)*, in press.

Johnson, E.M., Maeno, H. and Greengard, P. (1971) Phosphorylation of endogenous protein of rat brain by cyclic AMP-dependent protein kinase. *J. biol. Chem.*, 246: 7731–7739.

Kelly, P., Cotman, C. and Largen, M. (1979) Cyclic AMP-stimulated protein kinases at brain synaptic junctions. *J. biol. Chem.*, 254: 1564–1575.

Laemmli, U.K. (1970) Cleavage of structural proteins during the assembly of the head of bacteriophage T4. *Nature (Lond.)*, 227: 680–685.

Lagenauer, C., Sommer, I. and Schachner, M. (1980) Subclass of astroglia in rat cerebellum recognized by monoclonal antibody. *Dev. Biol.*, 79: 367–378.

Littlefield, J.W. (1964) Selection of hybrids from matings of fibroblasts in vitro and their presumed recombinants. *Science*, 145: 709.

Matus, A. (1978) Synaptic membranes and junctions from brain. *Methods Membr. Biol.*, 9: 203–236.

Matus, A., Ng, M.L. and Jones, D.H. (1979) Immunohistochemical localization of neurofilament antigen in rat cerebellum. *J. Neurocytol.*, 8: 513–525.

Matus, A., Pehling, G., Ackermann, M. and Maeder, J. (1980) Brain postsynaptic densities: their relationship to glial and neuronal filaments. *J. Cell Biol.*, 87: 346–359.

Morgan, D.G. and Routtenberg, A. (1980) Evidence that a 41,000 dalton brain phosphoprotein is pyruvate dehydrogenase. *Biochem. biophys. Res. Commun.*, 95: 569–576.

Neville, Jr., D.M. (1975) Isolation of cell surface membrane fractions from mammalian cells and organs. *Methods Membr. Biol.*, 3: 1–49.

Ng, M.L. and Matus, A. (1979a) Long duration phosphorylation of synaptic membrane proteins. *Neuroscience*, 4: 1265–1274.

Ng, M.L. and Matus, A. (1979b) Protein phosphorylation in isolated plasma membranes and postsynaptic junctional structures from brain synapses. *Neuroscience*, 4: 169–180.

Towbin, H., Staehelin, T. and Gordon, J. (1979) A procedure for the electrophoretic transfer of proteins from polyacrylamide gels to nitrocellulose sheets and some applications. *Proc. nat. Acad. Sci. (Wash.)*, 76: 4350–4354.

Trisler, D., Schneider, M.D. and Nirenberg, M. (1981) A topographic gradient of molecules in retina can be used to identify neuron position. *Proc. nat. Acad. Sci. (Wash.)*, 78: 2145–2149.

Ueda, T. and Greengard, P. (1977) Adenosine 3′:5′-monophosphate-regulated phosphoprotein system of neuronal membranes. *J. biol. Chem.*, 252: 5155–5163.

Ueda, T., Greengard, P., Berzins, K., Cohen, R.S., Blomberg, F., Grab, D.J. and Siekevitz, P. (1979) Subcellular distribution in cerebral cortex of two proteins phosphorylated by a cAMP dependent protein kinase. *J. Cell Biol.*, 83: 308–319.

Vulliamy, T., Rattray, S. and Mirsky, R. (1981) Cell surface antigen distinguishes sensory and autonomic peripheral neurones from central neurones. *Nature (Lond.)*, 291: 418–420.

Weller, M. and Rodnight, R. (1971) Turnover of protein-bound phosphoryserine in membrane preparations from ox brain catalysed by intrinsic kinase and phosphatase activity. *Biochem. J.*, 124: 393–406.

Williams, M. and Rodnight, R. (1977) Protein phosphorylation in nervous tissue: Possible involvement in nervous tissue function and relationship to cyclic nucleotide metabolism. *Progr. Neurobiol.*, 8: 183–250.

Wood, J.C., Wallace, R.W., Whitaker, J.N. and Cheung, W.Y. (1980) Immunocytochemical localization of calmodulin in regions of rodent brain. *Ann. N.Y. Acad. Sci.*, 356: 75–82.

# Specific Inhibition of the Phosphorylation of Protein I, a Synaptic Protein, by Affinity-Purified Anti-Protein I Antibody

TETSUFUMI UEDA and SHIGETAKA NAITO

*Mental Health Research Institute and Departments of Psychiatry and Pharmacology, University of Michigan, Ann Arbor, MI 48109, U.S.A.*

## BACKGROUND

The pioneering work of Sutherland and his colleagues has led to the concept that the physiological effects of certain hormones are initially mediated through formation of cyclic AMP (cAMP) and subsequent phosphorylation of appropriate enzymes in the target cells (Robison et al., 1971). Whether a similar mechanism underlies the synaptic effects of certain neurotransmitters, in particular, monoamine transmitters, has been an active subject of investigation (Bloom, 1975; Greengard, 1976, 1978, 1981; Daly, 1975; Kebabian, 1977; Klein and Kandel, 1978). Perhaps the first evidence to suggest that cAMP may play an important role in the nervous system is the observation that both adenylate cyclase and cAMP phosphodiesterase are most concentrated in the gray matter of the brain among the tissues examined (Sutherland et al., 1962; Butcher and Sutherland, 1962). These enzymes were shown to be enriched in those subcellular fractions derived from the synaptic region (De Robertis et al., 1967). Moreover, certain putative neurotransmitters such as norepinephrine and histamine were shown to increase levels of cAMP (Kakiuchi and Rall, 1968; Shimizu et al., 1970), possibly through activation of adenylate cyclase. Subsequently, the presence of various monoamine neurotransmitter-sensitive adenylate cyclases, which are blocked by respective antagonists, was demonstrated in cell-free preparations from several nervous tissues (Kebabian et al., 1972; Brown and Makman, 1972; Clement-Cormier et al., 1974; Karobath and Leitich, 1974; Nathanson and Greengard, 1974; Iversen, 1975; Hegstrand et al., 1976). Bloom and his colleagues provided electrophysiological evidence to suggest that cAMP mediates the inhibitory effect of norepinephrine on the spontaneous firing rate of cerebellar Purkinje cells (Siggins et al., 1969; Hoffer et al., 1969). In 1968, Krebs and his colleagues demonstrated that the action of cAMP is to activate a class of protein kinase referred to as cAMP-dependent protein kinase (Walsh et al., 1968; Rubin and Rosen, 1975; Krebs and Beavo, 1979; Glass and Krebs, 1980). This enzyme was found to be abundant in the brain (Miyamoto et al., 1969) and enriched in those subcellular fractions containing synaptic elements (Maeno et al., 1971). These studies led to the hypothesis (Greengard et al., 1972) that there must be a specific endogenous substrate for cAMP-dependent protein kinase in the synaptic region, which would mediate the electrophysiological responses elicited by those neurotransmitters which activate adenylate cyclase (Fig. 1). For these reasons, we searched for such an endogenous protein substrate. Using $[\gamma\text{-}^{32}P]ATP$ of high specific radioactivity, SDS–polyacrylamide gel electrophoresis, and autoradiography, we initially demonstrated that cAMP markedly stimulates the endogenous phosphorylation of one specific protein in a

88

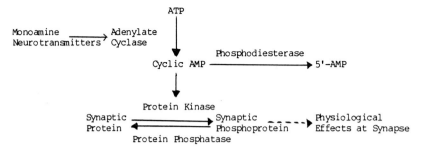

Fig. 1. Proposed molecular mechanism underlying some of the synaptic effects of monoamine neurotransmitters.

synaptic membrane fraction (Johnson et al., 1972). By choosing an appropriate incubation time, we found that two proteins serve as prominent endogenous substrates for cAMP-dependent (but not cGMP-dependent) protein kinase in the synaptic membrane fraction; these two phosphoproteins were designated protein I and protein II (Ueda et al., 1973). Subsequently, each of these protein bands was resolved into two bands: protein I into proteins Ia and Ib (Ueda and Greengard, 1977), and protein II into proteins IIa and IIb (Lohmann et al., 1978; Walter et al., 1979). Other investigators have also shown that specific proteins corresponding to protein I and protein II are phosphorylated by endogenous cyclic AMP-dependent protein kinase present in synaptic membrane fractions (Routtenberg and Ehrlich, 1975; Dunkley et al., 1976; Kelly and Cotman, 1979; DeBlas et al., 1979). In addition, microtubule-associated protein₂ (MAP₂) was found to serve as an endogenous substrate for cAMP-dependent protein kinase (Sloboda et al., 1975; Lohmann et al., 1980). Preliminary experiments indicated that protein I appeared to be specific to nervous tissues (Ueda et al., 1973). In view of the possibility that protein I might play an important role in synaptic events, research efforts were made to purify and characterize protein I, and study the immunocytochemical localization of protein I.

*Physicochemical properties*

It was found that protein I could be extracted at pH 3 from the membranes derived from the synaptic region without significant loss of the capability to serve as substrate for cAMP-dependent protein kinase. Protein I was purified to apparent homogeneity from pH 3 extract of membrane fractions from the bovine brain by adsorption chromatography on hydroxylapatite and gel filtration on Bio-Gel P-150 (Ueda and Greengard, 1977). Purified protein I contains two similar polypeptides, referred to as protein Ia and protein Ib. They have similar molecular weights ($M_r = 86\ 000$ and $80\ 000$, respectively), amino acid compositions, and isoelectric points (10.3 and 10.2, respectively). An interesting feature of their physicochemical properties is that they are rich in proline and glycine, and contain a domain which is susceptible to the action of highly purified collagenase; the serine residue which is phosphorylated by cAMP-dependent protein kinase occurs in the collagenase-resistant domain. Furthermore, their sedimentation coefficient (2.9 S) and Stokes radius (59 Å) values are unusually smaller and larger, respectively, than expected for a globular protein with molecular weights of 80 000 to 86 000, which indicates that proteins Ia and Ib have an extended structure. Further studies suggest that the collagenase-resistant fragment ($M_r = 48\ 000$) of proteins Ia and Ib is much more globular than intact proteins Ia and Ib; the sedimentation coefficient and Stokes radius have been shown to be 2.9 S and 30 Å, respectively (Ueda and Greengard, unpublished results). These physicochemical properties are all compatible with the structural model, in which protein Ia and protein Ib are both made up of a globular, collagenase-resistant region and an elongated, collagenase-sensitive region. Recent studies have suggested that the collagenase-sensitive region may be involved in the attachment of protein I to the membrane (Ueda, 1981).

*Distribution*

Protein I is exclusively present in the nervous system, and, in particular, highly enriched in the mammalian brain (Ueda and Greengard, 1977; De Camilli et al., 1979; Goelz et al., 1981). In the brain, it is most concentrated in the frontal cortex, hippocampal cortex and thalamus; it is also present in the cerebellar cortex, basal ganglia and substantia nigra, septal nucleus and hypothalamus in high concentrations (Bloom et al., 1979; Goelz et al., 1981). In the cerebellar cortex, it is particularly abundant in the molecular layer and in the glomeruli structure within the granule cell layer (Bloom et al., 1979; De Camilli et al., 1979). It also occurs in the spinal cord where it is more concentrated in the cervical and lumbar segments than in the thoracic segments, and, cross-sectionally, found more in the dorsal horn than in the ventral horn (Ueda et al., 1981). Outside the central nervous system, it has been found in the posterior pituitary, in the inner plexiform of the retina, in the superior cervical ganglion, in the ciliary ganglion, and in the innervated areas of smooth muscles and adrenal medulla (De Camilli et al., 1979). However, it is virtually absent in the regions which contain predominantly axons or in those tissues devoid of synapses (Ueda and Greengard, 1977; Bloom et al., 1979; De Camilli et al., 1979). In the nervous system, protein I is found only in neurons (Sieghart et al., 1978; Bloom et al., 1979; De Camilli et al., 1979), and within these neurons it is localized in the synaptic region, being associated primarily with presynaptic vesicles, and to some extent with postsynaptic densities and presynaptic membranes (Bloom et al., 1979; Ueda et al., 1979; Kelly and Cotman, 1979; DeBlas et al., 1979). This synaptic localization is in accord with the observation (Lohmann et al., 1978) that protein I appears in parallel to synapse formation during development.

*Calcium/calmodulin-dependent phosphorylation*

In the course of studies directed at finding some of the biochemical mechanisms underlying the physiological effects of calcium in the nerve terminal, Krueger et al. (1977) found that an influx of $Ca^{2+}$ into intact synaptosomes causes an increase in the state of phosphorylation of several proteins. The most marked effect was on two proteins which had electrophoretic mobilities indistinguishable from those of proteins Ia and Ib. These two proteins were shown to be identical to proteins Ia and Ib, which had previously been identified as endogenous substrates for cAMP-dependent protein kinase (Sieghart et al., 1979). The effect of calcium on the phosphorylation of these proteins was shown to be mediated by calmodulin (Schulman and Greengard, 1978) and calcium/calmodulin-dependent protein kinases (Kennedy and Greengard, 1981). These calcium/calmodulin-dependent protein kinases are distinct from other calcium/calmodulin-dependent protein kinases such as myosin light chain kinase and phosphorylase *b* kinase, and catalyze the phosphorylation of proteins Ia and Ib at multiple sites, two serine residues in the collagenase-sensitive region and one in the collagenase-resistant region (Huttner et al., 1981).

*Pharmacological agents which can regulate phosphorylation of protein I in intact neurons*

Depolarizing agents such as $K^+$ and veratridine were shown to cause an increase in the state of phosphorylation of protein I in slices of rat cerebral cortex in the presence of calcium in the medium (Forn and Greengard, 1978). The $K^+$-induced phosphorylation is a function of the membrane depolarization, and occurs at a reasonably rapid rate, reaching a maximal level within 20 sec, at 60 mM potassium ions, followed by gradual dephosphorylation. It is possible to rephosphorylate protein I by removing $K^+$ from, and subsequently adding it to, the incubation medium. The alternate phosphorylation and dephosphorylation can be repeatedly produced, which indicates that protein I is a dynamic protein, altering the state of phosphorylation in response to changes in the membrane potential.

Although the depolarizing agents (Forn and Greengard, 1978) and certain convulsants (Strömbom et al., 1979) were shown to increase the state of phosphorylation of protein I, direct evidence for the link between those neurotransmitters which activate adenylate cyclase and the phosphorylation of protein I had been lacking for some time. Recently, serotonin and dopamine were shown to increase, through activation of adenylate cyclase, the state of phosphorylation of protein I in slices of the facial motor nucleus (Dolphin and Greengard, 1981a,b) and in sections of the superior cervical ganglion (Nestler and Greengard, 1980),

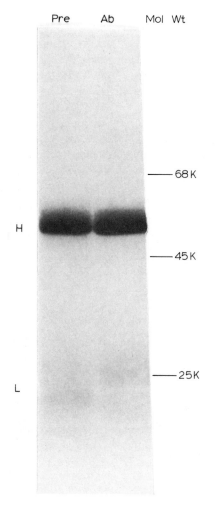

Fig. 2. Affinity-purified anti-protein I antibodies (Ab) and preimmune immunoglobulin G (Pre), stained with Coomassie brilliant blue, after each preparation (9.8 μg) had been subjected to SDS–polyacrylamide gel (10%) electrophoresis. H and L indicate the positions of the heavy and light chains of immunoglobulin G, respectively. (Naito and Ueda, 1981.)

respectively; the affected site of phosphorylation was in "peptide 1", which is phosphorylated by cAMP-dependent and calcium/calmodulin-dependent protein kinases, and not in "Peptides 2–5", which are phosphorylated by calcium/calmodulin-dependent protein kinases. In these regions of the nervous system, protein I appears to be localized almost exclusively in the nerve terminals from which serotonin and dopamine are absent. Therefore, Greengard and colleagues have postulated that these neurotransmitters not only act on classically defined postsynaptic receptors, but also diffuse over some distance to act on neighboring presynaptic terminals where adenylate cyclase is activated, and subsequently cAMP-dependent phosphorylation of protein I takes place. Based upon these presynaptic effects of the neurotransmitters and calcium ions and the predominant localization of protein I on synaptic vesicles, it has been postulated that protein I is involved in regulation of synaptic vesicle function (Greengard, 1981). However, it has been difficult to identify the precise role of the phosphorylation of protein I, partly due to the lack of a specific substrate-directed inhibitor of the phosphorylation.

## PURIFICATION AND IDENTIFICATION AS IMMUNOGLOBULIN G OF ANTI-PROTEIN I ANTIBODY

We have recently purified anti-protein I antibodies from rabbit antiserum by affinity column chromatography (Naito and Ueda, 1981). An affinity column was made by conjugating purified protein I to Affi-Gel 10 agarose beads, to which anti-protein I antiserum was then applied. Nonspecifically bound materials were desorbed with 2 M NaCl, and specifically bound antibodies were eluted with 0.1 M citric acid (pH 2.5). Normal immunoglobulin G was purified from preimmune or nonimmune rabbit serum by affinity chromatography on protein A-conjugated Sepharose. The purified antibody preparation contains essentially two polypeptides, which have electrophoretic mobilities similar to those of the heavy and light chains of immunoglobulin G (Fig. 2). Ouchterlony double immunodiffusion test showed that protein I reacted with the immunoglobulin G purified from antiserum but not with IgG from preimmune

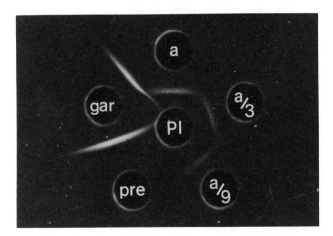

Fig. 3. Ouchterlony double immunodiffusion test of purified anti-protein I antibodies and preimmune immunoglobulin G. PI, protein I (1.4 μg); a, a/3, and a/9, 36, 12, and 4 μg, respectively, of purified anti-protein I antibodies; pre, preimmune immunoglobulin G (36 μg); gar, partially purified goat anti-rabbit IgG antibodies (36 μg). (Naito and Ueda, 1981.)

serum, whereas both types of rabbit IgG reacted with goat anti-rabbit IgG, as expected (Fig. 3). These results indicate that the affinity-purified anti-protein I antibodies are indeed a specific population of IgG.

### INHIBITION BY ANTI-PROTEIN I IgG OF PHOSPHORYLATION OF PROTEIN I IN A PURIFIED PREPARATION AND VARIOUS SUBCELLULAR FRACTIONS

We have found that the purified anti-protein I IgG inhibits the phosphorylation of purified protein I by exogenous cAMP-dependent protein kinase (Fig. 4). It also inhibited endogenous phosphorylation of Protein I in a synaptic vesicle fraction, in which protein I is the major substrate for cAMP-dependent protein kinase (Fig. 5). The anti-protein I IgG had no significant effect on the phosphorylation of other proteins, with the exception of two minor proteins.

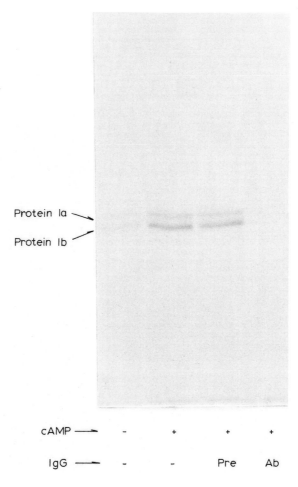

Fig. 4. Inhibition by anti-protein I IgG of the phosphorylation of purified protein I by cAMP-dependent protein kinase. The cAMP-dependent phosphorylation of protein I (1.1 $\mu$g) was carried out in the absence or presence of anti-protein I IgG (Ab; 16 $\mu$g), or of preimmune IgG (Pre; 16 $\mu$g), and the phosphorylated samples were subjected to SDS–polyacrylamide gel (6.9%) electrophoresis and autoradiography. (Naito and Ueda, 1981.)

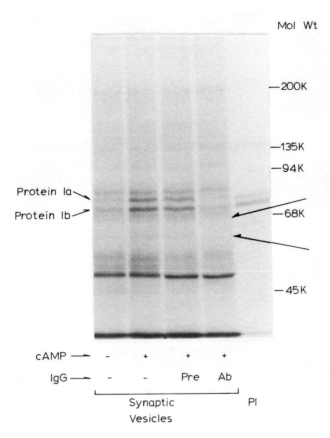

Fig. 5. Effect of anti-protein I IgG on cAMP-dependent endogenous phosphorylation of protein I in a synaptic vesicle fraction. The synaptic vesicle preparation was subjected to endogenous phosphorylation in the absence or presence of anti-protein I IgG (Ab; 33 μg) or preimmune IgG (Pre; 33 μg), followed by SDS–polyacrylamide gel (6.9%) electrophoresis and autoradiography. PI, phosphorylated purified protein I. (Naito and Ueda, 1981.)

Further studies have suggested that these phosphopolypeptides were derived from protein I by endogenous proteolysis, which may have occurred prior to, or during, the preparation of synaptic vesicles. When a crude synaptic vesicle fraction was incubated in the absence or presence of purified protein I, there was a time-dependent decrease in protein I, accompanied by an increase in two phosphoproteins corresponding to the arrow-indicated minor proteins. Moreover, these minor phosphoproteins were found to be sensitive to the action of highly purified bacterial collagenase, a unique proteolytic enzyme known to cleave protein I specifically among the phosphoproteins in the synaptosome (Sieghart et al., 1979) and synaptic membrane fractions (Ueda, 1981). Thus, we infer that the anti-protein I IgG can block phosphorylation not only of protein I but also of some of its digestion products such as those indicated by arrows.

Although protein I is most enriched in a highly purified synaptic vesicle fraction (Ueda et al., 1979), it is also present in other subcellular fractions such as synaptic plasma membrane and synaptic junctional complex fractions (Ueda et al., 1973; Routtenberg and Ehrlich, 1975; Dunkley et al., 1976; Kelly and Cotman, 1979; DeBlas et al., 1979). It is known that synaptic plasma membrane fractions contain other endogenous substrates for cAMP-dependent protein

94

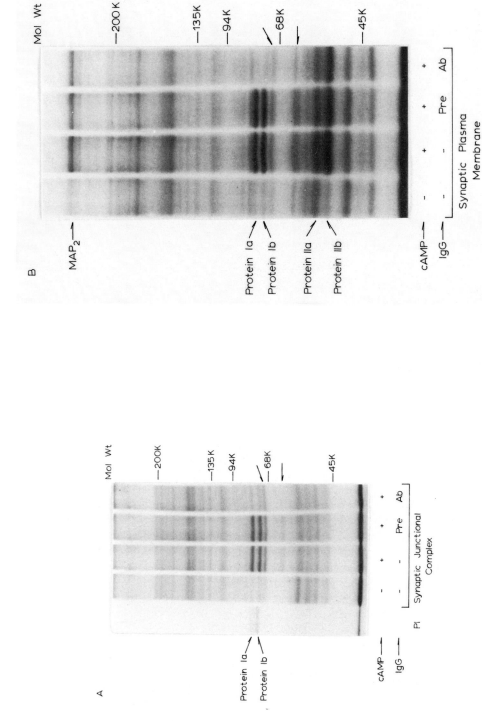

Fig. 6. Effect of anti-protein I IgG on endogenous phosphorylation of proteins present in synaptic junctional complex (A) and synaptic plasma membrane (B) fractions. Synaptic junctional complex (25 μg) and synaptic plasma membrane (50 μg) fractions were subjected to phosphorylation in the absence or presence of anti-protein I IgG (Ab; 4.9 μg in A and 19.6 μg in B), followed by SDS–polyacrylamide gel electrophoresis and autoradiography. PI, phosphorylated purified protein I.

kinase, such as protein IIa, protein IIb (Lohmann et al., 1978; Walter et al., 1979; DeBlas et al., 1979; Ueda, 1981), and microtubule-associated protein (MAP$_2$) (DeBlas et al., 1979; Lohmann et al., 1980). Therefore, we have examined the effect of the anti-protein I IgG on endogenous protein phosphorylation in synaptic junctional complex and synaptic plasma membrane fractions in order to determine the specificity of the specific IgG in its action to inhibit the phosphorylation of protein I. The anti-protein I IgG inhibited markedly the phosphorylation of protein I in both the synaptic junctional complex (Fig. 6A) and synaptic membrane fractions (Fig. 6B). It also inhibited the phosphorylation of two minor proteins, which are indistinguishable from those observed in the synaptic vesicle fraction. In contrast, the anti-protein I IgG had virtually no effect on the phosphorylation of the other proteins including protein IIa, protein IIb, and MAP$_2$. Thus, the anti-protein I IgG is highly specific to protein I and its degraded fragments in its action to inhibit protein phosphorylation.

## INHIBITION BY ANTI-PROTEIN I IgG OF cAMP-DEPENDENT AND CALCIUM-DEPENDENT PROTEIN KINASES IN THE HOMOGENATE OF CEREBRUM

The above observations have suggested the possibility that the anti-protein I IgG might be used as a unique probe in investigating the biological function of protein I phosphorylation. For this purpose, it would be crucial to establish firmly that the purified anti-protein I IgG blocks the phosphorylation of nothing but protein I and its degraded fragments. For this reason, we have examined the whole homogenate of rat cerebrum for the effect of the anti-protein I IgG on the endogenous phosphorylation of all possible substrate proteins in the tissue. As shown in Fig. 7A, only protein I and the arrow-indicated minor protein among approximately 30 visualized phosphoproteins were susceptible to the inhibitory action of the anti-protein I IgG. Similar to the case of the above subcellular fractions from bovine brain, we have obtained evidence to indicate that this minor phosphoprotein is also likely to be a polypeptide derived from protein I. Under the incubation conditions used, the anti-protein I IgG had essentially no effect on cAMP-dependent phosphorylation of protein IIa, protein IIb, or MAP$_2$, nor had any significant effect on phosphorylation of the smaller proteins which were separated on 12% gel (data not shown). This observation verifies the specific action of the purified anti-protein I IgG: inhibiting the phosphorylation of protein I.

As reviewed earlier, it is known that protein I is phosphorylated, not only by cAMP-dependent protein kinase, but also by calcium-dependent protein kinases; the former kinase phosphorylates a serine residue in the collagenase-resistant domain of the protein I molecule, and the latter phosphorylates two serine residues on the collagenase-sensitive domain and one on the collagenase-resistant domain. It would be of interest and importance to determine whether the anti-protein I IgG blocks the calcium-dependent phosphorylation of protein I, and has any effects on calcium-dependent phosphorylation of other proteins. For this purpose, the whole cerebral homogenate was used because it contains endogenous calmodulin and calcium/cal-modulin-dependent kinases, and all possible substrates for those kinases, so that the specificity of the anti-protein I IgG would be vigorously tested. As shown in Fig. 7B, calcium stimulated the phosphorylation of a great number of proteins, among which the phosphorylation of protein Ib was markedly inhibited by the anti-protein I IgG. It had no significant effect on the phosphorylation of the other proteins; the effect on protein Ia could not be determined, however, because large amounts of radioactive phosphate were incorporated into a protein(s) which had a highly similar electrophoretic mobility in SDS to protein Ia. To solve this

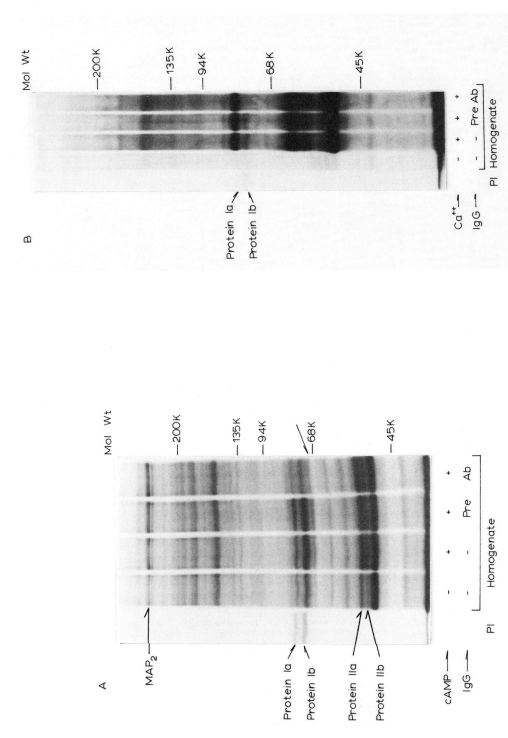

Fig. 7. Effect of anti-protein I IgG on cAMP-dependent (A) and calcium-dependent (B) endogenous phosphorylation of proteins in homogenates of rat cerebrum. Crude homogenates (25 μg) of rat cerebrum were subjected to cAMP-dependent and calcium-dependent phosphorylation in the absence or presence of anti-protein I IgG (Ab; 2.4 μg) or of preimmune IgG (Pre; 2.4 μg), followed by SDS–polyacrylamide gel electrophoresis and autoradiography. PI, phosphorylated purified protein I. (Naito and Ueda, 1981.)

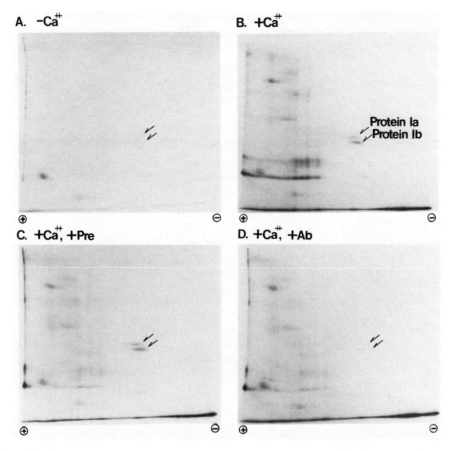

Fig. 8. Effect of anti-protein I IgG on calcium-dependent endogenous phosphorylation of protein I in homogenates of rat cerebrum, as analyzed by two-dimensional gel electrophoresis. Crude homogenates (25 μg) of rat cerebrum were subjected to calcium-dependent phosphorylation in the absence (A, B) or presence of anti-protein I IgG (Ab; 2.4 μg) (C), or of preimmune IgG (Pre; 2.4 μg) (D), followed by two-dimensional (non-equilibrium pH gradient and SDS) gel electrophoresis and autoradiography. (Naito and Ueda, 1981.)

problem, the phosphorylated proteins were analyzed by two-dimensional electrophoresis (O'Farrell et al., 1977). As shown in Fig. 8, this method permitted the separation of protein Ia from the otherwise electrophoretically similar protein(s); it appears that this contaminating protein of a similar molecular weight is acidic and did not enter the gel in the first dimensional pH gradient electrophoresis. Thus, Fig. 8 clearly shows that the anti-protein I IgG inhibits the calcium-dependent phosphorylation of protein Ia as well as that of protein Ib, without affecting the phosphorylation of the others.

Although cAMP-dependent and calcium-dependent kinases phosphorylate the distinct sites of protein I which are located in different regions of the molecule, the above observations indicate that the affinity-purified anti-protein I IgG is capable of blocking the phosphorylation of all of these sites. This has suggested the possibility that the purified anti-protein I IgG masks both the collagenase-resistant and -sensitive portions of protein I, or that it represents a mixture of microheterogeneous IgGs, which recognize various distinct sites of the protein I molecule. In the latter case, the anti-protein I IgG might inhibit the cAMP-dependent phosphorylation of

98

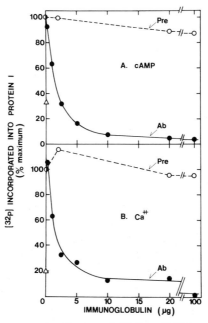

Fig. 9. Comparison of the inhibitory potencies of anti-protein I IgG in cAMP-dependent (A) and calcium-dependent (B) endogenous phosphorylation of protein I in homogenates of rat cerebrum. Crude homogenates of rat cerebrum (25 μg) were subjected to phosphorylation in the presence of various amounts of anti-protein I IgG (Ab, ●———●) or preimmune IgG (Pre, ○———○), followed by two-dimensional electrophoresis and autoradiography. The spots of protein Ia and protein Ib were identified with authentic protein I. The portion of the gel containing both protein Ia and protein Ib was cut out, and radioactivity determined in a scintillation spectrophotometer and expressed as % maximum. △, amounts of [$^{32}$P]phosphate incorporated in the absence of cAMP (A) or calcium (B), in the absence of IgG. The 100% maximum in A is 284 cpm, and the 100% maximum in B is 431 cpm. (Naito and Ueda, 1981.)

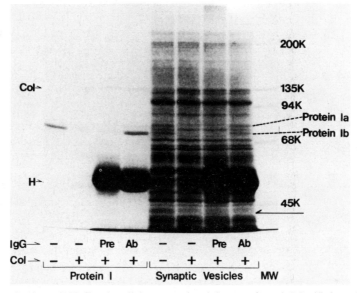

Fig. 10. Effect of anti-protein I IgG on the collagenase-catalyzed cleavage of protein I. Purified protein I (1.6 μg) or a synaptic vesicle fraction (50 μg) was first incubated in the absence or presence of anti-protein I IgG (Ab, 49 μg) or of preimmune IgG (Pre, 49 μg) at 0°C for 15 min, and then subjected to proteolysis by collagenase (Col, 50 units/0.1 ml) at 30°C for 30 min in the presence of 2 mM CaCl$_2$ and 4 mM Tris–HCl (pH 7.4), followed by SDS–polyacrylamide gel electrophoresis. The proteins in the gel were stained with Coomassie blue. Col and H indicate the positions of collagenase and the heavy chain of IgG, respectively. (Naito and Ueda, 1981.)

protein I with a different potency than might the calcium-dependent phosphorylation. However, the experimental results shown in Fig. 9 indicate that the anti-protein I IgG is equally potent in its inhibitory action on both types of phosphorylation. This still leaves the two possibilities that the anti-protein I IgG molecule interacts with both the collagenase-resistant and -sensitive regions of protein I, and that the IgG preparation contains a mixture of microheterogeneous IgGs which have similar titer.

In order to determine independently whether the anti-protein I IgG interacts with the collagenase-sensitive region of protein I, its effect on collagenase-catalyzed proteolysis of protein I was examined (Fig. 10). The anti-protein I IgG blocked the proteolytic action of collagenase not only on purified protein I but also on protein I which is bound to the synaptic vesicle. The bacterial collagenase used in this study showed a remarkable substrate specificity;

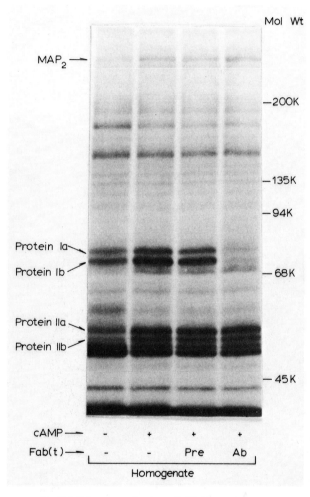

Fig. 11. Effect of the monovalent Fab(t) fragment of anti-protein I IgG on endogenous phosphorylation of proteins in homogenates of rat cerebrum. The Fab(t) fragments of anti-protein I IgG and preimmune IgG were prepared by treating the purified IgGs with trypsin. Crude homogenates of rat cerebrum (25 μg) were subjected to cAMP-dependent phosphorylation in the absence or presence of the Fab(t) fragment (7.4 μg) of anti-protein I IgG or that (8.5 μg) of preimmune IgG, followed by SDS–polyacrylamide gel electrophoresis and autoradiography. (Naito and Ueda, 1981.)

it cleaved only protein I and the arrow-indicated protein among the Coomassie-blue-stained proteins in the synaptic vesicle fraction. The anti-protein I IgG blocked the action of collagenase on protein I but not on the arrow-indicated protein, which further verifies its specific interaction with protein I.

## SPECIFIC INHIBITION OF ENDOGENOUS PHOSPHORYLATION OF PROTEIN I IN THE BRAIN HOMOGENATE BY MONOVALENT Fab FRAGMENT OF ANTI-PROTEIN I IgG

The above finding of the specific inhibitory action of the purified anti-protein I IgG on the phosphorylation of protein I is important because it raises the possibility that the anti-protein I IgG might be used as a powerful tool in the investigation of the physiological function of protein I. However, it would be conceivably difficult, in practice, to use intact IgG as an effective agent in physiological experiments; for instance, it may not be possible to introduce into neurons the intact IgG molecules which have a rather large molecular weight, either by an iontophoretic method or though a carrier such as liposomes, in an effort to observe an effect on synaptic events. Anticipating this difficulty, we have prepared monovalent Fab(t) fragments of both anti-protein I and preimmune IgGs by treating their intact IgGs with trypsin, and examined their effect on endogenous protein phosphorylation in a crude homogenate of cerebrum. The Fab(t) fragments have a much smaller molecular weight (46 000) than the intact molecules of IgG (154 000) (Edelman et al., 1968). As shown in Fig. 11, the Fab(t) fragment derived from anti-protein I IgG, not that from preimmune IgG, specifically inhibited the cAMP-dependent phosphorylation of protein I. The Fab(t) fragment also inhibited calcium-dependent phosphorylation of protein I without affecting the phosphorylation of other proteins (data not shown).

## CONCLUDING REMARKS

We have provided evidence that the affinity-purified anti-protein I IgG, either the intact molecule or its monovalent Fab fragment, inhibits specifically the phosphorylation of protein I without affecting the phosphorylation of other proteins, including those which are substrates for the cAMP-dependent protein kinase or calcium/calmodulin-dependent protein kinases. This indicates that the specific inhibition by the anti-protein I IgG probably has resulted from its blocking action on the phosphorylation sites of protein I rather than from its blocking action on the catalytic sites of the protein kinases. This substrate-directed specific inhibitor of the phosphorylation of protein I may provide a unique probe in the investigation of the precise synaptic function of protein I phosphorylation. In particular, the monovalent Fab(t) fragment which has a substantially lower molecular weight than the intact IgG, and yet is capable of causing the specific inhibition, will be amenable to certain experimentations. For instance, it is feasible to apply the Fab(t) fragment to the soma of identified large neurons in culture by iontophoresis or pressurephoresis, and monitor its electrophysiological effects in the neurons to determine whether protein I phosphorylation in these neurons has any postsynaptic function. To obtain a clue as to the presynaptic function of protein I, one might attempt to fuse synaptosomes with liposomes into which the Fab(t) fragment had been incorporated, and examine whether it has any effects on the neurotransmitter release from or uptake into the synaptosomes. It is also possible to test the Fab(t) fragment directly for an effect on neurotransmitter uptake into isolated synaptic vesicles.

It is not an easy task to identify the precise biological function of covalent modifications, such as phosphorylation, of newly discovered macromolecules, particularly those which are localized in the synaptic region. Correlative approaches are useful at early stages of the game; they often narrow down to certain possibilities and suggest some putative functions. However, evidence provided by these approaches is not adequate to establish a specific cause–effect relationship. Immunobiochemical and genetic approaches are considered to constitute more effective probes in this regard. Successful immunobiochemical approaches provide a tool which achieves the specific blockade of the biochemical reaction involving the macromolecule in question, in contrast to many of the pharmacological agents which often interact with more than one species of macromolecule. Until an appropriate genetic method becomes available, immunobiochemical approaches appear to be the methods best suited for experimentation aimed at determining the biological role of the covalent modification of the macromolecule. We have presented evidence here that we have obtained an immunobiochemical tool hopefully effective in identifying the precise function of the protein I phosphorylation in the synapse. However, it should be pointed out that the anti-protein I IgG used in this study did not distinguish between the cAMP-dependent phosphorylation site and the calcium-dependent phosphorylation sites of protein I. Therefore, successful production of monoclonal antibodies capable of site-specific inhibition is awaited.

## ACKNOWLEDGEMENTS

This work was supported by United States Public Health Service Grant NS 15113. We thank Mary Roth for excellent assistance in the preparation of the manuscript.

## REFERENCES

Bloom, F.E. (1975) The role of cyclic nucleotides in central synaptic function. In *Reviews of Physiology, Biochemistry and Pharmacology,* Springer-Verlag, Berlin, pp. 1–103.

Bloom, F.E., Ueda, T., Battenberg, E. and Greengard, P. (1979) Immunocytochemical localization, in synapses, of protein I, an endogenous substrate for protein kinases in mammalian brain. *Proc. nat. Acad. Sci. (Wash.),* 76: 5982–5986.

Brown, J.H. and Makman, M.H. (1972) Stimulation by dopamine of adenylate cyclase in retinal homogenates and of adenosine-3′,5′-cyclic monophosphate formation in intact retina. *Proc. nat. Acad. Sci. (Wash.),* 69: 539–543.

Butcher, R.W. and Sutherland, E.R. (1962) Adenosine 3′,5′-phosphate in biological materials. I. Purification and properties of cyclic 3′,5′-nucleotide phosphodiesterase and use of this enzyme to characterize adenosine 3′,5′-monophosphate in human urine. *J. biol. Chem.,* 237: 1244–1250.

Clement-Cormier, Y.C., Kebabian, J.W., Petzold, G.L. and Greengard, P. (1974) Dopamine-sensitive adenylate cyclase in mammalian brain: a possible site of action of antipsychotic drugs. *Proc. nat. Acad. Sci. (Wash.),* 71: 1113–1117.

Daly, J.W. (1975) Role of cyclic nucleotides in the nervous system. In *Handbook of Psychopharmacology,* Vol. 5, L.L. Iversen, S.D. Iversen and S.H. Snyder (Eds.), Plenum Press, New York, pp. 47–130.

DeBlas, A.L., Wang, Y.-J., Sorensen, R. and Mahler, H.R. (1979) Protein phosphorylation in synaptic membranes regulated by adenosine 3′:5′-monophosphate: regional and subcellular distribution of the endogenous substrates. *J. Neurochem.,* 33: 647–659.

De Camilli, P., Ueda, T., Bloom, F.E., Battenberg, E. and Greengard, P. (1979) Widespread distribution of protein I in the central and peripheral nervous systems. *Proc. nat. Acad. Sci. (Wash.),* 76: 5977–5981.

De Robertis, E., DeLores Arnaiz, G.R., Alberici, M., Butcher, R.W. and Sutherland, E.W. (1967) Subcellular distribution of adenyl cyclase and cyclic phosphodiesterase in rat brain cortex. *J. biol. Chem.,* 242: 3487–3493.

Dolphin, A.C. and Greengard, P. (1981a) Serotonin stimulates phosphorylation of protein I in the facial motor nucleus of rat brain. *Nature (Lond.)*, 289: 76–79.

Dolphin, A.C. and Greengard, P. (1981b) Neurotransmitter- and neuromodulator-dependent alterations in phosphorylation of protein I in slices of rat facial nucleus. *J. Neurosci.*, 1: 192–203.

Dunkley, P.R., Holmes, H. and Rodnight, R. (1976) Phosphorylation of synaptic-membrane proteins from ox cerebral cortex in vitro. *Biochem. J.*, 661–666.

Edelman, G.M., Gall, W.E., Waxdal, M.J. and Kornigsberg, W.H. (1968) The covalent structure of a human γG-immunoglobulin. I. Isolation and characterization of the whole molecule, the polypeptide chains, and the tryptic fragments. *Biochemistry*, 7: 1950–1958.

Forn, J. and Greengard, P. (1978) Depolarizing agents and cyclic nucleotides regulate the phosphorylation of specific neuronal proteins in rat cerebral cortex slices. *Proc. nat. Acad. Sci. (Wash.)*, 75: 5195–5199.

Glass, D.B. and Krebs, E.G. (1980) Protein phosphorylation catalyzed by cyclic AMP-dependent and cyclic GMP-dependent protein kinases. *Annu. Rev. Pharmacol. Toxicol.*, 20: 363–388.

Goelz, S.E., Nestler, E.J., Chehrazi, B. and Greengard, P. (1981) Distribution of protein I in mammalian brain as determined by a detergent-based radioimmunoassay. *Proc. nat. Acad. Sci. (Wash.)*, 78: 2130–2134.

Greengard, P. (1976) Possible role for cyclic nucleotides and phosphorylated membrane proteins in post-synaptic actions of neurotransmitters. *Nature (Lond.)*, 260: 101–108.

Greengard, P. (1978) *Cyclic Nucleotides, Phosphorylated Proteins and Neuronal Functions*, Raven Press, New York.

Greengard, P. (1981) Intracellular signals in the brain. *Harvey Lectures*, Series 75, Academic Press, New York, pp. 227–331.

Greengard, P., McAfee, D.A. and Kebabian, J.W. (1972) On the mechanism of action of cyclic AMP and its role in synaptic transmission. In *Advances in Cyclic Nucleotide Research*, Vol. 1, Raven Press, New York, pp. 337–355.

Hegstrand, L.R., Kanof, P.D. and Greengard, P. (1976) Histamine-sensitive adenylate cyclase in mammalian brain. *Nature (Lond.)*, 260: 163–165.

Hoffer, B.J., Siggins, G.R. and Bloom, F.E. (1969) Prostaglandins $E_1$ and $E_2$ antagonize norepinephrine effects on cerebellar Purkinje cells: microelectrophoretic study. *Science*, 166: 1418–1420.

Huttner, W.B. and Greengard, P. (1979) Multiple phosphorylation sites in protein I and their differential regulation by cyclic AMP and calcium. *Proc. nat. Acad. Sci. (Wash.)*, 76: 5402–5406.

Huttner, W.B., DeGennaro, L.J. and Greengard, P. (1981) Differential phosphorylation of multiple sites in purified protein I by cyclic AMP-dependent and calcium-dependent protein kinases. *J. biol. Chem.*, 256: 1482–1488.

Iversen, L.L. (1975) A dopamine-sensitive adenylate cyclase models synaptic receptors, illuminating antipsychotic drug action. *Science*, 188: 1084.

Johnson, E.M., Ueda, T., Maeno, H. and Greengard, P. (1972) Adenosine 3',5'-monophosphate-dependent phosphorylation of a specific protein in synaptic membrane fractions from rat cerebrum. *J. biol. Chem.*, 247: 5650–5652.

Kakiuchi, S. and Rall, T. (1968) Studies on adenosin 3',5'-phosphate in rabbit cerebral cortex. *Mol. Pharmacol.*, 4: 379–388.

Karobath, M. and Leitich, H. (1974) Antipsychotic drugs and dopamine-stimulated adenylate cyclase prepared from corpus striatum of rat brain. *Proc. nat. Acad. Sci. (Wash.)*, 71: 2915–2918.

Kebabian, J.W. (1977) Biochemical regulation and physiological significance of cyclic nucleotides in the nervous system. *Adv. cyclic Nucleotide Res.*, 8, pp. 421–508.

Kebabian, J.W., Petzold, G.L. and Greengard, P. (1972) Dopamine-sensitive adenylate cyclase in caudate nucleus of rat brain and its similarity to the "dopamine receptor." *Proc. nat. Acad. Sci. (Wash.)*, 69: 2145–2149.

Kelly, P.T. and Cotman, C.W. (1979) Cyclic AMP-stimulated protein kinases at brain synaptic junctions. *J. biol. Chem.*, 254: 1564–1575.

Kennedy, M.B. and Greengard, P. (1981) Two calcium/calmodulin-dependent protein kinases, which are highly concentrated in brain, phosphorylate protein I at distinct sites. *Proc. nat. Acad. Sci. (Wash.)*, 78: 1293–1297.

Klein, M. and Kandel, E.R. (1978) Presynaptic modulation of voltage-dependent $Ca^{2+}$ current: mechanism for behavioral sensitization in *Aplysia californica*. *Proc. nat. Acad. Sci. (Wash.)*, 75: 3512–3516.

Krebs, E.G. and Beavo, J.A. (1979) Phosphorylation–dephosphorylation of enzymes. *Annu. Rev. Biochem.*, 48: 923–959.

Krueger, B.K., Forn, J. and Greengard, P. (1977) Depolarization-induced phosphorylation of specific proteins, mediated by calcium ion influx, in rat brain synaptosomes. *J. biol. Chem.*, 252: 2764–2773.

Lohmann, S.M., Ueda, T. and Greengard, P. (1978) Ontogeny of synaptic phosphoproteins in brain. *Proc. nat. Acad. Sci. (Wash.)*, 75: 4037–4041.

Lohmann, S.M., Walter, U. and Greengard, P. (1980) Identification of endogenous substrate proteins for cAMP-dependent protein kinase in bovine brain. *J. biol. Chem.*, 255: 9985–9992.

Maeno, H., Johnson, E.M. and Greengard, P. (1971) Subcellular distribution of adenosine 3',5'-monophosphate-dependent protein kinase in rat brain. *J. biol. Chem.*, 246: 134–142.

Miyamoto, E., Kuo, J.F. and Greengard, P. (1969) Cyclic nucleotide-dependent protein kinases. III. Purification and properties of adenosine 3′,5′-monophosphate-dependent protein kinase from bovine brain. *J. biol. Chem.,* 244: 6395–6402.

Naito, S. and Ueda, T. (1981) Affinity-purified anti-protein I antibody. Specific inhibitor of phosphorylation of protein I, a synaptic protein. *J. biol. Chem.,* 256: in press.

Nathanson, J.A. and Greengard, P. (1974) Serotonin-sensitive adenylate cyclase in neural tissue and its similarity to the serotonin receptor: a possible site of action of lysergic acid diethylamide. *Proc. nat. Acad. Sci. (Wash.),* 71: 797–780.

Nestler, E.J. and Greengard, P. (1980) Dopamine and depolarizing agents regulate the state of phosphorylation of protein I in the mammalian superior cervical sympathetic ganglion. *Proc. nat. Acad. Sci. (Wash.)* 77: 7479–7483.

O'Farrell, P.Z., Goodman, H.M. and O'Farrell, P.H. (1977) High resolution two-dimensional electrophoresis of basic as well as acidic proteins. *Cell,* 12: 1133–1142.

Robison, G.A., Butcher, R.W. and Sutherland, E.W. (1971) *Cyclic AMP,* Academic Press, New York.

Routtenberg, A. and Ehrlich, Y.H. (1975) Endogenous phosphorylation of four cerebral cortical membrane proteins: role of cyclic nucleotides ATP and divalent cations. *Brain Res.,* 92: 415–430.

Rubin, C.S. and Rosen, O.M. (1975) Protein phosphorylation. *Annu. Rev. Biochem.,* 44: 831–887.

Schulman, H. and Greengard, P. (1978) Stimulation of brain membrane protein phosphorylation by calcium and endogenous heat-stable protein. *Nature (Lond.),* 271: 478–479.

Shimizu, H., Creveling, C.R. and Daly, J.W. (1970) Effect of membrane depolarization and biogenic amines on the formation of cyclic AMP in incubated brain slices. *Adv. Biochem. Psychopharmacol.,* 3: 135–154.

Sieghart, W., Forn, J., Schwarcz, R., Coyle, J.T. and Greengard, P. (1978) Neuronal localization of specific brain phosphoproteins. *Brain Res.,* 156: 345–350.

Sieghart, W., Forn, J. and Greengard, P. (1979) $Ca^{2+}$ and cyclic AMP regulate phosphorylation of same two membrane-associated proteins specific to nerve tissue. *Proc. nat. Acad. Sci. (Wash.),* 76: 2475–2479.

Siggins, G.R., Hoffer, B.J. and Bloom, F.E. (1969) Cyclic adenosine monophosphate: possible mediator for norepinephrine effects on cerebellar Purkinje cells. *Science,* 165: 1018–1020.

Sloboda, R.D., Rudolph, S.A., Rosenbaum, J.L. and Greengard, P. (1975) Cyclic AMP-dependent endogenous phosphorylation of a microtubule-associated protein. *Proc. nat. Acad. Sci. (Wash.),* 72: 177–181.

Strömbom, U., Forn, J., Dolphin, A.C. and Greengard, P. (1979) Regulation of the state of phosphorylation of specific neuronal proteins in mouse brain by in vivo administration of anesthetic and convulsant agents. *Proc. nat. Acad. Sci. (Wash.),* 76: 4687–4690.

Sutherland, E.W., Rall, T.W. and Menon, T. (1972) Adenylate cyclase. I. Distribution, preparation, and properties. *J. biol. Chem.,* 237: 1220–1227.

Ueda, T. (1981) Attachment of the synapse-specific phosphoprotein protein I to the synaptic membrane: a possible role of the collagenase-sensitive region of protein I. *J. Neurochem.,* 36: 297–300.

Ueda, T. and Greengard, P. (1977) Adenosine 3′:5′-monophosphate-regulated phosphoprotein system of neuronal membranes. I. Solubilization, purification, and some properties of an endogenous phosphoprotein. *J. biol. Chem.,* 252: 5155–5163.

Ueda, T., Maeno, H. and Greengard, P. (1973) Regulation of endogenous phosphorylation of specific proteins in synaptic membrane fractions from rat brain by adenosine 3′:5′-monophosphate. *J. biol. Chem.,* 248: 8295–8305.

Ueda, T., Greengard, P., Berzins, K., Cohen, R.S., Blomberg, F., Grab, D.J. and Siekevitz, P. (1979) Subcellular distribution in cerebral cortex of two proteins phosphorylated by a cAMP-dependent protein kinase. *J. Cell Biol.,* 83: 308–319.

Ueda, T., Stratford, C.A. and Larson, J. (1981) Distribution of protein I, a synapse-specific phosphoprotein, and adenylate cyclase in the rat spinal cord. *J. Neurochem.,* 36: 293–296.

Walsh, D.A., Perkins, J.P. and Krebs, E.G. (1968) An adenosine 3′,5′-monophosphate dependent protein kinase from rabbit skeletal muscle. *J. biol. Chem.,* 243: 3763–3765.

Walter, U., Lohmann, S.M., Sieghart, W. and Greengard, P. (1979) Identification of the cyclic AMP-dependent protein kinase responsible for endogenous phosphorylation of substrate proteins in synaptic membrane fraction from rat brain. *J. biol. Chem.,* 254: 12235–12239.

# Cyclic GMP-Dependent Protein Phosphorylation in Mammalian Cerebellum

DORIS J. SCHLICHTER

*Department of Biochemistry, University of Tennessee,*
*Knoxville, TN 37916, U.S.A.*

## CYCLIC GMP IN MAMMALIAN CEREBELLUM

The distribution and regulation of cyclic nucleotides in the central nervous system has been extensively reviewed (Bloom, 1975; Daly, 1977; Goldberg and Haddox, 1977; Nathanson, 1977; Bartfai, 1978, 1980; Ferrendelli, 1978; Greengard, 1978, 1979). Therefore discussion of this topic will be limited to a very brief summary focusing on cerebellar cyclic GMP (cGMP).

The level of cGMP in cerebellum (5–8 pmoles/mg protein) is 10–20 times that found in other regions of the brain (0.2–0.5 pmole/mg protein) (Daly, 1977). Despite the high concentration of cGMP present in cerebellum, basal soluble guanylate cyclase levels are not markedly higher in this brain region (approximately 0.02 pmole cGMP formed/min/mg protein in cerebellum as compared to 0.035–0.086 in other areas of the brain). The activity of cGMP phosphodiesterase in cerebellum (5 nmoles/min/mg) is, however, quite low compared to the rest of brain (25–40 nmoles/min/mg), suggesting that the non-stimulated level of this nucleotide is determined by the rate of degradation (Bartfai, 1980). Cerebellar cGMP levels are altered by numerous agents which affect neuronal function, particularly those which increase or decrease motor activity (see Ferrendelli, 1978). In cerebellar slices, cellular depolarization, induced by veratridine, ouabain or high $K^+$ levels, produces large elevations (25–30-fold) in cGMP (Ferrendelli et al., 1973; Ferrendelli et al., 1976) which are absolutely dependent upon extracellular $Ca^{2+}$.

It is probable that a large portion of cerebellar cGMP is localized in Purkinje cells, which constitute the sole neuronal output of the cerebellum. Mao et al. (1975) observed that a strain of neurological mutant mice, nervous, which are missing over 90% of cerebellar Purkinje cells, had an 80% loss of cGMP from the cerebellum. Intracerebellar injection of kainic acid, a neurotoxic analogue of gluamic acid, the probable excitatory neurotransmitter released upon Purkinje cells at afferent synapses, produces an initial elevation of cGMP, followed within 72 h by an 80% reduction in the level of this nucleotide (Biggio et al., 1978). Also, activation or inhibition of cerebellar Purkinje cells by drugs or putative neurotransmitters is correlated with an increase or decrease, respectively, in cerebellar cGMP (for review see Ferrendelli, 1978; Costa, 1978).

Thus it seems likely that in one type of neuron, the Purkinje cell, cGMP levels are closely linked to activity of the nerve cell. In various systems, cGMP elevations have been observed in response to the neurotransmitters acetylcholine, histamine and norepinephrine acting at muscarinic, $H_1$- and $\alpha$-adrenergic receptors respectively (Bartfai, 1978). In cat sensorimotor cortex (Swartz and Woody, 1979; Woody et al., 1978) intracellular iontophoresis of cGMP mimics the increase in neuronal resistance produced by extracellularly applied acetylcholine. However, whether cGMP plays a role directly in neuronal function, through the cGMP-dependent phosphorylation of proteins involved in control of membrane permeability as has been hypothesized (Greengard, 1976) or secondarily, perhaps through regulation of calcium levels (Woody, 1977) remains to be established.

## cGMP-DEPENDENT PROTEIN KINASE

Within nerve cells (and all other cell types) the mediator of the effects of cGMP is presumed to be the enzyme cGMP-dependent protein kinase (cGK) (Kuo and Greengard, 1969; Greengard, 1978). This enzyme, which appears to be the principal cGMP-binding protein in mammalian tissues, has recently been the subject of two thoughtful and comprehensive reviews (Gill and McCune, 1979; Glass and Krebs, 1980). Early reports on cGK suggested that upon binding cGMP the enzyme dissociated, releasing an active catalytic subunit (Van Leemput-Coutrez et al., 1973; Miyamoto et al., 1973; Kuo et al., 1974; Shoji et al., 1977) analogous to activation of the cyclic AMP-dependent protein kinases (cAK) (Walsh and Ashby, 1973; Rubin and Rosen, 1975; Nimmo and Cohen, 1977). However, the enzyme, purified to apparent homogeneity from bovine lung (Gill et al., 1976; Lincoln et al., 1977) and heart (Flockerzi et al., 1978), has been shown to be a dimer of identical subunits of molecular weight 74 000–81 000 (Lincoln et al., 1977; Gill et al., 1977) each of which possesses phosphotransferase and cyclic nucleotide-binding activity (Gill et al., 1976; Lincoln et al., 1978). The subunits are apparently linked by disulfide bridges (Gill et al., 1977; Rochette-Egly and Castagna, 1978) and activation of the enzyme occurs without dissociation (Gill et al., 1976; Takai et al., 1976). Limited proteolysis of cGK produces a fragment of the enzyme which is catalytically active in the absence of cGMP (Lincoln et al., 1978; Inoue et al., 1976) possibly explaining the apparent dissociation observed in early, partially purified preparations of the enzyme.

Amino acid analysis of cGK and the type II cAK indicates that significant sequence homology exists between the enzymes (Lincoln and Corbin, 1977) and the two types of kinase are similar in many physical properties (see Gill and McCune, 1979). It has been proposed that these enzymes are homologous proteins (Lincoln and Corbin, 1977; Gill et al., 1977), but many differences, in addition to specificity of cyclic nucleotide binding and mechanism of activation, exist between the cGMP-dependent and cAMP-dependent protein kinases. Both cGK (De Jonge and Rosen, 1977) and type II cAK (Erlichman et al., 1974; Rangel-Aldoa and Rosen, 1976b) demonstrate autophosphorylation. However, phosphorylation of the regulatory subunit of type II cAK by the catalytic subunit slows reassociation of the subunits, encouraging the net dissociation of the enzyme (Rangel-Aldoa and Rosen, 1976a). Autophosphorylation of cGK, which is inhibited by cGMP and stimulated by cAMP and histone (Lincoln et al., 1978; De Jonge and Rosen, 1977) has no apparent effect upon activity of the enzyme. The monomeric regulatory subunit of cAK apparently has two cAMP-binding sites (Corbin et al., 1978; Corbin and Lincoln, 1978) and, in the type II regulatory subunit, these sites are independent (Buss et al., 1979). (The cyclic nucleotide binding sites of the type I cAK holoenzyme may possess some positive cooperativity (Hoppe et al., 1978). cGMP-dependent protein kinase binds only one cGMP per monomer and the binding sites are positively cooperative (Buss et al., 1979; McCune and Gill, 1979). The two types of enzyme also appear to be immunologically distinct. Antibodies prepared by Walter et al. (1980) against cGK from bovine lung did not cross-react with type I or type II cAK or with catalytic subunit, nor did antisera against the type I or type II regulatory subunit show any detectable cross-reactivity with cGK.

*Quantitation of cGMP-dependent protein kinase*

Detection and accurate quantitation of cGK has presented numerous problems (see Gill and McCune, 1979) since in most tissues cAK is present in far higher concentrations (Casnellie et al., 1978). Recently a more specific assay technique, utilizing the rapid partial purification by anion exchange chromatography of cGK present in small tissue samples, has been developed (Bandle and Guidotti, 1980). Photoaffinity labeling of cyclic nucleotide-dependent protein kinases with 8-azido derivatives of cyclic nucleotides has also been successfully employed. The photoaffinity label 8-azidoadenosine 3′, 5′-monophosphate (8-$N_3$-cAMP) has been used to great advantage in studies on the distribution and properties of the cAMP-dependent protein kinases (Walter et al., 1977a,b; 1978). Specific photoactivated labeling of cGK with 8-azido-guanosine 3′,5′-monophosphate has been reported (Geahlen et al., 1979). However, the lability and poor synthetic yield of 8-azidoguanosine 3′,5′-monophosphate preclude its routine use. In view of the observation that 8-azidoinosine 3′,5′-monophosphate (8-$N_3$-cIMP) activates cGK with an apparent activation constant of $5 \times 10^{-6}$ M (Miller et al., 1973), this compound was investigated as a possible photoaffinity label for the enzyme (Casnellie et al., 1978).

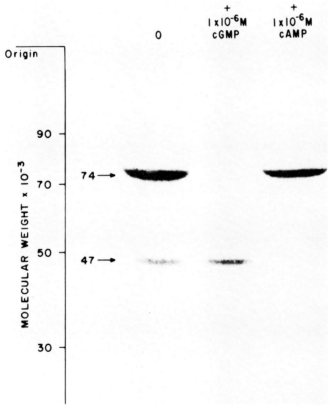

Fig. 1. Autoradiograph showing the photoactivated incorporation of 8-$N_3$-[$^{32}$P]cIMP into protein bands of partially purified cGK of bovine lung. Photoaffinity labeling was carried out under standard conditions and the proteins were separated by SDS–polyacrylamide gel electrophoresis. (From Casnellie et al., 1978. Reproduced by permission.)

In partially purified preparations of cGK from bovine lung, subjected to photoaffinity labeling with 8-N$_3$-[$^{32}$P]cIMP and then to SDS–polyacrylamide gel electrophoresis, the photoaffinity ligand was covalently incorporated into only two proteins of molecular weights 74 000 and 47 000 (Fig. 1). Incorporation of 8-N$_3$-[$^{32}$P]cIMP into the 74 000 dalton protein was completely abolished by the addition of 1 $\mu$M cGMP to the photoaffinity-labeling mixture. This inhibition by cGMP of the photoactivated incorporation of 8-N$_3$-[$^{32}$P]cIMP, together with the molecular weight of the labeled protein, strongly suggested that the labeled species was the monomer of cGK. In further experiments, the 74 000 dalton protein was demonstrated to co-purify with cGK activity and with the major peak of cGMP-binding activity from bovine lung. Half-maximal incorporation of 8-N$_3$-[$^{32}$P]cIMP into the 74 000 dalton monomer of cGK was observed at a concentration of 1.9 $\mu$M, in good agreement with the concentrations determined for activation of the enzyme and inhibition of [$^3$H]cGMP binding (Table I).

TABLE I

COMPARISON OF THE AFFINITY CONSTANTS OF 8-N$_3$-cIMP FOR cGMP-DEPENDENT PROTEIN KINASE*

| | |
|---|---|
| Kinase activation | $1.0 \times 10^{-6}$ M |
| Inhibition constant | $2.5 \times 10^{-6}$ M |
| Covalent incorporation | $1.9 \times 10^{-6}$ M |

* Data from Casnellie et al., 1978.

The 47 000 dalton protein labeled by photoactivated incorporation of 8-N$_3$-[$^{32}$P]-cIMP in partially purified preparations of cGK from bovine lung was determined to be the regulatory subunit of type I cAK. The inclusion of 1 $\mu$M cAMP in the photoaffinity-labeling mixture completely eliminated the incorporation of 8-N$_3$-[$^{32}$P]cIMP into this protein (Fig. 1). Type I cAK binds and is activated by cIMP (Walter et al., 1977a) and was present as a contaminant in the enzyme preparation. Although 8-N$_3$-[$^{32}$P]cIMP also labels cAMP-binding proteins in crude tissue extracts, this property does not limit the usefulness of the radioactive derivative for studying cGMP-binding proteins. By SDS–polyacrylamide gel electrophoresis, the 74 000 monomer of cGK can easily be separated from other proteins. The use of 8-N$_3$-[$^{32}$P]cIMP for quantitation of cGK is not as straightforward as the use of 8-N$_3$-[$^{32}$P]cAMP in quantitation of cAMP-binding proteins. Unlike the labeling of the cAMP-dependent protein kinases by 8-N$_3$-cAMP (Walter et al., 1977a), 8-N$_3$-cIMP is not incorporated into cGMP-binding proteins with 100% efficiency. However, in a study discussed in the next section (Schlichter et al., 1980), in which the efficiency of the photoactivated incorporation of 8-N$_3$-[$^{32}$P]cIMP into cGK was determined, it was possible to use this photoaffinity label to measure the absolute concentration of cGMP-binding proteins in crude tissue extracts.

*Localization of cGMP-dependent protein kinase in the central nervous system*

Early reports on cGK indicated that this enzyme was highly concentrated in mammalian cerebellum (Hofmann and Sold, 1972; Takai et al., 1975) and lung (Nakazawa and Sano, 1975). In a survey of rat tissues cGMP-binding and cGK activity were found to be highest in lung, cerebellum and heart (Lincoln et al., 1976). The distribution of cGK within mammalian brain has been examined by use of 8-N$_3$-[$^{32}$P]cIMP (Schlichter et al., 1980). For this study it was necessary to determine the efficiency of the photoactivated incorporation of 8-N$_3$-[$^{32}$P]cIMP into cGK (see the proceeding section). This was accomplished by measuring the incorporation of 8-N$_3$-[$^{32}$P]cIMP, under standard conditions, into apparently homogeneously

TABLE II

CONCENTRATION OF cGMP-DEPENDENT PROTEIN KINASE HO-
LOENZYME IN CYTOSOL OF VARIOUS BRAIN REGIONS OF THE CAT*

| Brain region | cGMP-dependent protein kinase (pmole/mg protein) |
|---|---|
| Cerebellar nuclei | 1,73 |
| Cerebellar vermis (cortex) | 1.20 |
| Cerebellar hemisphere (cortex) | 0.90 |
| Choroid plexus | 0.34 |
| Medulla | 0.11 |
| Temporal cortex | 0.08 |
| Hippocampus | 0.05 |
| Tectum | 0.04 |

\* Data from Schlichter et al., 1980.

pure, highly active cGK purified from bovine lung (specific activity, assayed according to Flockerzi et al. (1978) with histone H2b as a substrate, 3.2 $\mu$moles $^{32}$P transferred per min per mg protein). Under the conditions used, the incorporation of 8-N$_3$-[$^{32}$P]cIMP into the purified enzyme was $0.18 \pm 0.04$ mole per mole holoenzyme (145 000 dalton dimer). This efficiency of labeling of cGK was not altered by the addition of brain cytosol protein to the photoaffinity-labeling mixture, therefore absolute values for cGK in various brain regions were calculated by assuming the same efficiency of incorporation of 8-N$_3$-[$^{32}$P]cIMP into the enzyme present in crude tissue extracts. Using this technique, cerebellum was found to contain far more cGK than any other brain region examined (Table II). Regions of cat brain which contained low but significant amounts of cGK (0.02–0.04 pmole/mg protein) were: frontal cortex, occipital cortex, corpus callosum, basal ganglia, thalamus, hypothalamus, olfactory bulb, pons and pituitary. Assay of cGK concentration in various areas of rat brain by RIA (Lohmann et al., 1981) confirmed that the level in cerebellum (1.63 pmoles/mg protein) far exceeded that found in other brain regions. Small amounts of cGK were also found throughout the brain with this technique.

Within mammalian cerebellum it is probable that a substantial portion of the cGK present is localized in Purkinje cells. In nervous mutant mice, in which over 90% of cerebellar Purkinje cells are missing, cGK activity was reduced to 37%, and [$^3$H]-cGMP-binding activity to 33%, of levels found in control animals (Bandle and Guidotti, 1978). Developmental studies in rat (Bandle and Guidotti, 1979) revealed that cGK in the cerebellum, very low at birth, begins to increase at day 10 after birth and reaches adult levels at day 25; this period coincides with the formation of the Purkinje cell dendritic tree and the establishment of synapses between Purkinje cells and their major afferent inputs (Berry and Bradley, 1976; Shimono et al., 1976).

The localization of cGK within the cerebellum was also investigated by use of 8-N$_3$-[$^{32}$P]cIMP (Schlichter et al., 1980). Several strains of mutant mice possessing discrete cerebellar deficiencies were employed. Two of the strains of mutant mice, Purkinje cell degeneration (PCD; pcd/pcd) and nervous (nr/nr) lose more than 90% of cerebellar Purkinje cells with no significant loss of other cell types (Landis, 1973; Landis and Mullen, 1978). In weaver (wv/wv) mutants essentially all cerebellar granule cells are lost, again with no significant loss of other cell types (Rakic and Sidman, 1973a,b; Roffler-Tarlov and Sidman, 1978). The staggerer (sg/sg) mutation results in a loss of virtually all cerebellar granule cells

110

(Landis and Sidman, 1978) and a large deficit of Purkinje cells (Herrup and Mullen, 1979). Nervous, PCD and staggerer are autosomal recessive mutations; heterozygous animals are phenotypically normal. Heterozygous weaver mice lose a small fraction of cerebellar granule cells (Roffler-Tarlov and Sidman, 1978). In each case heterozygous and homozygous wild-type animals (refered to as +/?) of the appropriate strain were used as controls.

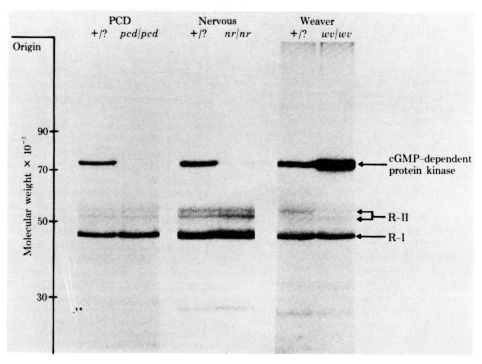

Fig. 2. Autoradiograph showing the photoactivated incorporation of 8-N$_3$-[$^{32}$P]cIMP into cytosol proteins of individual cerebella from various types of neurological mutant mice. Photoaffinity labeling was carried out under standard conditions and the proteins were separated by SDS–polyacrylamide gel electrophoresis. (From Schlichter et al., 1980. Reproduced by permission.)

The $150\,000 \times g$ supernatant fraction (cytosol) from individual cerebella of mutant or control mice was subjected to photoaffinity labeling with 8-N$_3$-[$^{32}$P]cIMP and SDS–polyacrylamide gel electrophoresis. The labeling of cytosol from cerebella of mice lacking Purkinje cells (PCD and nervous) demonstrated large reductions in the level of cGK (Fig. 2) suggesting that Purkinje cells are indeed highly enriched in this enzyme. Homozygous recessive PCD mice (pcd/pcd), in which Purkinje cells are almost completely absent, had a 96% reduction in cerebellar cGK as compared to normal (+/?) animals. This reduction was seen both when the data were expressed on the basis of enzyme per mg protein (Table III) and on the basis of enzyme per total cerebellum (Table IV). Type I cAK, which was also labeled by 8-N$_3$-[$^{32}$P]cIMP, was not reduced in pcd/pcd animals. (The loss of type I cAK per total cerebellum in the pcd/pcd animals was due to the reduction in mass of the cerebellum found in mutant animals.) Homozygous recessive nervous mutants (nr/nr), which lose 90% of their cerebellar Purkinje cells, had an 85% reduction in the concentration of cGK as compared to normal animals (Tables III and IV). A greater than 70% reduction in the amount of cGK in the cerebellum, and a small decrease in the amount of type I cAK was also found in the staggerer

TABLE III

LEVELS OF cGMP-DEPENDENT PROTEIN KINASE HOLOENZYME AND OF TYPE I cAMP-DEPENDENT PROTEIN KINASE HOLOENZYME IN CEREBELLAR CYTOSOL OF VARIOUS NEUROLOGICAL MUTANT MICE*

| Mutation | Genotype | Protein kinase (pmole/mg protein) | |
|---|---|---|---|
| | | cGMP-dependent | Type I cAMP-dependent |
| PCD | +/? | $0.60 \pm 0.08$ | $0.48 \pm 0.03$ |
| | pcd/pcd | $0.02 \pm 0.01$ | $0.49 \pm 0.07$ |
| Nervous | +/? | $0.55 \pm 0.01$ | $0.70 \pm 0.14$ |
| | nr/nr | $0.08 \pm 0.01$ | $0.97 \pm 0.06$ |
| Weaver | +/? | $0.48 \pm 0.13$ | $0.42 \pm 0.03$ |
| | wv/wv | $1.30 \pm 0.41$ | $0.30 \pm 0.10$ |

* Data from Schlichter et al., 1980. Photoaffinity labeling was carried out under standard conditions and the absolute amount of 8-$N_3$-[$^{32}$P]cIMP incorporated was corrected for the efficiency of incorporation as described. Data represent the mean $\pm$ S.D. for 4–6 samples of each genotype.

TABLE IV

LEVELS OF cGK HOLOENZYME AND TYPE I cAK HOLOENZYME PER CEREBELLUM IN VARIOUS NEUROLOGICAL MUTANT MICE*

| Mutation | Genotype | Cerebellar wt, % of control | Protein kinase (pmole/cerebellum) | |
|---|---|---|---|---|
| | | | cGMP-dependent | Type I cAMP-dependent |
| PCD | +/? | 100 | $0.64 \pm 0.11$ | $0.51 \pm 0.13$ |
| | pcd/pcd | 52 | $0.01 \pm 0.01$ | $0.26 \pm 0.07$ |
| Nervous | +/? | 100 | $0.45 \pm 0.05$ | $0.56 \pm 0.05$ |
| | nr/nr | 67 | $0.04 \pm 0.01$ | $0.44 \pm 0.03$ |
| Weaver | +/? | 100 | $0.34 \pm 0.10$ | $0.38 \pm 0.04$ |
| | wv/wv | 37 | $0.43 \pm 0.08$ | $0.08 \pm 0.02$ |

* Data from Schlichter et al., 1980. Photoaffinity labeling was carried out under standard conditions and the absolute amount of 8-$N_3$-[$^{32}$P]cIMP incorporated was corrected for the efficiency of incorporation. Data represent the mean $\pm$ S.D. for 4–6 samples of each genotype.

mutant which loses virtually all of its granule cells but also has a substantial (60–90 %) reduction in the number of cerebellar Purkinje cells.

Homozygous weaver animals, which lose virtually all cerebellar granule cells, demonstrated a more than 2-fold increase in cerebellar cGK (Fig. 2, Tables III and IV). Since granule cells make up a large portion of the cerebellar mass, the cerebellum in these animals is greatly reduced in weight. This loss of granule cells creates a relative enrichment in Purkinje and other cells in the remaining tissue and a concomitant increase in the concentration of cGK. A similar increase in cGK was observed in cerebella from rats in which complete elimination of cerebellar granule cells was achieved by postnatal X-irradiation (Altman and Anderson, 1972). The amount of cGK per total cerebellum was not significantly different for wv/wv and

112

control (+ / ?) animals (Tables III and IV). No difference in cGK concentration would be expected if the enzyme is located in a cell type other than granule cells.

Recent immunocytochemical studies (Lohmann et al., 1981) using antibodies to cGK support the conclusion that the enzyme is highly concentrated in Purkinje cells of the cerebellum. Immunoreactivity was observed on Purkinje cell parikarya in the Purkinje cell layer of the cerebellum (Fig. 3) and upon both Purkinje cell dentrites in the molecular layer and axons passing through the granule cell layer. Staining was observed throughout the cytoplasm of the Purkinje cell but was not present on the nucleus.

No other neuronal element was found to be immunoreactive in either cerebellum or brain. However, smooth muscle cells of the cerebral vasculature were lightly stained. This is consistent with the high level of cGK usually found in smooth muscle (Casnellie et al., 1978). Assay by photoaffinity label of microvessels prepared from whole rabbit brain demonstrated a cGK concentration of 0.16 pmole/mg protein (Schlichter et al., 1980). It is possible, therefore, that a portion of the low level of cGK found in brain regions other than cerebellum is derived from smooth muscle of blood vessels.

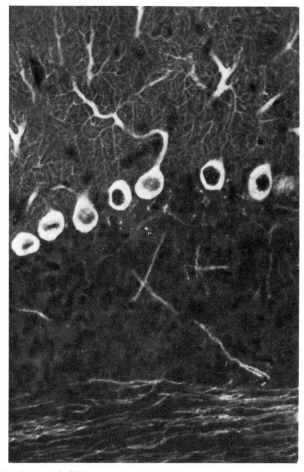

Fig. 3. Fluorescent localization of cGK immunoreactivity in the rat cerebellum. Immunoreactive material appears white. Bright immunoreactivity is visible throughout the Purkinje cells with the exception of the nuclei. (From Lohmann et al., 1981. Reproduced by permission.)

The characterization of cGK has progressed far faster than our knowledge about other elements of the cGMP-dependent protein phosphorylation system. Identification of endogenous substrates for cGK has proven particularly difficult. For this reason, most studies on cGK have relied on histone as a phosphate acceptor. cGMP-dependent protein kinase catalyzes the in vitro transfer of phosphate from ATP to histone fractions H1, H2A, and H2B (Yamamoto et al., 1977; Hashimoto et al., 1976; Flockerzi et al., 1978), however the interaction between histone and cGK may be atypical as unphysiologically high $Mg^{2+}$ concentrations are required for optimal activity with this substrate (Flockerzi et al., 1978). The $K_m$ of cGK for histone H2B (1.5 $\mu$M) is 3.5 times lower than that of cAK for this protein (5.3 $\mu$M) (Glass and Krebs, 1979). Both cGK and cAK catalyze the phosphorylation of two sites on histone H2B, Ser-32 and Ser-36, however phosphorylation of Ser-32 is more rapid with cGK and of Ser-36 with cAK (Hashimoto et al., 1976; Yamamoto et al., 1977). The preference of cGK for Ser-32 is apparently based on $K_m$ since, with synthetic peptides corresponding to the phosphorylation sites of histone H2B, the $V_{max}$ observed for Ser-36 was actually higher than that for Ser-32 (Glass and Krebs, 1979). The optimal primary sequence for cAK (X-Y-Ser where X corresponds to one or two basic residues (Kemp et al., 1975, 1976; Daile et al., 1975)) is also that preferred by cGK (Lincoln and Corbin, 1977) however it is probable that additional substrate specificity determinants exist for cGK.

*Phosphorylation of cAMP-dependent protein kinase substrates by cGMP-dependent protein kinase*

As numerous probable in vivo substrates for cAK have been identified, many investigations have focused on the efficacy of cGK in utilizing these cAK substrates (for review see Glass and Krebs, 1980; Krebs and Beavo, 1979). Phosphorylase *b* kinase (Lincoln and Corbin, 1977, 1978b; Khoo et al., 1977; Khoo and Gill, 1979), cardiac troponin I (Blumenthal et al., 1978; Lincoln and Corbin, 1978a), hormone sensitive lipase (Khoo et al., 1977), glycogen synthetase, pyruvate kinase, fructose-1,6-biphosphatase (Lincoln and Corbin, 1977, 1978b) and possibly cholesterol ester hydrolase (Khoo et al., 1977) can be phosphorylated by cGK, however in each case far higher amounts of cGK than of cAK were required. With cardiac troponin I the two types of kinase showed almost equal $K_m$ values, but the $V_{max}$ observed with cAK was over 10 times that with cGK (Lincoln and Corbin, 1978a). With the exception of cardiac troponin I, which was not found to be phosphorylated in vivo by cGK (England, 1977), it is unknown to what extent these proteins may serve as physiologically significant substrates for cGK.

*Specific substrates for cGMP-dependent protein kinase*

A few proteins have been identified which are phosphorylated in response to low concentrations of cGMP and are presumably specific cGK substrates. Casnellie and Greengard (1974) reported the cGMP-dependent incorporation of [$^{32}$P]phosphate into two proteins of molecular weight 130 000 and 100 000 in membrane fractions of small intestine, ductus deferens and uterus. A similar cGMP-dependent phosphorylation of proteins present in guinea pig vas deferens has also been described (Wallach et al., 1978). Membranes prepared from brush border of rat intestinal epithelium contain an 86 000 dalton protein which is phosphorylated in response to cGMP (De Jonge, 1976). Shaltz et al. (1978) also observed cGMP-stimulated phosphate incorporation into proteins in microvillus membranes from intestinal epithelium. In horse peripheral blood lymphocytes the phosphorylation of nuclear acidic proteins is ap-

114

parently increased in response to cGMP and cholinergic agents (Johnson and Hadden, 1975). Recently Geahlen and Krebs (1980) demonstrated that the regulatory subunit of type I cAK (which unlike the type II regulatory subunit, is not phosphorylated by the cAK catalytic subunit) can serve as a substrate for cGK ($K_m = 2.2 \; \mu$M). Interestingly, in this case only the type I regulatory subunit bearing bound cAMP was a substrate for the cGK catalyzed phosphotransferase reaction; in the absence of bound cyclic nucleotide the regulatory subunit functioned as a competitive inhibitor of cGK.

Eukaryotic ribosomal proteins, which are known to be phosphorylated in vitro by cAK and by cyclic-nucleotide-independent protein kinases (Wool, 1979) are also subject to phosphorylation by cGK (Chihara-Nakashima et al., 1977). Issinger et al (1980) compared the in vitro phosphorylation of eukaryotic ribosomal subunits catalyzed by cAK and cGK. Incubation of ribosomal subunits with $[\gamma\text{-}^{32}\text{P}]$ATP and catalytic subunit of cAK resulted in the incorporation of approximately 1.0 mole of $[^{32}\text{P}]$phosphate per mole of S6 and 0.1–0.2 mole of $[^{32}\text{P}]$phosphate per mole of several other proteins in both the large and small subunit. cGMP-dependent protein kinase catalyzed the incorporation of phosphate into these same proteins, but at a much lower efficiency. One protein, however, S2, was phosphorylated 4 times faster by cGK than by cAK. In vivo, only S6 has been shown to be phosphorylated and this phosphorylation has no apparent functional effect (Wool, 1979).

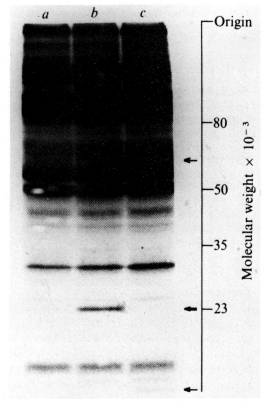

Fig. 4. Autoradiogram of endogenous protein phosphorylation in cerebellar cytosol. cGMP, but not cAMP, stimulated the phosphorylation of a protein with an apparent molecular weight of 23 000 as indicated by the heavy arrow. cAMP stimulated phosphate incorporation into several proteins of lower and higher molecular weight (light arrows). a, control; b, $+ 1 \times 10^{-6}$ M cGMP; c, $+ 1 \times 10^{-6}$ M cAMP. (From Schlichter et al., 1978. Reproduced by permission.)

In neuronal tissue the cGMP-dependent phosphorylation of only a few proteins has been reported. cGMP stimulates the incorporation of phosphate into several proteins in synaptic membranes of human putamen and frontal cortex (Boehme et al, 1978); the major phosphorylated species had a molecular weight of 60 000. Membranes of nerve roots from *Aplysia* contain two proteins, molecular weight 68 000 and 62 000, which show increased phosphorylation in response to low concentrations of cGMP (Ram and Erlich, 1978). In mammalian cerebellum, which has high concentrations of cGMP (Daly, 1977) and cGK (Lohmann et al., 1981; Schlichter et al., 1980), a 23 000 dalton soluble substrate for cGK has been identified (Schlichter et al., 1978). The addition of 1 $\mu$M cGMP and [$\gamma$-$^{32}$P]ATP to the 100 000 × $g$ supernatant fraction from rabbit cerebellum resulted in the phosphorylation of this 23 000 dalton protein (Fig. 4). The phosphorylation was rapid, reaching half-maximal in approximately 15 sec. An equal concentration of cAMP failed to stimulate the incorporation of [$^{32}$P]phosphate into this protein.

*Characterization of the cerebellar cGMP-dependent protein kinase substrate*

The 23 000 dalton cerebellar substrate for cGK (termed G substrate) has recently been purified 8 000-fold to apparent homogeneity from rabbit cerebellum and the physical properties of the protein examined (Aswad and Greengard, 1981a). cGMP-dependent protein kinase catalyzes the incorporation of two phosphates into this protein, both on threonine residues. The amino acid sequences of the two phosphorylation sites have been determined (Aitken et al., 1981). Purified $^{32}$P-labeled G substrate demonstrated three spots on isoelectric focusing with isoelectric points of 5.2, 5.3 and 5.6 (Fig. 5). All three forms resolved by isoelectric focusing

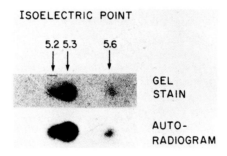

Fig. 5. Isoelectric focusing pattern of purified G substrate. (From Aswad and Greengard, 1981a. Reproduced by permission.)

contained [$^{32}$P]phosphate. The multiple isoelectric forms did not appear to be due to differing levels of phosphorylation as the nonphosphorylated protein also exhibited three isoelectric forms (pI. 5.6, 5.8 and 6.0) and treatment with beef heart phosphoprotein phosphatase did not change the isoelectric focusing pattern. G substrate is heat stable, high in charged amino acids and apparently possesses little ordered structure. The properties of this cerebellar protein are summarized in Table V.

The cellular function of G substrate is not known, however the physical properties of this protein (low molecular weight, heat stability, lack of ordered structure) are shared by several proteins which have been shown to function as modulators of the activity of various kinases and phosphatases: calmodulin (Cheung, 1980; Means and Dedman, 1980), cAMP-dependent protein kinase inhibitor (Walsh et al., 1971; Demaille et al., 1977) and phosphatase inhibitor-I (Huang and Glinsmann, 1976; Nimmo and Cohen, 1978a). The ressemblance to phosphatase

TABLE V

SUMMARY OF PHYSICAL PROPERTIES OF G SUBSTRATE*

| Property | Method of determination | Value |
|---|---|---|
| | SDS/polyacrylamide gel electrophoresis | 23 000 |
| | Amino acid composition | 23 500 |
| | Strokes radius and sedimentation coefficient | 21 700 |
| Isoelectric point | Two-dimensional gel electrophoresis | |
| | Phospho form | 5.2, 5.3, 5.6 |
| | Dephospho form | 5.6, 5.8, 6.0 |
| Stokes radius | Gel filtration | 31 A |
| Sedimentation coefficient ($s_{20,w}$) | Sucrose gradient | 1.7S |
| Frictional ratio ($f/f_0$) | Stokes radius and sedimentation coefficient | 1.7 |

* From Aswad and Greengard, 1981a. Reproduced by permission.

inhibitor-I, a small molecular weight inhibitor of phosphorylase phosphatase (Nimmo and Cohen, 1978b) is particularly strong. Both proteins are heat and acid stable, have little or no tertiary structure and demonstrate multiple isoelectric forms. Phosphatase inhibitor-I is phosphorylated by cAK on a single threonine residue; the amino acid sequence of this phosphorylation site is very similar to the sequence of the two phosphorylation sites on G substrate (Aitken et al., 1981). Preliminary experiments with G substrate suggest that this protein may have some activity as a phosphatase inhibitor (Aswad and Greengard, 1981a).

The kinetics of the phosphorylation of G substrate by cGK and cAK have also been examined by Aswad and Greengard (1981b). Both cGK and cAK catalyzed the incorporation of approximately 2 moles of [$^{32}$P]phosphate per mole of G substrate. Phosphorylation by a combination of both enzymes resulted in the corporation of 2.4 moles [$^{32}$P]phosphate per mole G substrate, suggesting that the enzymes phosphorylate essentially the same two sites. Analysis of the protein maximally phosphorylated by cAK revealed small amounts of

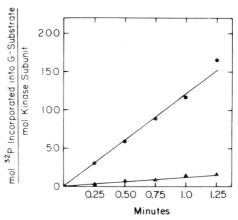

Fig. 6. Initial rate kinetics for phosphorylation of G substrate. Phosphorylation assays were carried out with 0.5 $\mu$M G substrate, 100 $\mu$M [$\gamma$-$^{32}$P]ATP and either 0.025 $\mu$g/ml of cGK plus 1 $\mu$M cGMP (●———●) or 0.025 g/ml of cAK catalytic subunit (▲———▲) for the times indicated. The rates have been normalized to equal concentrations of catalytic subunits. (From Aswad and Greengard, 1981b. Reproduced by permission.)

[$^{32}$P]phosphoserine. As no phosphoserine was observed when phosphorylation of the protein was carried out with cGK (Aswad and Greengard, 1981a), it was concluded that some other sites may be slowly phosphorylated by high levels of cAK. Both phosphorylation sites are utilized at equal rates by cGK while with cAK the phosphorylation of site 1 proceeds 4 times faster than that of site 2 (Aitken et al., 1981).

Initial rate kinetics forphos phorylation of G substrate indicated that the protein was phosphorylated approximately 9 times faster by cGK than by cAK (Fig. 6). The preferential phosphorylation of G substrate by cGK was apparently due to the difference in $K_m$ demonstrated by the two enzymes for this protein (0.21 $\mu$M for cGK and 5.8 $\mu$M for cAK) as very little difference in $V_{max}$ was observed (2.2 $\mu$moles/min/mg for cGK and 1.9 $\mu$moles/min/mg for cAK). A similar, though less marked, $K_m$ difference has been reported for the two enzymes with histone H2B (Glass and Krebs, 1979).

An interesting finding in early reports on cGK was the high $Mg^{2+}$ concentration (50–100 mM) required for maximal activity of the enzyme (Gill et al., 1976; Lincoln et al., 1977; Takai et al., 1975, 1976; Nakazawa and Sano, 1975; Kuo et al., 1976; Nishiyama et al., 1975). This unphysiologically high $Mg^{2+}$ requirement was apparently due to the use of histone as a substrate and not an inherent property of the enzyme (Flockerzi et al., 1978). Khoo and Gill (1979) demonstrated that the $Mg^{2+}$ concentration required with non-histone substrates was 2–5 mM. Using a synthetic peptide corresponding to the prefered cGK phosphorylation site on histone H2B Glass and Krebs (1979) found that the $Mg^{2+}$ concentration necessary for maximal cGK phosphotransferase activity was 1–3 mM. The optimal $Mg^{2+}$ concentration for phosphorylation of G substrate by cGK was approximately 1 mM (Fig. 7). At this $Mg^{2+}$ concentration, the activity of cGK was stimulated approximately 20-fold by cGMP.

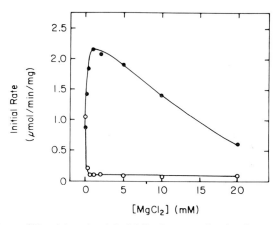

Fig. 7. Effect of MgCl$_2$ on cGK activity using 1.0 $\mu$M G substrate as the phosphate acceptor. Initial rates were measured. Assays were carried out in the presence (●———●) and absence (○———○) of 1 $\mu$M cGMP. (From Aswad and Greengard, 1981b. Reproduced by permission.)

*Cellular localization of the cerebellar cGMP-dependent protein kinase substrate*

G substrate was first identified in rabbit cerebellar cytosol (Schlichter et al., 1978). Since cGK in mouse cerebellum appeared to be highly concentrated in Purkinje cells (Schlichter et al., 1980) it was of interest to determine if G substrate showed a similar distribution. Mouse cerebellum contains a similar 23 000 dalton cGK substrate, although the level in mouse is only 10–20 % of that in rabbit. Therefore, it was possible to examine the level of this substrate in

118

various strains of mutant mice missing specific cerebellar cell types (Schlichter et al., 1980). Cerebellar cytosol from mutant mice (pcd/pcd and wv/wv) and age-matched control mice (+/?) was subjected to phosphorylation and the phosphorylated proteins separated by SDS–polyacrylamide gel electrophoresis and visualized by autoradiography. Substrate levels were then measured by scanning the autoradiograms with a densitometer.

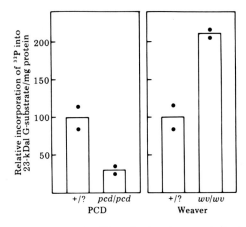

Fig. 8. Level of the 23 000 dalton G substrate in PCD (pcd/pcd) and weaver (wv/wv) cerebellar mutants. Each bar represents the average of two samples, with two cerebella pooled per sample. ●, actual values for the pooled cerebella. The mean value of the controls (+/?) for each strain of mice was arbitrarily set at 100 units. (From Schlichter et al., 1980. Reproduced by permission.)

The apparent amount of the 23 000 dalton G substrate in PCD mutants, which have lost greater than 90% of cerebellar Purkinje cells, was found to be 70% lower than that in age-matched control mice (Fig. 8), suggesting that Purkinje cells are highly enriched in this substrate. In the homozygous recessive weaver mutants, in which granule cells are essentially absent, the level of the 23 000 dalton G substrate was 2-fold higher than that in the control mice. This 2-fold increase in the 23 000 dalton G substrate in the weaver mutant was similar to the increase in cGK observed in this mutant and was presumably due to the relative enrichment in other cell types resulting from the loss of granule cells. Changes in the level of the 23 000 dalton G substrate qualitatively paralleled changes in the concentration of cGK in both PCD and weaver mice. The reduction in the apparent amount of G substrate in the PCD mutant mice was `substantial, but less than the reduction observed in the concentration of the enzyme. However, preliminary experiments indicate that the 30% of substrate apparently remaining in the PCD mutants may be largely due to a contaminating phosphoprotein in the 23 000 dalton region of the gels used to measure substrate levels. Immunoprecipitation of proteins phosphorylated by cGK in PCD and control cerebellar cytosol with specific antibodies to rabbit G substrate revealed a greater than 90% reduction in G substrate in the homozygous recessive PCD animals (J. Detre and A. Nairn, personal communication). Therefore it seems likely that both cerebellar cGK and the 23 000 G substrate are highly enriched in Purkinje cells.

## SUMMARY

Numerous questions remain to be answered about the possible involvement of the cGMP-dependent protein phosphorylation system in neuronal function. Cerebellum, with high cGMP levels responsive to various agents which alter neuronal activity and a uniquely high cGK content, appeared to be the tissue of choice for approaching some of these problems. Two questions were addressed in these studies: first, what reactions occur subsequent to the activation of cGK, specifically, what are the endogenous substrate proteins of this enzyme in cerebellum and second, what is the cellular localization of the various elements of the cGMP system in this tissue? There is now strong evidence that the 23 000 dalton G substrate is indeed an endogenous substrate for cerebellar cGK. Purified G substrate is preferentially phosphorylated by cGK at a rapid rate and at a physiologically appropriate $Mg^{2+}$ concentration. In cerebellar cytosol, G substrate is endogenously phosphorylated in response to low concentrations of cGMP. Finally, cerebellar cGK and G substrate appear to be highly concentrated in one cell type, the Purkinje cell. The uniquely high concentration of these two elements of the cGMP-dependent phosphorylation system in Purkinje cells suggests that the cGMP-dependent phosphorylation of specific proteins may have an important function in this type of neuronal cell.

## REFERENCES

Aitken, A., Bilham, T., Cohen, P., Aswad, D. and Greengard, P. (1981) A specific substrate from rabbit cerebellum for guanosine 3':5'-monophosphate-dependent protein kinase. III. Amino acid sequences at the two phosphorylation sites. *J. biol. Chem.*, 256: 3501–3506.

Altman, J. and Anderson, W.J. (1972) Experimental reorganization of the cerebellar cortex. I. Morphological effects of elimination of all microneurons with prolonged X-irradiation started at birth. *J. comp. Neurol.*, 146: 355–406.

Aswad, D.W. and Greengard, P. (1981a) A specific substrate from rabbit cerebellum for guanosine 3':5'-monophosphate-dependent protein kinase. I. Purification and characterization. *J. biol. Chem.*, 256: 3487–3493.

Aswad, D.W. and Greengard, P. (1981b) A specific substrate from rabbit cerebellum for guanosine 3':5'-monophosphate-dependent protein kinase. II. Kinetic studies on its phosphorylation by guanosine 3':5'-monophosphate-dependent and adenosine 3':5'-monophosphate-dependent protein kinases. *J. biol. Chem.*, 256: 3494–3500.

Bandle, E. and Guidotti, A. (1978) Studies on the cell location of cyclic 3', 5'-guanosine monophosphate-dependent protein kinase in cerebellum. *Brain Res.*, 156: 412–416.

Bandle, E. and Guidotti, A. (1979) Ontogenetic studies of cGMP-dependent protein kinase in rat cerebellum. *J. Neurochem.*, 32: 1343–1347.

Bandle, E. and Guidotti, A. (1980) A simple and rapid method for the assay of cyclic GMP-dependent protein kinase. *J. Neurosci. Methods*, 2: 419–427.

Bartfai, T. (1978) Cyclic nucleotides in the central nervous system. *Trends biochem. Sci.*, 3: 121–124.

Bartfai, T. (1980) Cyclic nucleotides in the central nervous system. *Curr. Top. Cell. Regul.*, 16: 226–269.

Berry, M. and Bradley, P. (1976) The growth of the dendritic trees of Purkinje cells in the cerebellum of the rat. *Brain Res.*, 112: 1–35.

Biggio, G., Corda, M.G., Casu, M., Salis, M. and Gessa, G.L. (1978) Disappearance of cerebellar cyclic GMP induced by kainic acid. *Brain Res.*, 154: 203–208.

Bloom, F.E. (1975) The role of cyclic nucleotides in central synaptic function. *Rev. Physiol. Biochem. Pharmacol.*, 74: 1–103.

Blumenthal, D.K., Stull, J.T. and Gill, G.N. (1978) Phophorylation of cardiac troponin by guanosine 3':5'-monophosphate-dependent protein kinase. *J. biol. Chem.*, 253: 334–336.

Boehme, D.H., Kosecki, R. and Marks, N. (1978) Protein phosphorylation in human synaptosomal membranes. Evidence for the presence of substrates for cyclic nucleotide guanosine 3':5'-monophosphate dependent protein kinases. *Brain Res. Bull.*, 3: 697–700.

Buss, J.E., McCune, R.W. and Gill, G.N. (1979) Comparison of cyclic nucleotide binding to adenosine 3':5'-monophosphate and guanosine 3',5'-monophosphate-dependent protein kinases. *J. cyclic Nucl. Res.*, 5: 225–237.

Casnellie, J.E. and Greengard, P. (1974) Guanosine 3':5'-cyclic monophosphate-dependent phosphorylation of endogenous substrate proteins in membranes of mammalian smooth muscle. *Proc. nat. Acad. Sci. (Wash.)*, 71: 1891–1895.

Casnellie, J.E., Schlichter, D.J., Walter, U. and Greengard, P. (1978) Photoaffinity labeling of a guanosine 3′:5′-monophosphate-dependent protein kinase from vascular smooth muscle. *J. biol. Chem.*, 253: 4771–4776.

Cheung, W.Y. (1980) Calmodulin plays a pivotal role in cellular regulation. *Science*, 207: 19–27.

Chihara-Nakashima, M., Hashimoto, E. and Nishizuka, Y. (1977) Intrinsic activity of guanosine 3′:5′-monophosphate-dependent protein kinase similar to adenosine 3′:5′-monophosphate-dependent protein kinase. II. Phosphorylation of ribosomal proteins. *J. Biochem.*, 81: 1863–1867.

Corbin, J.D. and Lincoln, T.M. (1978) Comparison of cAMP- and cGMP-dependent protein kinases. *Adv. cyclic Nucl. Res.*, 9: 159–170.

Corbin, J.D., Sugden, P.H., West, L., Flockhart, D.A., Lincoln, T.M. and McCarthy D. (1978) Studies on the properties and mode of action of the purified regulatory subunit of bovine heart adenosine 3′:5′-monophosphate-dependent protein kinase. *J. biol. Chem.*, 253: 3997–4003.

Costa, E. (1978) Some new vistas on neuronal communication mechanisms: Impact on the neuropharmacology of GABA transmission. In *Interactions between Putative Neurotransmitters in the Brain*, S. Garattini, J.F. Pujol and R. Samanin (Eds.), Raven Press, New York, pp. 75–87.

Daile, P., Carnegie, P.R. and Young, J.D. (1975) Synthetic substrate for cyclic AMP-dependent protein kinase. *Nature (London)*, 257: 416–418.

Daly, J. (1977) *Cyclic Nucleotides in the Nervous System*, Plenum Press, New York, pp. 33–34.

De Jonge, H.R. (1976) Cyclic nucleotide-dependent phosphorylation of intestinal epithelium proteins. *Nature (London)*, 262: 590–592.

De Jonge, H.R. and Rosen, O.M. (1977) Self-phosphorylation of cyclic guanosine 3′:5′-monophosphate-dependent protein kinase from bovine lung. *J. biol. Chem.*, 252: 2780–2783.

Demaille, J.G., Peters, K.A. and Fischer, E.H. (1977) Isolation and properties of the rabbit skeletal muscle protein inhibitor of adenosine 3′,5′-monophosphate dependent protein kinases. *Biochemistry*, 16: 3080–3086.

England, P.J. (1977) Phosphorylation of the inhibitory subunit of troponin in perfused hearts of mice deficient in phosphorylase kinase. Evidence for the phosphorylation of troponin by adenosine 3′:5′-phosphate-dependent protein kinase in vivo. *Biochem. J.*, 168: 307–310.

Erlichman, J., Rosenfeld, R. and Rosen, O.M. (1974) Phosphorylation of a cyclic adenosine 3′:5′-monophosphate-dependent protein kinase from bovine cardiac muscle. *J. biol. Chem.*, 249: 5000–5003.

Ferrendelli, J.A. (1978) Distribution and regulation of cyclic GMP in the central nervous system. *Adv. cyclic Nucl. Res.*, 9: 453–464.

Ferrendelli, J.A., Kinscherf, D.A. and Chang, M.M. (1973) Regulation of levels of guanosine 3′:5′-monophosphate in the central nervous system: Effects of depolarizing agents. *Mol. Pharmacol.*, 9: 445–454.

Ferrendelli, J.A., Rubin, E.H. and Kinsherf, D. (1976) Influence of divalent cations on regulation of cyclic GMP and cAMP levels in brain tissue. *J. Neurochem.*, 26: 741–748.

Flockerzi, V., Speichermann, N. and Hofmann, F. (1978) A guanosine 3′:5′-monophosphate-dependent protein kinase from bovine heart muscle. *J. biol. Chem.*, 253: 3395–3399.

Geahlen, R.L. and Krebs, E.G. (1980) Regulatory subunit of the type I cAMP-dependent protein kinase as an inhibitor and substrate of the cGMP-dependent protein kinase. *J. biol. Chem.*, 255: 1164–1169.

Geahlen, R.L., Haley, B.E. and Krebs, E.G. (1979) Synthesis and use of 8-azidoguanosine 3′:5′-cyclic monophosphate as a photoaffinity label for cyclic GMP-dependent protein kinase. *Proc. nat. Acad. Sci. (Wash.)*, 76: 2213–2217.

Gill, G.N. and McCune, R.W. (1979) Guanosine 3′,5′-monophosphate-dependent protein kinase. *Curr. Top. cell. Regul.*, 15: 1–45.

Gill, G.N., Holdy, K.E., Walton, G.M. and Kanstein, C.B. (1976) Purification and characterization of 3′:5′-cyclic GMP-dependent protein kinase. *Proc. nat. Acad. Sci. (Wash.)*, 73: 3918–3922.

Gill, G.N., Walton, G.M. and Sperry, P.J. (1977) Guanosine 3′:5′-monophosphate-dependent protein kinase from bovine lung: Subunit structure and characterization of the purified enzyme. *J. biol. Chem.*, 252: 6443–6449.

Glass, D.B. and Krebs, E.G. (1979) Comparison of the substrate specificity of adenosine 3′:5′-monophosphate- and guanosine 3′:5′-monophosphate-dependent protein kinases. Kinetic studies using synthetic peptides corresponding to phosphorylation sites in histone H2B. *J. biol. Chem.*, 254: 9728–9738.

Glass. D.B. and Krebs, E.G. (1980) Protein phosphorylation catalyzed by cyclic AMP-dependent and cyclic GMP-dependent protein kinases. *Annu. Rev. Pharmacol. Toxicol.*, 20: 363–388.

Goldberg, N.D. and Haddox, M.K. (1977) Cyclic GMP metabolism and involvement in biological regulation. *Annu. Rev. Biochem.*, 46: 823–896.

Greengard, P. (1976) Possible role for cyclic nucleotides and phosphorylated membrane proteins in postsynaptic actions of neurotransmitters. *Nature (London)*, 260: 101–108.

Greengard, P. (1978) *Cyclic Nucleotides, Phosphorylated Proteins, and Neuronal Function*, Raven Press, New York, pp. 67–97.

Greengard, P. (1979) Cyclic nucleotides, phosphorylated proteins and the nervous system. *Fed. Proc.*, 38: 2208–2217.

Hashimoto, E., Takeda, M., Nishizuka, Y., Hamana, K. and Iwai, K. (1976) Studies on the sites of histone phosphorylated by adenosine 3′:5′-monophosphate-dependent and guanosine 3′:5′-monophosphate-dependent protein kinases. *J. biol. Chem.*, 251: 6287–6293.

Herrup, K. and Mullen, R.J. (1979) Regional variation and absence of large neurons in the cerebellum of the staggerer mousse. *Brain Res.*, 172: 1–12.

Hofmann, F. and Sold, G. (1972) A protein kinase activity from rat cerebellum stimulated by guanosine-3′:5′-monophosphate. *Biochem. biophys. Res. Commun.*, 49: 1100–1107.

Hoppe, J., Lawaczeck, R., Rieke, E. and Wagner, K.G. (1978) Mechanism of activation of protein kinase I from rabbit skeletal muscle. The equilibrium parameters of ligand interaction and protein dissociation. *Eur. J. Biochem.*, 90: 585–593.

Huang, F.L. and Glinsmann, W.H. (1976) Separation and characterization of two phosphorylase phosphatase inhibitors from rabbit skeletal muscle. *Eur. J. Biochem.*, 70: 419–426.

Inoue, M., Kishimoto, A., Takai, Y. and Nishizuka, Y. (1976) Guanosine 3′:5′-monophosphate-dependent protein kinase from silkworm: Properties of a catalytic fragment obtained by limited proteolysis. *J. biol. Chem.*, 251: 4476–4478.

Issinger, O.-G., Beier, H., Speichermann, N., Flockerzi, V. and Hofmann, F. (1980) Comparison of phosphorylation of ribosomal proteins from HeLa and Krebs II ascites-tumor cells by cyclic AMP-dependent and cyclic GMP-dependent protein kinases. *Biochem. J.*, 185: 89–99.

Johnson, E.M. and Hadden, J.W. (1975) Phosphorylation of lymphocyte nuclear acidic proteins: regulation by cyclic nucleotides. *Science*, 187: 1198–1200.

Kemp, B.E., Byland, D.B., Huang, T.-S. and Krebs, E.G. (1975) Substrate specificity of the cyclic AMP-dependent protein kinase. *Proc. nat. Acad. Sci. (Wash.)*, 72: 3448–3452.

Kemp, B.E., Benjamin, E. and Krebs, E.G. (1976) Synthetic hexapeptide substrates and inhibitors of 3′:5′-cyclic AMP-dependent protein kinase. *Proc. nat. Acad. Sci. (Wash.)*, 73: 1038–1042.

Khoo, J.C. and Gill, G.N. (1979) Comparison of cyclic nucleotide specificity of guanosine 3′,5′-monophosphate-dependent protein kinase and adenosine 3′,5′-monophosphate-dependent protein kinase. *Biochim. biophys. Acta*, 584: 21–32.

Khoo, J.C., Sperry, P.J., Gill, G.N. and Steinberg, D. (1977) Activation of hormone-sensitive lipase and phosphorylase kinase by pourified cyclic GMP-dependent protein kinase. *Proc. nat. Acad. Sci. (Wash.)*, 74: 4843–4847.

Krebs, E.G. and Beavo, J.A. (1979) Phosphorylation–dephosphorylation of enzymes. *Annu. Rev. Biochem.*, 48: 923–959.

Kuo, J.F. and Greengard, P. (1969) Cyclic nucleotide-dependent protein kinases IV. Widespread occurrence of adenosine 3′,5′-monophosphate-dependent protein kinase in various tissues and phyla of the animal kingdom. *Proc. nat. Acad. Sci. (Wash.)*, 64: 1349–1355.

Kuo, J.F., Miyamoto, E. and Reyes, P. (1974) Activation and dissociation of adenosine 3′-5′-monophosphate-dependent and guanosine 3′-5′-monophosphate-dependent protein kinases by various cyclic nucleotide analogues. *Biochem. Pharmacol.*, 23: 2011–2021.

Kuo, J.F., Kuo, W.-N., Shoji, M., Davis, C.W., Seery, V.L. and Donnelly, Jr., T.E. (1976) Purification and general properties of guanosine 3′:5′-monophosphate-dependent protein kinase from guinea pig fetal lung. *J. biol. Chem.*, 251: 1759–1766.

Landis, S.C. (1973) Ultrastructural changes in the mitochondria of cerebellar Purkinje cells of nervous mutant mice. *J. Cell Biol.*, 57: 782–797.

Landis, S.C. and Mullen, R.J. (1978) The development and degeneration of Purkinje cells in pcd mutant mice. *J. comp. Neurol.*, 177: 125–144.

Landis, D.M.D. and Sidman, R.L. (1978) Electron microscopic analysis of postnatal histogenesis in the cerebellar cortex of staggerer mutant mice. *J. comp. Neurol.*, 179: 831–864.

Lincoln, T.M. and Corbin, J.D. (1977) Adenosine 3′:5′-monophosphate-dependent and guanosine 3′:5′-monophosphate dependent protein kinases: Possible homologous proteins. *Proc. nat. Acad. Sci. (Wash.)*, 74: 3239–3243.

Lincoln, T.M. and Corbin, J.D. (1978a) Purified cyclic GMP-dependent protein kinase catalyzes the phosphorylation of cardiac troponin inhibitory subunit (TN-I). *J. biol. Chem.*, 253: 337–339.

Lincoln, T.M. and Corbin, J.D. (1978b) On the role of the cAMP and cGMP-dependent protein kinases in cell function. *J. cyclic Nucl. Res.* 4: 3–14.

Lincoln, T.M., Hall, C.L., Park, C.R. and Corbin, J.D. (1976) Guanosine 3′:5′-cyclic monophosphate binding proteins in rat tissues. *Proc. nat. Acad. Sci. (Wash.)*, 73: 2559–2563.

Lincoln, T.M., Dills, Jr., W.L. and Corbin, J.D. (1977) Purification and subunit composition of guanosine 3′:5′-monophosphate-dependent protein kinase from bovine lung. *J. biol. Chem.*, 252: 4269–4275.

Lincoln, T.M., Flockhart, D.A. and Corbin, J.D. (1978) Studies on the structure and mechanism of activation of the guanosine 3′:5′-monophosphate-dependent protein kinase. *J. biol. Chem.*, 253: 6002–6009.

Lohmann, S.M., Walter, U., Miller, P.E., Greengard, P. and De Camilli, P. (1981) Immunohistochemical localization of cyclic GMP-dependent protein kinase in mammalian brain. *Proc. nat. Acad. Sci. (Wash.)*, 78: 653–657.

Mao, C.C., Guidotti, A. and Landis, S. (1975) Cyclic GMP: reduction of cerebellar concentrations in "nervous" mutant mice. *Brain Res.*, 90: 335–339.

McCune, R.W. and Gill, G.N. (1979) Positive cooperativity in guanosine 3′:5′-monophosphate binding to guanosine 3′:5′-monophosphate-dependent protein kinase. *J. biol. Chem., 254: 5083*–5091.

Means, A.R. and Dedman, J.R. (1980) Calmodulin — an intracellular calcium receptor. *Nature (Lond.)*, 285: 73–77.

Miller, J.P., Boswell, K.H., Muneyama, K., Simon, L.N., Robins, R.K. and Schuman, D.A. (1973) Synthesis and biochemical studies of various 8-substituted derivatives of guanosine 3′,5′-cyclic phosphate, inosine 3′,5′-cyclic phosphate, and xanthosine 3′,5′-cyclic phosphate. *Biochemistry*, 12: 5310–5319.

Miyamoto, E., Petzold, G.L., Kuo, J.F. and Greengard, P. (1973) Dissociation and activation of adenosine 3′,5′-monophosphate-dependent and guanosine 3′,5′-monophosphate-dependent protein kinases by cyclic nucleotides and substrate proteins. *J. biol. Chem.*, 248: 179–189.

Nakazawa, K. and Sano, M. (1975) Partial purification and properties of guanosine 3′:5′-monophosphate-dependent protein kinase from pig lung. *J. biol. Chem.*, 250: 7415–7419.

Nathanson, J.A. (1977) Cyclic nucleotides and nervous system function. *Physiol. Rev.*, 57: 157–256.

Nimmo, H.G. and Cohen, P. (1977) Hormonal control of protein phosphorylation. *Adv. cyclic Nucl. Res.*, 8: 145–266.

Nimmo, H.G. and Cohen, P. (1978a) The regulation of glycogen metabolism: Purification and characterization of protein phosphatase inhibitor-I from rabbit skeletal muscle. *Eur. J. Biochem.*, 87: 341–351.

Nimmo, H.G. and Cohen, P. (1978b) The regulation of glycogen metabolism. Phosphorylation of inhibitor-I from rabbit skeletal muscle and its interaction with protein phosphatases-III and -II. *Eur. J. Biochem.*, 87: 353–365.

Nishiyama, K., Katakami, H., Yamamura, H., Takai, Y., Shimomura, R. and Nishizuka, Y. (1975) Functional specificity of guanosine 3′:5′-monophosphate-dependent and adenosine 3′:5′-monophosphate-dependent protein kinases from silkworm. *J. biol. Chem.*, 250: 1297–1300.

Rakic, P. and Sidman, R.L. (1973a) Sequence of developmental abnormalities leading to granule cell deficit in cerebellar cortex of weaver mutant mice. *J. comp. Neurol.*, 152: 103–132.

Rakic, P. and Sidman, R.L. (1973b) Organization of cerebellar cortex secondary to deficit of granule cells in weaver mutant mice. *J. comp. Neurol.*, 152: 133–162.

Ram, J.L. and Erlich, Y.H. (1978) Cyclic GMP-stimulated phosphorylation of membrane-bounds proteins from nerve roots of *Aplysia californica*. *J. Neurochem.*, 30: 487–491.

Rangel-Aldoa, R. and Rosen, O.M. (1976a) Dissociation and reassociation of the phosphorylated and nonphosphorylated forms of adenosine 3′:5′-monophosphate-dependent protein kinase from bovine cardiac muscle. *J. biol. Chem.*, 251: 3375–3380.

Rangel-Aldao, R. and Rosen, O.M. (1976b) Mechanism of self-phosphorylation of adenosine 3′:5′-monophosphate-dependent protein kinase from bovine cardiac muscle. *J. biol. Chem.*, 251: 7526–7529.

Rochette-Egly, C. and Castagna, M. (1978) Evidence for a role of sulfhydryl groups in catalytic activity and subunit interaction of the cyclic GMP-dependent protein kinase from silkworm. *Biochim. biophys. Acta*, 526: 107–15.

Roffler-Tarlov, S. and Sidman, R.L. (1978) Concentrations of glutamic acid in cerebellar cortex and deep nuclei of normal mice and weaver, staggerer and nervous mutants. *Brain Res.*, 142: 269–283.

Rubin, C.S. and Rosen, O.M. (1975) Protein phosphorylation. *Annu. Rev. Biochem.*, 44: 831–887.

Schlichter, D.J., Casnellie, J.E. and Greengard, P. (1978) An endogenous substrate for cGMP-dependent protein kinase in mammalian cerebellum. *Nature (Lond.)*, 273: 61–62.

Schlichter, D.J., Detre, J.A., Aswad, D.W., Chehrazi, B. and Greengard P. (1980) Localization of cyclic GMP-dependent protein kinase and substrate in mammalian cerebellum. *Proc. nat. Acad. Sci. (Wash.)*, 77: 5537–5541.

Shaltz, L.J., Kimberg, D.V. and Cattieu, K.A. (1978) Cyclic nucleotide-dependent phosphorylation of rat intestinal microvillus and basal-lateral membrane proteins by an endogenous protein kinase. *Gastroenterology*, 75: 838–846.

Shimono, T., Nosaka, S. and Saski, K. (1976) Electrophysiological study on the postnatal development of neuronal mechanisms in the rat cerebellar cortex. *Brain Res.*, 108: 279–294.

Shoji, M., Patrick, J.G., Tse, J. and Kuo, J.F. (1977) Studies on the cyclic GMP-dependent protein kinase from bovine aorta. Possible existence of a catalytic subunit. *J. biol. Chem.*, 252: 4347–4353.

Swartz, B.E. and Woody, C.D. (1979) Correlated effects of acetylcholine and cyclic guanosine monophosphate on membrane properties of mammalian neocortical neurons. *J. Neurobiol.*, 10: 465–488.

Takai, Y., Nishiyama, K., Yamamura, H. and Nishizuka, Y. (1975) Guanosine 3':5'-monophosphate-dependent protein kinase from bovine cerebellum. Purification and characterization. *J. biol. Chem.* 250, 4690–4695.

Takai, Y., Nakaya, S., Inoue, M., Kishimoto, A., Nishiyama, K., Yamamura, H. and Nishizuka, Y. (1976) Comparison of mode of activation of guanosine 3':5'-monophosphate-dependent and adenosine 3':5'-monophosphate-dependent protein kinases from silkworm. *J. biol. Chem.*, 251: 1481–1487.

Van Leemput-Coutrez, M., Camus, J. and Christophe, J. (1973) Cyclic nucleotide-dependent protein kinases of the rat pancreas. *Biochem. biophys. Res. Commun.*, 54: 182–190.

Wallach, D., Davies, P.J.A. and Pastan, I. (1978) Cyclic AMP-dependent phosphorylation of filamin in mammalian smooth muscle. *J. biol. Chem.*, 253: 4739–4745.

Walsh, D.A. and Ashby, C.D. (1973) Protein kinases: Aspects of their regulation and diversity. *Recent Progr. Hormone Res.*, 29: 329–359.

Walsh, D.A., Ashby, C.D., Gonzalez, C., Calkins, D., Fischer, E.H. and Krebs, E.G. (1971) Purification and characterization of a protein inhibitor of adenosine 3',5'-monophosphate-dependent protein kinases. *J. biol. Chem.*, 246: 1977–1985.

Walter, U., Uno, I., Liu, A.Y.-C. and Greengard, P. (1977a) Identification, characterization, and quantitative measurement of cyclic AMP receptor proteins in cytosol of various tissues using a photoaffinity ligand. *J. biol. Chem.*, 252: 6494–6500.

Walter, U., Uno, I., Liu, A.Y.-C. and Greengard (1977b) Study of autophosphorylation of isoenzymes of cyclic AMP-dependent protein kinases. *J. biol. Chem.*, 252: 6588–6590.

Walter, W., Kanof, P., Schulman, H. and Greengard, P. (1978) Adenosine 3':5'-monophosphate receptor proteins in mammalian brain. *J. biol. Chem.*, 253: 6275–6280.

Walter, U., Miller, P., Wilson, F., Menkes, D. and Greengard, P. (1980) Immunological distinction between guanosine 3':5'-monophosphate-dependent and adenosine 3':5'-monophosphate-dependent protein kinases. *J. biol. Chem.*, 255: 3757–3762.

Woody, C.D. (1977) If cyclic GMP is a neuronal second messenger what is the message? In *Cholinergic Mechanisms and Psychopharmacology*, D.J. Jenden (Ed.), Plenum Press, New York, pp. 253–260.

Woody, C.D., Swartz, B.E. and Gruen, E. (1978) Effects of acetylcholine and cyclic GMP on input resistance of cortical neurons in awake cats. *Brain Res.*, 158: 373–395.

Wool, I.G. (1979) The structure and function of eukaryotic ribosomes. *Annu. Rev. Biochem.*, 48: 719–754.

Yamamoto, M., Takai, Y., Hashimoto, E. and Nishizuka, Y. (1977) Intrinsic activity of guanosine 3':5'-monophosphate-dependent protein kinase similar to adenosine 3':5'-monophosphate-dependent protein kinase. I. Phosphorylation of histone fractions. *J. Biochem.*, 81: 1857–1862.

# Calcium Ion Stimulated Protein Kinases in Myelin

ELENA H. PETRALI and PRAKASH V. SULAKHE

*Department of Physiology, College of Medicine, University of Saskatchewan,*
*Saskatoon, S7N OWO Canada*

## INTRODUCTION

It is now established that several distinct protein kinases are present in mammalian tissues. Of these, some are activated by cyclic AMP (cAMP) (kinase A) or by cyclic GMP (cGMP) (kinase G) while some do not require either nucleotide for activity. Recently, two additional $Ca^{2+}$-stimulated kinases have been described — one of these requires calmodulin (hereafter called $Ca^{2+}$ kinase) (see review by Schulman et al., 1980) and the other, requires phospholipids such as phosphatidyl serine (hereafter called kinase C) (Takai et al., 1979; Kuo et al., 1980). All these kinases reportedly phosphorylate a large number of protein substrates. Further, there exist many discrepancies between the results of in vitro and in vivo phosphorylation of substrate proteins especially if such substrates are normally present in organized structures such as membrane, microfilaments and myofibrils. Thus, only a few protein substrates have been established as specific substrates for the above-mentioned kinases. Myelin basic protein (MBP) is interesting since both in vivo and in vitro studies show its phosphorylation (Carnegie et al., 1974; Miyamoto and Kakiuchi, 1974a,b; Steck and Appel, 1974). Further, earlier studies showed that myelin-associated protein kinases (Miyamoto, 1975, 1976; Miyamoto et al., 1978) as well as exogenously added kinase A phosphorylated this major protein constituent of myelin membrane. We were intrigued by the reported high capacity of MBP to incorporate $^{32}P$, at least under in vitro conditions (Carnegie et al., 1974; Miyamoto and Kakiuchi, 1974a,b; Yourist et al., 1978). We thus undertook a systematic study of protein kinases in myelin. This led to the discovery of a $Ca^{2+}$-stimulatable kinase activity in myelin (Petrali et al., 1978; Sulakhe et al., 1978). We now provide evidence that myelin contains $Ca^{2+}$ kinase as well as kinase C and for both these kinases, MBP is an excellent substrate. In contrast, MBP is a poor substrate for kinase A, which is also present in myelin preparations. In this article, we describe the properties of myelin-associated $Ca^{2+}$ kinase, kinase C and kinase A deduced from studying the phosphorylation of MBP. The likely significance of MBP phosphorylation in myelin function is also briefly discussed.

## MATERIALS AND METHODS

Several types of rat brain myelin preparations (from male Wistar rat) were used in the present study. Myelin isolated according to Petrali et al. (1980) was used in most of the kinetic studies. Highly purified myelin as well as myelin-like membrane ($SN_4$) were prepared by the method of Waehneldt et al. (1977). Isolation of myelin subfractions by sucrose density gradient centrifugation was carried out as described by Sulakhe et al. (1980a). Myelin from sciatic nerve, spinal cord and cauda equina was isolated essentially according to Petrali et al. (1980).

Determination of myelin phosphorylation was carried out as previously described (Petrali et al., 1980; Sulakhe et al., 1980a,b). Separation of myelin polypeptides by sodium dodecyl sulphate–polyacrylamide gel electrophoresis was carried out by the method of Laemmli (1970). Autoradiographic detection of phosphorylated polypeptides and other details have been described in earlier publications from this laboratory (Petrali et al., 1980; Sulakhe et al., 1980a). Photoaffinity labelling of cAMP kinase with 8-azido[2-$^3$H]cAMP or 8-azido[$^{32}$P]cAMP was carried out by the method of Pomerantz et al. (1975).

We arbitrarily define basal kinase and total kinase when the assay mixture contains $Mg^{2+}$ and $Mg^{2+}$ plus $Ca^{2+}$ respectively. $Ca^{2+}$-stimulated kinase activity is determined as the difference between basal and total kinase activities.

## RESULTS

### Stimulation by $Ca^{2+}$

Myelin isolated from rat brain white matter contained an endogenous $Mg^{2+}$-dependent protein kinase which effected the phosphorylation of serine and threonine residues of MBPs, both small (SBP) and large (LBP). In fresh membrane preparations, $Ca^{2+}$, in micromolar concentrations, augmented (up to 2-fold) the phosphorylation of MBPs with the half-maximal and maximal effect seen at 5–7 $\mu$M and $25 \pm 2$ $\mu$M $Ca^{2+}$ (Table I). Addition of Triton X-100, a

TABLE I

DEPENDENCE ON $Ca^{2+}$ OF $Ca^{2+}$-STIMULATED PHOSPHORYLATION OF MBP

| Myelin fraction | $V_{max}$ (pmole/mg protein/2 min | | $K_a$ for $Ca^{2+}$ ($\mu$M) | |
|---|---|---|---|---|
| | − Triton | + Triton | − Triton | + Triton |
| Fresh | $143 \pm 7$ | $143 \pm 6$ | $5.5 \pm 0.3$ | $7.6 \pm 0.5$ |
| Stored | $71 \pm 3$ | $137 \pm 5$ | $5.2 \pm 0.2$ | $7.4 \pm 0.4$ |

non-ionic detergent, to assay mixture did not appreciably increase the $Ca^{2+}$-stimulatable phosphorylation (shown as Difference in Fig. 1) of fresh myelin when the detergent was present in low concentrations (less than 0.1%); at high concentrations, the detergent inhibited the rate of $Ca^{2+}$-dependent myelin phosphorylation. On the other hand, Triton X-100 did increase the $Ca^{2+}$-stimulated phosphorylation of myelin that was stored for 1–3 days at 4°C prior to assay. At the same time, storage of isolated myelin decreased the $Ca^{2+}$-stimulated phosphorylation assayed in the absence of the detergent. It is intriguing that Triton X-100 almost fully restored the decreased $Ca^{2+}$-stimulated phosphorylation of the stored myelin fraction to the level seen in fresh preparation assayed without Triton X-100 or with low concentrations of the detergent (less than 0.1%). The basal phosphorylation showed a progressive increase with increasing concentrations of Triton X-100 and such an increase was marked following storage of myelin.

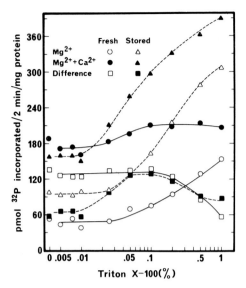

Fig. 1. Effect of varying Triton X-100 on basal and $Ca^{2+}$-stimulatable phosphorylation of myelin. Rat brain myelin isolated according to Petrali et al. (1980) was phosphorylated for 2 min at 30°C. When present, $MgCl_2$ was 1 mM, $CaCl_2$, 1.05 mM and $[\gamma-^{32}P]$ATP, 50 $\mu$M. 1 mM EGTA was present in all assays and membrane protein was 46$\mu$g. Myelin was assayed immediately (fresh) or following its storage for 3 days at 4°C (stored). Difference represents $Ca^{2+}$-stimulated phosphorylation.

*Inhibitory action of EGTA — its dependence on the nature of membrane preparations and assay conditions*

In order to demonstrate the presence of a $Mg^{2+}$-dependent $Ca^{2+}$-stimulatable kinase in myelin, it was necessary to establish the level of basal $Mg^{2+}$-dependent activity which was obtained by addition of EGTA to the assay mixture. Since only micromolar concentrations of $Ca^{2+}$ were necessary for optimal activity of $Ca^{2+}$ kinase, we routinely added 1 mM EGTA to attain the basal level of phosphorylation. We also noted that the assay mixture contained about 10–20 $\mu$M $Ca^{2+}$ present as contaminant of assay reagents, including that introduced with the membrane fraction. Thus, when added to the assay, EGTA in a concentration-dependent manner decreased the phosphorylation of myelin until the level of ionized $Ca^{2+}$ was below 0.1 $\mu$M. Such an inhibitory response, however, depended on whether the fraction assayed was fresh or stored. For example, in fresh and stored membranes, the maximal inhibitory effect of EGTA amounted to $70 \pm 2\%$ and $27 \pm 1\%$, respectively. Interestingly, when the phosphorylation was carried out in the presence of Triton X-100 (0.05%), the maximal inhibitory effect of the chelator was essentially similar ($65 \pm 2\%$) for both fresh and stored membranes. These and other results described later in this article indicate that a calmodulin-like protein participates in the $Ca^{2+}$-stimulatable phosphorylation of fresh myelin. However, calmodulin-requiring kinase appears to be labile and its activity decreases nearly 70–80% by storage of the membranes for 1–3 days at 4°C. At the same time, following storage of the membranes, $Ca^{2+}$-stimulated phosphorylation observed with Triton X-100 present in the assay appears to be due to a separate $Ca^{2+}$ kinase, which does not require calmodulin. This latter enzyme in many regards resembles a newly discovered multifunctional protein kinase, called kinase C (Takai et al., 1979). In fact, it seems that when phosphorylation is determined in the presence of Triton X-100, two major effects of the detergent become evident. (1) The detergent in low concentrations does not influence calmodulin-requiring $Ca^{2+}$ kinase and inhibits it at higher

128

concentrations. (2) The detergent promotes the activity of kinase C with the stimulatory effect being much greater in stored myelin fractions. Thus, myelin provided an interesting model with which to study two separate $Ca^{2+}$-stimulated kinases, especially since MBP was an excellent substrate for either kinase.

*Regulatory role of* $Mg^{2+}$

The nucleotide substrate for myelin protein kinases appears to be $Mg-ATP^{2-}$ (and not $Ca-ATP^{2-}$) and in this form, $Mg^{2+}$ interacted with the catalytic site with an apparent affinity of about 0.07 mM (Petrali et al., 1980). $Mg^{2+}$ concentrations much higher than ATP were required for maximal phosphorylation determined with or without $Ca^{2+}$ in the assays (Fig. 2).

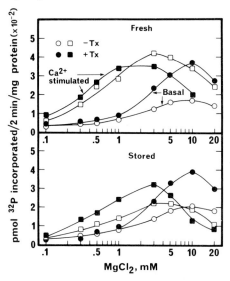

Fig. 2. Effect of varying $MgCl_2$ on basal and $Ca^{2+}$-stimulated phosphorylation. With the exception of the indicated $MgCl_2$ concentrations, all other details were similar to Fig. 1. When present, Triton X-100 was 0.05%.

There must be an additional site(s) to which $Mg^{2+}$ and other divalent cations bind. For $Mg^{2+}$, the binding affinity of such sites (site II) on the kinase in the absence of $Ca^{2+}$ was in the millimolar range (3–5 mM) and when $Mg^{2+}$ interacted with this site, the catalytic reactivity (i.e. $V_{max}$) was markedly increased. Interestingly, Triton X-100 augmented the site II-dependent stimulatory effect of $Mg^{2+}$, an observation true for both fresh and stored myelin preparations. The $Ca^{2+}$ kinase appeared to have a different $Mg^{2+}$ dependence. For example, half-maximal increases were obtained at 0.3–0.5 mM $Mg^{2+}$ irrespective of whether the phosphorylation was determined with and without Triton X-100. A noteworthy finding was that the detergent augmented the $Mg^{2+}$-dependent increase in $Ca^{2+}$ kinase in stored, but not fresh, myelin preparations.

*$Ca^{2+}$-calmodulin-dependent protein kinase is present in fresh myelin preparations*

That $Ca^{2+}$-stimulated phosphorylation of MBPs requires calmodulin was supported by several lines of evidence (Sulakhe et al., 1980a,b, 1981). (1) Isolated myelin contained about 1 $\mu$g calmodulin-like protein/mg myelin protein. Of this, about 40% was easily removed from the membrane by exposure to EGTA. (2) The EGTA extract of myelin contained calmodulin-like protein, a conclusion based on the ability of the extract to restore the activity of calmodulin-deficient phosphodiesterase to the same extent as purified, exogenously added calmodulin. (3) EGTA treatment of myelin selectively decreased $Ca^{2+}$-stimulatable phosphorylation of MBP and this was restored by addition of the EGTA extract. (4) When EGTA was added to the assay mixture, it decreased (70%) the phosphorylation of myelin in a concentration-dependent manner. Further, this decrease amounted to only 25% when stored myelin preparations were tested, again indicating the lability of the calmodulin-sensitive enzyme system. (5) EGTA extract contained a polypeptide band which comigrated with a purified sample of calmodulin. (6) A heat-stable calmodulin-binding protein ($BP_{70}$) markedly inhibited the $Ca^{2+}$-stimulated phosphorylation of MBP; $BP_{70}$ did not inhibit basal phosphorylation. Recently, Endo and Hidaka (1980) showed the presence of a calmodulin-dependent $Ca^{2+}$ kinase in myelin isolated from rabbit brain.

*Triton X-100 inhibits $Ca^{2+}$calmodulin-dependent phosphodiesterase and stimulates $Ca^{2+}$ kinase of stored myelin preparations*

In order to know whether Triton X-100 augmented the $Ca^{2+}$-stimulatable phosphorylation of myelin peptides (when a stored membrane fraction was assayed) by augmenting interactions between $Ca^{2+}$, calmodulin, kinase and substrate proteins — the minimum four essential components of the phosphorylation system —, or by some alternate mechanisms, we tested the effect of the detergent on partially purified $Ca^{2+}$-calmodulin-dependent cAMP phosphodiesterase activity. The results indicated a marked concentration-dependent inhibitory effect

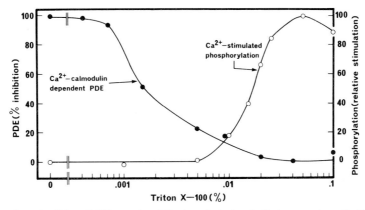

Fig. 3. Effect of varying Triton X-100 on calmodulin-dependent phosphodiesterase and myelin $Ca^{2+}$-stimulated kinase. Partially purified calmodulin-deficient cAMP phosphodiesterase was incubated in the presence of 100 $\mu$M $CaCl_2$ and 100 ng calmodulin without and with varying Triton X-100. For $Ca^{2+}$-stimulated phosphorylation, stored myelin was phosphorylated for 15 min at 30°C. Other assay conditions were similar to those described in Fig. 1.

of Triton X-100 (Fig. 3). For comparison, stimulation of myelin $Ca^{2+}$ kinase, at various detergent concentrations, is shown in Fig. 3. There was a clear separation in the dependence on the detergent concentrations between the inhibition of the phosphodiesterase and the stimulation of $Ca^{2+}$ kinase. This observation supported the view that the detergent-dependent augmentation of $Ca^{2+}$ kinase is due to the stimulatory effect of Triton X-100 on calmodulin-independent kinase of myelin, especially when the stored membrane fraction was used in the phosphorylation assay. In synaptic membranes prepared from rat cerebral cortex (gray matter), $Ca^{2+}$-calmodulin-dependent protein kinase is present, selectively phosphorylating two polypeptides ($M_r$ 65 K and 55 K). Triton X-100 (0.05%) markedly inhibited the $Ca^{2+}$-stimulated phosphorylation of these peptides (Sulakhe et al., 1981). This finding further supports the view that the detergent inhibits membrane-associated, $Ca^{2+}$-calmodulin-regulatable, enzyme systems.

### Likely mechanismes of calmodulin insensitivity of $Ca^{2+}$-stimulated kinase of stored myelin preparations

The following discussion assumes that the reported information of calmodulin-regulated enzyme (cAMP phosphodiesterase and $Mg^{2+}$-$CA^{2+}$- ATPase) is applicable to myelin $Ca^{2+}$ kinase. Cheung (1971) reported that limited proteolysis causes a marked and irreversible activation of cAMP phosphodiesterase and renders the enzyme insensitive to $Ca^{2+}$ and calmodulin. Recently it has been shown (Klee, 1980) that such proteolytic activation depends on the removal of a 22 000 dalton peptide from the enzyme. Also, the proteolyzed diesterase is unable to bind calmodulin. The proteolytic activation, in many regards, produces effects on the enzyme which are similar to those seen with calmodulin activation. The major difference is that following proteolytic activation the enzyme is $Ca^{2+}$-insensitive. Klee (1980) suggests that calmodulin binding and limited proteolysis displace an inhibitory domain of the enzyme that exhibits higher but similar $V_{max}$. The observed phospholipid activation of cAMP phosphodiesterase by Wolff and Brostrom (1976) might result from a similar mechanism. Amongst phospholipids, lysolecithin was most potent and Lubrol PX (a non-ionic detergent), but not EGTA, reversed the phospholipid activation of the enzyme. Myelin fractions are known to possess proteolytic activity (Rumsby et al., 1970). Thus it is likely that during isolation and/or storage of myelin, some proteolysis may have taken place. The decreased $Ca^{2+}$ kinase and EGTA inhibition following storage thus could be accounted for by proteolytic alterations in the calmodulin-requiring myelin kinase. However, it is important to note that even if such proteolysis took place during myelin storage, $Ca^{2+}$-dependent stimulation of MBP phosphorylation was still demonstrable, albeit to a decreased level compared to that of the fresh membrane. Highly purified myelin is reportedly devoid of any demonstrable phospholipase C activity (Gwarsha et al., 1980). Thus, it is unlikely that lysolecithin was formed during storage. Further, EGTA did inhibit $Ca^{2+}$ kinase of stored myelin, especially when phosphorylation was determined in the presence of Triton X-100. This detergent as well as deoxycholate increased the activity of $Ca^{2+}$ kinase in stored myelin. With regard to phosphodiesterase, Lubrol PX antagonized the lysolecithin-dependent activation of the enzyme. This makes it difficult to conclude that during storage calmodulin-requiring kinase was converted to a calmodulin-independent form. Thus other possibilities, especially the presence in myelin of a $Ca^{2+}$-sensitive, calmodulin-independent kinase, need serious consideration.

### Effect of phenothiazines on myelin kinases

Weiss and Levin (1978) showed that trifluoperazine (TFP) and other phenothiazines markedly inhibited calmodulin-dependent cAMP phosphodiesterase. Such an inhibition resulted from the $Ca^{2+}$-dependent binding of TFP to calmodulin. Since then, many investigators have used TFP and other phenothiazines as probes in the study of calmodulin-mediated processes. We found that in stored myelin, TFP (Sulakhe et al., 1981) and chlorpromazine (Fig. 4) inhibited $Ca^{2+}$ kinase only at high concentrations ($> 200\ \mu M$) of these agents. On the other hand, in a rat cerebral cortex synaptic membrane fraction, TFP (Sulakhe et al., 1981) and chlorpromazine (CPZ) (Fig. 4) caused complete inhibition of $Ca^{2+}$ kinase at 100 $\mu M$. We know that synaptic membrane-associated $Ca^{2+}$ kinase requires calmodulin (Sulakhe et al., in preparation). At high concentrations, TFP and CPZ are known to interact with membrane lipids (Mori et al., 1980). Thus, the inhibitory effect of TFP and CPZ on myelin $Ca^{2+}$ kinase could likely result from the interaction of these with myelin phospholipids. This implies that

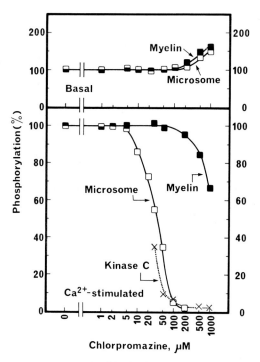

Fig. 4. Effect of chlorpromazine on basal and $Ca^{2+}$-stimulated phosphorylation in myelin and microsomes. Rat cerebral cortex microsomal fraction (enriched in synaptic membrane) and myelin were phosphorylated in the absence or presence of varying amounts of chlorpromazine. The results on kinase C are taken from the publication by Mori et al. (1980). In assays for microsomal fraction, a cytosolic fraction (100 000 × $g$ supernatant fluid) was added, which contained calmodulin and was necessary for the maximal $Ca^{2+}$-stimulated phosphorylation of microsomal polypeptides of $M_r$ 65 000 and 55 000 (Sulakhe et al., in preparation). Isolated myelin was stored overnight at 4°C prior to its assay.

$Ca^{2+}$ kinase of stored myelin depends upon phospholipids for its activity. Also the lack of inhibitory effect of low concentrations of TFP or CPZ on $Ca^{2+}$-stimulated phosphorylation of stored myelin further suggests that calmodulin-requiring kinase is either absent or contributes little to the observed phosphorylation. At high concentrations, TFP or CPZ increased the basal kinase activity both in the case of myelin and synaptic membrane fraction. These results thus suggest that basal kinase activity does not depend on membrane lipids and is an activity of the enzyme separate from $Ca^{2+}$ kinase(s) in either membrane tested. It is interesting that CPZ inhibitory response of kinase C and $Ca^{2+}$ kinase (of synaptic membrane) were quite similar. It is thus possible that besides $Ca^{2+}$ kinase synaptic membranes contain kinase C. Recent observation by Wrenn et al. (1980) supports this view.

*Detergent-dependent stimulation of $Ca^{2+}$ kinase is not due to increased accessibility of substrate and co-factors*

It is known that isolated membrane fractions generally comprise of heterogenous populations of vesicles in terms of their orientation (sideness). When we tested the effects of ionophores (A23187 or alamethicin), they only moderately increased (30–40%) the $Ca^{2+}$-dependent phosphorylation of MBP (Sulakhe et al., 1981). Also, such increase could not be seen when Triton X-100 was included in the assays. We have earlier found that alamethicin

132

increased by nearly 3-fold the basal adenylate cyclase activity in a rat brain particulate fraction. In this fraction, about 70% of vesicles were of the right-side out orientation (unpublished observations).

## Distribution of $Ca^{2+}$ kinase and cAMP kinase amongst myelin subfractions

When myelin was centrifuged on a discontinuous sucrose density gradient, five subfractions were isolated. Based on their densities, these were termed light (L), light-medium (LM), medium (M), medium-heavy (MH) and heavy (H). $Ca^{2+}$ kinase as well as MBPs were enriched in lighter fractions (L and LM) whereas cAMP kinase sedimented in heavier fractions (Sulakhe et al., 1980a). The latter fractions were also enriched in polypeptides of $M_r > 45\ 000$, including Wolfgram peptides (WP) and myelin-associated glycoproteins (MGP). Proteolipid protein (PLP) was more concentrated in the lighter fractions. Similar findings were obtained when myelin subfractions, prepared by continuous sucrose density gradient centrifugation, were analyzed for their polypeptide compositions and assayed for endogenous kinase-catalyzed phosphorylation (Sulakhe et al., 1980a, 1981).

## cAMP kinase is enriched in myelin-like membrane $(SN_4)$

We observed that cAMP stimulated rather modestly (20%) the phosphorylation of MBP and only when Triton X-100 was present. It thus appeared that the cAMP binding site on the regulatory subunit of cAMP kinase in myelin was buried in the membrane matrix and/or that the cAMP kinase activity of myelin preparations might be due to the presence of non-myelin contaminants. Both of these possibilities were supported by further study. As shown in Fig. 5, in a highly purified myelin, cAMP kinase was barely detectable whereas in a myelin-like membrane fraction, termed $SN_4$, it was readily demonstrated. On the other hand, $Ca^{2+}$ kinase showed the reverse pattern. Incorporation of 8-azido[2-$^3$H]cAMP was much higher in $SN_4$

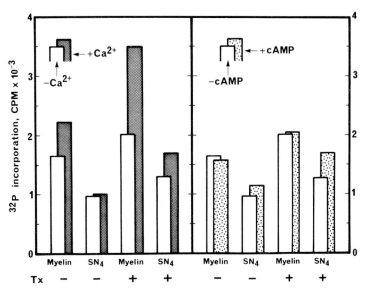

Fig. 5. Comparison between $Ca^{2+}$-stimulated and cAMP-stimulated phosphorylation of highly purified myelin and $SN_4$. Myelin (30 μg/assay) and $SN_4$ (20 μg/assay) isolated according to Waehneldt et al. (1977) were phosphorylated for 15 min. $MgCl_2$ was 1 mM; $CaCl_2$, 1.05 mM. All assays contained 1 mM EGTA. When present, Triton X-100 (Tx) concentration was 0.025%. Membrane fractions were stored overnight prior to assay.

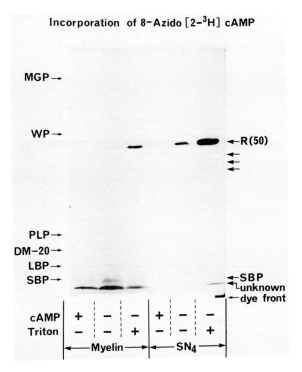

Fig. 6. Fluorographic detection and quantitation of regulatory subunit of kinase A in myelin and $SN_4$. Myelin (120 $\mu g$) and $SN_4$ (40 $\mu g$) were photolyzed in the presence of 0.80 $\mu M$ of 8-azido[2-$^3$H]cAMP. In some incubations, cAMP (1 mM, non-radioactive) and/or Triton X-100 (0.05%) were present. Membranes were then solubilized with sodium dodecyl sulphate (SDS) and subjected to electrophoresis according to the Laemmli procedure. Incorporation of 8-azido[2-$^3$H]cAMP was detected by the fluorographic method of Bonner and Laskey (1974). X-ray film was exposed to slab for 60 days. MGP, myelin-associated glycoprotein; WP, Wolfgram peptides; PLP, proteolipid protein; DM-20, intermediate protein; SBP, small basic protein; LBP, large basic protein.

relative to myelin when determined in the absence and presence of Triton X-100 (Fig. 6). We estimated that the content of cAMP kinase in $SN_4$ is about 15-fold higher compared to purified myelin. Interestingly, even in the case of $SN_4$, cAMP binding site(s) were buried in the membrane matrix. While cGMP stimulated the phosphorylation in $SN_4$ to the same extent as cAMP, it exhibited considerably lower affinity (Fig. 7). The results also suggested that cGMP promoted the activity of the cAMP kinase rather than that of a cGMP kinase. In other words, it is unlikely that $SN_4$ or myelin possess cGMP kinase.

*Phosphorylation in regions with $M_r$ less than 14 000*

Three distinct regions of proteins migrating faster than SBP, showed $^{32}$P incorporation both in the case of myelin and $SN_4$ (Fig. 8). Coomassie blue staining of the slab gel failed to show the presence of polypeptide bands corresponding to (or in) these regions (A to C). $Ca^{2+}$, but not cAMP, increased, whereas Triton X-100 decreased the phosphorylation of region A (Fig. 8A). On the other hand, the detergent and/or $MgCl_2$ promoted the phosphorylation of region C (Fig. 8B). It is likely that $^{32}$P incorporation into these regions represents lipid phosphorylation. We have as yet not identified which of the myelin lipids are phosphorylated under the assay conditions used. We do know, however, that such phosphorylation is catalyzed by an

134

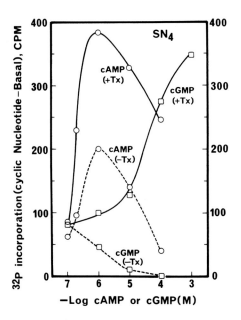

Fig. 7. Stimulatory effect of cAMP and cGMP on phosphorylation of SN$_4$. SN$_4$ (20 $\mu g$/assay) was phosphorylated by incubating for 15 min at 30°C in the assay mixture containing 1 mM MgCl$_2$, 1 mM EGTA, 50 $\mu$M ATP and varying amounts of cAMP or cGMP. Triton X-100 (Tx) concentration was 0.025%, when present.

enzymatic reaction, since in the absence of Mg$^{2+}$ (but with [$\gamma$-$^{32}$P]ATP present), radioactivity in these regions could not be detected (Fig. 8B).

*Is MBP a calmodulin-binding protein?*

We observed that MBP prepared by the method of Golds and Braun (1978) produced inhibitory effects on several calmodulin-dependent enzymes. The enzymes tested included rat brain adenylate cyclase, partially purified cAMP phosphodiesterase from bovine brain and Ca$^{2+}$ kinase of a rat brain synaptic membrane fraction. Further, phosphorylation of MBP did not alter its inhibitory character. Also thermal exposure (70°C, 10 min) of the MBP preparation did not abolish its inhibitory character. While it has been shown that a number of basic proteins can bind calmodulin and thereby inhibit the activities of calmodulin-requiring enzymes (e.g. Itano et al., 1980), it is not as yet clear whether MBP itself or a minor contaminant in the MBP preparation possesses this inhibitory activity (Sulakhe et al., 1980c).

*Stimulation and solubilization by deoxycholate of myelin kinase*

Besides non-ionic detergents (e.g. Triton X-100), ionic detergents (e.g. deoxycholate, DOC) stimulated both basal and Ca$^{2+}$-stimulated protein kinase of stored myelin (Fig. 9); the stimulation by DOC of Ca$^{2+}$-stimulated kinase (2.5-fold) was greater relative to basal activity (30%). When myelin was exposed to varying amounts of DOC, there appeared to be solubilization of Ca$^{2+}$-kinase at higher DOC concentrations (Fig. 10). However, it is important to note that MBPs were also solubilized with higher DOC concentrations (results not shown). In these and other experiments we obtained evidence that DOC solubilized Ca$^{2+}$ kinase as enzyme substrate complex. Triton X-100 also solubilized the enzyme, but again along with its substrate proteins (unpublished observations). With either DOC or Triton

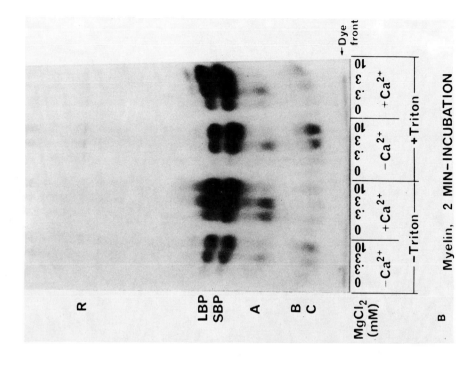

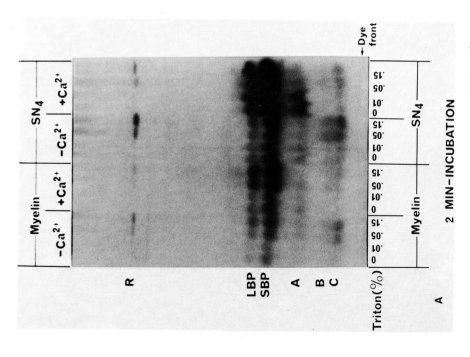

Fig. 8. Phosphorylation of basic proteins and lipids in myelin and SN$_4$: autoradiographic detection. A: Following phosphorylation ($\pm$ Ca$^{2+}$ and in the presence of indicated amounts of Triton X-100), myelin and SN$_4$ were solubilized and electrophoresed on slab gel (see Sulakhe et al., 1980a). Phosphorylated proteins and lipids were detected by autoradiography. SBP, small basic protein; LBP, large basic protein; R, regulatory subunit of cAMP kinase in membrane. A, B and C show the regions that likely represent lipid phosphorylation. B: Similar to A, except that myelin phosphorylation ($\pm$ Ca$^{2+}$) was carried out in the presence of varying amounts of MgCl$_2$ in assay. When present, Triton X-100 was 0.05%.

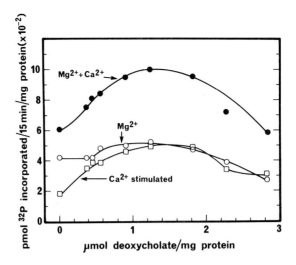

Fig. 9. Stimulation by deoxycholate of myelin phosphorylation. Myelin isolated according to Waehneldt et al. (1977) was phosphorylated in the absence and presence of varying amounts of deoxycholate. Membrane fraction was stored for 3 days at 4°C prior to assay.

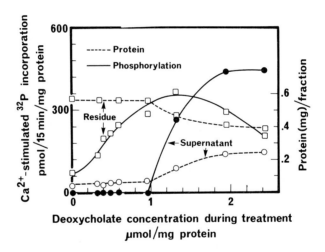

Fig. 10. Solubilization of $Ca^{2+}$-stimulated kinase by deoxycholate. Myelin was isolated according to Waehneldt et al. (1977) and after overnight storage at 4°C was exposed at 4°C to varying amounts of deoxycholate (600 $\mu$g protein, final volume of 0.15 ml). The tubes were then centrifuged (Beckman Airfuge), and the supernatant fluids and residues were assayed in the presence (50 $\mu$M) and absence of $Ca^{2+}$.

X-100, we have so far been able to solubilize only 30% of the total $Ca^{2+}$-stimulated kinase activity. This indicated that the enzyme is rather tightly bound to myelin and may in fact be an integral myelin protein.

*Protein kinase in peripheral nerve myelin*

Myelin-enriched fractions and myelin isolated from rat and mouse sciatic nerve (and cauda equina) showed the presence of basal and $Ca^{2+}$-stimulated protein kinase activities (Petrali and

Sulakhe, 1979; Sulakhe et al., 1980b). Triton X-100 markedly increased the kinase activity, especially that stimulated by $Ca^{2+}$ (Fig. 11). Amongst the membrane polypeptides $P_0$ ($M_r\, 28\,000$), which is a major glycoprotein, was mainly phosphorylated and $^{32}P$ incorporation into $P_0$ accounted for nearly 60% of the total incorporation. Other peptides, Y ($M_r\, 26\,000$), $P_1$ ($M_r\, 20\,000$) and $P_2$ ($M_r\, 16\,000$) were also phosphorylated. $Ca^{2+}$, in $\mu$M concentrations, augmented phosphorylation of these polypeptides. cAMP, on the other hand, failed to stimulate the phosphorylation of peripheral nerve myelin.

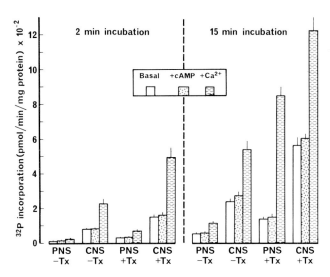

Fig. 11. Comparison of endogenous protein kinases in central and peripheral nerve myelin. Myelin preparations from rat brain stem white matter (CNS) and sciatic nerve (PNS) were phosphorylated in the absence and presence of Triton X-100 (Tx). When added, cAMP and $Ca^{2+}$ were 5 and 50 $\mu$M respectively. Phosphorylation was determined either by 2 min or 15 min incubation of the membrane fractions.

*Alterations in the phosphorylation of myelin from peripheral nervous system of genetically dystrophic mouse*

Besides abnormalities of skeletal muscle in genetically dystrophic mouse (dy/dy), abnormalities in some specific regions of the peripheral nervous system (PNS) have been recognized in this animal model of muscular dystrophy (e.g. Bradley and Jenkison, 1973). Myelin isolated from dorsal and ventral roots, but not from the sciatic nerve, of the dystrophic mouse shows a marked decrease in the glycoprotein, $P_0$ (Wiggins and Morell, 1978). We confirmed this observation. Additionally, we found marked decreases in the $Ca^{2+}$-stimulated phosphorylation of dystrophic myelin peptides, notably $P_0$, Y, $P_1$ and $P_2$. Such decreases could be detected in the myelin prepared from cauda equina (Fig. 12) but not from sciatic nerve, spinal cord or brain (Petrali and Sulakhe, 1980). Lower levels of $^{32}P$ incorporation in these peptides from the dystrophic myelin were seen even after taking into account the lowered contents of these polypeptides (Petrali and Sulakhe, 1980). This finding thus suggests that in the dy/dy mouse, besides its substrate proteins, the $Ca^{2+}$ kinase is also affected by the dystrophic process, at least in the later stages of the disease.

138

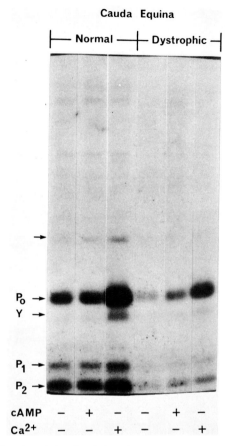

Fig. 12. Autoradiographic detection of phosphorylation of cauda equina myelin: comparison between normal and dystrophic mouse. Myelin was phosphorylated in the absence and presence of cAMP (5 $\mu$M) or Ca$^{2+}$ (50 $\mu$M). Note that P$_0$, a glycoprotein, and other myelin proteins (P$_1$, P$_2$ and Y) were phosphorylated. Ca$^{2+}$ but not cAMP promoted the phosphorylation. In dystrophic myelin, a much lower level of phosphorylation of these peptides was present.


## DISCUSSION

Two novel and potentially important observations concerning myelin protein kinases were made in this study: (1) the presence of Ca$^{2+}$-stimulatable kinase(s) in myelin prepared from the central and peripheral nervous systems of rodents and (2) low levels of cAMP kinase in multilamellar myelin, but higher levels in SN$_4$, isolated from rat brain white matter. The former observation deserves special comment.

Several lines of evidence indicate that, in freshly prepared myelin, stimulation by Ca$^{2+}$ of MBP phosphorylation is catalyzed by an endogenous kinase and requires the participation of calmodulin-like proteins that are also present in myelin. Thus a likely mechanism underlying the stimulatory action of Ca$^{2+}$ implicates the binding of Ca$^{2+}$ to calmodulin-like proteins. Ca$^{2+}$ then presumably alters the conformation of these proteins such that kinase activity is increased. This postulate is analogous to the postulated mechanism for Ca$^{2+}$-calmodulin-dependent stimulation of cAMP phosphodiesterase and many other recently discovered calmodulin-regulatable enzymes (see reviews by Cheung, 1980; Wang and Waisman, 1979). We noted that the calmodulin-requiring myelin kinase is labile such that its activity was markedly decreased (50–60%) by storage of the membranes for 1–3 days at 4°C. In fresh myelin, Triton X-100, in low concentrations, did not increase the activity of calmodulin-requiring kinase and, in high concentrations, was inhibitory. Interestingly, basal kinase was markedly stimulated by the detergent with the degree of stimulation dependent on the concentration of Triton X-100. Following storage of the membrane fraction, low concentrations of Triton X-100 did augment the intial rate of $Ca^{2+}$-stimulatable phosphorylation with the degree of stimulation depending on the concentrations of $Mg^{2+}$, ATP and $Ca^{2+}$ in the assay as well as the temperature and pH of the assay mixture. Basal kinase activity was stimulated, in fact, to a greater degree by the detergent in stored myelin preparations. Sodium deoxycholate also increased basal and $Ca^{2+}$-stimulatable kinase of stored myelin. An additional interesting finding was that in stored myelin membrane Triton X-100 restored the rate of $Ca^{2+}$-stimulated phosphorylation essentially to that observed in fresh myelin (assayed with or without the detergent present). However, it is difficult to explain the detergent-dependent increase in $Ca^{2+}$ kinase activity as resulting from higher activity of calmodulin-requiring kinase. For example, the detergent decreased the calmodulin-dependent stimulation of cAMP phsophodiesterase. Sharma (1981) recently suggested that Triton X-100 binds to calmodulin in the presence of $Ca^{2+}$ and thus likely inhibits the stimulation by calmodulin of cAMP phosphodiesterase. We further observed that Triton X-100 decreased the activity of $Ca^{2+}$-calmodulin-dependent protein kinase in synaptic membranes from rat cerebral cortex (Sulakhe et al., 1980c, 1981). In stored myelin preparations, a variety of inhibitors of calmodulin were either ineffective or their effects were detected only at higher concentrations in terms of inhibition of $Ca^{2+}$ kinase. These included (1) a heat-labile calmodulin binding protein ($BP_{80}$) (Wang et al., 1980); (2) EGTA; (3) phenothiazines (Weiss and Levin, 1978); and (4) W-7 (Hidaka et al., 1980). Additionally, Triton X-100-dependent stimulation of myelin $Ca^{2+}$ kinase was seen at the detergent concentrations > 0.01%, the concentrations which were inhibitory for calmodulin-dependent stimulation of cAMP phosphodiesterase. Thus, the possibility must be considered that in stored myelin preparations the detergent increases $Ca^{2+}$ kinase activity in a calmodulin-independent manner.

The properties of $Ca^{2+}$ kinase of stored myelin resembled in many regards the properties of a newly discovered, multifunctional $Ca^{2+}$ kinase that requires phospholipids for its activity. In rat brain, this kinase, termed kinase C (Takai et al., 1979), exists as an inactive proenzyme of $M_r$ 77 000. The active form of the kinase C is obtained by a controlled proteolytic cleavage (catalyzed by a specific $Ca^{2+}$-dependent protease) of the proenzyme and is of $M_r$ 55 000. In the presence of $Ca^{2+}$, kinase C is activated by reversible attachment to the membrane that contains the essential activating factor — namely phosphatidyl serine and phosphatidyl inositol (Nishizuka, this volume). Very recent work by Nishizuka and associates (Minakuchi et al., 1982) and Kuo and associates (personal communication) shows that isolated MBP is an excellent substrate for partially purified kinase C (prepared from rat brain and guinea pig heart). A further interesting finding is that kinase C shows no requirement for calmodulin but instead requires acidic phospholipids.

Several recent observations show that calmodulin-regulatable enzyme systems can be made calmodulin-independent by certain treatments. For example, the tryptic proteolysis of calmodulin-dependent cAMP phosphodiesterase converts it to $Ca^{2+}$-calmodulin-independent form (see review by Klee, 1980). Incorporation of solubilized $Mg^{2+}$-$Ca^{2+}$-ATPase into phosphatidyl serine vesicles also renders the enzyme calmodulin-independent (Penniston et al., 1980). Thus it is possible that during storage of myelin, some proteolysis may have taken place, especially since myelin preparations are known to contain proteinase(s). This could explain the decreased activity of $Ca^{2+}$ kinase in stored myelin. Alternatively, the stimulatory effect of Triton X-100 on $Ca^{2+}$ kinase of stored myelin may result from interaction of the detergent with the myelin lipids. Since $Ca^{2+}$ binding to calmodulin reportedly increases the hydrophobicity of calmodulin and this, according to some investigators, mediates calmodulin-dependent activation of enzymes such as cAMP phosphodiesterase or $Mg^{2+}$-$Ca^{2+}$-ATPase. It may be then that Triton X-100 or exogenous phospholipids provide the necessary hydrophobic environment and render calmodulin-dependent enzymes either $Ca^{2+}$ and/or calmodulin-independent. Thus the lability of calmodulin-sensitive $Ca^{2+}$ kinase following myelin storage could well be due to decreased ability of $Ca^{2+}$ to augment hydrophobicity of myelin-associated calmodulin rather than the lability of the enzyme itself. Does this mean that stored myelin does not contain kinase C? While no clear-cut answer is available at present, inhibitory effects of high concentrations of phenothiazines would support the notion that kinase C is present in myelin. These drugs are known to bind to membrane phospholipids and thus could interfere with the phospholipid dependence of membrane enzymes such as kinase C of myelin. Table II

TABLE II

COMPARISON BETWEEN $Ca^{2+}$-STIMULATED PHOSPHORYLATION OF MBP IN FRESH AND STORED MYELIN AND PARTIALLY PURIFIED KINASE C

|  | Fresh myelin | Stored myelin | Kinase C |
|---|---|---|---|
| Triton X-100 |  |  |  |
| low concentrations | Marginal or no stimulation | Stimulation | Stimulation * |
| high concentrations | Inhibition | Inhibition | Not known |
| Trifluoperazine or chlorpromazine |  |  |  |
| low concentrations | Not known | No effect | No effect |
| high concentrations | Not known | Inhibition | Inhibition |
| Exogenous calmodulin | Stimulation | No effect | No effect |
| Heat-labile calmodulin-binding protein | Not known | No effect | No effect |
| EGTA | Inhibition | Marginal inhibition or no effect | No effect |
| MBP | Excellent substrate (endogenous) | Excellent substrate (endogenous) | Excellent substrate (exogenous) |
| Affinity for $Ca^{2+}$ | 6–8 $\mu$M | 6–8 $\mu$M | 3–5 $\mu$M |
| Phospholipids | Already present | Already present | Required |

* Data on kinase C are taken from various publications by Nishizuka and associates and Kuo and associates.

provides the comparison between the kinase C and $Ca^{2+}$ kinases of fresh and stored myelin. It is interesting that $Ca^{2+}$ kinase of stored myelin resembles the kinase C in many of its properties. Thus, it is indeed difficult to exclude the presence of kinase C in myelin preparations. Further work is undoubtedly required to establish this view.

In our study, we determine the phosphorylation of MBP by endogenous kinase activity. Thus, the rates and maximal capacity of MBP phosphorylation assume that serine and/or threonine residues of MBP are "vacant", i.e. in unphosphorylated from (also see Petrali et al., 1980). However, this may not be correct since isolated MBP contains phosphorus (Mc Namara and Appel, 1977). Further, there are differences in the location of phosphorylated serines, when in vivo and in vitro phosphorylation of MBP is compared (Carnegie et al., 1974; Chou et al., 1976). While MBP contains about 26 phosphorylatable amino acid residues (serines and threonines), only one (Ser-55) is phosphorylated by endogenous kinase(s) (Carnegie et al., 1974). On the other hand a large amount of phosphorylation (up to 30 moles/mole) of isolated (soluble) basic protein is catalyzed by exogenous kinase A (Yourist et al., 1978), which undoubtedly must be due to phosphorylation of serines, threonines, as well as some other amino acid residues (Smith et al., 1976). In addition, the possibility exists that different serine residues of MBP undergo phosphorylation by various myelin-associated kinases.

Our study shows a much lower content of kinase A in typical multilamellar myelin fractions whereas it is considerable in myelin-like membrane ($SN_4$). These and other observations (e.g. marginal stimulation of MBP phosphorylation by cyclic nucleotides) support the view that MBP is a poor substrate for myelin-associated kinase A. Recently, Kuo and associates (personal communication) arrived at a similar conclusion. It is still possible that in the cell kinase A phosphorylates MBP, however, our in vitro studies so far do not lend support to this view.

While MBP is a major protein constituent of brain myelin, its exact location in myelin and its role in myelin structure or function are clearly speculative at this time. A number of excellent reviews address this issue (e.g. see Morell, 1977, and articles therein). Extensive work documents that MBP does interact with myelin lipids as well as another major protein of myelin — namely the proteolipid protein (PLP). Thus a number of studies have examined the amounts of MBP and PLP as well as their interaction in myelin obtained from various experimental and human diseases that involve or affect myelin (see Baumann, 1980, and articles therein). We have considered that MBP and PLP control the compaction of multilamellar myelin, assembly of myelin from its precursor membrane and permeability characteristics of myelin at least in some specific regions of axons. Any one or all of these regulatory functions of MBP can conceivably be influenced by the $Ca^{2+}$-stimulated phosphorylation of this critical protein. Further studies of myelin protein kinases thus should provide information of considerable potential value.

## SUMMARY

Myelin isolated from rat brain stem white matter contained endogenous $Mg^{2+}$-dependent protein kinase which selectively phosphorylated small (SBP) and large (LBP) myelin basic protein (MBP). $Ca^{2+}$, in $\mu$M concentrations, augmented the kinase-catalyzed phosphorylation of MBP. In freshly prepared myelin, calmodulin-like proteins, which are present in the membrane, are required for the stimulatory effect of $Ca^{2+}$ on MBP phosphorylation. Triton X-100 increased the $Ca^{2+}$-stimulated MBP phosphorylation, especially in stored myelin preparations. Several lines of evidence suggested that in stored membrane fractions $Ca^{2+}$-stimulated kinase, which is calmodulin-independent, is present. The properties of such kinase resembled in many regards a newly discovered phospholipid-dependent $Ca^{2+}$-stimulated kinase (kinase C) by Nishizuka and associates from rat brain cytosolic fraction. Thus, myelin appears to contain two types of $Ca^{2+}$-stimulated kinases that utilize the same substrate protein, namely MBP. Many characteristics of the two $Ca^{2+}$-stimulated kinases are described. In a multilamellar myelin, cAMP-stimulated kinase is barely detectable; this kinase, however, is considerably enriched in a myelin-like membrane, termed $SN_4$. Both in myelin and $SN_4$, cAMP kinase appears to be buried in the membrane matrix. Peripheral nerve myelin also

142

contained $Mg^{2+}$-dependent protein kinase, two types of $Ca^{2+}$-stimulated kinases and low amount of cAMP kinase. In this case, $P_0$, a glycoprotein, and other basic proteins ($P_1$ and $P_2$) served as substrates for peripheral nerve myelin kinases. In later stages of genetic muscular dystrophy in dy/dy mouse, there was a marked and selective reduction in the $Ca^{2+}$-stimulated phosphorylation of peripheral nerve proteins in cauda equina myelin preparations.

## ACKNOWLEDGEMENTS

This work is supported by a grant (to PVS) from the Medical Research Council of Canada. Dr. E. Petrali was a post-doctoral fellow of the Canadian Muscular Dystrophy Association. Many thanks are due to Ms. Brenda Thiessen, Ms. Barbara Raney and Ms. Rose Wsiaki for their able assistance in various aspects of this study and to Mr. Robert Hutchinson, for illustrations. We are grateful to Drs. J.H. Wang and R.K. Sharma (University of Manitoba, Winnipeg) for the generous supply of calmodulin-deficient cAMP phosphodiesterase, calmodulin and calmodulin-binding proteins.

## REFERENCES

Baumann, N. (1980) *Neurological Mutations Affecting Myelination,* INSERM Symp. No. 14, Elsevier/North-Holland, Amsterdam.

Bonner, W.M. and Laskey, R.A. (1974) A film detection method for tritium labelled proteins and nucleic acids in polyacrylamide gels. *Eur. J. Biochem.,* 46: 83–88.

Bradley, W.G. and Jenkison, M. (1973) Abnormalities of peripheral nerves in murine muscular dystrophy. *J. neurol. Sci.,* 18: 227–247.

Carnegie, P.R., Dunkley, P.R., Kemp, B.E. and Murray, A.W. (1974) Phosphorylation of selected serine and threonine residues in myelin basic protein by endogenous and exogenous protein kinases. *Nature (Lond.),* 249: 147–150.

Cheung, W.Y. (1971) Cyclic 3',5'-nucleotide phosphodiesterase: Evidence for the properties of a protein activator. *J. biol. Chem.,* 246: 2859–2869.

Cheung, W.Y. (1980) Calmodulin plays a pivotal role in cellular regulation. *Science,* 207: 19–27.

Chou, F.C.H., Chou, C.H.J., Shapira, R. and Kibler, R.F. (1976) Basis of microheterogeneity of myelin basic protein. *J. biol. Chem.,* 251: 2671–2679.

Endo, T. and Hidaka, H. (1980) $Ca^{2+}$-calmodulin dependent phosphorylation of myelin isolated from rabbit brain. *Biochem. biophys. Res. Commun.,* 97: 553–558.

Golds, E.E. and Braun, P.E. (1978) Cross-linking studies on the conformation and dimerization of myelin basic protein in solution. *J. biol. Chem.,* 253: 8171–8177.

Gwarsha, K., Rumsby, M.G. and Little, C. (1980) Phospholipase C *(Bacillus cereus)* digestion of phospholipids in myelin isolated from central nervous tissue: Removal of myelin basic protein increase exposure of lipids to the enzyme. *Biochem. Soc. Trans.,* 8: 601–602.

Hidaka, H., Yamaki, T., Naka, M., Tanaka, T., Hayashi, H. and Kobayashi, R. (1980) Calcium-regulated modulator protein interacting agents inhibit smooth muscle calcium-stimulated protein kinase and ATPase. *Mol. Pharmacol.,* 17: 66–72.

Itano, T., Itano, R. and Penniston, J.T. (1980) Interactions of basic polypeptides and proteins with calmodulin. *Biochem. J.,* 189: 455–459.

Klee, C. (1980) Calmodulin: Structure: function relationships. In *Calcium and Cell Function,* W.Y. Cheung (Ed.), Academic Press, New York, pp. 59–77.

Kuo, J.F., Andersson, R.G.G., Wise, B.C., Mackerlova, L., Salomonsson, I., Brackett, N.L., Katoh, N., Shoji, M. and Wrenn, R.W. (1980) Calcium-dependent protein kinase: Widespread occurrence in various tissues and phyla of the animal kingdom and comparison of effects of phospholipid, calcium and trifluoperazine. *Proc. nat. Acad. Sci. (Wash.),* 77: 7039–7043.

Laemmli, U.K. (1970) Cleavage of structural proteins during the assembly of the head of bacteriophage T4. *Nature (Lond.),* 227: 680–685.

McNamara, J.O. and Appel, S.H. (1977) Myelin basic protein phosphatase activity in rat brain. *J. Neurochem.*, 29: 27–35.

Minakuchi, R., Takai, Y., Yu, B. and Nishizuka, Y. (1981) Widespread occurrence of calcium-activated, phospholipid-dependent protein kinase in mammalian tissues. *J. Biochem.*, 89: 1651–1654.

Miyamoto, E. (1975) Protein kinases in myelin of rat brain: solubilization and characterization. *J. Neurochem.*, 24: 503–512.

Miyamoto, E. (1976) Phosphorylation of endogenous proteins in myelin of rat brain. *J. Neurochem.*, 26: 573–577.

Miyamoto, E. and Kakiuchi, S. (1974a) In vitro and in vivo phosphorylation of myelin basic protein by cerebral protein kinase. *Nature (Lond.)*, 249: 150–151.

Miyamoto, E. and Kakiuchi, S. (1974b) In vitro and in vivo phosphorylation of myelin basic protein by exogenous and endogenous adenosine 3′:5′-monophosphate-dependent protein kinase in brain. *J. biol. Chem.*, 249: 2769–2777.

Miyamoto, E., Miyazaki, K., Hirose, R. and Kashiba, A. (1978) Multiple forms of protein kinases in myelin and microsomal fractions of boveine brain. *J. Neurochem.*, 31: 269–275.

Morell, P. (1977) *Myelin,* Plenum Press, New York.

Mori, T., Takai, Y., Minakuchi, R., Yu, B. and Nishizuka, Y. (1980) Inhibitory action of chlorpromazine, dibucaine, and other phospholipid-interacting drugs on calcium-activated, phospholipid-dependent protein kinase. *J. biol. Chem.*, 255: 8378–8380.

Penniston, J.T., Graf, E., Niggli, V. Verma, A.K. and Carafoli, E. (1980) The plasma membrane calcium ATPase. In *Calcium Binding Proteins: Structure and Function,* F.L. Siegel, E. Carafoli, R.H. Kretsinger, D.H. MacLennan and R.H. Wasserman (Eds.), Elsevier/North-Holland, New York, pp. 23–30.

Petrali, E.H. and Sulakhe, P.V. (1979) Calcium ion stimulated endogenous protein kinase catalyzed phosphorylation of peripheral nerve myelin proteins. *Can. J. Physiol. Pharmacol.*, 57: 1200–1204.

Petrali, E.H. and Sulakhe, P.V. (1980) Calcium ion stimulated endogenous protein kinase catalyzed phosphorylation of peripheral and central nerve myelin proteins: Comparison between normal and genetically dystrophic mouse. *Enzyme*, 25: 102–105.

Petrali, E.H., Thiessen, B.J. and Sulakhe, P.V. (1978) Phosphorylation of myelin basic proteins. (Abstr.). In *Proc. 23rd Ann. Psych. Res. Meeting,* pp. 33–34.

Petrali, E.H., Thiessen, B.J. and Sulakhe, P.V. (1980) Characteristics of magnesium-dependent $Ca^{2+}$-stimulated endogenous protein kinase-catalyzed phosphorylation of basic proteins in myelin isolated from rat brain stem white matter. *Arch. Biochem. Biophys.*, 205: 520–535.

Pomerantz, A.H., Rudolph, S.A., Haley, B.E. and Greengard, P. (1975) Photoaffinity labeling of a protein kinase from bovine brain with 8-azidoadenosine 3′,5′-monophosphate. *Biochemistry*, 14: 3858–3862.

Rumsby, M.G., Riekkinen, P.J. and Arstila, A.V. (1970) A critical evaluation of myelin preparations. Non-specific esterase activity associated with central nerve myelin preparations. *Brain Res.*, 24: 495–516.

Schulman, H., Hunter, W.B. and Greengard, P. (1980) Calcium-dependent protein phosphorylation in mammalian brain and other tissues. In *Calcium and Cell Function,* Vol. I, W.Y. Cheung (Ed.), Academic Press, New York, pp. 219–252.

Sharma, R.K. (1981) Inhibition of cyclic nucleotide phosphodiesterase by calmodulin and Triton X-100 complex. *Fed. Proc.*, 40: 1739 (Abstr.).

Smith, L.S., Kern, C.W., Halpern, R.M. and Smith, R.A. (1976) Phosphorylation on basic amino acids in myelin basic protein. *Biochem. biophys. Res. Commun.*, 71: 459–465.

Steck, A.J. and Appel, S.H. (1974) Phosphorylation of myelin basic protein. *J. biol. Chem.*, 249: 5416–5420.

Sulakhe, P.V., Petrali, E.H. and Thiessen, B.J. (1978) Calcium ion-stimulated endogenous protein kinase catalyzed phosphorylation of myelin and its basic proteins. *Soc. Neurosci. Abstr.*, 4: 249.

Sulakhe, P.V., Petrali, E.H., Davis, E.R. and Thiessen, B.J. (1980a) Calcium ion stimulated endogenous protein kinase catalyzed phosphorylation of basic proteins in myelin subfractions and myelin-like membrane fraction from rat brain. *Biochemistry*, 19: 5363–5371.

Sulakhe, P.V., Petrali, E.H., Thiessen, B.J. and Davis, E.R. (1980b) Calcium ion-stimulated phosphorylation of myelin proteins. *Biochem. J.*, 186: 469–473.

Sulakhe, P.V., Petrali, E.H. and Harley, D.L. (1980c) Is myelin basic protein a calmodulin binding protein? In *Calcium-Binding Proteins: Structure and Function,* Vol. 14, F.L. Siegel, E. Carafoli, R.H. Kretsinger, D.H. MacLennan and R.H. Wasserman (Eds.), Elsevier/North-Holland, New York, pp. 239–240.

Sulakhe, P.V., Petrali, E.H. and Raney, B.L. (1981) A highly active calcium ion stimulated endogenous protein kinase in myelin: Kinetic and other characteristics, calmodulin dependence and comparison with other brain kinase(s). In *Calmodulin and Intracellular $Ca^{2+}$-receptors,* H. Hidaka and S. Kakiuchi (Eds.), Plenum Press, New York, in press.

Takai, Y., Kishimoto, A., Ionue, M. and Nishizuka, Y. (1979) Calcium-dependent activation of a multifunctional protein kinase by membrane phospholipids. *J. biol. Chem.*, 254: 3692–3695.

Waehneldt, T.V., Matthieu, J.-M. and Neuhoff, V. (1977) Characterization of a myelin-related fraction (SN₄) isolated from rat forebrain at two developmental stages. *Brain Res.,* 138: 29–43.

Wang, J.H. and Waisman, D.M. (1979) Calmodulin and its role in the second messenger system. *Curr. Top. cell. Regul.,* 15, 47–107.

Wang, J.H., Sharma, R.K. and Tam, S.W. (1980) Calmodulin-binding proteins. In *Calcium and Cell Function,* Vol. I, W.Y. Cheung (Ed.), Academic Press, New York, pp. 305–328.

Weiss, B. and Levin, R.M. (1978) Mechanism for selectively inhibiting the activation of cyclic nucleotide phosphodiesterase and adenylate cyclase by antipsychotic agents. *Adv. cyclic Nucleot. Res.,* 9: 285–303.

Wiggins, R.C. and Morell, P. (1978) Myelin of the peripheral nerve of the dystrophic mouse. *J. Neurochem.,* 31: 1101–1105.

Wolff, D.J. and Brostrom, C.O. (1976) $Ca^{2+}$-dependent cyclic nucleotide phosphodiesterase from brain: Identification of phospholipids as calcium-independent activators. *Arch. Biochem. Biophys.,* 173: 720–731.

Wrenn, R.W., Katoh, N., Wise, B.C. and Kuo, J.F. (1980) Stimulation by phosphatidylserine and calmodulin dependent phosphorylation of endogenous proteins from cerebral cortex. *J. biol. Chem.,* 255: 12042–12046.

Yourist, J.E., Ahmad, F. and Brady, A.H. (1978) Solubilization and partial characterization of a phosphoprotein phosphatase from human myelin. *Biochim. biophys. Acta,* 522: 452–464.

# The Regulation of Enzyme Activity by Reversible Phosphorylation

D. GRAHAME HARDIE and PAUL S. GUY

*Department of Biochemistry, University of Dundee, Medical Sciences Institute, Dundee, DD1 4HN, Scotland*

## INTRODUCTION

It will be evident from an inspection of the other articles in this volume that protein phosphorylation is a regulatory mechanism which is of great significance to brain function. The various cell types in the brain contain very active protein kinases and phosphatases, some of which appear to be brain-specific, and others of which are present in much higher concentration in brain than in other tissues. It is also clear that the state of phosphorylation of many brain proteins changes in a physiologically relevant manner. However, in most cases the function of these protein phosphorylation events in the brain is not understood. This is undoubtedly due to the inherent technical difficulty in reconstituting in vitro complex processes such as neurotransmission. By contrast, the experimenter working in intermediary metabolism has a much easier task, since it is usually straightforward to study the activity of a soluble enzyme in vitro. It is therefore not surprising that our understanding of the role of protein phosphorylation is most advanced in this area, and that the regulation of intermediary metabolism serves as a model which guides the study of other systems in which protein phosphorylation may play a regulatory role.

In this article we will very briefly review the scope and importance of protein phosphorylation in metabolism, and will then discuss in more detail the experimental criteria which should be met to establish the role of reversible phosphorylation in a particular regulatory system. We will consider in particular some of the techniques that may be used, and also some of the problems that may be encountered. The discussion will be illustrated with examples drawn mainly from our own system, which is the regulation of fatty acid synthesis, but we shall refer to other systems, where appropriate, to indicate the generality of a particular phenomenon. It is hoped that experience gained in the study of a relatively simple system such as ours will be of value to experimenters working in the more technically demanding area of brain function.

Readers who require a more comprehensive treatment of enzyme regulation by protein phosphorylation should refer to the excellent review by Krebs and Beavo (1979), and to articles in the recent volume edited by Cohen (1980a).

## PROTEIN PHOSPHORYLATION AND ITS ROLE IN INTERMEDIARY METABOLISM

Table I gives a list of enzymes in intermediary metabolism which have now been shown to be regulated by reversible phosphorylation. The list is not intended to be comprehensive and

TABLE I

EXAMPLES OF ENZYMES OF INTERMEDIARY METABOLISM REGULATED BY REVERSIBLE PHOSPHORYLATION IN RESPONSE TO EXTRACELLULAR SIGNALS

| Enzyme | Extracellular signal(s) | Multiple phosphorylation? | Effect | References |
|---|---|---|---|---|
| Phosphorylase (muscle) | Nervous impulse, β-agonists | − | $K_a\downarrow K_i\uparrow$ | Fletterick and Madsen (1980) |
| Phosphorylase kinase (muscle) | Nervous impulse, β-agonists | ✓ | $K_a\downarrow V_{max}\uparrow$ | Cohen (1980b) |
| Glycogen synthase | Insulin, Glucagon, β-agonists, α-agonists, vasopressin | ✓ | $K_a\uparrow$ | Embi et al. (1980) |
| Pyruvate kinase (L) | Glucagon, α-agonists | − | $K_m\uparrow, K_a\uparrow, K_i\downarrow$ | Engström (1980) |
| Pyruvate dehydrogenase | Insulin | ✓ | $V_{max}\downarrow$ | Denton and Hughes (1978) |
| Acetyl-CoA carboxylase | Insulin, glucagon, β-agonists, α-agonists, vasopressin | ✓ | $K_a\uparrow, V_{max}\downarrow$ | Hardie and Guy (1980) |
| Glycerol phosphate acyltransferase | β-agonists | ? | ↓ | Nimmo and Houston (1978) |
| Hormone sensitive lipase | β-agonists, insulin | ? | ↑ | Nilsson et al. (1980) |
| Hydroxymethylglutaryl-CoA reductase | Insulin, glucagon | ? | $V_{max}\downarrow$ | Ingebritsen and Gibson (1980) |
| Hydroxymethylglutaryl-CoA reductase kinase | Insulin, glucagon | ? | ↑ | Ingebritsen and Gibson (1980) |
| Phenylalanine hydroxylase | Glucagon | ? | ↑ | Donlon and Kaufman (1978) |

Where detailed kinetics have not been carried out, the effect on enzyme activity is indicated by an arrow (↑, activation; ↓, inactivation).

mainly reflects our own interest in the metabolism of body fuels. We have also omitted certain enzymes which are known to be phosphorylated in vivo but where the function of this modification is not yet clear. We would like to make several general points from this table. Firstly, it is now very clear that protein phosphorylation as a regulatory device is ubiquitous in nature, at least in metabolism. Table I includes examples of enzymes in carbohydrate, lipid and amino acid metabolism. Protein phosphorylation is as general a mechanism as allosteric regulation, and usually the key regulatory enzyme in a pathway is subject to both types of control. Allosteric regulation is the mechanism by which the pathway responds to purely local changes in metabolite levels. By contrast, all of the protein phosphorylation systems in Table I are triggered by a hormonal or nervous stimulus, i.e. by information initiated at a site remote from the target cell itself.

The allosteric and covalent levels of control may interact, as is revealed by the final column of Table I. In some cases the effect of protein phosphorylation is to change the maximum velocity ($V$) for the reaction catalysed, in which case an effect will be observed no matter what the concentration of allosteric effectors. Perhaps more common is the other case in which $V$ is unchanged but there exists what may be called a "$K$ effect". Thus, phosphorylation may affect the $K_m$ for a substrate, e.g. phosphoenolpyruvate and liver pyruvate kinase (Ekman et al., 1976); the $K_A$ for an allosteric activator, e.g. glucose 6-phosphate and glycogen synthase (Larner and Villar-Palasi, 1971); or the $K_I$ for an allosteric inhibitor, e.g. ATP and phosphorylase (Fischer et al., 1970). If protein phosphorylation acts via a $K$ effect, then the overall result of phosphorylation will depend on the levels of substrate and/or allosteric effectors within the cell. A second type of interaction between allosteric and covalent modification is the case where the presence of an allosteric effector may modulate the rate of phosphorylation or dephosphorylation of the enzyme. A good example here is the inhibition of the phosphorylation of liver pyruvate kinase by its allosteric activator, fructose-1,6-bisphosphate (El-Maghrabi et al., 1980).

Another observation one may make from the data summarised in Table I is the frequency with which multiple phosphorylation occurs. In many cases a single protein kinase may phosphorylate more than one site, with phosphorylation of the additional sites having no direct effect on enzyme activity, e.g. phosphorylation of phosphorylase kinase by cyclic AMP-(cAMP) dependent protein kinase (Cohen, 1973) and phosphorylation of pyruvate dehydrogenase by pyruvate dehydrogenase kinase (Yeaman et al., 1978; Sugden et al., 1979). Alternatively, a particular enzyme may be phosphorylated by more than one protein kinase at different sites. The classic example of this is muscle glycogen synthase which can be phosphorylated by five distinct protein kinases at up to seven sites (Cohen et al., 1982). While the phosphorylation of all of these sites has not yet been demonstrated in vivo, this extreme case of multiple phosphorylation may represent the means by which a series of different extracellular signals can independently regulate the activity of a single enzyme.

In view of the common occurrence of multiple phosphorylation among the enzymes of intermediary metabolism, it seems reasonable to expect its occurrence among other classes of protein. It certainly occurs in the brain, as the chapter in this volume on the protein 1 system will indicate. The moral to be drawn from this observation is that measurement of the total level of phosphorylation of a protein may only represent a crude reflection of the phosphorylation state of individual sites.

# CRITERIA FOR ESTABLISHING THE ROLE OF PROTEIN PHOSPHORYLATION IN A PHYSIOLOGICAL EFFECT

If one had to summarise in one sentence the role of protein phosphorylation in the regulation of intermediary metabolism, one might say that it represents a means by which an extracellular signal (e.g. a hormone) can modulate or override the cell's internal control systems. This appears to be true of all the examples listed in Table I, although the mechanisms by which the hormones elicit the change in phosphorylation have not in every case been clarified. However, it must be said that just because a protein has been shown to be phosphorylated reversibly, either in vivo or in vitro, one cannot automatically ascribe to this event the function given above. Other possibilities must also be considered, including the rather unsatisfactory conclusion that the phosphorylation event has no function. One common occurrence which must be considered is the formation of a phosphorylated intermediate in a reaction pathway. Unlike regulatory protein phosphorylations, these phosphorylated intermediates are usually acid-labile, but there are exceptions to this rule. Phosphoglucomutase has serine phosphate as a reaction intermediate, and therefore becomes phosphorylated to form an acid-stable derivative (Ray and Roscelli, 1964).

How then does one set about testing the hypothesis that a protein phosphorylation event is involved in the effect of an extracellular signal? Krebs (1973) proposed six criteria which should be met to establish the role of protein phosphorylation in an effect of cAMP. In the light of experience these criteria were later revised by Nimmo and Cohen (1977) and by Krebs and Beavo (1979). For the remainder of this article we will discuss the application of these criteria. Since cAMP represents only one of a family of second messengers which may mediate the effect of an extracellular signal, and bearing in mind the prevalence of multiple phosphorylation by multiple protein kinases, these criteria perhaps need restating in a more general form. We have, therefore, adapted the criteria of Nimmo and Cohen, which may be restated as follows:

A protein kinase/phosphatase system may be considered to be involved in the effect of an extracellular signal if: (1) the extracellular signal produces a reversible change in the function of a protein in vivo or in an intact cell system; (2) the protein kinase/phosphatase produces a similar reversible change in function of the protein in a reconstituted system in vitro; (3) the protein kinase or phosphatase phosphorylates or dephosphorylates the protein in vitro at a rate sufficient to explain the effect of the extracellular signal in vivo or in an intact cell system; (4) the protein is phosphorylated or dephosphorylated in vivo or in an intact cell system, in response to the extracellular signal, at the same site phosphorylated or dephosphorylated by the protein kinase or phosphatase in vitro.

How then does one apply these criteria? For the remainder of this article we will discuss the techniques that may be used, their advantages and drawbacks, and some of the problems that may be encountered. The points that are discussed reflect our own experiences in studies of the effect of adrenaline on fatty acid synthesis in adipose tissue.

## THE FIRST CRITERION

*The extracellular stimulus produces a reversible change in the function of a protein in vivo or in an intact cell system*

This may at first sight seem the easiest of the four criteria to satisfy, but often the reverse is true. It may perhaps be relatively straightforward to demonstrate an effect of an extracellular signal on an intracellular process, e.g. fatty acid synthesis. The difficulty, of course, lies in pinning the effects of an extracellular signal down to a particular protein, or combination of proteins. The rate of fatty acid synthesis in a tissue may be reliably estimated by measuring the rate of incorporation of tritium from $^3H_2O$ into total fatty acid, a method which provides an absolute measure of the rate of fatty acid synthesis from any precursor (Jungas, 1968). The effects of various hormones on fatty acid synthesis are summarised in Table II, with all of these

TABLE II

EFFECTS OF HORMONES ON THE RATE OF FATTY ACID SYNTHESIS IN VIVO OR IN INTACT CELLS

| Hormone | Experimental system | Effect | References |
|---------|--------------------|--------|-----------|
| Glucagon | Rat liver in vivo | ↓ | Cook et al. (1977) |
| | Chicken liver cells | ↓ | Watkins et al. (1977) |
| | Rat liver cells | ↓ | Geelen et al. (1978) |
| Adrenaline | Perfused mouse liver | ↓ | Ma et al. (1977) |
| | Rat adipose tissue pieces | ↓ | Cahill et al. (1960) |
| Insulin | Rat liver in vivo | ↑ | Stansbie et al. (1976) |
| | Rat liver cells | ↑ | Geelen et al. (1978) |
| | Rat adipose tissue in vivo | ↑ | Stansbie et al. (1976) |
| | Rat brown adipose tissue in vivo | ↑ | McCormack and Denton (1977) |
| Vasopressin | Perfused mouse liver | ↓ | Ma and Hems (1975) |
| Angiotensin II | Perfused mouse liver | ↓ | Ma et al. (1977) |

effects being observed within minutes of addition of hormone to the tissue. These conclusions are drawn from numerous experiments either in vivo, with perfused organs, with tissue slices, or with isolated cells, and a discussion of the relative merits of these experimental systems is beyond the scope of this article. Although we are working in this laboratory on all of these hormonal effects, we will concentrate in this article on the effect of adrenaline in adipose tissue, for which the most complete information is available. How does one determine the site of action of adrenaline on fatty acid synthesis within the adipose cell? In studies of intermediary metabolism, three general approaches have been used to identify sites of regulation. The first is to measure the levels of intermediates in the pathway under the different regulatory states. Newsholme and Gevers (1967) and Newsholme (1980) have discussed this approach in detail. An enzyme is considered to be regulated if it catalyses a non-equilibrium step in the cell and if the concentration of its substrates changes in the opposite direction to a change in flux through the pathway. While this approach can provide perhaps the most rigorous evidence for regulation of a particular step, there are often major technical difficulties in the determination of metabolite levels. Thus the major metabolites of fatty acid synthesis, e.g. acetyl-CoA, are distributed between different cell compartments, and some may also be largely protein bound, which makes it currently impossible to estimate their free concentration in the relevant cell compartment with any certainty.

A second approach is to provide an intact cell system with metabolites which occur at various points along the metabolic pathway, and see if the effect of the extracellular signal still occurs. If the effect no longer occurs, then regulation must be exerted at a point preceding that metabolite in the pathway. The major problem with this approach is the lack of permeability of intact plasma membrane to most metabolites, which severely restricts its use.

A third approach is to treat intact cells with the extracellular signal, homogenise, and determine the activity of individual enzymes in the cell-free extract. This approach has been used successfully to identify one site of action of adrenaline on fatty acid synthesis in adipose tissue as the enzyme acetyl-CoA carboxylase. Table III shows the effect of adrenaline treatment of isolated adipocytes on the kinetic properties of acetyl-CoA carboxylase measured in a cell-free extract. It seems reasonable to conclude that adrenaline also affects the activity of the enzyme in the intact cell, although one must be aware that changes in the properties of the enzyme may easily occur during or after homogenisation. It can also be seen from the data in Table III that incubation of the cell-free extracts with magnesium and calcium ions entirely reverses the effects of adrenaline on enzyme activity. This reversal is almost certainly the result of activation of endogenous protein phosphatases by the divalent cations. The important point in this context is that these data show that the apparent effect of adrenaline on enzyme activity is not due simply to different recoveries of acetyl-CoA carboxylase activity during preparation of the extract, or to some irreversible process such as proteolysis.

TABLE III

REVERSIBLE EFFECT OF ADRENALINE ON ACETYL-CoA CARBOXYLASE ACTIVITY IN ISOLATED ADIPOCYTES

|  |  | $V$ (mU/g wet wt.) | $K_A$ citrate (mM) |
|---|---|---|---|
| Fresh extract | Control | $114 \pm 3$ | $0.77 \pm 0.15$ |
|  | Adrenaline | $85 \pm 2$ | $1.53 \pm 0.17$ |
| After incubation with $Mg^{2+}$ and $Ca^{2+}$ | Control | $116 \pm 3$ | $0.32 \pm 0.09$ |
|  | Adrenaline | $113 \pm 2$ | $0.43 \pm 0.06$ |

Results are expressed as mean $\pm$ S.E.M. of 30 observations.
Date reproduced from Brownsey et al. (1979).

While these results establish that adrenaline inactivates acetyl-CoA carboxylase reversibly in isolated adipocytes, they do not of course prove that a protein phosphorylation is involved. They do not even prove that a covalent modification is involved. One might argue that a non-covalent (i.e. allosteric) effect would be lost by dilution during homogenisation and enzyme assay, especially in the case of adipocytes where homogenisation dilutes the cell contents by several 100-fold. However, the effects of a tight-binding allosteric effector can survive such treatment. Glucagon brings about phosphorylation of the enzyme phosphofructokinase in the liver (Kagimoto and Uyeda, 1979) and also inactivates the enzyme by increasing the $K_m$ for the substrate, fructose 6-phosphate (Castano et al., 1979; Pilkis et al., 1979). It would be logical to connect these two events: however it is now clear that the effects of glucagon are mediated by a novel allosteric effector, fructose 2,6-bisphosphate (Van Schaftingen et al., 1980; Pilkis et al., 1981). This allosteric effector activates the enzyme at sub-micromolar concentrations, and the effects of glucagon treatment of isolated liver cells are not readily reversed by desalting either by dialysis or gel filtration. In order to establish that a covalent modification such as phosphorylation is involved in the effect of an extracellular signal, it is therefore necessary to apply the remaining three criteria.

# THE SECOND CRITERION

*The protein kinase/phosphatase produces a similar reversible change in function of the protein in a reconstituted system in vitro*

A direct demonstration of a change in function of the protein concomitant with phosphorylation or dephosphorylation in a cell-free system is clearly essential. This is usually achieved initially in a crude or partially purified system, as was the case with acetyl-CoA carboxylase (Carlson and Kim, 1973). The effect should be time-dependent and, for a putative phosphorylation event, should be Mg-ATP-dependent. One complication of a crude or partially purified system is that phosphorylation may occur on addition of Mg-ADP due to the presence of contaminating adenylate kinase.

A time-dependent and Mg-ATP-dependent effect on the function of a protein in a crude or partially purified system represents a preliminary indication that a protein phosphorylation may be involved, but there are often other explanations for such an effect. Acetyl-CoA carboxylase, for example, is under certain conditions inactivated in a time-dependent manner on incubation with Mg-ATP, due to the formation of the carboxylated enzyme intermediate, which readily dissociates to inactive subunits in the absence of the allosteric activator, citrate (Lane et al., 1974). This occurs even with the homogenous enzyme in the complete absence of any protein phosphorylation. It is therefore essential that the effect is shown to occur only in the presence of the protein fraction containing the putative protein kinase or phosphatase. If the protein kinase or phosphatase involved has a specific inhibitor, then a further control experiment should show that the effect is blocked by the presence of the inhibitor. For example, the activation of rabbit mammary acetyl-CoA carboxylase produced by addition of rabbit muscle protein phosphatase-1 is blocked by inhibitor-2, a heat-stable protein that is a very potent and specific inhibitor of this protein phosphatase (Hardie and Cohen, 1979).

To study phosphorylation and dephosphorylation directly, incorporation of $^{32}$P from [$\gamma$-$^{32}$P]ATP into the protein or release of [$^{32}$P]phosphate from $^{32}$P-labelled protein must be measured. To explain a large effect on the function of the protein, phosphate must be incorporated in stoichiometric amounts. Since the stoichiometry will be affected by the number of phosphorylation sites, the possibility of multiple phosphorylation (see Section 2) should also be investigated. To obtain definitive answers, these studies must be carried out with the homogeneous protein, although less quantitative results may be obtained by isolating the protein from a cruder mixture using either an antibody, or some analytical procedure such as polyacrylamide gel electrophoresis in sodium dodecyl sulphate.

Fig. 1 shows results obtained in our laboratory using acetyl-CoA carboxylase purified to homogeneity from lactating rat mammary gland (Hardie and Guy, 1980). If the enzyme is incubated with [$\gamma$-$^{32}$P]ATP and the catalytic subunit of cAMP-dependent protein kinase, $^{32}$P is rapidly incorporated up to 1 molecule of phosphate per subunit of acetyl-CoA carboxylase, followed by a slower incorporation which approaches 2 molecules of phosphate per subunit. There is also a 60–70 % decrease in the activity of the enzyme which correlates with the rapid phase of phosphorylation. In the control experiment, the heat-stable protein inhibitor of cAMP-dependent protein kinase (Walsh et al., 1971) was added. This almost completely prevents both phosphorylation and inactivation (Fig. 1).

An important component of criterion 2 is the fact that the effect should be reversible. This is especially important in cases such as ours where phosphorylation leads to inactivation. There are many reasons, other than phosphorylation, why a protein should become inactivated, e.g. proteolysis, denaturation, oxidation of sulphhydryls, dissociation or aggregation of subunits.

152

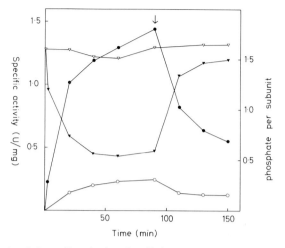

Fig. 1. Reversible phosphorylation and inactivation of purified rat mammary acetyl-CoA carboxylase by cAMP-dependent protein kinase and protein phosphatase-1. Acetyl-CoA carboxylase (0.82 mg/ml) was incubated with $[\gamma$-$^{32}$P]ATP and the catalytic subunit of cAMP-dependent protein kinase (7 U/ml). At the point indicated by the arrow, phosphorylation was blocked by the addition of excess protein kinase inhibitor, and protein phosphatase-1 was added to a final concentration of 20 U/ml. At various times aliquots were removed for estimation of $^{32}$P incorporation into protein (circles), and assay of acetyl-CoA carboxylase at 0.5 mM citrate (triangles). In the control experiment (open symbols) protein kinase inhibitor was added at zero time. Data reproduced from Hardie and Guy (1980).

One can rule out most of these other possibilities by demonstrating that one can reverse the effect by adding a protein phosphatase. Both the inactivation and the phosphorylation of acetyl-CoA carboxylase are reversed by addition of protein phosphatase-1 (Fig. 1). For laboratories which do not have access to purified protein phosphatases, it should be noted that commercial alkaline phosphatases are often effective in this regard, as was demonstrated by Nimmo and Houston (1978) for the enzyme glycerol phosphate acyl transferase.

The overall stoichiometry of phosphorylation, and the fact that complete reactivation is achieved without complete removal of $^{32}$P from the protein (Fig. 1) both suggest that acetyl-CoA carboxylase is phosphorylated at more than one site by cAMP-dependent protein kinase. This hypothesis was confirmed by peptide mapping (Fig. 2). If the amount of $^{32}$P radioactivity in the protein is determined by Cerekov counting of acid-insoluble pellets in microcentrifuge tubes, one can recover the samples after counting, digest with a proteolytic enzyme, and run peptide maps (Hardie and Guy, 1980). For $^{32}$P-labelled peptides, isoelectric focussing in thin-layer polyacrylamide gels, with detection by autoradiography, is an excellent technique which gives high resolution in a single dimension (Fig. 2). The results show that acetyl-CoA carboxylase is phosphorylated in one major site contained in a tryptic peptide of isoelectric point (pI) about 7, with several minor sites. The activity of the enzyme correlates inversely with the state of phosphorylation of the pI 7 peptide (cf. Figs. 1 and 2).

For proteins phosphorylated by cAMP-dependent protein kinase, trypsin is perhaps the best proteolytic enzyme to use for peptide mapping. This is because all known sites of phosphorylation for this protein kinase contain one or, more usually, two adjacent basic residues immediately N-terminal to the phosphorylated residues (Krebs and Beavo, 1979). It is therefore not possible to have two or more phosphorylation sites on the same tryptic peptide. This latter possibility may occur, however, with other protein kinases, e.g. pyruvate dehydrogenase kinase (Yeaman et al., 1978; Sugden et al., 1979) and glycogen synthase kinase-3

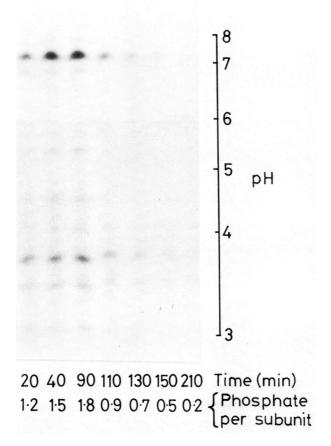

Fig. 2. Isoelectric focussing of tryptic peptides derived from purified rat mammary acetyl-CoA carboxylase during phosphorylation by cAMP-dependent protein kinase and dephosphorylation by protein phosphatase-1. Trichloroacetic acid-insoluble pellets of $^{32}$P-labelled protein were obtained from an experiment identical to that shown in Fig. 1. The pellets were performic acid oxidised, digested with trypsin, and subjected to isoelectric focussing in a 0.5 mm thin-layer polyacrylamide gel. The photograph shows an autoradiograph of the dried gel. The pH gradient was determined using a surface electrode immediately on completion of isoelectric focussing. The phosphatase was added immediately after the 90 min sample was taken.

(Rylatt et al., 1980). It is also worth noting that trypsin can generate more than one labelled peptide from a single site due to incomplete cleavage at a double basic sequence such as lys-arg (Parker et al., 1981).

While the above comments describe the ideal that should be attained to satisfy the second criterion, there are many problems and artifacts awaiting the experimenter who attempts to study the effect of phosphorylation or dephosphorylation in a highly purified system. There are several potential reasons why an effect observed in an intact cell system should apparently be lost on purification.

One possibility that may easily be tested is the common finding that an effect of phosphorylation is not observed under optimal assay conditions. As discussed in Section 2, in many cases phosphorylation acts via a "$K$ effect" and has no effect on maximal velocity. Fig. 3 shows the

154

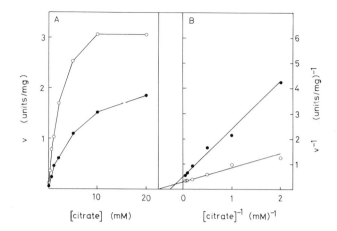

Fig. 3. Effect of phosphorylation by cAMP-dependent protein kinase on the citrate dependence of acetyl-CoA carboxylase. Acetyl-CoA carboxylase (0.82 mg/ml) was incubated with [γ-³²P]ATP and the catalytic subunit of cAMP-dependent protein kinase (7 U/ml) either with (open symbols) or without (closed symbols) excess protein kinase inhibitor. After 90 min at 30° C, the reaction was stopped by adding EDTA in slight excess of the total magnesium, and acetyl-CoA carboxylase activity was assayed at different citrate concentrations. (A) Direct plot; (B) reciprocal plot. Data reproduced from Hardie and Guy (1980).

dependence on the allosteric activator citrate of acetyl-CoA carboxylase which has been treated with or without cAMP-dependent protein kinase. Phosphorylation by the kinase produces a 2-fold increase in the $K_A$ for citrate, while only depressing maximal velocity slightly. It should be noted that this is very similar to the effect of adrenaline on acetyl-CoA carboxylase activity in isolated adipocytes (Table 3). In order to see a significant change in activity it is therefore necessary to use suboptimal citrate concentrations, as in Fig. 1. In other cases it may be necessary to use suboptimal substrate concentrations (e.g. pyruvate kinase; Ekman et al., 1976). Another important factor is pH — many enzyme assays are carried out at non-physiological pH. Thus muscle phosphorylase kinase is activated 40-fold by phosphorylation if the assay is carried out at the 'physiological'' pH of 6.8 but only 1.4-fold at the 'optimal'' pH of 8.2 (Cohen, 1973).

Another reason why phosphorylation may have no effect on the purified protein is the possibility that a change has occurred to the protein during purification. This may be a subtle change, such as oxidation of a sulphydryl, which may be very difficult to pin down. A very common problem with regulatory enzymes is the occurrence of limited proteolysis during the isolation of the enzyme. This often produces a form of the enzyme that is fully active, but has lost its regulatory potential. Muscle phosphorylase kinase is activated by limited proteolysis of the α subunit (Cohen, 1973). Since activation by phosphorylation is due to phosphorylation of the β subunit, it is possible to prepare a form of the enzyme which can still be phosphorylated but which is already fully activated. Limited proteolysis also mimics the effect of phosphorylation on glycogen synthase (Takeda and Larner, 1975) and liver pyruvate kinase (Bergström et al., 1978). In the latter case the proteolysis does not produce a visible change in the mobility of the subunit on polyacrylamide gel electrophoresis in sodium dodecyl sulphate. We have found that limited proteolysis of acetyl-CoA carboxylase has the opposite effect, i.e. it mimics dephosphorylation. Fig. 4 shows the effect of trypsin on the activity of acetyl-CoA carboxylase isolated from rabbit mammary gland in the presence of fluoride (Guy and Hardie, 1981). This preparation of the enzyme contains 6 moles of phosphate per mole of enzyme subunit and can

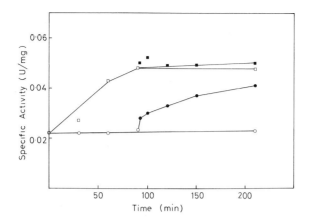

Fig. 4. Effect of protein phosphatase-1 and/or trypsin on acetyl-CoA carboxylase activity. Acetyl-CoA carboxylase was purified from rabbit mammary gland in the presence of fluoride, as described by Hardie and Cohen (1979). The enzyme (0.5 mg/ml) was incubated with or without protein phosphatase-1 (10 U/ml) and at 90 min trypsin was added to a portion of both incubations to a final concentration of 25 ng/ml. Aliquots were removed at various times for assay of acetyl-CoA carboxylase at 1 mM citrate. ○, control; □, + protein phosphatase-1; ●, control + trypsin; ■, + protein phosphatase-1 + trypsin. Data reproduced from Guy and Hardie (1981).

be activated by treatment with protein phosphatase-1 (Fig. 4), which reduces the phosphate to 4 moles per mole of subunit (Hardie and Cohen, 1979). Trypsin activates the enzyme in an identical manner to dephosphorylation (Fig. 4) and concomitantly cleaves off a fragment from one end of the polypeptide chain (Guy and Hardie, 1981). This fragment would appear to be a regulatory region of polypeptide which inhibits the enzyme only when it is phosphorylated.

The technical problems described above are likely to be magnified severalfold when more complex systems which involve interaction of many proteins are studied. A case in point is protein synthesis: there is abundant circumstantial evidence, obtained from crude reticulocyte lysates, which suggests that phosphorylation of initiation factor EIF-2 prevents re-initiation of protein synthesis. However, as yet, no-one has satisfactorily demonstrated an effect of phosphorylation on EIF-2 in a reconstituted system (Hunt, 1980).

## THE THIRD CRITERION

*The protein kinase or phosphatase should phosphorylate or dephosphorylate the protein in vitro at a rate sufficient to explain the effect of the extracellular signal in vivo or in an intact cell system*

It is necessary to insert this criterion because the specificity of protein kinases and phosphatases tends to be relative rather than absolute. If enough protein kinase is added almost any protein may become phosphorylated. It has been shown, for example, that cAMP-dependent protein kinase will phosphorylate denatured lysozyme in vitro even though the native enzyme is not a substrate (Bylund and Krebs, 1975) and at high concentration the protein kinase will even phosphorylate hydroxyproline residues (Feramisco et al., 1979). The important question is — is the rate of phosphorylation rapid enough to be physiologically significant in vivo?

The effect of adrenaline on fatty acid synthesis in adipose cells can be observed within 10 min of addition of the hormone (Brownsey et al., 1979). The detailed time course at shorter intervals is not known. The experiment shown in Fig. 1 was carried out at a concentration of the protein kinase which we estimate to be approximately one third of the physiological concentration (Hardie and Guy, 1980; Guy et al., 1980). The concentration of cAMP-dependent protein kinase in vivo is, in fact, surprisingly high: Hofmann et al. (1977) estimated its concentration in several tissues, including brain, to be 0.2–0.4 $\mu$moles/kg wet weight. This is comparable to the concentration of many of its known substrates. The rate of phosphorylation of acetyl-CoA carboxylase by cAMP-dependent protein kinase is therefore sufficient to explain an effect of adrenaline occurring within minutes in adipose tissue. The rates of phosphorylation of other proteins may have to be much more rapid than this to explain physiological effects. The rate of phosphorylation of muscle phosphorylase kinase by cAMP-dependent protein kinase is at least one order of magnitude faster than that of acetyl-CoA carboxylase (Hardie and Guy, 1980). This rate is consistent with the increased breakdown of muscle glycogen which occurs within seconds of addition of adrenaline. Such rapid phosphorylation events may also be very important in the brain.

## THE FOURTH CRITERION

*The protein is phosphorylated or dephosphorylated in vivo or in an intact cell system in response to the extracellular signal, at the same site phosphorylated or dephosphorylated by the protein kinase or phosphatase in vitro*

Establishment of this criterion puts the whole hypothesis on solid ground. However, in view of the common occurrence of multiple phosphorylation by multiple protein kinases (Table I), a demonstration that the protein is phosphorylated in vivo is not enough: it is essential to study the phosphorylation of individual sites.

The choice of experimental material with which to test this criterion is very important. While the whole animal seems an obvious choice, this usually requires injection of very large quantities of $^{32}$P. In addition, interpretation of results is often difficult when hormones, agonists or antagonists are injected into whole animals. An in vitro tissue or cell system is usually preferable.

If the protein under study is present in the tissue in very large amounts, it may be possible to study phosphorylation in vivo or in intact cells without using radioactive labelling. This was achieved in the case of muscle phosphorylase kinase, where it was established that adrenaline treatment in vivo caused phosphorylation at the same site as cAMP-dependent protein kinase in vitro (Yeaman and Cohen, 1975). The phosphopeptides were isolated and quantitated using tracer amounts of $^{32}$P-labelled phosphopeptides, prepared in vitro, as markers.

In most cases shortage of material will preclude detection of unlabelled phosphopeptides and will necessitate the use of $^{32}$P-labelled cells. To study a change in phosphorylation, it is important that the cells are completely equilibrated with $^{32}$P *before* addition of the hormone or agonist, otherwise an observed effect could merely be the result of a change in specific radioactivity of the intracellular ATP. This equilibration can be readily achieved using tissue culture, or isolated cells, e.g. adipocytes (Avruch et al., 1976). However, equilibration often occurs very slowly with tissue pieces or slices, or even with perfused organs such as the Langendorff heart preparation (England and Walsh, 1976).

Once the cells are equilibrated with $^{32}$P, the extracellular signal is added and after a suitable time interval the protein under study is isolated. It is obviously essential that this is carried out under conditions which do not allow a change in the phosphorylation state of the protein. For experiments involving large pieces of tissue, the incubation should be stopped whenever possible using freeze-clamping, and homogenisation and purification should be carried out using media which preclude phosphorylation and dephosphorylation. Unfortunately the ideal medium has yet to be devised. Addition of acid will in most cases render impossible the isolation of the protein. The method usually adopted is to add inhibitors of protein phosphatases such as fluoride which will convert most, but not all, protein phosphatases into forms dependent on divalent cations (Mackenzie et al., 1980). EDTA is also added to prevent further phosphorylation by chelating magnesium, and to inhibit divalent cation-dependent protein phosphatases. Wherever possible the state of phosphorylation should be assessed at every stage during the purification. For an enzyme where phosphorylation acts via a $K$ effect, this can be achieved by measuring the relevant $K$ value at each stage during the isolation. It is, of course, difficult to rule out that a change has occurred during the preparation of the initial cell-free extract.

In many cases the low abundance of the protein or the small amount of tissue that can be incubated will preclude a conventional isolation procedure. To study the phosphorylation of individual sites on acetyl-CoA carboxylase in isolated adipocytes, we developed a method

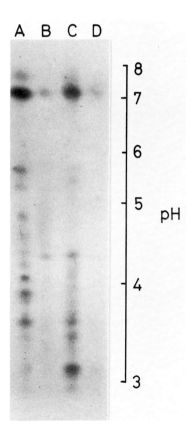

Fig. 5. Comparison of sites phosphorylated on purified acetyl-CoA carboxylase by cAMP-dependent protein kinase and sites phosphorylated in intact, isolated adipocytes. The photograph shows an autoradiograph of a dried gel after isoelectric focussing of $^{32}$P-labelled tryptic peptides. (A) enzyme phosphorylated by cAMP-dependent protein kinase in vitro; (B) enzyme isolated from $^{32}$P-labelled adipocytes incubated without hormone; (C) enzyme isolated from $^{32}$P-labelled adipocytes after incubation for 10 min with adrenaline (1 $\mu$M); (D) as (C), but extract incubated for 30 min with MgCl$_2$ (5 mm) at 37° C before isolation of enzyme. Data reproduced from Brownsey and Hardie (1980).

involving immunoprecipitation and isoelectric focussing in collaboration with Dr. Roger Brownsey at the University of Bristol. Isolated adipocytes were equilibrated in a medium containing [$^{32}$P]phosphate, incubated with or without adrenaline, and acetyl-CoA carboxylase was isolated by immunoprecipitation using a monospecific antibody. The immunoprecipitates were performic acid oxidised, digested with trypsin, and analysed by isoelectric focussing (Fig. 5). It can be seen that adrenaline produces a large increase in radioactivity in several tryptic peptides which comigrate with peptides prepared from enzyme labelled with [$\gamma$-$^{32}$P]ATP and cAMP-dependent protein kinase in vitro, including the major pI 7 peptide which we believe to regulate the enzyme activity (see Section 4).

This approach should be applicable to almost any protein and, with the advent of the technique of monoclonal antibody production, it is no longer necessary to have a homogeneous protein for antibody production. Another approach, which does not include complete purification of the protein, is to measure the activity of the protein in a crude or partially purified extract, before and after complete phosphorylation and complete dephosphorylation, preferably using added protein kinases and phosphatases. This method is much less direct and does not usually give information about phosphorylation of individual sites. A particular problem is the necessity to ensure that the phosphorylation and dephosphorylation reactions have gone to completion. However, it has been used successfully to access changes of phosphorylation of phosphatase inhibitor-1 in vivo (Foulkes and Cohen, 1979) and hydroxymethylglutaryl-CoA reductase, and its associated protein kinase, in isolated hepatocytes (Ingebritsen et al., 1979).

## CONCLUDING REMARKS

Of the eleven enzymes listed in Table I, the four criteria have been satisfied in their entirety for only four of them, and in each of these cases for only one hormone. These rigorously demonstrated examples of protein phosphorylation are the effect of adrenaline on muscle phosphorylase kinase (Yeaman and Cohen, 1975), the effect of glucagon on liver pyruvate kinase (Engstrom, 1980), the effect of insulin on pyruvate dehydrogenase in adipose tissue (Hughes et al., 1980) and the effect of adrenaline on acetyl-CoA carboxylase in adipose tissue (Brownsey and Hardie, 1980). In most other cases the role of protein phosphorylation is well established except that the phosphorylation of individual sites has not been examined both in vivo and in vitro. In view of the fact that multiple phosphorylation is turning out to be the rule rather than the exception (Table I), this is a serious omission.

When one comes to study brain functions such as the regulation of neurotransmission, there will clearly be major technical obstacles in the application of the four criteria. It is difficult to develop crude cell-free systems which carry out such complex processes, let alone to reconstitute them from purified components. However, while the application of the second and third criteria is much simpler if it can be carried out with a homogeneous protein, some progress can be achieved using cruder systems. It would merely be necessary to have a method for the rapid isolation of the protein from a mixture, so that its phosphate content could be estimated and peptide mapping could be carried out. Perhaps the ideal technique for this isolation, which is almost universally applicable, is the use of a monospecific antibody for immunoprecipitation or affinity chromatography. Peptide mapping can then be carried out using almost any technique, with isoelectric focussing being a very sensitive method which only requires tracer amounts of the protein (Brownsey and Hardie, 1980). An alternative method which does not require an antibody is the isolation of the protein by a one-dimensional or, if necessary, two-dimensional gel electrophoresis procedure. Since the protein is usually obtained as a dodecyl sulphate–protein complex, the choice of peptide mapping procedures is rather restricted. However some information about the identity of phosphorylation sites can still be obtained using a limited proteolysis technique such as that described by Cleveland et al. (1977).

Readers from the neurochemical field who have persevered to the end of this article are to be thanked for their patience. Our one hope is that some of the ideas we have discussed will be applicable to brain research and will stimulate progress in this fascinating but demanding field.

## ACKNOWLEDGEMENTS

Studies in our laboratory, some of which are described in this article, were carried out with the support of Project Grants from the Medical Research Council and the British Diabetic Association.

## REFERENCES

Avruch, J. Leone, G.R. and Martin, D.B. (1976) Identification and subcellular distribution of adipocyte peptides and phosphopeptides. *J. biol. Chem.*, 251: 1505–1510.

Bergström, G., Ekman, P., Humble, E. and Engström, L. (1978) Proteolytic modification of pig and rat liver pyruvate kinase type L including phosphorylatable site. *Biochim. biophys. Acta*, 532: 259–267.

Brownsey, R.W. and Hardie, D.G. (1980) Regulation of acetyl-CoA carboxylase: identity of sites phosphorylated in intact cells treated with adrenaline and in vitro by cyclic AMP-dependent protein kinase. *FEBS Lett.*, 120: 67–70.

Brownsey, R.W., Hughes, W.A. and Denton, R.M. (1979) Adrenaline and the regulation of acetyl-CoA carboxylase in rat epididymal adipose tissue. Inactivation of the enzyme is associated with phosphorylation and can be reversed on dephosphorylation. *Biochem. J.*, 184: 23–32.

Bylund, D.B. and Krebs, E.G. (1975) Effect of denaturation on the susceptibility of proteins to enzymic phosphorylation. *J. biol. Chem.*, 250: 6355–6361.

Cahill, G.F., LeBœuf, B. and Flinn, R.B. (1960) Studies on rat adipose tissue in vitro. VI. Effect of epinephrine on glucose metabolism. *J. biol. Chem.*, 235: 1246–1250.

Carlson, C.A. and Kim, K.H. (1973) Regulation of hepatic acetyl coenzyme A carboxylase by phosphorylation and dephosphorylation. *J. biol. Chem.*, 250: 6355–6361.

Castaño, J.G., Nieto, A. and Felíu, J.E. (1979) Inactivation of phosphofructokinase by glucagon in rat hepatocytes. *J. biol. Chem.*, 254: 5576–5579.

Cleveland, D.W., Fischer, S.G., Kirschner, M.W. and Laemmli, U.K. (1977) Peptide mapping by limited proteolysis in sodium dodecyl sulphate and analysis by gel electrophoresis. *J. biol. Chem.*, 252: 1102–1106.

Cook, G.A., Nielsen, R.C., Hawkins, R.A., Mehlman, M.A., Lakshmanan, M.R. and Veech, R.L. (1977) Effect of glucagon on hepatic malonyl coenzyme A concentration and on lipid synthesis. *J. biol. Chem.*, 252: 4421–4424.

Cohen, P. (1973) The subunit structure of rabbit skeletal muscle phosphorylase kinase, and the molecular basis of its activation reactions. *Eur. J. Biochem.*, 34: 1–14.

Cohen, P. (Ed.) (1980a) Newly discovered systems of regulation by reversible phosphorylation. In *Molecular Aspects of Cellular Regulation*, Vol. 1, Elsevier/North-Holland, Amsterdam.

Cohen, P. (1980b) The role of calcium ions, calmodulin, and troponin on the regulation of phosphorylase kinase from rabbit skeletal muscle. *Eur. J. Biochem.*, 111: 563–574.

Cohen, P., Yellowlees, D., Aitken, A., Donella-Deana, A., Hemmings, B.A. and Parker, P. (1981) Separation and characterisation of glycogen synthase kinase-3, glycogen synthase kinase-4 and glycogen synthase kinase-5 from rabbit skeletal muscle. *Eur. J. Biochem.*, in press.

Denton, R.M. and Hughes, W.A. (1978) Pyruvate dehydrogenase and the hormonal regulation of fat synthesis in mammalian tissues. *Int. J. Biochem.*, 9: 545–572.

Donlon, S. and Kaufman, S. (1978) Glucagon stimulation of rat hepatic phenylalanine hydroxylase through phosphorylation in vivo. *J. biol. Chem.*, 253: 6657–6659.

Ekman, P., Dahlqvist, U., Humble, E. and Engström, L. (1976) Comparative kinetic studies on the L-type pyruvate

160

kinase from rat liver and the enzyme phosphorylated by cyclic 3',5'-AMP stimulated protein kinase. *Biochim. biophys. Acta*, 429: 374–382.

El-Maghrabi, M.R., Haston, W.S., Flockhart, D.A., Claus, T.H. and Pilkis, S.J. (1980) Studies on the phosphorylation and dephosphorylation of L-type pyruvate kinase by the catalytic subunit of cyclic AMP-dependent protein kinase. *J. biol. Chem.*, 255: 668–675.

Embi, N., Rylatt, D.B. and Cohen, P. (1980) Glycogen synthase kinase-3 from rabbit skeletal muscle. Separation from cyclic AMP-dependent protein kinase and phosphorylase kinase. *Eur. J. Biochem.*, 107: 519–527.

England, P.J. and Walsh, D.A. (1976) A rapid method for the measurement of $[\gamma\text{-}^{32}P]ATP$ specific radioactivity in tissue extracts and its application to the study of $^{32}Pi$ uptake in perfused rat heart. *Anal. Biochem.*, 75: 429–493.

Engström, L. (1980) Regulation of liver pyruvate kinase by phosphorylation-dephosphorylation. In *Molecular Aspects of Cellular Regulation*, Vol. 1, P. Cohen (Ed.), Elsevier/North-Holland, Amsterdam, pp. 11–31.

Feramisco, J.R., Kemp, B.E. and Krebs, E.G. (1979) Phosphorylation of hydroxyproline in a synthetic peptide catalysed by cyclic AMP-dependent protein kinase. *J. biol. Chem.*, 254: 6987–6990.

Fischer, E.H., Pocker, A. and Saari, J.C. (1970) The structure, function and control of glycogen phosphorylase. *Essays Biochem.*, 6: 23–68.

Fletterick, R.J. and Madsen, N.B. (1980) The structures and related functions of phosphorylase *a*. *Annu. Rev. Biochem.*, 49: 31–61.

Foulkes, J.G. and Cohen, P. (1979) The hormonal control of glycogen metabolism. Phosphorylation of protein phosphatase-1 in vivo in response to adrenaline. *Eur. J. Biochem.*, 97: 251–256.

Geelen, M.J.H., Beynen, A.C., Christiansen, R.Z., Lepreau-Jose, M.J. and Gibson, D.M. (1978) Short-term effects of insulin and glucagon on lipid synthesis in isolated rat hepatocytes. Covariance of acetyl-CoA carboxylase activity and the rat of $^{3}H_2O$ incorporation into fatty acids. *FEBS Lett.*, 95: 326–330.

Guy, P.S. and Hardie, D.G. (1981) Regulation of mammalian acetyl-CoA carboxylase. Limited proteolysis mimics dephosphorylation. *FEBS Lett.*, 132: 67–70.

Guy, P.S., Cohen, P. and Hardie, D.G. (1980) Rat mammary gland ATP-citrate lyase is phosphorylated by cyclic AMP-dependent protein kinase. *FEBS Lett.*, 109: 205–208.

Hardie, D.G. and Cohen, P. (1979) Dephosphorylation and activation of acetyl-CoA carboxylase from lactating rabbit mammary gland. *FEBS Lett.*, 103: 333–338.

Hardie, D.G. and Guy, P.S. (1980) Reversible phosphorylation and inactivation of acetyl-CoA carboxylase from lactating rat mammary gland by cyclic AMP-dependent protein kinase. *Eur. J. Biochem.*, 110: 167–177.

Hofmann, F., Bechtel, P.J. and Krebs, E.G. (1977) Concentrations of cyclic AMP-dependent protein kinase subunits in various tissues. *J. biol. Chem.*, 252: 1441–1447.

Hughes, W.A., Brownsey, R.W. and Denton, R.M. (1980) Studies on the incorporation of $[^{32}P]$phosphate into pyruvate dehydrogenase in intact rat fat cells. *Biochem. J.*, 192: 479–481.

Hunt, T. (1980) Phosphorylation and the control of protein synthesis in reticulocytes. In *Molecular Aspects of Cellular Regulation*, Vol. 1, P. Cohen (Ed.), Elsevier/North-Holland, Amsterdam, pp. 175–202.

Ingebritsen, T.S. and Gibson, D.M. (1980) Reversible phosphorylation of hydroxymethylglutaryl-CoA reductase. In *Molecular Aspects of Cellular Regulation*, Vol. 1, P. Cohen (Ed.), Elsevier/North-Holland, Amsterdam, pp. 63–94.

Ingebritsen, T.S., Geelen, M.J.H., Parker, R.A., Evenson, K.J. and Gibson, D.M. (1979) Modulation of hydroxymethylglutaryl-CoA reductase activity, reductase kinase activity, and cholesterol synthesis in rat hepatocytes in response to insulin and glucagon. *J. biol. Chem.*, 254: 9986–9989.

Jungas, R.L. (1968) Fatty acid synthesis in adipose tissue incubated in tritiated water. *Biochemistry*, 7, 3708–3717.

Kagimoto, T. and Uyeda, K. (1979) Hormone-stimulated phosphorylation of liver phosphofructokinase in vivo. *J. biol. Chem.*, 254: 5584–5587.

Krebs, E.G. (1973) The mechanism of hormonal regulation by cyclic AMP. In *Endocrinology, Proceedings of the 4th International Congress*, Excerpta Medica, Amsterdam, pp. 17–29.

Krebs, E.G. and Beavo, J.A. (1979) Phosphorylation–dephosphorylation of enzymes. *Annu. Rev. Biochem.*, 48: 923–959.

Lane, M.D., Moss, J. and Polakis, S.E. (1974) Acetyl coenzyme A carboxylase. *Curr. Top. cell. Regul.*, 8: 139–195.

Larner, J. and Villar-Palasi, C. (1971) Glycogen synthesis and its control. *Curr. Top. cell. Regul.*, 3: 195–236.

Ma, G.Y. and Hems, D.A. (1975) Inhibition of fatty acid synthesis and stimulation of glycogen breakdown by vasopressin in the perfused mouse liver. *Biochem. J.*, 152: 389–392.

Ma, G., Gove, C.D. and Hems, D.A. (1977) Inhibition of fatty acid synthesis and stimulation of glucose release by angiotensin II and adrenaline in the perfused mouse liver. *Biochem. Soc. Trans.*, 5: 986–989.

Mackenzie, C.W., Bulbulian, G.J. and Bishop, J.S. (1980) Use of fluoride to inactivate phosphorylase *a* phosphatases from rat liver cytosol. Presence of fluoride-insensitive glycogen synthase-specific phosphatase. *Biochim. biophys. Acta*, 614: 413–424.

McCormack, J.G. and Denton, R.M. (1977) Evidence that fatty acid synthesis in the interscapular brown adipose tissue of cold-adapted rats is increased in vivo by insulin by mechanisms involving parallel activation of pyruvate dehydrogenase and acetyl-CoA carboxylase. *Biochem. J.*, 166: 627–630.

Newsholme, E.A. (1980) Reflections on the mechanisms of action of hormones. *FEBS Lett.*, 117, Suppl., K121–K134.

Newsholme, E.A. and Gevers, W. (1967) Control of glycolysis and gluconeogenesis in liver and kidney cortex. *Vitam. Horm.*, 25: 1–87.

Nilsson, N.O., Stralfors, P., Fredrickson, G. and Belfrage, P. (1980) Regulation of adipose tissue lipolysis: effects of noradrenaline and insulin on phosphorylation of hormone-sensitive lipase and on lipolysis in intact rat adipocytes. *FEBS Lett.*, 111: 125–130.

Nimmo, H.G. and Cohen, P. (1977) Hormonal control of protein phosphorylation. *Adv. cyclic Nucleot. Res.*, 8: 145–266.

Nimmo, H.G. and Houston, B. (1978) Rat adipose tissue glycerol phosphate acyl transferase can be inactivated by cyclic AMP-dependent protein kinase. *Biochem. J.*, 176: 607–610.

Parker, P., Aitken, A., Bilham, T., Embi, N. and Cohen, P. (1981) Amino acid sequence of a region in rabbit skeletal muscle glycogen synthase phosphorylated by cyclic AMP-dependent protein kinase. *FEBS Lett.*, 123: 332–336.

Pilkis, S.J., Schlumpf, J., Pilkis, J. and Claus, T.H. (1979) Regulation of phosphofructokinase activity by glucagon in isolated rat hepatocytes. *Biochem. biophys. Res. Commun.*, 88: 960–967.

Pilkis, S.J., El-Maghrabi, M.R., Pilkis, J., Claus, T.H. and Cumming, D.A. (1981) Fructose-2,6-bisphosphate, a new activator of phosphofructokinase. *J. biol. Chem.*, 256: 3171–3174.

Ray, W.J. and Roscelli, G.A. (1964) A kinetic study of the phosphoglucomutase pathway. *J. biol. Chem.*, 239: 1228–1236.

Rylatt, D.B., Aitken, A., Bilham, T., Condon, G.D., Embi, N. and Cohen, P. (1980) Glycogen synthase from rabbit skeletal muscle. Amino acid sequence at the sites phosphorylated by glycogen synthase kinase-3, and extension of the *N*-terminal sequence containing the site phosphorylated by phosphorylase kinase. *Eur. J. Biochem.*, 107: 528–537.

Stansbie, D., Brownsey, R.W., Crettaz, M. and Denton, R.M. (1976) Acute effects in vivo of anti-insulin serum on rates of fatty acid synthesis and activities of acetyl-coenzyme A carboxylase and pyruvate dehydrogenase in liver and epididymal adipose tissue of fed rats. *Biochem. J.*, 160: 413–416.

Sugden, P.H., Kerbey, A.L., Randle, P.J., Waller, C.A. and Reid, K.B.M. (1979) Amino acid sequences around the sites of phosphorylation in the pig heart pyruvate dehydrogenase complex. *Biochem. J.*, 181: 419–426.

Takeda, Y. and Larner, J. (1975) Structural studies on rabbit muscle glycogen synthase. *J. biol. Chem.*, 250: 8951–8956.

Van Schaftingen, E., Hue, L. and Hers, H.G. (1980) Fructose-2,6-bisphosphate, the probable structure of the glucose- and glucagon-sensitive stimulator of phosphofructokinase. *Biochem. J.*, 192: 897–901.

Walsh, D.A., Ashby, C.D., Gonzalez, C., Calkins, D., Fischer, E.H. and Krebs, E.G. (1971) Purification and characterisation of a protein inhibitor of adenosine-3′,5′-monophosphate dependent protein kinases. *J. biol. Chem.*, 246: 1977–1985.

Watkins, P.A., Tarlow, D.M. and Lane, M.D. (1977) Mechanism for acute control of fatty acid synthesis by glucagon and 3′,5′ cyclic AMP in the liver cell. *Proc. nat. Acad. Sci. (Wash.)*, 74: 1497–1501.

Yeaman, S.J. and Cohen, P. (1975) The hormonal control of activity of skeletal muscle phosphorylase kinase. Phosphorylation of the enzyme at two sites in vivo in response to adrenalin. *Eur. J. Biochem.*, 51: 93–104.

Yeaman, S.J., Hutcheson, E.T., Roche, T.E., Pettit, F.H., Brown, J.R., Reed, L.J., Watson, D.C. and Dixon, G.H. (1978) Sites of phosphorylation on pyruvate dehydrogenase from bovine kidney and heart. *Biochemistry*, 17: 2364–2370.

# Substrates of Nuclear Protein Kinases in Rat C6 Glial Cell Cultures

RICHARD A. JUNGMANN, JANIE J. HARRISON, DEBORAH MILKOWSKI,
SEUNG-KI LEE, JOHN S. SCHWEPPE and MICHAEL F. MILES

*Cancer Center and Department of Molecular Biology, Northwestern University Medical School,
303 East Chicago Avenue, Chicago, IL 60611, U.S.A.*

## INTRODUCTION

Cyclic nucleotides participate in the development, differentiation, and proper functioning of the central nervous system (Bloom, 1975; Nathanson, 1977). The molecular mechanism(s) by which hormones, through adenosine $3',5'$-monophosphate (cAMP), regulate the activity of specific genes in nervous tissue is, however, unknown. Clonal cell lines growing in culture which continue to exhibit differentiated functions have proven useful for studying the biosynthesis of specialized cell products. The rat C6 glial cell line responds to $\beta$-adrenergic agonists with an activation of its adenyl cyclase and a rapid transient rise of cAMP levels (Gilman and Nirenberg, 1971), followed by the increased activity of lactate dehydrogenase and other enzymes such as phosphodiesterase (Schwartz and Passonneau, 1974) and ornithine decarboxylase (Bachrach, 1975). Additionally, there is a catecholamine-induced increase of $\beta$-nerve growth factor (Schwartz et al., 1977; Schwartz and Costa, 1977). Other differentiated characteristics of the C6 glial cell line include several glial markers such as the brain-specific induction of glycerol phosphate dehydrogenase by hydrocortisone (McGinnis and DeVellis, 1978), S-100 protein (Benda et al., 1971), $2',3'$-cAMP $3'$-phosphohydrolase (Zanetta et al., 1972), and glial fibrillary acidic protein (Bissell et al., 1974). However, no neuronal markers have been identified in C6 cells. Thus, the C6 cells offer the advantage of serving as a useful glial model for evaluating the effects of putative neurotransmitters on cAMP levels, nuclear protein phosphorylation and their possible relationship to lactate dehydrogenase induction.

In the rat C6 glial cell a causal relationship between initial $\beta$-adrenergic receptor activation by catecholamines and the subsequent induction of lactate dehydrogenase has been postulated (DeVellis and Brooker, 1973). An elevated level of cAMP appears to be a prerequisite for the induction, and $\beta$-adrenergic blockers successfully inhibit it. It is a generally held view that the molecular mechanism of cAMP action involves the activation of cAMP-dependent protein kinase and the subsequently ensuing phosphorylative modification of regulatory proteins. To test the validity of this idea, our laboratory has recently investigated isoproterenol-mediated changes of the glial cell cAMP–protein kinase system during the preinduction phase of lactate dehydrogenase. Stimulation of glial cells with isoproterenol leads to a rapid increase (up to 250-fold) of cAMP levels (within 2–5 min after application of the effector agent) and to a concomitant dissociation of the type I cAMP-dependent protein kinase for the duration of 2–60 min after isoproterenol stimulation (Jungmann et al., 1979). Additionally, nuclear cAMP-dependent protein kinase activity becomes increased at about 5 min and lasts for periods of up to 90 min after $\beta$-adrenergic receptor stimulation (Jungmann et al., 1979; Schwartz and Costa,

164

1980). This phenomenon of increased nuclear protein kinase activity which follows the increase of intracellular cAMP levels has been interpreted as translocation of cytoplasmic cAMP-dependent protein kinase (Jungmann and Kranias, 1977). Whether the increased nuclear protein kinase activity is due to a shift of cytoplasmic cAMP-dependent protein kinase to the nucleus is likely but remains to be examined in more detail. Other feasible mechanisms could, at least in part, account for the increase of nuclear protein kinase activity.

As a continuation of our studies on the action of nuclear protein kinase in C6 glial cells, we will summarize in this report our findings dealing with the identification of C6 glial cell nuclear proteins which are substrates for the nuclear protein kinases. It should be pointed out that these studies have been carried out during the preinduction phase of lactate dehydrogenase hoping to ultimately correlate these findings and to determine the role of the isoproterenol-mediated phosphorylative modification of nuclear proteins in the induction process of lactate dehydrogenase.

## MODULATION OF C6 GLIAL CELL CYCLIC AMP LEVELS

The $\beta$-adrenergic agonist isoproterenol increases intracellular cAMP levels by at least two orders of magnitude within 15 min after the exposure of glial cells to the stimulant (Fig. 1). In the experiments glial cells were grown to confluency in a serum-containing medium (Derda et al., 1980) which was changed to a serum-free medium 48 h prior to isoproterenol stimulation. When the culture medium is additionally changed to a phosphate-free medium 20 h prior to

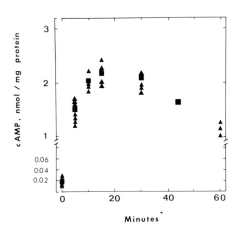

Fig. 1. Time course of glial cell intracellular cAMP levels after isoproterenol ($10^{-5}$ M) stimulation. ▲, glial cells cultured in serum-free medium 48 h prior to isoproterenol stimulation; ■, glial cells cultured in serum-free medium replaced with phosphate-free medium 20 h prior to stimulation.

stimulation, isoproterenol is equally effective in increasing intracellular cAMP levels. The finding that deletion of phosphate from the culture medium does not significantly affect stimulation of cAMP levels by isoproterenol is critical to our subsequent phosphorylation experiments which were carried out in phosphate-free culture medium.

## PHOSPHORYLATIVE MODIFICATION OF C6 GLIAL CELL HISTONES

The involvement of histones together with DNA in forming the nucleosomal structure is now well established (McGhee and Felsenfeld, 1980), although the packing of nucleosomes to a higher order of structure, the chromatin, still remains to be precisely elucidated. Nevertheless, it is clear that structural modifications of histones, accompanied by changes of their charge, can markedly affect histone–DNA interaction with resulting structural and functional modifications of chromatin. With these considerations in mind we have asked the question whether or not C6 glial cell histones become structurally modified by nuclear protein kinase(s) as the result of isoproterenol stimulation and whether these phosphorylations are mediated by cAMP.

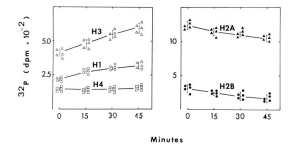

**Minutes**

Fig. 2. Time course of isoproterenol-mediated phosphorylative modification of glial cell histones in vivo. Rat C6 glial cells were labeled with $Na_2H^{32}PO_4$ and then stimulated for the indicated times in the presence of $10^{-5}$ M isoproterenol. Separation of the individual histones by SDS–polyacrylamide gel electrophoresis and analysis of radioactivity in the histones was performed as described previously (Harrison et al., 1980). The individual points at the given times have been slightly spread along the $x$-axis to allow for better graphical representation. Error bars indicate the standard deviation of the means of all points at a given time. H, histone.

The data of Fig. 2 illustrate that [$^{32}$P]phosphate incorporation into several histones is altered by isoproterenol. Not only are there significant increases of the degree of $^{32}$P labeling of histones H1 and H3, but the incorporation of [$^{32}$P]phosphate into histones H2A and H2B is slightly but significantly decreased. The level of phosphorylation of histone H4 is not affected. There is no change of $^{32}$P incorporation into histones in unstimulated control cells (data not shown), thus indicating that the observed phosphorylative modifications are due to the presence of isoproterenol.

Since the histone fraction H1 isolated by acid extraction is heterogeneous and consists of several subspecies (Kinkade, 1969), we undertook a detailed investigation of the phosphorylation of the individual subspecies and the effect of isoproterenol on these phosphorylations. Histone H1 can be separated by sodium dodecyl sulfate electrophoresis into three subspecies e.g. H1-1, H1-2, and H1-3 (Kinkade, 1969). Quantitatively in rat C6 glial cells histone H1 is composed of 68.5% H1-1, 24.0% H1-2, and 7.6% H1-3 (Harrison et al., 1980). When histone H1 is isolated from [$^{32}$P]phosphate-labeled cells before and after isoproterenol treatment and separated by electrophoresis into subspecies H1-1, H1-2, and H1-3, various amounts of $^{32}$P radioactivity are associated with the histones. As shown in Table I, the extent of [$^{32}$P]phosphate incorporation into total histone H1 fraction is increased by about 37% in stimulated cells (see also Fig. 2). However, the analysis of the individual subspecies indicates that the increased phosphorylation is confined to the H1-1 subspecies. Incorporation of [$^{32}$P]phosphate into histone H1-2 is not significantly modified as determined by $t$ test analysis. Additionally,

TABLE I

PHOSPHORYLATIVE MODIFICATION OF HISTONE H1 SUBSPECIES IN
ISOPROTERENOL-STIMULATED RAT C6 GLIAL CELLS

| | Specific activity $\times 10^{-7}$* | | Specific activity ratio ** |
|---|---|---|---|
| | Isoproterenol | | |
| | − | + | |
| Total H1 | 3.25 | 4.45 | 1.37 ± 0.13 *** |
| H1-1 | 3.36 | 5.12 | 1.52 ± 0.15 |
| H1-2 | 3.30 | 3.83 | 1.16 ± 0.12 |
| H1-3 | 2.65 | 2.22 | 0.84 ± 0.08 |

Rat C6 glioma cells were labeled with $Na_2H^{32}PO_4$ and then stimulated for 1 h in the presence of 10 $\mu$M isoproterenol. Total histone fraction H1 was isolated, separated into its subspecies by electrophoresis, and $^{32}P$ radioactivity in each subspecies was determined.
* Specific activity = moles [$^{32}P$]phosphate incorporated/mole histone.
** Ratio = specific activity of stimulated cells/specific activity of control cells.
*** Values are given as means ± standard deviation of the mean ($n = 4$).

the degree of phosphorylation of histone H1-3 is slightly but significantly decreased in stimulated cells. It appears then, that the observed increased phosphorylation of total histone H1 fraction is primarily due to the increased selective phosphorylation of the H1-1 subspecies. We have identified that the altered $^{32}P$ levels of histones H1-1 and H1-3 after stimulation are not caused by differences in the amount of total extractable histone H1 between unstimulated and stimulated cells, since the extracted amounts of histone H1 are identical in both cell preparations. Also, the differences cannot be explained on the basis that the relative subspecies composition of histone H1 is quantitatively changed after isoproterenol stimulation. The relative amounts of subspecies are identical in histone H1 extracted from stimulated and unstimulated cells.

The above findings, namely the increased incorporation of [$^{32}P$]phosphate into phosphorylation sites of histones H1-1 and H3 and the dephosphorylation of sites in histones H1-3, H2A and H2B, suggest a rather complex control mechanism involving the interaction of not only protein kinase(s) but of phosphoprotein phosphatase(s) as well. Additional complexity is added by the fact that histones possess multiple sites at which phosphorylation and dephosphorylation can occur. Therefore, the state of phosphorylation of each of these sites must be investigated in order to gain information on the over-all extent of phosphorylative modification. Since it is well established that histone H1 possesses multiple intramolecular phosphate acceptor amino acids (serines and threonines) (Langan, 1978; Gurley et al., 1977), and since these amino acids are potential substrates for nuclear protein kinases and phosphatases, we examined the extent of phosphorylative modification of each histone H1 subfraction after its proteolytic cleavage by chymotrypsin. The $NH_2$-terminal and COOH-terminal fragments were analyzed for [$^{32}P$]phosphate content and for the presence of [$^{32}P$]phosphoserine and [$^{32}P$]phosphothreonine. Table II illustrates that the increased phosphorylation of histone H1-1 is caused mainly by a modification of the $NH_2$-terminal fragment. On the other hand, isoproterenol-mediated dephosphorylation of histone H1-3 occurs in both the $NH_2$-terminal and the COOH-terminal fragments. An interesting observation is made when the phosphorylation sites of histone H1-2 are examined. Histone H1-2, which does not exhibit a net change of [$^{32}P$]phosphate

TABLE II

EFFECT OF ISOPROTERENOL ON PHOSPHATE INCORPORATION INTO NH$_2$-TERMINAL
AND COOH-TERMINAL HISTONE H1 FRAGMENTS OBTAINED AFTER
PROTEOLYTIC CLEAVAGE

| Histone | Specific activity ratio * ± S.D. | | |
|---------|---------------|------------------------|--------------------------|
|         | Intact molecule | NH$_2$-terminal fragment | COOH-terminal fragment |
| H1-1 | 1.32 ± 0.13 | 1.38 ± 0.08 | 1.23 ± 0.23 |
| H1-2 | 0.91 ± 0.07 | 1.23 ± 0.08 | 0.76 ± 0.06 |
| H1-3 | 0.71 ± 0.11 | 0.72 ± 0.08 | 0.69 ± 0.16 |

Rat C6 glial cell cultures were labeled with Na$_2$H$^{32}$PO$_4$ and stimulated with isoproterenol as described in Table I. Total histone fraction was isolated from intact cells with 0.4 N H$_2$SO$_4$, separated into its subspecies by electrophoresis (Bonner and Pollard, 1975), and electrophoretically separated after cleavage with chymotrypsin according to Cleveland et al. (1977).
* Ratio = specific activity of intact histone, respectively terminal fragment from isoproterenol-stimulated cells/specific activity of control cells.

incorporation after isoproterenol stimulation (see Table I), undergoes increased phosphorylation of the NH$_2$-terminal fragment concomitantly with a dephosphorylation in the COOH-terminal fragment. Thus, the phosphorylative changes of the NH$_2$-terminal and COOH-terminal fragments in opposite directions of about equal magnitude obscure the structural modifications of histone H1-2, when only the over-all net phosphorylation of the intact molecule is examined. Analysis of the NH$_2$-terminal and COOH-terminal fragments as well as of the intact histone subspecies for the presence of phosphoserine and phosphothreonine indicates that at least 93 % of the [$^{32}$P]phosphate is present in the form of [$^{32}$P]phosphoserine, with only minor quantities of [$^{32}$P]phosphothreonine.

The $\beta$-adrenergic agonist isoproterenol is known to exert its action by binding to $\beta$-adrenergic receptors (Maguire et al., 1976; Lucas and Bockaert, 1977; Terasaki and Brooker, 1978) thereby activating adenyl cyclase and causing increased intracellular cAMP levels. Whether this mechanism of isoproterenol action is also involved in and leads to the phosphorylative modification of C6 glial cell histones can be tested by blocking the binding of isoproterenol to the $\beta$-adrenergic receptor sites. This can be accomplished by using DL-propranolol, a $\beta$-ad-

TABLE III

PHOSPHORYLATIVE MODIFICATIONS OF HISTONE H1 SUBSPECIES AFTER
TREATMENT OF RAT C6 GLIAL CELLS WITH ISOPROTERENOL OR
ISOPROTERENOL/DL-PROPRANOLOL

| Histone | Specific activity ratio * ± S.D. | |
|---------|--------------|------------------------------|
|         | Isoproterenol | Isoproterenol + DL-propranolol |
| H1-1 | 1.52 ± 0.15 | 0.98 ± 0.03 |
| H1-2 | 1.16 ± 0.12 | 1.03 ± 0.11 |
| H1-3 | 0.84 ± 0.08 | 1.09 ± 0.08 |

Rat C6 glial cell cultures were labeled with Na$_2$H$^{32}$PO$_4$ and stimulated with isoproterenol ($10^{-5}$ M) or with isoproterenol ($10^{-5}$ M) + DL-propranolol ($10^{-5}$ M) as described in Table I. Total histone H1 and its subspecies were isolated and radioactivity was determined as described in Table I.
* Ratio = specific activity of stimulated cells/specific activity of control cells.

renergic antagonist, and its addition to C6 glial cell cultures prior to isoproterenol stimulation. The results are shown in Table III. Addition of DL-propranolol to the cell cultures successfully prevents the phosphorylative modification of total histone H1 and its subfractions mediated by isoproterenol.

The above results with DL-propranolol suggest that the phosphorylation and dephosphorylation reactions achieved by isoproterenol treatment of C6 cells are mediated via binding of isoproterenol to $\beta$-adrenergic receptor sites and generation of cAMP. Hence it follows that by addition of cAMP to C6 cell cultures the effect of isoproterenol on histone phosphorylation should be mimicked and that similar phosphorylative modifications should be observed. The use of cAMP itself as a stimulant is, however, complicated by its relative instability toward phosphodiesterase which prevents the intracellular accumulation of the cyclic nucleotide at a concentration sufficient to accomplish its action. The cyclic nucleotide analogue, dibutyryl cAMP, is generally used instead of cAMP because of its greater stability toward phosphodiesterase. Thus, we have incubated C6 glial cells with dibutyryl cAMP to test whether it would mimick the action of isoproterenol on the phosphorylation of C6 glial cell histones. The results are shown in Table IV. Similar to the action of isoproterenol, dibutyryl cAMP causes

TABLE IV

EFFECT OF DIBUTYRYL cAMP ON PHOSPHATE INCORPORATION INTO HISTONE H1 SUBFRACTIONS AND THEIR $NH_2$-TERMINAL AND COOH-TERMINAL FRAGMENTS OBTAINED AFTER PROTEOLYTIC CLEAVAGE

| *Histone* | *Specific activity ratio* * $\pm$ *S.D.* | | |
|---|---|---|---|
| | *Intact molecule* | *$NH_2$-terminal fragment* | *COOH-terminal fragment* |
| H1-1 | 1.48 $\pm$ 0.18 | 1.38 $\pm$ 0.11 | 1.81 $\pm$ 0.71 |
| H1-2 | 1.09 $\pm$ 0.10 | 0.92 $\pm$ 0.03 | 1.24 $\pm$ 0.18 |
| H1-3 | 1.84 $\pm$ 0.19 | 1.74 $\pm$ 0.21 | 1.95 $\pm$ 0.20 |

Rat C6 glial cell cultures were labeled with $Na_2H^{32}PO_4$ and stimulated for 1 h with $10^{-3}$ M dibutyryl cAMP under the conditions described in Table I. Total histone and its subfractions were isolated and chymotryptic cleavage was carried out as described in Table II.
* Ratio = specific activity of intact histone, respectively terminal fragment from isoproterenol-stimulated cells/specific activity of control cells.

slight but significant increases of $^{32}$P incorporation into total histone H1 fraction and into histone subfraction H1-1. Additionally, it appears that the overall net [$^{32}$P]phosphate incorporation into H1-2 is not changed by dibutyryl cAMP.

An interesting and marked difference between the action of isoproterenol and dibutyryl cAMP is identified when the phosphorylative change of histone H1-3 is analyzed. Whereas isoproterenol causes a decrease of [$^{32}$P]phosphate incorporation into H1-3 (see Tables I and II), dibutyryl cAMP markedly increases H1-3 phosphorylation by about 84% over control levels. This action of dibutyryl cAMP, seemingly inconsistent with the action of isoproterenol, could be explained in several ways. Firstly, the increased phosphorylation of H1-3 may be an artifactual reaction due to the effect of butyrate which can form from dibutyryl cAMP by the action of deacylase (Castagna et al., 1977). There is evidence that sodium butyrate selectively increases the phosphorylation of high mobility group proteins 14 and 17 (Levy-Wilson, 1981) and of histone H3 (Whitlock et al., 1980). Secondly, dibutyryl cAMP causes the activation of nuclear protein kinase(s) other than the kinase(s) which is activated by that fraction of cAMP generated by isoproterenol via $\beta$-adrenergic receptor activation. An example of this action of dibutyryl cAMP is provided by Byus et al. (1977) who investigated the effects of concanavalin A and dibutyryl cAMP on the dissociation of the type I and II cAMP-dependent protein kinase isozymes in human peripheral lymphocytes. Concanavalin A promoted the dissociation of only the type I isozyme. Addition of dibutyryl cAMP to lymphocytes, on the other hand, led to the dissociation and activation of both the type I and II isozymes. cAMP-dependent protein kinases are postulated to exhibit marked specificity in their mode of action (Jungmann and Russell, 1977). Hence, it is conceivable that a different pattern of H1-3 phosphorylation is obtained depending upon the type of isozyme being activated. Should this be the case, considerable caution needs to be exercised when studying and interpreting phosphorylation patterns mediated by dibutyryl cAMP. It cannot be assumed automatically that these phosphorylation patterns are identical to those mediated by the primary effector agents even though dibuturyl cAMP may mimick the ultimate physiologic response of the effector agent.

## PHOSPHORYLATION OF HIGH MOBILITY GROUP PROTEINS 14 AND 17

During the course of study of the phosphorylation of C6 glial cell histone H1, we consistently observed the association of considerable amounts of $^{32}$P radioactivity with the high mobility group proteins (HMG) 14 and 17. These $^{32}$P levels were markedly higher than those associated with histone H1. This is a potentially interesting observation, since HMG 14 and 17 are preferentially associated with the transcriptionally active regions of the chromatin (Weisbrod and Weintraub, 1979; Bakayev et al., 1979; Weisbrod et al., 1980; Albanese and Weintraub, 1980; Gazit et al., 1980) and have been found to be phosphorylated in vivo to a higher degree in the transcriptionally active than inactive chromatin (Levy-Wilson, 1981). Although the function of HMG 14 and 17 is not known, it is believed that they may be active in maintaining the conformation of transcriptionally active genes (Gazit et al., 1980). Since phosphorylation of nuclear proteins results in a modification of their charge properties and hence binding properties to DNA, phosphorylative modification of HMG 14 and 17 is of paramount interest.

When histone H1 is prepared by selective acid extraction of C6 glial cells, HMG proteins are coextracted with the histone H1 fraction (Harrison and Jungmann, 1981). HMG 14 and 17 can be separated from histone H1 either by CM–Sephadex chromatography which, however, does not separate HMG 14 from 17, or by SDS–polyacrylamide gel electrophoresis which also separates HMG 14 from 17 (see Fig. 3). Using these separation procedures, we have studied the phosphorylation of HMG 14 and 17 in C6 glial cells and have evaluated a potential effect of isoproterenol on these modifications. When C6 glial cells are incubated with $Na_2H^{32}PO_4$, [$^{32}$P]phosphate is incorporated into the HMG proteins (fractions 48–55) as shown in Fig. 3A. Separation of the HMG proteins in these fractions by SDS–polyacrylamide gel electrophoresis and subsequent autoradiography reveals the presence of $^{32}$P-labeled HMG 14 and 17 (Fig. 3B). Quantitation of $^{32}$P incorporation indicates consistently higher $^{32}$P labeling (by about 50%) of HMG 17 than 14 (Table V). Determination of the phosphate acceptor amino acids shows that 40% of the total $^{32}$P radioactivity incorporated into HMG 14 is present in the form of phosphothreonine. The remainder of the $^{32}$P label is identified as phosphoserine. Some phosphothreonine is also found in HMG 17. In contrast to histone phosphorylation, the presence of isoproterenol does not cause a modulation of HMG 14 and 17 phosphorylation. Despite our failure to demonstrate an effect of isoproterenol, we cannot rule out such an effect on the modification of intramolecular phosphorylation sites in HMG 14 and 17. This judg-

170

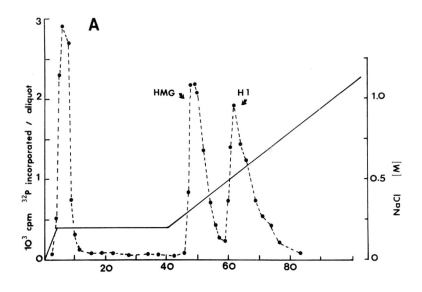

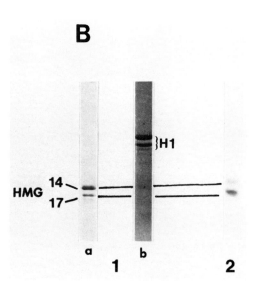

Fig. 3. Chromatographic and electrophoretic separation of [32]P-labeled HMG 14 and 17 from rat C6 glial cells. A: CM–Sephadex chromatography of a 5% trichloroacetic acid-soluble fraction containing histone H1 and HMG 14 and 17. ●–––●, [32]P radioactivity; ─────, NaCl (M). B: Separation of histone H1 and HMG 14 and 17 by SDS–polyacrylamide gel electrophoresis. Lanes 1a, b: HMG 14 and 17 and histone H1 subfractions after staining with amido black dye; lane 2: autoradiogram of electrophoretically separated, [32]P-labeled HMG 14 and 17.

ement is based on the previous finding (see Table II) that isoproterenol mediates an increased phosphorylation of the $NH_2$ terminus with a concomitant dephosphorylation of equal magnitude of the COOH-terminal fragment of histone H1-2 resulting in no apparent net change of phosphorylation of the intact H1-2 molecule. A similar detailed analysis of the individual intramolecular phosphorylation sites has to be carried out to delineate the potential effect of isoproterenol more precisely.

TABLE V

PHOSPHORYLATION OF HMG 14 AND 17 IN RAT C6 GLIAL CELLS

| HMG | Specific activity* | | Specific activity ratio** | Phosphoserine | Phosphothreonine |
|---|---|---|---|---|---|
| | Isoproterenol | | | % of total phosphoamino acid | |
| | − | + | | | |
| 14 | 5432 | 5758 | 1.06 ± 0.13*** | 60 ± 2 | 40 ± 2 |
| 17 | 8058 | 8863 | 1.10 ± 0.13 | 88 ± 2 | 12 ± 1 |

Rat C6 glial cells were labeled with $Na_2H^{32}PO_4$ and then stimulated for 1 h with isoproterenol ($10^{-5}$ M). HMG 14 and 17 were isolated, separated by electrophoresis, and $^{32}P$ radioactivity in each HMG was determined.
* Specific activity = cpm [$^{32}P$]phosphate incorporated/$\mu$g HMG.
** Ratio = specific activity of stimulated cells/specific activity of control cells.
*** Values are given as means ± standard deviation of the mean ($n$ = 4).

## PHOSPHORYLATIVE MODIFICATION OF HISTONE H1 AND HMG 14 AND 17 IN TRANSCRIPTIONALLY ACTIVE REGIONS OF THE CHROMATIN

Although the isoproterenol-mediated phosphorylative changes of histones H1-1, H1-2 and H1-3 are significant, the magnitude of the changes is small particularly in view of the large quantities of histones in the nucleus. It can be calculated that isoproterenol stimulation involves the transfer of only one molecule of phosphate per $10^7$ molecules of histone H1-1. Possibly, the distribution of the structurally modified histone molecules occurs randomly throughout the chromatin. Buf if we assume a regulatory function of the phosphorylations, it is more likely that the modified histones are located at functionnally and/or structurally key points of the chromatin, for example in transcriptionally active regions. To test this idea we have subjected nuclei of C6 glial cells to micrococcal nuclease digestion which yields a chromatin that can be separated into fractions enriched in transcriptionally active chromatin (released fraction) and chromatin which is depleted in these transcriptionally active regions (pellet fraction). If the structural modifications occur on protein molecules located selectively in either of these chromatin regions, the quantitative extent of the phosphorylation/dephosphorylation should be magnified in these fractions. Otherwise random distribution of the modified molecules may be assumed.

In the experiment from which we have obtained the data listed in Table VI, nuclei of control and isoproterenol-stimulated $^{32}P$-labeled C6 glial cells were subjected to limited digestion with micrococcal nuclease. After separation of the digested chromatin into released and pellet fractions, histone H1 subfractions and HMG 14 and 17 were isolated and the degree of $^{32}P$ labeling in each fraction was determined. To allow for a more uniform expression of the data and better comparison, the relative amount of $^{32}P$ labelling is expressed as the ratio of the amount of $^{32}P$ in the released fraction versus amount of $^{32}P$ label in the pellet fraction. Several important findings become evident from the data of Table VI. Firstly, although the phosphorylation of HMG 14 and 17 is apparently not affected by isoproterenol, the relatively high

TABLE VI

PHOSPHORYLATION OF HISTONE H1 SUBFRACTIONS AND OF HMG 14 AND 17
ISOLATED FROM MICROCOCCAL NUCLEASE-TREATED C6 GLIAL CHROMATIN FRACTIONS

| Nuclear protein | Specific activity of released fraction/specific activity of pellet ± S.D. | |
|---|---|---|
| | Isoproterenol | |
| | − | + |
| H1-1 | 1.19 ± 0.12 | 1.42 ± 0.16 |
| H1-2 | 1.39 ± 0.14 | 1.22 ± 0.15 |
| H1-3 | 2.05 ± 0.28 | 1.84 ± 0.44 |
| HMG 14 | 2.33 ± 0.52 | 2.21 ± 0.30 |
| HMG 17 | 1.75 ± 0.23 | 1.74 ± 0.04 |

Rat C6 glial cells were labeled with $Na_2H^{32}PO_4$ and then stimulated for 1 h with isoproterenol ($10^{-5}$ M). Nuclei were isolated, subjected to micrococcal nuclease digestion and released and pellet chromatin fractions were prepared according to Levy-Wilson and Dixon (1979). Histones and HMG proteins were isolated and their $^{32}P$ radioactivity was determined as described in Tables I and V.

specific activity ratios indicate that HMG 14 and 17 in the transcriptionally active (released) chromatin fraction are more highly phosphorylated than in the relatively inactive chromatin of the pellet fraction. Secondly, among the histone H1 subspecies $^{32}P$-labelled H1-3 is present in larger amounts in the released fraction. Thirdly, phosphorylated histones H1-1 and H1-2 are more evenly distributed between released and pellet fractions. However, in untreated cells, there is about 19% respectively 39% more $^{32}P$ label associated with H1-1 and H1-2 of the released fractions than with the pellet. After isoproterenol stimulation the relative degree of H1-1 phosphorylation in the released fraction increases from about 19% to 42%, whereas no significant change of distribution of $^{32}P$-labeled H1-2 occurs after isoproterenol stimulation.

## PHOSPHORYLATION OF RNA POLYMERASE II IN C6 GLIAL CELLS

A number of laboratories have reported the phosphorylation of mammalian RNA polymerase I and II subunits either in vitro (Jungmann et al., 1974; Hirsch and Martelo, 1976; Kranias et al., 1977) or in vivo (Dahmus, 1981). The functional significance of this structural modification is, however, unknown. It has been postulated that phosphorylation of polymerase will lead to its functional modifications (Jungmann and Kranias, 1977). Functional modulation of the enzyme responsible for structural gene transcription, RNA polymerase II, constitutes an attractive model for the direct control of transcriptional events by nuclear protein kinases. Following isoproterenol stimulation, C6 cells respond with an alteration of transcriptional activity resulting in a modulation of general RNA synthesis (DeVellis and Brooker, 1973) and increased levels of lactate dehydrogenase M subunit mRNA (Derda et al., 1980; Miles et al., 1981). It was therefore of interest to identify potential phosphorylative modifications of RNA polymerase II after isoproterenol stimulation.

When RNA polymerase II from control and isoproterenol-stimulated $^{32}P$-labeled C6 glial cells is immunoprecipitated with chicken anti-calf RNA polymerase II antiserum and subjected to SDS–polyacrylamide gel electrophoresis, the autoradiographic patterns shown in Fig. 4 (lanes B and D) are obtained. In spite of the relatively high background of $^{32}P$ in the lower

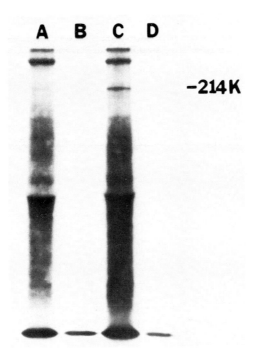

Fig. 4. Autoradiograms of immunoprecipitated RNA polymerase II isolated from [32]P-labeled C6 glial cells before and after isoproterenol ($10^{-5}$ M) stimulation. Immunoprecipitated RNA polymerase was subjected to SDS–polyacrylamide gel electrophoresis. Lanes A and C show autoradiograms of RNA polymerase immunoprecipitated with chicken anti-calf RNA polymerase II antiserum; lanes B and D show autoradiograms of RNA polymerase immunoprecipitated with pre-immune chicken serum. Lanes A, B: unstimulated samples; lanes C and D: RNA polymerase from isoproterenol-stimulated cells.

two-thirds of the gels, it can be seen that a protein band corresponding to the 214 000 dalton subunit of RNA polymerase II is markedly phosphorylated in the polymerase obtained from isoproterenol-stimulated glial cells (Fig. 4, lane C). Immunoprecipitation of RNA polymerase II from control and stimulated cells using preimmune chicken serum, electrophoresis of the immunoprecipitate and autoradiography reveal no significant amounts of [32]P-labeled protein (Fig. 4, lanes B and D).

Densitometric scanning of the autoradiographs allows a semi-quantitative assessment of the extent of phosphorylation as shown in Fig. 5. The peak corresponding to the 214 000 dalton subunit is clearly visible in the densitometric scan of RNA polymerase from stimulated cells (Fig. 5A) but not in control cells. Determination of the ratio of the optical densities of polymerase from stimulated cells versus non-stimulated cells (Fig. 5B) indicates a relatively unchanged ratio throughout the scans with the exception of the ratio determined for the 214 000 dalton subunit which is selectively increased by about 2–3-fold. Recovery of the gel section containing the 214 000 dalton subunit and partial acid hydrolysis of the [32]P-labeled subunit resulted in the identification of only [32P]phosphoserine (Fig. 6). No [32P]phosphothreonine was identified. The amount of [32P]phosphoserine identified in the subunit isolated from stimulated cells is about 2-fold higher than from control cells.

Based on previous findings that isoproterenol stimulation of C6 glial cells leads to increased intracellular cAMP levels (see Fig. 1) and increased nuclear cAMP-dependent protein kinase

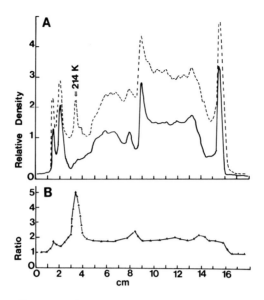

Fig. 5. Densitometric scans of immunoprecipitated RNA polymerase II from unstimulated cells (———) and from stimulated C6 glial cells (– – – –). These scans were taken from the autoradiograms shown in Fig. 4, lanes A and C. The position of the 214 000 dalton RNA polymerase II subunit is indicated. B: Ratio of optical densities (relative density of scan from stimulated cells/relative density of scan from unstimulated cells) calculated from the scans of A.

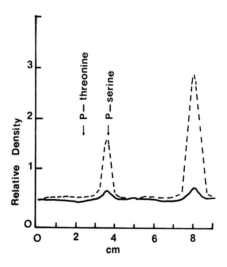

Fig. 6. Analysis of [³²P]phosphoamino acids by paper electrophoresis. Partial acid hydrolysates of gel slices containing the 214 000 dalton subunit were fractionated by paper electrophoresis at pH 2.4 (1 % formic acid 4 % acetic acid; 500 V; 16 h. ³²P acceptor amino acids were visualized by autoradiography and identified by co-migration of authentic phosphoserine and phosphothreonine. The figure depicts densitometric scans of the autoradiographs obtained from samples of unstimulated cells (———) and from stimulated cells (– – – –).

activity (Jungmann et al., 1979; Schwartz and Costa, 1980), it is likely that the phosphorylative modification of the subunit is a cAMP-mediated event. Previously, we have demonstrated the in vitro phosphorylation of the 180 000 and 25 000 dalton subunits of calf thymus RNA polymerase II by highly purified homologous cAMP-dependent protein kinase (Kranias et al., 1977). Our previous failure to identify in vitro phosphorylation of the 214 000 dalton subunit can be best explained considering that the 180 000 dalton subunit arises after proteolytic modification of the larger subunits of the polymerase, especially during extensive purification procedures. Immunoprecipitation of the polymerase from nuclear protein extracts is fast and may eliminate or reduce proteolysis.

## CONCLUSION

Nuclear proteins of confluent rat C6 glial cell cultures are very highly phosphorylated. Their separation after labeling with $Na_2H^{32}PO_4$ by SDS–polyacrylamide gel electrophoresis and identification by autoradiography has allowed us to identify between 250 and 300 individual phosphorylated peptides. The chemical nature and function of most of these peptides are unknown and it can be assumed that most of the phosphorylations are of constitutive nature. In this report we have identified a number of the better characterized nuclear proteins as phosphoproteins, e.g. histones, HMG 14 and 17, and RNA polymerase II, and we have

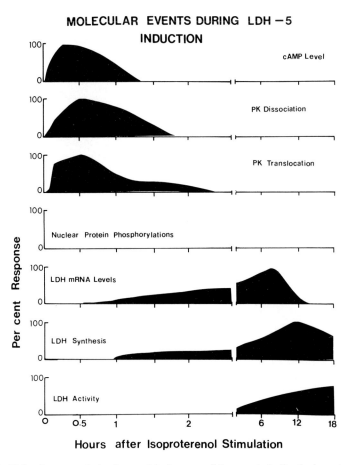

Fig. 7. Molecular events during lactate dehydrogenase-5 isozyme induction by isoproterenol.

presented evidence that the phosphorylation/dephosphorylation state of these proteins is either subject to effector agent regulation or occurs preferentially at certain loci of the chromatin which differ in their transcriptional activities. The isoproterenol-mediated phosphorylative changes occur relatively rapidly (within 1 h after isoproterenol treatment) and our data are consistent with, but do not prove, the notion that these phosphorylations structurally alter chromatin and result in a modulation of chromatin function. Since under our experimental conditions isoproterenol treatment of C6 glial cells leads to the nuclear synthesis of lactate dehydrogenase M subunit mRNA and subsequent synthesis of lactate dehydrogenase M subunit (Derda et al., 1980; Miles et al., 1981), we believe that some of the observed phosphorylative changes are part of the mechanism whereby isoproterenol, via cAMP, regulates the de novo synthesis of lactate dehydrogenase mRNA and lactate dehydrogenase protein. The temporal correlation of the various molecular events observed during lactate dehydrogenase induction are not inconsistent with this view. This has to be stressed, since the activities of several other proteins, such as phosphodiesterase (Schwartz and Passonneau, 1974) and ornithine decarboxylase (Bachrach, 1975), are also induced by catecholamines in C6 glial cells, although the precise mechanisms of their induction has not been elucidated. It is especially important to note that the induction time courses of proteins other than lactate dehydrogenase do not correlate precisely with the time course of lactate dehydrogenase induction and its associated molecular events. The molecular events elicited by isoproterenol in C6 glial cells and their temporal correlation are graphically shown in Fig. 7. Following the isoproterenol-mediated elevation of cAMP concentration, a cascade of molecular events ensues over a 24-h period culminating in increased activity levels of glial cell lactate dehydrogenase-5 isozyme (Derda et al., 1980). Intermediate events are the dissociation and translocation of glial cell cAMP-dependent protein kinase (Jungmann et al., 1979; Schwartz and Costa, 1980), and the nuclear phosphorylation events described in this report. Again it should be pointed out that although a correlation of some of the events has been established on a molecular level, e.g. the isoproterenol- (and cAMP-) mediated phosphorylative modification of several histones and of RNA polymerase II on one hand, and the increased levels of lactate dehydrogenase mRNA and accelerated synthesis of lactate dehydrogenase on the other hand, the involvement and precise role of the phosphorylative changes of these nuclear proteins in lactate dehydrogenase induction still have to be determined and is the subject of our future research.

## ACKNOWLEDGEMENTS

Research described in this report has been supported by NIH grant GM 23895, and by the Research and Education Fund, Northwestern Memorial Hospital.

## REFERENCES

Albanese, I. and Weintraub, H. (1980) Electrophoretic separation of a class of nucleosomes enriched in HMG 14 and 17 and actively transcribed globin genes. *Nucleic Acids Res.,* 8: 2787–2805.

Bachrach, U. (1975) Cyclic AMP-mediated induction of ornithine decarboxylase of glioma and neuroblastoma cells. *Proc. nat. Acad. Sci. (Wash.),* 73: 3087–3091.

Bakayev, V.V., Schmatchenko, V.V. and Georgiev, G.P. (1979) Subnucleosome particles containing high mobility group proteins HMG-E and HMG-G originate from transcriptionally active chromatin. *Nucleic Acids Res.,* 7: 1525–1540.

Benda, P., Someda, K., Messer, J. and Sweet, W. (1971) Morphological and immunochemical studies of rat glial tumors and clonal strains propagated in culture. *J. Neurosurg.*, 34: 310–323.

Bissell, M., Rubinstein, L., Bignami, A. and Herman, M. (1974) Characteristics of the rat C6 glioma maintained in organ culture system. Production of glial fibrillary acid protein in the absence and gliafibrillogenesis. *Brain Res.*, 82: 77–89.

Bloom, F.E. (1975) The role of cyclic nucleotides in central synaptic function. *Rev. Physiol. Biochem. Pharmacol.*, 74: 1–103.

Bonner, W.M. and Pollard, H.B. (1975) The presence of F3-Fa$_1$ dimers and oligomers in chromatin. *Biochem. biophys. Res. Commun.*, 64: 282–288.

Byus, C.V., Klimpel, G.R., Lucas, D.O. and Russell, D.H. (1977) Type I and type II cyclic AMP-dependent protein kinase as opposite effectors of lymphocyte mitogenesis. *Nature (Lond.)*, 268: 63–64.

Castagna, M., Palmer, W.K. and Walsh, D.A. (1977) Metabolism of N$^6$, O$^{2'}$-[$^3$H]dibutyryl cyclic adenosine 3',5'-monophosphate and macromolecular interaction of the products in perfused rat liver. *Arch. Biochem. Biophys.*, 181: 46–60.

Cleveland, D.W., Fischer S.G., Kirschner, M.W. and Laemmli, U.K. (1977) Peptide mapping by limited proteolysis in sodium dodecyl sulfate and analysis by gel electrophoresis. *J. biol. Chem.*, 252: 1102–1106.

Dahmus, M.E. (1981) Phosphorylation of eukaryotic DNA-dependent RNA polymerase. Identification of calf thymus RNA polymerase subunits phosphorylated by two purified protein kinases, correlation with in vivo sites of phosphorylation in HeLa cell RNA polymerase. *J. biol. Chem.*, 256: 3332–3339.

Derda, D.F., Miles, M.F., Schweppe, J.S. and Jungmann, R.A. (1980) Cyclic AMP regulation of lactate dehydrogenase. Isoproterenol and N$^6$,O$^{2'}$-dibutyryl cyclic AMP increase the levels of lactate dehydrogenase-5 isozyme and its messenger RNA in rat C6 glioma cells. *J. biol. Chem.*, 255: 11112–11121.

DeVellis, J. and Brooker, G. (1973) Induction of enzymes by glucocorticoids and catecholamines in a rat glial cell line. In *Tissue Culture of the Nervous System*, G. Sato (Ed.), Plenum Press, New York, pp. 231–245.

Gazit, B., Panet, A. and Cedar, H. (1980) Reconstitution of a deoxyribonuclease I-sensitive structure on active genes. *Proc. nat. Acad. Sci. (Wash.)*, 77: 1787–1790.

Gilman, A.G. and Nirenberg, M. (1971) Effect of catecholamines on the adenosine 3',5'-cyclic monophosphate concentrations of clonal satellite cells of neurons. *Proc. nat. Acad. Sci. (Wash.)*, 68: 2165–2168.

Gurley, L.R., Walters, R.A., Hildebrand, C.E., Ratliff, R.L., Hohmann, P.G. and Tobey, R.A. (1977) Sequential biochemical events related to cell proliferation. In *Mechanisms and Control of Cell Division*, T.L. Rost and E.M. Gifford, Jr. (Eds.), Dowden, Hutchison and Ross, Inc., Stroudsburg, PA, pp. 3–43.

Harrison, J.J. and Jungmann, R.A. (1981) Phosphorylative modification of rat C6 glioma cell high mobility group proteins 14 and 17. *Biochem. biophys. Res. Commun.*, submitted for publication.

Harrison, J.J., Suter, P., Suter, S. and Jungmann, R.A. (1980) Isoproterenol-induced phosphorylative modification in vivo of rat C6 glioma cell histones. *Biochem. biophys. Res. Commun.*, 96: 1253–1260.

Hirsch, J. and Martelo, O.J. (1976) Phosphorylation of rat liver ribonucleic acid polymerase I by nuclear protein kinases. *J. biol. Chem.*, 251: 5408–5413.

Jungmann, R.A. and Kranias, E.G. (1977) Nuclear phosphoprotein kinases and the regulation of gene transcription. *Int. J. Biochem.*, 8: 819–830.

Jungmann, R.A. and Russell, D.H. (1977) Cyclic AMP, cyclic AMP-dependent protein kinase, and the regulation of gene expression. *Life Sci.*, 20: 1787–1789.

Jungmann, R.A., Hiestand, P.C. and Schweppe, J.S. (1974) Adenosine 3':5'-monophosphate-dependent protein kinase and the stimulation of ovarian nuclear ribonucleic acid polymerase activities *J. biol. Chem.*, 249: 5444–5454.

Jungmann, R.A., Christensen, M.L. and Derda, D.F. (1979) Isoproterenol-stimulated induction of lactate dehydrogenase and modulation of nuclear protein kinase activity in C6 rat glioma cells. In *Effects of Drugs on the Cell Nucleus*, H. Busch, S.T. Crooke and Y. Daskal (Eds.), Academic Press, New York, pp. 507–519.

Kinkade, Jr., J.M. (1969) Qualitative species differences and quantitative tissue differences in the distribution of lysine-rich histones. *J. biol. Chem.*, 244: 3375–3386.

Kranias, E.G., Schweppe, J.S. and Jungmann, R.A. (1977) Phosphorylative and functional modifications of nucleoplasmic RNA polymerase II by homologous 3':5'-monophosphate dependent protein kinase from calf thymus and by heterologous phosphatase. *J. biol. Chem.*, 252: 6750–6758.

Langan, T.A. (1978) Methods for the assessment of site-specific histone phosphorylation. *Methods Cell Biol.*, 19: 127–142.

Levy-Wilson, B. (1981) Enhanced phosphorylation of high-mobility-group proteins in nuclease-sensitive mononucleosomes from butyrate-treated HeLa cells. *Proc. nat. Acad. Sci. (Wash.)*, 78: 2189–2193.

Levy-Wilson, B. and Dixon, G.H. (1979) Limited action of micrococcal nuclease on trout testis nuclei generates two mononucleosome subsets enriched in transcribed DNA sequences. *Proc. nat. Acad. Sci. (Wash.)*, 76: 1682–1686.

178

Lucas, M. and Bockaert, J. (1977) Use of (−)-[³H]dihydroalprenolol to study beta adrenergic receptor-adenylate cyclase coupling in C6 glioma cells: Role of 5'-guanylylimidodiphosphate. *Mol. Pharmacol.*, 13: 314–329.

Maguire, M.E., Wiklund, R.A., Anderson, H.J. and Gilman, A.G. (1976) Binding of [¹²⁵I]iodohydroxybenzylpindolol to putative $\beta$-adrenergic receptors of rat glioma cells and other cell clones. *J. biol. Chem.*, 251: 1121–1231.

McGhee, J.D. and Felsenfeld, G. (1980) Nucleosome structure. *Annu. Rev. Biochem.*, 94: 1115–1156.

McGinnis, J.F. and DeVellis, J. (1978) Glucocorticoid regulation in rat brain cultures. Hydrocortisone increases the rate of synthesis of glycerol phosphate dehydrogenase in C6 glioma cells. *J. biol. Chem.*, 253: 8483–8492.

Miles, M.F., Hung, P. and Jungmann, R.A. (1981) Cyclic AMP regulation of lactate dehydrogenase. Quantitation of lactate dehydrogenase M-subunit messenger RNA in isoproterenol- and N⁶, O²'-dibutyryl cyclic AMP-stimulated rat C6 glioma cells by hybridization analysis using a cloned cDNA probe. *J. biol. Chem.*, 256: 12545–12552.

Nathanson, J.A. (1977) Cyclic nucleotides and nervous system function. *Physiol. Rev.*, 57: 157–256.

Schwartz, J.P. and Costa, E. (1977) Regulation of nerve growth factor content in C6 glioma cells by $\beta$-adrenergic receptor stimulation. *Naunyn-Schmiedeberg's Arch. Pharmakol. exp. Pathol.*, 300: 123–129.

Schwartz, J.P. and Costa, E. (1980) Protein kinase translocation following $\beta$-adrenergic receptor activation in C6 glioma cells. *J. biol. Chem.*, 255: 2943–2948.

Schwartz, J.P. and Passonneau, J.V. (1974) Cyclic AMP-mediated induction of cAMP phosphodiesterase of the C6 glioma cells. *Proc. nat. Acad. Sci. (Wash.)*, 71: 3844–3848.

Schwartz, J.P., Chuang, D.-M. and Costa, E. (1977) Increase in nerve growth factor content of C6 glioma cells by the activation of a $\beta$-adrenergic receptor. *Brain Res.*, 137: 369–375.

Teresaki, W.L. and Brooker, G. (1978) [¹²⁵I]iodohydroxybenzylpindolol binding sites on intact rat glioma cells. Evidence for $\beta$-adrenergic receptors of high coupling efficiency. *J. biol. Chem.*, 253: 5418–5425.

Weisbrod, S. and Weintraub, H. (1979) Isolation of a subclass of nuclear proteins responsible for conferring a DNase I-sensitive structure on globin chromatin. *Proc. nat. Acad. Sci. (Wash.)*, 76: 630–634.

Weisbrod, S., Groudine, M. and Weintraub, H. (1980) Interaction of HMG 14 and 17 with actively transcribed genes. *Cell*, 19: 289–301.

Whitlock, Jr., J.P., Augustine, R. and Schulman, H. (1980) Calcium-dependent phosphorylation of histone H3 in butyrate-treated HeLa cells. *Nature (Lond.)*, 287: 74–76.

Zanetta, J., Benda, P., Gombos, G. and Morgan, I. (1972) The presence of 2',3'-cAMP 3'-phosphohydrolase in glial cells in tissue culture. *J. Neurochem.*, 19: 881–883.

# Activation of Multiple S6 Phosphorylation and its Possible Role in the Alteration of mRNA Expression

G. THOMAS

*Friedrich Miescher-Institut, P.O. Box 273, CH 4002, Basel, Switzerland*

## INTRODUCTION

Stimulation of cell growth in culture by serum (Bürk, 1966; Hershko et al., 1971; Holley 1975), low concentrations of polypeptide growth factors (Gospodarowics, 1974; Rinderknecht and Humbel, 1976; Carpenter and Cohen, 1979) or prostaglandis (Jimenez de Asua et al., 1975) leads to the activiation of a number of seemingly unrelated metabolic processes. However, because these processes appear to be activated in a coordinate manner it led Tomkins and co-workers to collectively refer to them as the "pleitotypic response" (Hershko et al., 1971). More recent studies carried out with individual growth factors and hormones by Jimenez de Asua and co-workers have more clearly demonstrated that the initiation of DNA synthesis and cell proliferation in culture are dependent on a sequence of events which are expressed in an orderly manner as cells progress through the pre-replicative or lag phase (Jimenez de Asua et al., 1979). One of the most important events activated in this pathway is protein synthesis. It is required throughout lag phase for the initiation of DNA synthesis (Brooks, 1977) and throughout the S and $G_2$ phases for mitosis and cell division (Tobey et al., 1971).

The increase in protein synthesis has been shown to be 2–3-fold within the first 2 h following serum stimulation (Stanners and Becker, 1971; Rudland, 1974). This increase is most easily observed as a large shift of inactive 80S ribosomes and stored non-polysomal mRNA into actively translating polysomes (Rudland et al., 1975). As expected from these observations the increase in the rate of protein synthesis is due to an increase in the rate of initiation (Stanners and Becker, 1971). Though the activation of protein synthesis is well documented, along with the activation of a number of other cellular events during this time, we have as yet little understanding of the underlying biochemical processes involved in regulating its expression. In the case of protein synthesis, however, many of the translational components involved have been structurally well characterized and in many instances we know their functions in vitro. Therefore we have argued that protein synthesis may serve as a useful model for determining how a growth factor acting on the cell surface is able to turn on a process within the cell (reviewed by Thomas and Gordon, 1979).

Because of the large number of components involved in protein synthesis (over 400) we have limited our studies to ribosomal protein phosphorylation–dephosphorylation reactions. We made this choice for two reasons: (1) because phosphorylation and dephosphorylation of cellular proteins are known to serve as mediators of cellular regulatory signals (Tomkins, 1975; Greengard, 1978), and (2) because ribosomal proteins are phosphorylated under a variety of growth conditions (Wool, 1979; Traugh, 1981). In this paper we review our findings to date concerning the role of ribosomal protein phosphorylation in the activation of protein synthesis and discuss the direction of future studies.

## MATERIALS AND METHODS

### Cell culture and radioactive labelling

Cells were grown and maintained as previously described (Thomas et al., 1979). Cultures were judged quiescent at 7 days after seeding when no mitotic cells were observed. Radioactive labelling of ribosomal proteins or total cytoplasmic proteins with $^{35}$S-methionine (Amersham) was carried out as before (Thomas et al., 1980, 1981, respectively).

### Polysome gradients

A portion, approximately 200–250 $\mu$l, of cell lysate was layered directly on a 17.1–41% isokenetic sucrose gradient followed by centrifugation at 485 000 $\times$ G (Ti 60 rotor, Beckman L5-65 centrifuge) for 55 min at 2° C (Thomas et al., 1977). The gradients were collected and absorbance at 260 nm was monitored as previously described (Thomas et al., 1977).

### Polyacrylamide gel electrophoresis

Analysis of ribosomal proteins on two-dimensional urea polyacrylamide gels was as previously described (Thomas et al., 1980). Analysis of cytoplasmic proteins by nonequilibrium pH gradient two-dimensional polyacrylamide gel electrophoresis was as described by O'Farrell et al. (1977) with the modifications of Thomas et al. (1981).

## RESULTS

### Increase in ribosomal protein phosphorylation

The activation of protein synthesis in quiescent 3T3 cells has been most easily observed as a large shift of inactive 80S ribosomes into actively translating polysomes (Fig. 1). Previously we have shown that during the time these inactive 80S ribosomes are shifting into actively translating polysomes there is a 100-fold increase in the amount of $^{32}$P incorporated into the protein fraction of 40S ribosomal subunits (Thomas et al., 1979). Further experiments, employing one-dimensional SDS and two-dimensional urea polyacrylamide gels also showed that the increase was due to the phosphorylation of a single 40S ribosomal protein, designated S6 (Haselbacher et al., 1979; Thomas et al., 1979). No corresponding increase was seen in 60S ribosomal proteins. Because serum stimulation also leads to a large increase in phosphate uptake (Cunningham and Pardee, 1969; Jimenez de Asua et al., 1974) and intracellular ATP content (Grummt et al., 1977) the increase in S6 phosphorylation may simply be ascribed to an increase in the specific activity of intracellular [$\gamma$-$^{32}$P]ATP. To test this possibility cells were stimulated with serum for 30 min in the presence of $^{32}$PO$_4$ and the $^{32}$P specific activity of S6, [$\gamma$-P]ATP and free Pi was determined. The results show that in the first 30 min following stimulation there is a 30-fold increase in the amount of $^{32}$P incorporated into S6 (Table I). In contrast, there is only a 2-fold increase in the specific activity of [$\gamma$-$^{32}$P]ATP and virtually no change in the specific activity of free $^{32}$Pi (Table I). Thus the increase in the amount of $^{32}$Pi incorporated into S6 cannot be simply attributable to an increase in the specific activity of [$\gamma$-$^{32}$P]ATP.

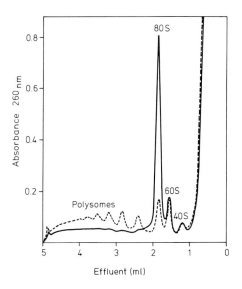

Fig. 1. Effect of serum on polysome formation. Parallel cultures of quiescent Swiss 3T3 cells were treated with NaCl (—) or 10% serum (--) for 2 h. The cells were then harvested and the polysomes analyzed as previously described (Thomas et al., 1977).

TABLE I

DETERMINATION OF S6-$^{32}$P, [$\gamma$-$^{32}$P]ATP AND $^{32}$Pi SPECIFIC ACTIVITIES IN QUIESCENT AND SERUM-STIMULATED CULTURES

|  | Quiescent (cpm/pmole) | Stimulated (cpm/pmole) | Stimulated/quiescent ratio |
|---|---|---|---|
| S6 | 0.31 | 8.62 | 27.75 |
| ATP-$\gamma$-phosphate | 1.97 | 4.17 | 2.11 |
| Pi | 12.60 | 12.80 | 1.02 |

Quiescent cultures of 3T3 cells, prepared as described in Materials and Methods, were treated with 0.15 M NaCl (quiescent) or 15% (by vol.) fetal calf serum (stimulated), in the presence of 0.11 mCi per ml $^{32}$PO$_4$ (Amersham). Analysis of S6, ATP-$\gamma$-PO$_4$ and Pi were carried out as described in Materials and Methods. For the determination of the specific activity of S6-$^{32}$P an 80S monosome molecular weight of $4.5 \times 10^6$ dalton, an extinction coefficient of $11.3 A_{260}$ per mg of 80S monosome and 1 mole of S6 per mole of 80S monosome were employed. Each value represents the average of 2 separate determinations. (Reprinted from Thomas et al., 1979.)

The absolute level of S6 phosphorylation can be measured by the extent to which its mobility changes on two-dimensional polyacrylamide gels (Gressner and Wool, 1974). The more phosphorylated the protein becomes the more slowly it migrates in both dimensions of electrophorisis. Therefore, to ensure that the increase in the amount of $^{32}$Pi incorporated into S6 accurately reflected an increase in the extent of phosphorylation, the level of S6 phosphorylation was also monitored on two-dimensional polyacrylamide gels. To carry out these studies cells were labelled to equilibrium with [$^{35}$S]menthionine and then treated for 30 min with 10% serum or an equal volume of NaCl. The ribosomal proteins were then separated by two-dimensional gel electrophoresis and analyzed by fluorography. The results show that in quiescent cells treated with NaCl most of S6 resides in the native unphosphorylated position (Fig. 2A). In contrast, treatment with 10% serum for 1 h leads to a marked shift of S6 to the most highly phosphorylated derivatives S6b and c (Fig. 2B). Treatment of a portion of either sample with alkaline phosphatase shifts all of S6 back to the native unphosphorylated position (inserts Fig. 2). Thus the increase in $^{32}$Pi content in S6 accurately demonstrates an increase in the extent of S6 phosphorylation.

*Serum withdrawal*

The increase in S6 phosphorylation correlates very closely with the activation of protein synthesis, either measured by the amount of [$^{35}$S]methionine incorporated into protein or the percentage of ribosomes as polysomes (Thomas et al., 1979). Therefore, we have concluded that the two events are tightly coupled. It is also known that the removal of serum from stimulated cells leads to an inhibition of protein synthesis (Soeiro and Amos, 1966; Hershko et al., 1971). Thus if the two events are coupled one would expect that S6 would become dephosphorylated when serum was removed from serum-stimulated cells. To test this possibility cells which had been pre-labelled with [$^{35}$S]methionine were stimulated for 60 min with serum, then washed 2 times with serum-free media and then incubated an additional 30 or 60 min in the absence of serum. The results show that in resting cells most of the S6 resided in the native dephosphorylated from and in phosphorylated derivatives S6a and b (Fig. 3A). Following serum stimulation for 60 min most of S6 shifted to derivatives S6c, d and e (Fig.

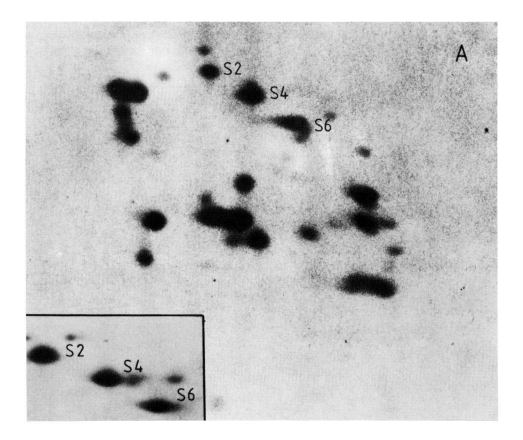

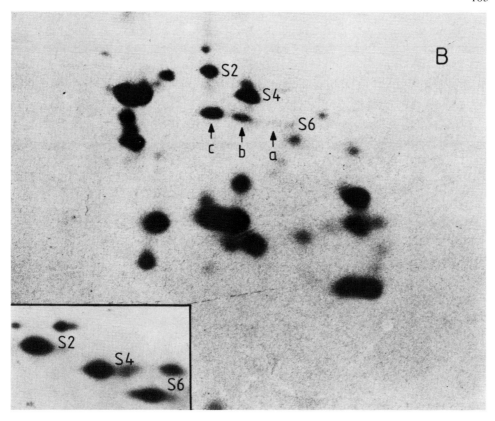

Fig. 2. Effect of serum on the extent of S6 phosphorylation. Parallel cultures of quiescent 3T3 cells which were pre-labelled to equilibrium with [$^{35}$S]methionine were treated for 30 min with NaCl (A) or 15% serum (B). After extraction of the ribosomal proteins they were either analyzed directly by fluorography or treated with alkaline phosphatase (inserts) and then analyzed by fluorography (reprinted from Thomas et al., 1979).

3B). Removal of serum for 30 min led to little change in the distribution of the S6 phosphory-lated derivatives (Fig. 3C). However, by 60 min serum withdrawal S6 was becoming de-phosphorylated and shifting back to the unphosphorylated form (Fig. 3D). Thus the results are consistent with the hypothesis that the phosphorylation of S6 and the activation of protein synthesis are two tightly coupled events during the early stages of lag phase.

*Role of S6 phosphorylation in polysome assembly*

What was important to determine now was whether or not the activation of protein synthesis, within the intact cell, was dependent on the multiple phosphorylation of S6. To examine this question cells were stimulated with serum in the presence of cycloheximide, a potent inhibitor of protein synthesis, or the methylxanthine SQ 20006, which is known to inhibit the phos-phorylation of S6. In the presence of cycloheximide (100 $\mu$g/M) the serum-induced shift of inactive 80S ribosomes into polysomes was inhibited by greater than 95%, however, there was no effect on the extent of S6 phosphorylation as compared to control cells (Fig. 4A, B). Thus the phosphorylation of S6 does not require protein synthesis. In contrast, if cells were stimulated with serum in the presence of SQ 20006 (1.2 mM) both the shift of 80S ribosomes

184

into polysomes (Fig. 5) and the multiple phosphorylation of S6 (Fig. 4C) were completely inhibited. If it is true that the methylxanthines are blocking the activation of protein synthesis via inhibiting the phosphorylation of S6 then, if the concentration of SQ 20006 is lowered so that there is only a partial inhibition of S6 phosphorylation, one should see a corresponding effect on the activation of protein synthesis. Indeed at 0.6 mM SQ 20006 both the phosphorylation of S6 (Fig. 4D) and the activation of protein synthesis (Fig. 5) are inhibited to approximately the same extent. The results, taken together, suggest that the phosphorylation of S6 is a prerequisite for the activation of protein synthesis and not a consequence of it.

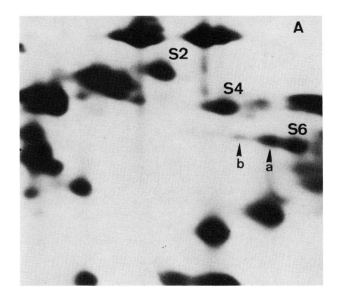

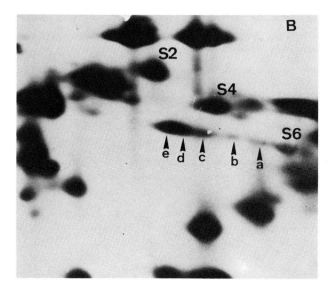

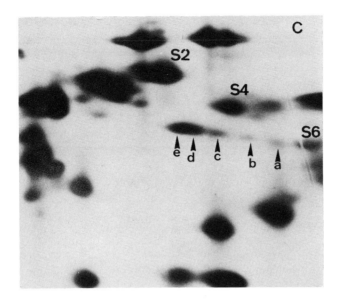

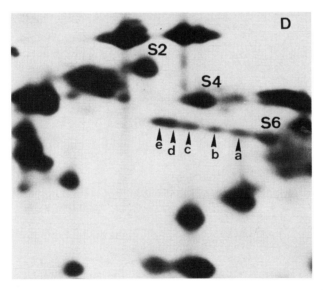

Fig. 3. Effect of serum withdrawal on S6 phosphorylation. Parallel cultures of quiescent 3T3 cells which were pre-labelled to equilibrium with [$^{35}$S]methionine were treated for 60 min with NaCl (A), 15% serum (B), 15% serum and then fresh media for 30 min (C), or 60 min (D). Ribosomal proteins were then analyzed by fluorography (reprinted from Thomas et al., 1980).

*Pattern of translation*

The results above and other experiments suggest that the phosphorylation of S6 facilitates some step in the process of initiation of protein synthesis. One possibility is that the phosphorylation of S6 may differentially change the affinity of the 40S ribosomal subunit for messenger RNA and thus lead to a change in the pattern of translation (Thomas et al., 1979,

186

1980; Wool, 1979; Gressner and Van de Leur, 1980; Traugh, 1981). In order to explore this possibility it was first asked whether the pattern of translation changed during the time S6 was becoming phosphorylated. Thus quiescent and serum-stimulated cells were pulse labelled with [$^{35}$S]methionine and the proteins which became labelled were analyzed by NEPHGE two-dimensional polyacrylamide gel electrophoresis. The most notable difference in the pattern of translation following serum stimulation (Fig. 6B) was the de novo appearance of cytoplasmic proteins of $M_r$ 26 000, 28 000, 45 000 and 47 000, designated $N_{26}$, $N_{28}$, $N_{45}$ and $N_{47}$. There

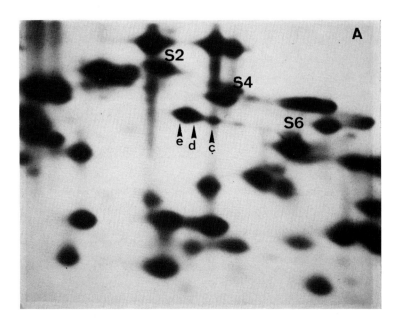

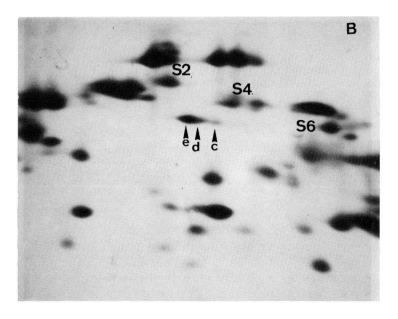

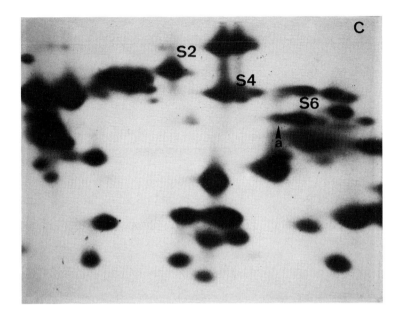

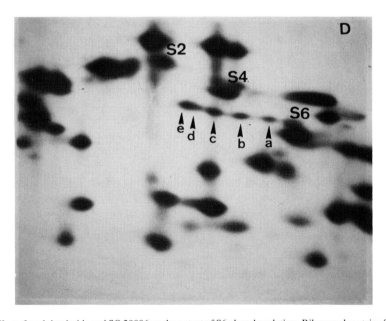

Fig. 4. Effect of cycloheximide and SQ 20006 on the extent of S6 phosphorylation. Ribosomal proteins from parallel cultures of quiescent 3T3 cells were labelled and analyzed as described in Fig. 3. (A) 15 % serum; (B) 15 % serum plus 100 $\mu$g/ml cycloheximide; (C) 15 % serum plus 1.2 mM SQ 20006; or (D) 0.6 mM SQ 20006 (reprinted from Thomas et al., 1980).

synthesis was not detectable in quiescent cells (Fig. 6A). In addition to these proteins four other proteins, designated $Q_{23}$, $Q_{49}$, $Q_{72}$ and $Q_{98}$, increased significantly as a fraction of the total labelled protein applied to the gel. Others, such as $Q_{31}$ and $Q_{42}$, $Q_{43}$, $Q_{53}$, $Q_{54}$ and $Q_{69}$

188

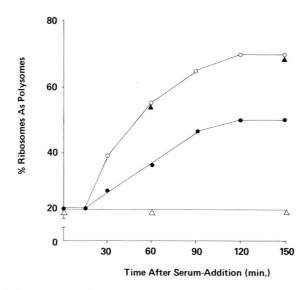

**Time After Serum-Addition (min.)**

Fig. 5. The effect of SQ 20006 and PGE₁ on serum-induced polysome formation. Resting cultures of Swiss 3T3 cells were treated with (○)15% serum alone, or together with (●) 0.6 mM SQ 20006, (△) 1.2 mM SQ 20006 or (▲) 50 μg/ml PGE₁. The percentage of ribosomes as polysomes was measured as described in the legend to Table 2. SQ 20006 and PGE₁ were added 15 min prior to the addition of serum. (Reprinted from Thomas et al., 1980).

increased to a lesser extent. In contrast, the synthesis of at least three proteins, $Q_{145}$, $Q_{176}$ and $Q_{178}$, appeared to decrease and that of $Q_{34}$, $Q_{45}$ and $Q_{46}$ appeared to change little. To ensure that these changes are not simply ascribable to differences in the ability of these proteins to enter the gel (Garrels, 1979; Bravo et al., 1981) we performed a double-label experiment. A lysate from a culture which had been stimulated for 2 h in the presence of [³H]isoleucine was mixed with an equal amount (in radioactivity) of [³⁵S]methionine protein from quiescent or 60 min stimulated culture. The samples were then separated by two-dimensional gel electrophoresis, the protein spots indicated in Fig. 6A, B were cut-out, and the ratio of [³⁵S]methionine/[³H]isoleucine for each spot was determined. The ratios for stimulated cells were then divided by the ratios for quiescent cells. As can be seen in Table II, the results agree quite closely with those in Fig. 6A, B.

To resolve the question of whether the synthesis of these proteins is under translational or transcriptional control the cells were next stimulated with serum for 60 min in the presence of actinomycin D and the proteins were analysed by two-dimensional gel electrophoresis (Fig. 7). As can be seen the increased incorporation of [³⁵S]methionine into proteins $N_{26}$, $N_{45}$, $N_{47}$, $Q_{31}$, $Q_{42}$, $Q_{53}$ and $Q_{72}$ was completely inhibited by the drug (Fig. 6). In contrast, the increased incorporation of [³⁵S]methionine into proteins $N_{28}$, $Q_{23}$, $Q_{45}$, $Q_{54}$, $Q_{69}$ and $Q_{98}$ was unaffected, and $Q_{49}$ appeared to be induced to an even higher level. Decreases observed in proteins $Q_{145}$, $Q_{176}$ and $Q_{178}$ were also unaffected by actinomycin D. Thus the data indicate that approximately one-half of the increases are due to alterations in mRNA expression at the translational level and one-half to alterations in mRNA expression at the transcriptional level. The results, which are summarized in Table III, are compatible with the possibility that S6 phosphorylation could alter the affinity of the ribosome for mRNA.

TABLE II

CHANGES IN THE AMOUNT OF [$^{35}$S]METHIONINE IN CYTOPLASMIC PROTEINS
AFTER SERUM STIMULATION

| Protein | Ration of [$^{35}$S]methionine/[$^{3}$H]isoleucine | | Amount change |
|---------|-----------|------------------|---------------|
| | Quiescent | Serum-stimulated | |
| Q$_{23}$ | 0.5 | 2.5 | 5.0 |
| Q$_{31}$ | 2.4 | 4.0 | 1.7 |
| Q$_{34}$ | 1.5 | 1.8 | 1.2 |
| Q$_{42}$ | 1.2 | 3.1 | 2.6 |
| Q$_{45}$ | 2.9 | 3.4 | 1.2 |
| Q$_{46}$ | 4.1 | 3.9 | 1.0 |
| Q$_{49}$ | 0.3 | 1.7 | 5.7 |
| Q$_{54}$ | 1.3 | 3.3 | 2.5 |
| Q$_{69}$ | 0.9 | 1.9 | 2.1 |
| Q$_{72}$ | 1.3 | 5.4 | 4.2 |
| Q$_{98}$ | 0.8 | 2.9 | 3.6 |
| Q$_{145}$ | 2.7 | 1.7 | 0.6 |
| Q$_{176}$ | 2.6 | 1.2 | 0.5 |
| Q$_{178}$ | 2.5 | 1.5 | 0.6 |

An equivalent amount ($1 \times 10^6$ cpm) of [$^{35}$S]methionine pulse-labelled extract from either quiescent cells or 60 min serum-stimulated cells was mixed with an equal amount ($1 \times 10^6$ cpm) of [$^{3}$H]isoleucine-labelled extract from cells which had been stimulated for 2 h in the continuous presence of [$^{3}$H]isoleucine. The quiescent cells and 60 min serum-stimulated cells were pulse-labelled with [$^{35}$S]methionine as described in Fig. 5. After two-dimensional polyacrylamide gel electrophoresis individual proteins were located by fluorography and those indicated above were eluted from the gel and the amounts of [$^{35}$S]methionine and [$^{3}$H]isoleucine present in each spot determined. The amounts of radioactivity incorporated into Q$_{43}$ and Q$_{53}$ were not determined. (Reprinted from Thomas et al., 1981.)

# DISCUSSION

The phosphorylation of S6 is not confined to the activation of 3T3 cells in culture but appears to be common to all eukaryotic systems whose direction of growth has been shifted from

TABLE III

EFFECT OF ACTINOMYCIN D ON SPECIFIC CYTOPLASMIC PROTEINS

| | | | |
|---|---|---|---|
| Q$_{23}$ | 0 | Q$_{54}$ | 0 |
| N$_{26}$ | + | N$_{56}$ | +(NS) |
| N$_{28}$ | 0 | Q$_{69}$ | 0 |
| Q$_{31}$ | + | Q$_{72}$ | + |
| Q$_{42}$ | + | Q$_{98}$ | 0 |
| Q$_{43}$ | 0 | Q$_{121}$ | +(NS) |
| N$_{45}$ | + | Q$_{145}$ | 0 |
| N$_{47}$ | + | Q$_{176}$ | 0 |
| Q$_{49}$ | 0 | Q$_{178}$ | 0 |
| Q$_{53}$ | + | | |

The results are summarized as described in the text. +, actinomycin D sensitive; 0, actinomycin D insensitive. NS, data not shown. (Reprinted from Thomas et al., 1981.)

relative quiescence to active proliferation. It was first observed in regenerating rat liver following partial hepatectomy, in concert with a large increase in protein synthesis (Gressner and Wool, 1974; Anderson et al., 1975). Similarly we have recently shown that following denervation of rat hemidiaphragm there is a large increase in the extent of S6 phosphorylation which correlates with a marked increase in protein synthesis and hypertrophy (Nielsen, Manchester, Towbin, Gordon and Thomas, in press). S6 has also been shown recently to become phosphorylated following fertilization of sea urchin eggs (Ballinger and Hunt, 1981) and during maturation of Xenopus oocytes (Nielsen, Thomas and Maller, 1981). Finally it has also been demonstrated that when Rous sarcoma temperature-sensitive transformed secondary chicken embryo fibroblasts are shifted from the non-permissive to the permissive temperature S6 becomes maximally phosphorylated (Decker, 1981). These results are consistent with the hypothesis that phosphorylation of S6 plays a central role in regulating the activation of protein synthesis during early times of marked cellular proliferation.

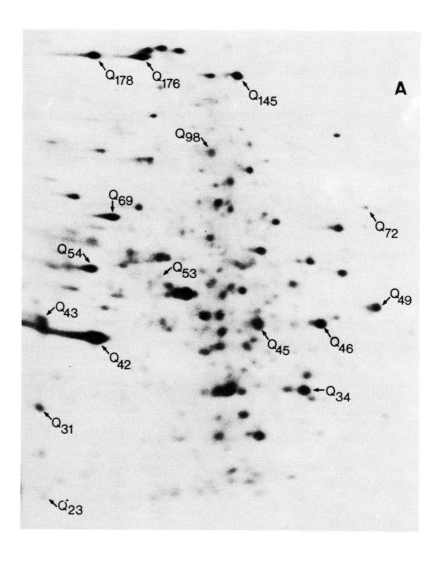

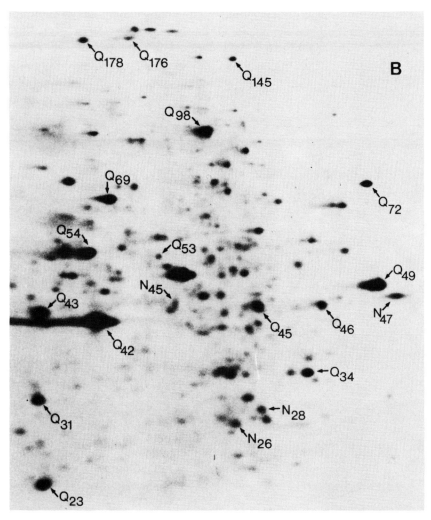

Fig. 6. Effect of serum on the pattern of translation. Total [$^{35}$S]methionine-labelled cytoplasmic proteins from quiescent cells (A) or quiescent cells stimulated with 15% serum for 60 min (B) were analyzed by nonequilibrium pH-gradient two-dimensional polyacrylamide gel electrophoresis (reprinted from Thomas et al., 1981).

The finding that cycloheximide has no effect on the extent of S6 phosphorylation, while SQ 20006 blocks both S6 phosphorylation and protein synthesis to approximately the same level, argues that S6 phosphorylation is a requirement of the activation of protein synthesis. It may also be argued that methylxanthines, such as SQ 20006, are blocking both events independently, and it is only a coincidence that they are inhibited to the same level. There are two lines of evidence against this possibility. First, Frenandez-Puentes et al. (1974) have shown that methylxanthines, at similar concentrations as used here, had no inhibitory effect on the rate of protein synthesis in an in vitro system derived from reticulocytes and using polyuridylic acid as messenger RNA. Indeed, at slightly higher concentrations they found a marked stimulation of protein synthesis. Thus the methylxanthines do not appear to block any

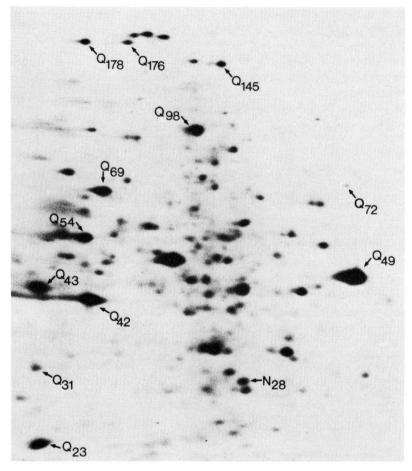

Fig. 7. Effect of actinomycin D on the pattern of translation. Same as Fig. 6B except cells were stimulated in the presence of actinomycin D (reprinted from Thomas et al., 1981).

specific step in protein synthesis. The reason that Fernandez-Puentes et al. (1974) saw no inhibitory effect was probably due to the fact that either S6 was already phosphorylated in their system or that it is only required for the activation of protein synthesis, such as in 3T3 cells, but not required for its maintenance. The second line of evidence against the possibility that the two events are not coupled is that increasing concentrations of serum and epidermal growth factor (EGF) affect both processes in an identical manner (Thomas et al., in press). Indeed with EGF there is no change in either process until the concentration is raised from $10^{-10}$ to $10^{-9}$ M. At this point there is a sharp burst in the rate of protein synthesis and S6 phosphorylation. However, increasing the concentration a 100-fold to $10^{-7}$ M leads to no further increase in either process. Thus the results, to date, support the view that the phosphorylation of S6 is a requirement for the activation of protein synthesis and not a consequence of it.

It is clear from earlier studies by Stanners and Becker (1971) and Rudland et al. (1975) that the increase in protein synthesis is due to an increase in the rate of initiation. S6 is an integral protein of the 40S ribosomal subunit which plays a central role in the process of initiation. Recently it has been shown by immune electron microscopy that S6 is largely located in the tRNA and mRNA binding site of the 40S subunit (Bommer et al., 1980). These results fit well with the studies of Terao and Ogata (1979a, b) showing that polyuridylic acid (poly(U)) protects S6 from chemical modification by auxintricarboxylic acid and can also be crosslinked to S6 by UV radiation. Consistent with these studies are results of Gressner and Van de Leur (1980) demonstrating that dissociation of poly(U) from 40S subunits containing highly phosphorylated S6 is much slower than from 40S subunits which contain little or no phosphorylated S6. The results then are compatible with S6 phosphorylation taking place in 3T3 cells during the time a large pool of stored non-polysomal mRNA is becoming associated with actively translating polysomes. Because the pattern of protein synthesis is changing during this time and because at least half the protein changes appear to be under translational control it is tempting to speculate that the phosphorylation of S6 could be involved in altering the affinity of the 40S ribosomal subunits for the large pool of stored non-polysomal mRNA and helping in sequestering it into actively translating polysomes (Thomas et al., 1979, 1980, 1981; Wool, 1979; Traugh, 1981). Experiments carried out in vitro with non-polysomal and polysomal mRNA should help to resolve this question.

The role of S6 phosphorylation in protein synthesis is far from understood, however, evidence is accumulating to suggest that S6 is located in an important functional site within the 40S ribosomal subunit and that the phosphorlylation of S6 may modulate this function.

REFERENCES

Anderson, W., Grundholm, A. and Sells, B. (1975) Modification of ribosomal proteins during liver regeneration. Biochem. biophys. Res. Commun., 62: 669–676.
Ballinger, D. and Hunt, T. (1981) Fertilization of sea urchin eggs is accompanied by 40S ribosomal subunit phosphorylation. Dev. Biol., in press.
Baserga, R. and Wiebel, F. (1969) The cell cycle of mammalian cells. Int. Rev. exp. Pathol., 7: 1–30.
Bommer, U.-A., Noll, F., Lutsch, G. and Bielka, H. (1980) Immunochemical detection of proteins in the small subunit of rat liver ribosomes involved in binding of the ternary initiation complex. FEBS Lett., 111: 171–174.
Bravo, R., Bellatin, J. and Celis, J.E. (1981) [35]S-Methionine labelled polypeptides from Hela cells, coordinates and percentages of some major polypeptides. Cell Biol. int. Rep., 5: 93–96.
Brooks, R.F. (1977) Continuous protein synthesis is required to maintain the probability of entry into S phase. Cell, 12: 311–317.
Bürk, R.R. (1966) Growth inhibitor of hamster fibroblast cells. Nature (Lond.), 212: 1261–1262.
Carpenter, G. and Cohen, S. (1979) Epidermal growth factor. Annu. Rev. Biochem., 48: 193–198.
Cunningham, D. and Pardee, A. (1969) Transport changes rapidly initiated by serum addition to "contact inhibited" cells. Progr. Biochem. Sci., 64: 1049–1056.
Decker, St. (1981) Phosphorylation of ribosomal protein S6 in avian sarcoma virus-transformed chicken embryo fibroblasts. Proc. nat. Acad. Sci (Wash.), 78: 4112–4115.
Fernandéz-Puentes, C., Carrasco, L. and Vazquez, D. (1974) The enhancement of polypeptide synthesis in mammalian systems by methylxanthines. FEBS Lett., 45: 132–135.
Garrels, J. (1979) Two-dimensional gel electrophoresis and computer analysis of proteins synthesized by clonal cell lines. Biochemistry, 254: 7961–7977.
Gospodarowicz, D. (1974) Localisation of a fibroblast growth factor and its effect alone and with hydrocortisone on 3T3 cell growth. Nature (Lond.), 249: 123–127.
Greengard, P. (1978) Phosphorylated proteins as physiological effectors. Science, 199: 146–152.
Gressner, A.M. and Van de Leur, E. (1980) Interaction of synthetic polynucleotides with small rat liver ribosomal subunits possessing low and highly phosphorylated protein S6. Biochim. biophys. Acta, 608: 459–468.
Gressner, A.M. and Wool, I.G. (1974) The phosphorylation of liver ribosomal proteins in vivo. J. biol. Chem., 249: 6917–6925.
Grummt, F., Dieter, P. and Grummt, I. (1977) Regulation of ATP pools, rRNA and DNA synthesis in 3T3 cells in response to serum or hypoxanthine. Eur. J. Biochem., 76: 7–12.

194

Haselbacher, G.K., Humbel, R.E. and Thomas, G. (1979) Insulin-like growth factor: Insulin or serum increase phosphorylation of ribosomal protein S6 during transition of stationary chick embro fibroblasts into early $G_1$ phase of the cell cycle. *FEBS Lett.*, 100: 185–190.

Hershko, A., Mamont, P., Shields, R. and Tomkins, G.M. (1971) Pleitotypic response. *Nature New Biol.*, 232: 206–211.

Holley, R.W. (1975) Control of growth of mammalian cells in cell culture. *Nature (Lond.)*, 258: 487–490.

Jimenez de Asua, L., Rozengurt, E. and Dulbecco, R. (1974) Kinetics of early changes in phosphate and uridine transport and cyclic AMP levels stimulated by serum in density-inhibited 3T3 cells. *Proc. nat. Acad. Sci. (Wash.)*, 71: 96–98.

Jimenez de Asua, L., Clingan, D. and Rudland, P.S. (1975) Initiation of cell proliferation in cultured mouse fibroblasts by prostaglandin $F_2$. *Proc. nat. Acad. Sci. (Wash.)*, 72: 2724–2728.

Jimenez de Asua, L., Richmond, K.M.V., Otto, A.M., Kubler, A.M., O'Farrell, M.K. and Rudland, P.S. (1979) Growth factors and hormones interact in a series of temporal steps to regulate the rate of initiation of DNA synthesis in mouse firbroblasts. In *Hormones and Cell Culture*, Cold Spring Harbor Conference on Cell Proliferation, Vol. 6, Cold Spring Harbor Laboratory, New York, pp. 403–422.

Nielsen, P.J., Thomas, G. and Maller, J.L. (1982) Increased phosphorylation of ribosomal protein S6 during maturation of Xenopus oocytes, *Proc. nat. Acad. Sci. (Wash.)*, 79: 2937–2941.

Nielsen, P.J., Manchester, K.L., Tombin, H., Gordon, J. and Thomas, G., The phosphorylation of ribosomal protein S6 in rat tissues following cycloheximide injection, in diabetes, and after denervation of diaphragm, *J. biol. Sci.*, in press.

O'Farrell, P.Z., Goodman, H.M. and O'Farrell, P.H. (1977) High resolution two-dimensional electrophoresis of basic as well as acid proteins. *Cell*, 12: 1133–1142.

Rinderknecht, E. and Humbel, R.E. (1976) Polypeptides with non-suppressible insulin-like and cell-growth promoting activities in human serum: Isolation, chemical characterization, and some biological properties of forms I and II. *Proc. nat. Acad. Sci. (Wash.)*, 73: 2365–2369.

Rudland, P.S. (1974) Control of translation in cultured cells: Continued synthesis and accumulation of messenger RNA in non-dividing cultures. *Proc. nat. Acad. Sci. (Wash.)*, 71: 750–754.

Rudland, P.S., Weil, S. and Hunter, A.R. (1975) Changes in RNA metabolism and accumultion of presumptive messenger RNA during transition from the growing to the quiescent state of cultured mouse fibroblasts. *J. mol. Biol.*, 96: 745–766.

Soeiro, R. and Amos, H. (1966) Arrested protein synthesis on polysomes of cultured chick embryo cells. *Science*, 154: 662–665.

Stanners, C.P. and Becker, H. (1971) Control of macromolecular synthesis in proliferating and resting Syrian hamster cells in monolayer culture. I. Ribosome function. *J. cell. Physiol.*, 77: 31–42.

Terao, K. and Ogata, K. (1979a) Proteins of small subunits of rat liver ribosomes that interact with poly(U). I. Effects of preincubation of poly(U) with 40S subunits on the interactions of 40S subunit proteins with aurintricarboxylic acid and with $NN'$-$p$-phenylenedimaleimide. *J. Biochem.*, 86: 597–603.

Terao, K. and Ogata, K. (1979b) Proteins of small subunits of rat liver ribosomes that interact with poly(U). II. Cross-links between poly(U) and ribosomal proteins in 40S subunits induced by UV irradiation. *J. Biochem.*, 86: 605–617.

Thomas, G. and Gordon, J. (1979) Regulation of protein synthesis during the shift of quiescent animal cells into the proliferative state. *Cell Biol. int. Rep.*, 3: 307–320.

Thomas, G., Siegmann, M., Bowman, P.D. and Gordon, J. (1977) The isolation and analysis of polysomes and ribosomal RNA from cells growing in monolayer culture. *Exp. Cell Res.*, 108: 253–258.

Thomas, G., Siegmann, M. and Gordon, J. (1979) Multiple phosphorylation of ribosomal protein S6 during transition of quiescent 3T3 cells into early $G_1$ and cellular compartmentalization of the phosphate donor. *Proc. nat. Acad. Sci. (Wash.)*, 76: 3952–3956.

Thomas, G., Siegmann, M., Kubler, A.M., Gordon, J. and Jimenez de Asua, L. (1980) Regulation of 40S ribosomal protein S6 phosphorylation in Swiss mouse 3T3 cells. *Cell*, 19: 1015–1023.

Thomas, G., Thomas, G. and Luther, H. (1981) Transcriptional and translational control of cytoplasmic proteins following serum stimulation of quiescent Swiss 3T3 cells. *Proc. nat. Acad. Sci. (Wash.)*, in press.

Thomas, G., Martin-Pérez, J., Siegmann, M. and Otto, A., The effect of serum, EGF, PGF2α and insulin on S6 phosphorylation and the initiation of protein and DNA synthesis, *Cell*, in press.

Tobey, R.A., Petersen, D.F. and Anderson, E.C. (1971) Biochemistry of $G_1$ and mitosis. In *Cell Cycle and Cancer*, R. Baserga (Ed.), Marcel Decker, New York, pp. 409–452.

Traugh, J.A. (1981) Regulation of protein synthesis by phosphorylation. In *Biochemical Actions of Hormones*, Academic Press, New York, pp. 167–208.

Wool, I. (1979) The structure and function of eukaryotic ribosomes. *Annu. Rev. Biochem.*, 48: 719–754.

# Ribosomal Protein Phosphorylation and Protein Synthesis in the Brain

SIDNEY ROBERTS

*Department of Biological Chemistry, School of Medicine, and Brain Research Institute, University of California Center for the Health Sciences, Los Angeles, CA 90024, U.S.A.*

## INTRODUCTION

Research on protein synthesis in the brain has focused mainly on two closely related problems: (1) the nature and properties of proteins formed in neural tissue which may serve specific brain functions, and (2) the mechanisms involved in regulation of the biosynthesis and function of these proteins. These regulatory processes appear to be concentrated at translational and post-translational sites of protein synthesis. A comprehensive overview of earlier research on these topics has been published (Roberts et al., 1977).

Considerable evidence supports the concept that protein phosphorylation plays a major role in the control of translational and post-translational events in eukaryotic cells (for recent reviews, see Weller, 1979; Cohen, 1980). An important aspect of this phenomenon is illustrated by the fact that several components of the translational process, including certain protein initiation factors, as well as specific constitutive proteins of the ribosome, exhibit variations in phosphorylation which appear to be correlated with alterations in protein synthesis.

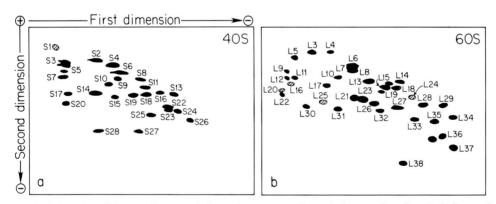

Fig. 1. Schematics of the two-dimensional electrophoretograms of constitutive proteins of cerebral ribosomal subunits. Ribosomal proteins were isolated from purified 40S and 60S subunits prepared from cerebral cortices of 7-day-old infant rats. The purified proteins were subjected to two-dimensional electrophoresis on polyacrylamide gels containing urea. The resulting gel electrophoretograms were stained with Coomassie brilliant blue. Ribosomal proteins are labeled according to the nomenclature of Sherton and Wool (1972, 1974). Several protein spots actually contained two or more components; e.g., protein S3 is composed of S3 and S3a (and possibly S3b). [Reprinted from Roberts and Ashby (1978).]

Our investigations have dealt primarily with ribosomal protein phosphorylation in the brain, physiological and pathological factors which alter this phenomenon, and the possible relationship of variations in the phosphorylation of specific brain ribosomal phosphoproteins to sequential steps in protein synthesis at the translational level. Evidence in support of the hypothesis that ribosomal protein phosphorylation is involved in the regulation of eukaryotic protein synthesis has recently come from several directions. Thus, cross-linking studies suggest that the S6 protein (Fig. 1a), which is the major phosphorylated protein of the 40S ribosomal subunit, participates in the binding of messenger RNA to this subunit (Terao and Ogata, 1979a). Other ribosomal proteins which are phosphorylated in vivo bind strongly to other translational components; e.g., protein S3a to eukaryotic initiation factor, eIF-2 (Westermann et al., 1979); protein L6 to tRNA (Ulbrich et al., 1980); and proteins L6 and L19 ro 5S and 5.8S ribosomal RNA (Ulbrich and Wool, 1978; Todokoro et al., 1981). A phosphorylated acidic protein of the 60S subunit appears to be required for the function of the eukaryotic elongation factor, EF-1 (Möller et al., 1975). In addition, several investigations have revealed that alterations in protein synthesis induced in eukaryotic cells in vitro are accompanied by parallel variations in phosphorylation of protein S6 (Martini and Kruppa, 1979; Terao and Ogata, 1979b; Wettenhall and Howlett, 1979; Thomas et al., 1980). However, previous efforts to determine whether experimentally induced alterations in phosphorylation of eukaryotic ribosomes are accompanied by variations in the translational activities of these ribosomes have not produced definitive results (Krystosek et al., 1974; Wool and Stöffler, 1974; Grankowski and Gasior, 1975; Kramer et al., 1977). Among the limitations of these earlier studies is the fact that the phosphorylation states of several ribosomal proteins which have not been shown to be phosphorylated in vivo were altered in the isolated ribosome-protein kinase systems employed to produce variations in phosphorylation in vitro. Moreover, the crude preparations of protein synthesis factors used to assess polypeptide synthesis in most of these studies, and in some cases, the ribosomes per se, contained sufficient protein kinase and protein phosphatase activities to alter ribosomal protein phosphorylation as polypeptide synthesis proceeded (Wool and Stöffler, 1974; Genot et al., 1978; S. Roberts, T.A. Francis and B.S. Morelos, unpublished observations). Recent advances in the isolation of soluble protein components of eukaryotic protein-synthesizing systems (Moldave and Grossman, 1979), coupled with procedures for selective alterations in the phosphorylation state of cerebral ribosomal proteins in vivo and in vitro (Francis and Roberts, 1978, 1980; Roberts and Ashby, 1978; Roberts and Morelos, 1979, 1980), provide the methodology required for more definitive investigations of the relationship between variations in ribosomal protein phosphorylation and ribosomal function in brain protein synthesis.

## RIBOSOMAL PROTEIN PHOSPHORYLATION IN RAT BRAIN

We have investigated ribosomal protein phosphorylation in rat brain cells in vivo and in vitro (Ashby and Roberts, 1975; Roberts and Ashby, 1978; Roberts and Morelos, 1979, 1980). In addition, this phosphorylation process has been studied in isolated brain ribosome-protein kinase systems (Francis and Roberts, 1978, 1980; Francis, 1980). Under appropriate circumstances, comparable results can be obtained with each of these preparations.

The investigations of ribosomal protein phosphorylation in rat cerebral cortex in vivo demonstrated for the first time that several structural proteins of both ribosomal subunits undergo phosphorylation in mammalian cells in situ (Roberts and Morelos, 1979). Thus, the roster of constitutive ribosomal proteins of rat cerebral 40S subunits which incorporated

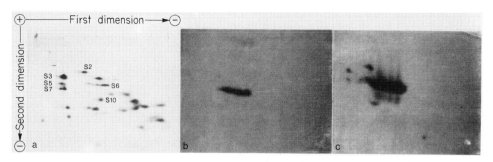

Fig. 2. Two-dimensional electrophoresis of proteins isolated from 40S subunits of rat cerebral cortex. Proteins extracted from the small subunit were subjected to two-dimensional electrophoresis on polyacrylamide gels containing urea. The amounts of protein applied to the first-dimensional gels were (a) 259 μg, (b) 312 μg and (c) 352 μg. (a) Electrophoretogram from untreated rats, stained with Coomassie brilliant blue. (b) Radioautograph, exposed for 1 day, of 40S proteins from rats given 2 mCi of [$^{32}$P]orthophosphate intracisternally 1 h before decapitation. (c) Radioautograph, exposed for 2 weeks, of a two-dimensional gel similar to that in (b). Magnifications of the electrophoretogram and the radioautographs are similar. [Reprinted from Roberts and Morelos (1979).]

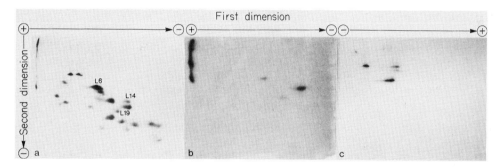

Fig. 3. Two-dimensional electrophoresis of proteins isolated from 60S ribosomal subunits of rat cerebrum. Infant rats were each given 2 mCi of [$^{32}$P]orthophosphate intracisternally in 20 μl of 0.9% NaCl. The animals were killed by decapitation 1 h later. Proteins extracted from the large subunit were subjected to two-dimensional electrophoresis on polyacrylamide gels containing urea. The amounts of protein applied to the first-dimensional gels were (a) 275 μg, (b) 368 μg and (c) 346 μg. (a) Two-dimensional electrophoretogram stained with Coomassie brilliant blue; the 60S proteins were applied to the anode in the first dimension. (b) Radioautograph of a similar two-dimensional gel of 60S proteins exposed for 3 weeks. (c) Radioautograph of a two-dimensional gel obtained when the 60S proteins were applied to the cathode in the first dimension; exposure time was 3 weeks. The 60S acidic proteins corresponding to the radioactive spots on reversed polarity gels stained too weakly to provide a useful photograph. [Reprinted from Roberts and Morelos (1979).]

radioactivity from [$^{32}$P]Pi in vivo included basic proteins with the electrophoretic mobility of S2, S3a, S5, S6 and S10 on two-dimensional gels (Fig. 2c). Ribosomal proteins of the cerebral 60S subunit which were actively phosphorylated in vivo included the basic proteins L6, L14 and L19 (Fig. 3b), as well as several acidic proteins (Fig. 3c). The phosphorylated derivatives of basic ribosomal proteins of both cerebral subunits could frequently be detected in spots or tails closely following the non-phosphorylated species on stained two-dimensional electrophoretograms (Figs. 2a and 3a). Earlier efforts to detect phosphorylation of ribosomal proteins other than protein S6 in rat liver in situ were unsuccessful (Gressner and Wool, 1974a,b, 1976; Treloar et al., 1977). These results indicate that ribosomal protein phosphory-

198

lation may be unusually active in the brain. This phenomenon may reflect the relatively high activity of protein kinase systems in the brain associated with ongoing neural activity (Daly, 1977), as well as the rapid turnover of polyribosomes in this organ (Zomzely et al., 1968).

The ribosomal phosphoprotein which undergoes most rapid phosphorylation in cerebral cortex in situ, as in other eukaryotic cells, is protein S6 of the small subunit (Roberts and Morelos, 1979; Wool, 1979; Leader, 1980). The cerebral S6 ribosomal protein has a molecular weight of approximately 32 000 and contains several serine residues which are phosphorylated in vivo (Fig. 2a, b). Administration of dibutyryl cyclic AMP (cAMP) intraperitoneally or intracisternally selectively increased phosphorylation of the more highly phosphorylated congeners of the S6 protein which traveled more slowly in the first dimension than did the non-phosphorylated form (Fig. 4b, e). Since the total incorporation of radiocactivity into the cerebral 40S ribosomal proteins was significantly increased under these circumstances (Roberts and Morelos, 1979), it is unlikely that the differences between the profiles of control and cAMP-treated animals can be ascribed to variations in the rate of protein S6 dephosphorylation. Administration of 3-isobutyl-1-methylxanthine also increased phosphorylation of the S6 protein (not shown). The effective dose of this potent inhibitor of cyclic nucleotide phosphodiesterases was considerably lower than that of dibutyryl cAMP (about one-fourth). Dibutyryl cyclic GMP (cGMP) did not stimulate phosphorylation of protein S6 (Fig. 4c, f). These results suggest that neurotransmitters and other agents that stimulate adenylate cyclase activity in specific areas of the brain (Von Hungen and Roberts, 1974; Daly, 1977) may produce effects on brain maturation and function partly by altering ribosomal protein phosphorylation.

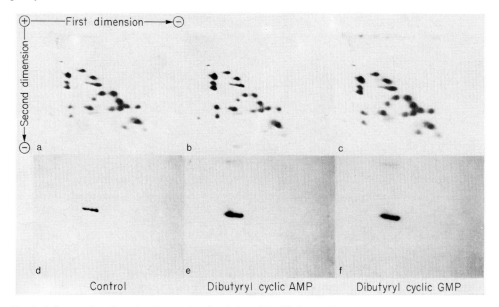

Fig. 4. Influence of cyclic nucleotides on phosphorylation of the S6 ribosomal protein of rat cerebral cortex in vivo. Infant rats were each given 2 mCi of [$^{32}$P]orthophosphate intracisternally in 20 $\mu$l of 0.9% NaCl. In two groups of animals, the intracisternal solution also contained either 25 $\mu$g of dibutyryl cAMP or 25 $\mu$g of dibutyryl cGMP. All rats were killed by decapitation 60 min later. Proteins extracted from the small subunit were subjected to two-dimensional electrophoresis on polyacrylamide gels containing urea. The amounts of protein applied to the first-dimensional gels were: control, 423 $\mu$g; dibutyryl cAMP, 397 $\mu$g; dibutyryl cGMP, 452 g. (a), (b) and (c) Electrophoretograms stained with Coomassie brilliant blue; (d), (e) and (f) radioautographs exposed for 1 day. [Reprinted from Roberts and Morelos (1979).]

The finding that cAMP stimulated phosphorylation of protein S6, but apparently no other ribosomal protein in rat cerebrum, in vivo or in vitro (Roberts and Ashby, 1978; Roberts and Morelos, 1979), suggests that phosphorylation of cerebral ribosomal proteins other than S6 may be directed by cAMP-independent protein kinases. Alternatively, cyclic nucleotide-induced alterations in phosphorylation of other cerebral ribosomal proteins might be obscured by the relatively slow turnover of phosphate groups in these proteins. In efforts to resolve this question, several investigators have characterized the spectrum of ribosomal proteins phosphorylated in isolated eukaryotic ribosomes in the presence of different purified protein kinases (for reviews, see Wool, 1979; Leader, 1980; Traugh, 1981).

We have investigated the phosphorylation of cerebral ribosomal proteins in reconstituted systems consisting of isolated ribosomal subunits or polyribosomes, $[\gamma\text{-}^{32}P]ATP$, and purified preparations of the catalytic subunit of cAMP-dependent protein kinase from rat cerebral cortex. Although protein S6 appeared to be the only cerebral ribosomal protein to respond to elevated concentrations of cAMP with increased phosphorylation in vivo, numerous additional ribosomal proteins could also be phosphorylated in isolated 40S or 60S subunits exposed to the protein kinase preparation (Francis and Roberts, 1978, 1980; Francis, 1980). In contrast, extensive exposure of purified cerebral polyribosomes to the catalytic subunit resulted in phosphorylation of only those ribosomal proteins of the 40S subunit that were most readily labeled in vivo: proteins S2, S6 and S10. Two other proteins of the 40S ribosomal subunit that were phosphorylated in vivo (S3a and S5) were labeled only in isolated 40S subunits in the reconstituted systems. These results suggest that phosphorylation of the latter two ribosomal proteins may also be limited to free 40S ribosomal subunits in vivo. The possible relationship between the state of ribosome association, ribosomal protein phosphorylation and ribosomal protein synthesis will be discussed below.

It should be emphasized that these observations with reconstituted ribosome-protein kinase systems do not necessarily signify that cAMP is the only physiological determinant of ribosomal protein phosphorylation in the brain. Thus, other investigators have shown that cGMP, as well as cyclic nucleotide-independent protein kinases, can catalyze phosphorylation of certain ribosomal proteins in other eukaryotic systems (Wool and Stöffler, 1974; Ventimiglia and Wool, 1974; Traugh and Porter, 1976; Issinger, 1977; Kudlicki et al., 1980; Issinger et al., 1980). Moreover, processes which do not appear to involve alterations in cyclic nucleotide metabolism, including phenomena that are accompanied by variations in protein synthesis, can alter ribosomal protein phosphorylation (Martini and Kruppa, 1979; Terao and Ogata, 1979b; Wettenhall and Howlett, 1979; Thomas et al., 1980). In fact, evidence has recently been presented that only certain sites in protein S6 may be phosphorylated under the influence of cAMP, whereas others appear to be phosphorylated only during stimulation of protein synthesis (Lastick and McConkey, 1981).

## HYPERPHENYLALANINEMIA AND BRAIN RIBOSOMAL PROTEIN PHOSPHORYLATION

Our investigations of the relationship between ribosomal protein phosphorylation and the regulation of protein synthesis in the brain have dealt with the model system of experimental hyperphenylalaninemia in infant rats. This condition results in alterations in brain protein synthesis, including abnormal myelination in the central nervous system, as well as behavioral modifications reminiscent of changes observed in human phenylketonuria (Gaull et al., 1975). Administration of a loading dose of L-phenylalanine (1 mg/g body wt.) intraperitoneally to

TABLE I

INFLUENCE OF PHENYLALANINE LOADING ON KINETICS OF UPTAKE OF [$^{32}$P]-ORTHOPHOSPHATE
INTO THE CEREBRAL CYTOSOL AND PHOSPHORYLATION OF PROTEINS IN RIBOSOMAL SUBUNITS
OF RAT CEREBRAL CORTEX IN VIVO

Infant rats were injected intraperitoneally with 2.5% L-phenylalanine (1 mg/g body wt.) in 0.45% NaCl, or an equivalent volume of 0.9% NaCl. Immediately thereafter, 2 mCi of [$^{32}$P]orthophosphate was administered intracisternally to each animal in 20 $\mu$l of 0.9% NaCl. The animals were killed at the intervals indicated. Each analysis represents the cytosol or ribosomes pooled from 8 animals. The results shown are means ± S.E.M. of 4 separate experiments. [Reprinted from Roberts and Morelos (1980).]

| Time after injection (min) | $10^{-5} \times {}^{32}P$ uptake (c.p.m./g of cortex) | Radioactivity in ribosomal proteins (c.p.m./$\mu$g) | |
|---|---|---|---|
| | | 40S | 60S |
| Saline-injected | | | |
| 30 | 2188 ± 161 | 63.7 ± 5.3 | 6.0 ± 0.9 |
| 60 | 2922 ± 140 | 90.4 ± 6.3 | 9.1 ± 1.2 |
| 120 | 4305 ± 149 | 137.4 ± 8.4 | 11.3 ± 1.5 |
| Phenylalanine-injected | | | |
| 30 | 2459 ± 184 | 46.2 ± 4.5 | 6.8 ± 1.0 |
| 60 | 3196 ± 229 | 56.0 ± 5.5 | 8.3 ± 0.8 |
| 120 | 4353 ± 270 | 59.0 ± 6.6 | 9.5 ± 0.9 |

infant rats decreased incorporation of radioactivity from intracisternally administered [$^{32}$P]orthophosphate into cerebral 40S ribosomal proteins (Table I). Only minor changes in phosphorylation of 60S ribosomal proteins were observed. Changes in phosphorylation of 40S ribosomal proteins after phenylalanine treatment were not associated with significant variations in uptake of intracisternally administered $^{32}$P into the cerebral cytosol.

The apparent inhibitory effect of phenylalanine loading on phosphorylation of 40S ribosomal proteins in cerebral cortices of infant rats was principally or entirely localized to the S6 protein of this tissue. 1 h after phenylalanine treatment, the more acidic components of this protein were markedly depleted on Coomassie blue-stained electrophoretograms (Fig. 5b). The control pattern of phosphorylation of the cerebral S6 ribosomal protein was reestablished within about 3 h of intraperitoneal administration of phenylalanine (Fig. 5c). Comparable changes in phosphorylation of the cerebral S6 protein after phenylalanine loading were detected on radioautographs of the two-dimensional electrophoretograms of cerebral 40S ribosomal proteins from infant rats given [$^{32}$P]orthophosphate intracisternally (Fig. 5d,e,f).

Earlier investigations have shown that the moderate excess of L-phenylalanine employed in these experiments resulted in a maximal increase in plasma phenylalanine values in infant rats within about 30 min of administration by the intraperitoneal route (Siegel et al., 1971; Bogucki and Roberts, 1979). The increase in plasma phenylalanine content was comparable with that observed in human phenylketonuria (Scriver and Rosenberg, 1973), and was accompanied by a 20-fold increase in the cerebral concentration of phenylalanine (Roberts and Morelos, 1976). In contrast, marked decreases were seen in brain concentrations of several neutral amino acids including threonine, valine, leucine, isoleucine, methionine and tryptophan (Roberts, 1968; Roberts and Morelos, 1976; Bogucki and Roberts, 1979). Perhaps the most striking effect of experimental hyperphenylalaninemia on brain protein-synthesizing mechanisms is the profound disaggregation of brain polyribosomes which occurs within 30 min of phenylalanine

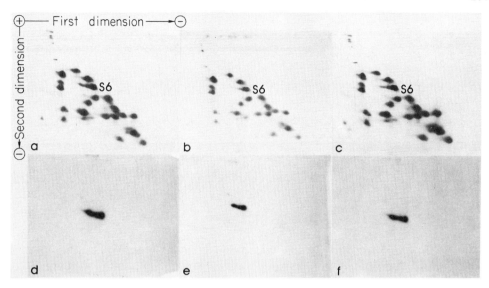

Fig. 5. Influence of phenylalanine loading on two-dimensional electrophoretograms of proteins isolated from 40S ribosomal subunits of rat cerebral cortex. Infant rats were injected intraperitoneally with 2.5% L-phenylalanine (1 mg/g body wt.) in 0.45% NaCl, or an equivalent volume of 0.9% NaCl. Either immediately thereafter, or 2 h later the animals received 2 mCi of [$^{32}$P]orthophosphate intracisternally in 20 $\mu$l of 0.9% NaCl. All animals were killed 1 h after the last injection. Cerebral ribosomes were isolated in the presence of 40 mM NaF to inhibit protein phosphatase activity. Proteins extracted from the small cerebral subunit were subjected to two-dimensional electrophoresis on polyacrylamide gels containing urea. (a), (b) and (c) show electrophoretograms stained for protein with Coomassie brilliant blue; (d), (e) and (f) show radioautographs exposed for 1 day. The amounts of ribosomal protein applied to the first-dimensional gels were: (a) and (d), 429 $\mu$g; (b) and (e), 409 $\mu$g; (c) and (f), 433 $\mu$g. In (a) and (d), rats were given [$^{32}$P]orthophosphate immediately after saline; in (b) and (e), rats were given [$^{32}$P]orthophosphate immediately after phenylalanine; in (c) and (f), rats were given [$^{32}$P]orthophosphate 2 h after phenylalanine. The position of S6 protein is marked on the electrophoretograms. [Reprinted from Roberts and Morelos (1980).]

administration (Fig. 6b). Parenteral administration of a mixture of the six neutral amino acids listed above plus tyrosine, subsequent to the injection of phenylalanine, tended to inhibit or reverse brain polyribosome disaggregation (Fig. 6f vs. e; see also, Hughes and Johnson (1977a, 1978b)). The amount of phenylalanine administered intraperitoneally in these latter experiments (2 mg/g body wt.) was twice the load used in the preceding investigations, in order to produce more extensive polyribosome disaggregation and clearer evidence of the reversal of this phenomenon by subsequent administration of the amino acid mixture (Roberts and Morelos, 1980).

In common with the results of studies with the smaller loading dose of phenylalanine, intraperitoneal administration of this amino acid to infant rats in amounts equivalent to 2 mg/g body wt. produced a marked decrease in the more highly phosphorylated species of the S6 protein in cerebral polyribosomes (Fig. 7b vs. a). Phenylalanine loading not only decreased the relative amounts of the phosphorylated congeners of the S6 protein in polyribosomes compared with the unlabeled non-phosphorylated species, but also decreased the total amount of radioactivity from [$^{32}$P]orthophosphate incorporated into the phosphorylated congeners. Subsequent administration of a mixture of seven neutral acids, which resulted in partial recovery of cerebral polyribosomes, also tended to restore the more highly phosphorylated congeners of the polyribosomal S6 protein and increased the total amount of radioactivity incorporated into

202

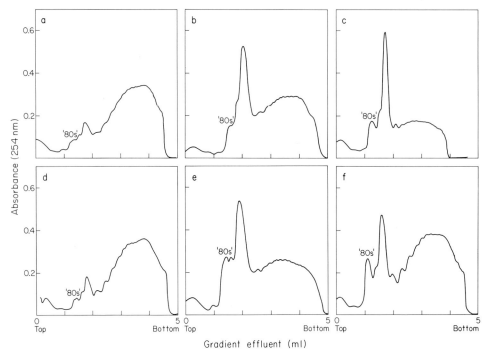

Fig. 6. Reversal of phenylalanine-induced disaggregation of cerebral polyribosomes by a mixture of seven neutral amino acids. Infant rats were each injected intraperitoneally with 3.0% L-phenylalanine (2 mg/g body wt.) in 0.45% NaCl, or an equivalent volume of 0.9% NaCl. Some animals from each of these two groups were killed after 30 or 60 min. At the later time interval, the remaining animals in each group received either a mixture of seven neutral amino acids (2 ml/100 g body wt.), or an equivalent volume of 0.9% NaCl, by the same route. The mixture of amino acids was composed of the L-isomers of leucine, isoleucine, valine, threonine, tyrosine, tryptophan and methionine, each present at a concentration of 3.75 mg/ml of 0.9% NaCl (Hughes and Johnson, 1978b). These animals were killed 1 h after the second injection. Ribosomes were isolated from the pooled cerebral cortices of three animals in each group by centrifugation for 20 h through medium containing 2 M sucrose. Sucrose-density-gradient analyses of the purified polyribosomes were carried out. The monoribosome peaks are indicated as 80S. (a) Animals given saline 1 h earlier; (b) animals given phenylalanine 30 min earlier; (c) animals given phenylalanine 1 h earlier; (d) animals given saline followed 1 h later by a second injection of saline and then killed after an additional hour; (e) animals given phenylalanine followed by saline 1 h later; (f) animals given phenylalanine followed by the amino acid mixture 1 h later. [Reprinted from Roberts and Morelos (1980).]

these congeners (Fig. 7c). It should also be noted that the S6 protein of rat cerebral cortex is normally much more highly phosphorylated in polyribosomes than in monoribosomes (Fig. 7a vs. d). A similar phenomenon has been noted in baby hamster kidney fibroblasts in culture (Leader and Coia, 1978). In the present investigations, phenylalanine administration decreased phosphorylation of protein S6 in separated cerebral polyribosomes (Fig. 7b), but simultaneously increased phosphorylation in the corresponding monoribosomes (Fig. 7e). The result was that the monoribosome and polyribosome populations contained the S6 protein in essentially equivalent states of phosphorylation. Subsequent treatment with the amino acid mixture tended to restore the control patterns of phosphorylation of the S6 protein (Fig. 7c, f). Although the phenylalanine-induced disaggregation of cerebral polyribosomes may be responsible for the altered distribution of phosphorylated congeners of the S6 ribosomal protein between polyribosomes and monoribosomes in hyperphenylalaninemia, other explanations

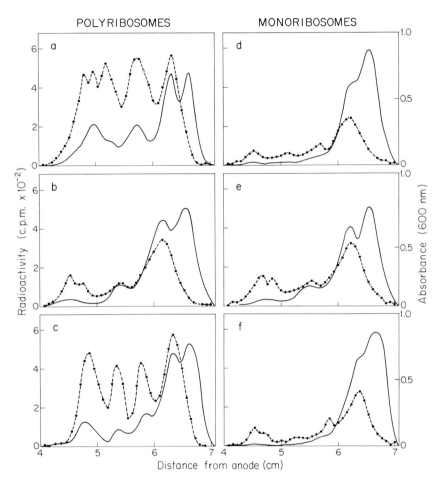

Fig. 7. Reversal of phenylalanine-induced alterations in phosphorylation of the S6 protein in separated cerebral polyribosomes and monoribosomes by a mixture of seven neutral amino acids. Infant rats were injected intraperitoneally with 3.0% L-phenylalanine (2 mg/g body wt.) in 0.45% NaCl, or an equivalent volume of 0.9% NaCl. After 45 min, the animals were each given 2 mCi of [$^{32}$P]orthophosphate intracisternally in 20 $\mu$l of 0.9% NaCl. After an additional 15 min, the animals were injected intraperitoneally with either 0.9% NaCl or a mixture of seven neutral amino acids as described in the legend to Fig. 6. The animals were killed 1 h after the second intraperitoneal injection. Purified cerebral ribosomes were prepared in the presence of 20 mM sodium molybdate to inhibit protein phosphatase activity and were then fractionated into polyribosomes and monoribosomes on sucrose density gradients. Proteins extracted from the 40S ribosomal subunit were subjected to two-dimensional electrophoresis. The amounts of protein applied to the first-dimensional gels were (in $\mu$g): (a) 396; (b) 402; (c) 415; (d) 399; (e) 422; (f) 406. After the two-dimensional gels were stained with Coomassie brilliant blue, a horizontal rectangular section corresponding to the S6 protein and its more acidic phosphorylated derivatives was cut out and scanned for absorbance at 600 nm (———). This section of the gel was then divided into 1 mm slices for determination of radioactivity (●– – –●). (a) and (d), animals given saline followed by a second injection of saline 1 h later; (b) and (e), animals given phenylalanine followed by saline 1 h later; (c) and (f), animals given phenylalanine followed by the amino acid mixture 1 h later. [Reprinted from Roberts and Morelos (1980).]

are possible. Thus, the finding that the S6 protein is normally more highly phosphorylated in cerebral polyribosomes than monoribosomes suggests that phosphorylation of this ribosomal protein occurs at some stage of polypeptide synthesis, whereas dephosphorylation occurs after termination of this process. If the observed reduction in brain polyribosomes after phenylalanine loading is due to a blockade of initiation processes as has been suggested by other investigators (Hughes and Johnson, 1976, 1977b), 40S subunits undergoing phosphorylation prior to initiation may accumulate and expand the pool of phosphorylated monoribosomes, while simultaneously decreasing the proportion of phosphorylated polyribosomes. However, this scenario seems unlikely in view of the fact that the total content of phosphorylated species of protein S6 in cerebral ribosomes was decreased in hyperphenylalaninemia (Table II).

TABLE II

INFLUENCE OF CYCLIC NUCLEOTIDES AND PHENYLALANINE LOADING ON PHOSPHORYLATION OF 40S RIBOSOMAL PROTEIN IN RAT CEREBRAL CORTEX IN VIVO

Infant rats were injected intraperitoneally with 2.5% L-phenylalanine (2 mg/g body wt.) in 0.45% NaCl, or an equivalent volume of 0.9% NaCl. Immediately thereafter, 2 mCi of [$^{32}$P]orthophosphate was administered intracisternally to each animal in 20 $\mu$l of 0.9% NaCl. The cyclic nucleotides (25 $\mu$g/rat) were administered intracisternally in conjunction with the radioactive isotope. The animals were killed 1 h later. The values shown are means ($\pm$ S.E.M., where indicated) for 20 animals in each group (Reprinted from Roberts and Morelos, 1982).

| Treatment | $10^{-5} \times {}^{32}P$ uptake (c.p.m./g of cortex) | Specific radioactivity (c.p.m./$\mu$g 40S protein) |
|---|---|---|
| Expt. 1 | | |
| Control | $3406 \pm 302$ | 132.0 |
| Dibutyryl cAMP | $3396 \pm 366$ | 170.3 |
| Phenylalanine | $3363 \pm 351$ | 73.6 |
| Phenylalanine + dibutyryl cAMP | $3187 \pm 149$ | 63.9 |
| Expt. 2 | | |
| Control | $2918 \pm 285$ | 118.2 |
| Dibutyryl cGMP | $3222 \pm 332$ | 99.1 |
| Phenylalanine | $2695 \pm 264$ | 65.5 |
| Phenylalanine + dibutyryl cGMP | $2836 \pm 345$ | 57.7 |

## ROLE OF cAMP-DEPENDENT PROTEIN KINASES IN CONTROL OF BRAIN RIBOSOMAL PROTEIN PHOSPHORYLATION

The mechanisms involved in the phenylalanine-induced decrease in phosphorylated congeners of the cerebral S6 protein have been investigated further. Intracisternal administration of dibutyryl cAMP or 3-isobutyl-1-methylxanthine, which increased phosphorylation of the S6 protein of cerebral 40S ribosomal subunits in control infant rats (Fig. 4), did not counteract the decreased phosphorylation of cerebral 40S ribosomal protein resulting from intraperitoneal administration of a loading dose of L-phenylalanine (Table II, Expt. 1). Dibutyryl cGMP was without effect on phosphorylation of cerebral 40S ribosomal protein in either group of animals (Table II, Expt. 2). After intracisternal injection of [$^{32}$P]Pi, about 95% of the radioactivity associated with cerebral 40S ribosomal protein in infant rats is present in serine hydroxyl residues of protein S6 (Roberts and Morelos, 1979).

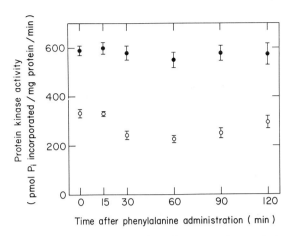

Fig. 8. Kinetics of alterations in protein kinase activity in crude extracts of rat cerebral cortex after phenylalanine administration in vivo. Infant rats were injected intraperitoneally with L-phenylalanine (2 mg/g body wt.) in 0.45% NaCl. The animals were killed at the intervals shown. Cerebral postmitochondrial supernatant fractions were prepared and assayed for protein kinase activity as described by Hofmann et al. (1977). Means ± S.E.M. for 4 determinations are shown. ○ , basal histone kinase activity measured in the absence of added cAMP; ● , histone-kinase activity measured in the presence of 2 μM cAMP.

TABLE III

INFLUENCE OF PRIOR ADMINISTRATION OF CYCLIC NUCLEOTIDES AND PHENYLALANINE LOADING ON cAMP-DEPENDENT HISTONE KINASE ACTIVITY IN CRUDE EXTRACTS OF RAT CEREBRAL CORTEX

Infant rats were injected intraperitoneally with 3.0% L-phenylalanine (2 mg/g body wt.) in 0.45% NaCl, or an equivalent volume of 0.9% NaCl. The dibutyryl derivative of the cyclic nucleotides (25 μg/rat) in 0.9% NaCl, or 0.9% NaCl, was given intracisternally in 20 μl 30 min later. All animals were killed 30 min after this second injection. Cerebral postmitochondrial supernatant fractions were prepared and assayed for protein kinase activity in the presence and absence of 10 μM cAMP, essentially as described by Palmer et al. (1980). Means ± S.E.M. for 4 determinations are shown.

| Treatment | Histone kinase activity (pmoles Pi/mg protein/min) | | Activity ratio |
|---|---|---|---|
| | − cAMP | + cAMP | |
| Control | 240 ± 7 | 493 ± 10 | 0.49 |
| Dibutyryl cAMP | 294 ± 7 | 478 ± 17 | 0.62 |
| Dibutyryl cGMP | 236 ± 10 | 472 ± 13 | 0.50 |
| Phenylalanine | 190 ± 5 | 463 ± 19 | 0.41 |
| Phenylalanine + dibutyryl cAMP | 200 ± 8 | 464 ± 15 | 0.43 |
| Phenylalanine + dibutyryl cGMP | 188 ± 9 | 470 ± 14 | 0.40 |

Diminished phosphorylation of the cerebral S6 protein in hyperphenylalaninemic animals was accompanied by decreased basal protein kinase activity in cerebral extracts from these animals (Fig. 8). Parenteral administration of dibutyryl cAMP or 3-isobutyl-1-methylxanthine, in doses which increased basal protein kinase activity in cerebral extracts from control infant rats, had no effect on this activity in phenylalanine-treated rats (Table III). Since the protein kinase response to an optimal dose of cAMP added in vitro to these various extracts was unaffected by the type of pretreatment of the animals, the protein kinase activity ratio

(− cAMP/ + cAMP) increased with administration of dibutyryl cAMP, decreased with phenylalanine loading, and was not restored in the latter instance by dibutyryl cAMP. Dibutyryl cGMP given intracisternally did not stimulate cerebral protein kinase activity. About 85 % of the histone kinase activity measured in the presence of cAMP could be eliminated by the specific protein inhibitor of the cAMP-dependent protein kinases (S. Roberts and B.S. Morelos, unpublished observations). The protein inhibitor also reduced basal protein kinase activity in cerebral extracts from control and hyperphenylalaninemic animals. Comparable results were obtained with separated cytosolic and microsomal preparations from infant rat cerebral cortex. The latter findings are consistent with evidence that cytosolic and microsomal cAMP-dependent protein kinases from rat brain are very similar or identical (Rubin et al., 1979).

L-Phenylalanine, added in vitro, also inhibited the basal activity of cerebral protein kinases in infant rats. The effective concentration of this amino acid was approximately 2.5 mM (S. Roberts and B.S. Morelos, unpublished observations). This concentration of L-phenylalanine is of the same order of magnitude as peak levels of the amino acid in brains or sera of infant animals after phenylalanine loading (Siegel et al., 1971; Roberts and Morelos, 1976; Hughes and Johnson, 1978b; Bogucki and Roberts, 1979), as well as in the sera of phenylketonuric human patients (Rosenberg and Scriver, 1980).

## RIBOSOMAL PROTEIN PHOSPHORYLATION AND BRAIN PROTEIN SYNTHESIS

The results described above imply that phenylalanine inhibition of cerebral ribosomal protein phosphorylation in vivo is due mainly to a direct or indirect action of this amino acid on cAMP-dependent protein kinases. cAMP, by virtue of its capacity to alter the structure and function of numerous phosphoproteins, is involved in the regulation of many phases of metabolic activity, including protein synthesis at both transcriptional and translational sites (Wicks, 1974; Weller, 1979). The specific contributions of phenylalanine-induced alterations in phosphorylation of brain S6 ribosomal protein to the neuropathology of hyperphenylalaninemia and phenylketonuria remain to be elucidated. Our laboratory is presently concerned with efforts to delineate possible alterations in initiation and elongation reactions of brain protein synthesis which may occur in hyperphenylalaninemic animals as a result of variations in phosphorylation of this or other cerebral ribosomal proteins. These investigations require the isolation of highly purified components of the translational process in protein synthesis. The use of impure preparations in earlier studies of environmentally induced or developmental variations in brain protein synthesis in vitro have been difficult to interpret because of the possible presence of protein kinases, protein phosphatases, ribonucleases and proteases in these preparations which could alter the structure and function of components of the reconstituted systems (Roberts, 1977).

In our earlier experiments with partially purified preparations of the soluble components of brain protein-synthesizing systems, highly purified cerebral ribosomal subunits from phenylalanine-treated and saline-treated infant rats were recombined in mix-and-match studies of their capacity for polypeptide synthesis in the presence or absence of the synthetic messenger RNA, poly(U) (Roberts, 1977). The results indicated that prior phenylalanine loading may actually enhance the capacity of cerebral ribosomes for polyphenylalanine synthesis (Table IV). The observed increase in poly(U)-directed polypeptide synthesis was localized in the cerebral 40S subunit. Functioning of the 60S subunit in poly(U)-directed polypeptide synthesis was not affected by phenylalanine treatment.

TABLE IV

INFLUENCE OF PHENYLALANINE LOADING ON poly(U)-DIRECTED POLYPEPTIDE SYNTHESIS BY
CEREBRAL RIBOSOMAL SUBUNITS FROM INFANT RATS

Infant rats were injected intraperitoneally with 2.5% L-phenylalanine (1 mg/g body wt.) in 0.45% NaCl, or an
equivalent volume of 0.9% NaCl. They were killed 30 min later and ribosomal subunits were prepared from pooled
cerebral cortices. The assay for polypeptide synthesis was carried out for 30 min at 37°C. The incubation medium
(0.5 ml) contained $0.04 A_{260}$ unit of 40S subunits, $0.08 A_{260}$ unit of 60S subunits, 50 μg of poly(U) and 0.5 μCi of
L-[U-14c]phenylalanine, as well as a complete amino acid-incorporating system (Zomzely-Neurath et al., 1973).
[Reprinted with modifications from Roberts (1977).]

| Source of ribosomal subunit | | Radioactivity incorporated (c.p.m. ±S.E.M.) | Percent change * |
|---|---|---|---|
| 40S | 60S | | |
| Saline | Saline | 10 920 ± 625 | |
| Phenylalanine | Phenylalanine | 13 900 ± 312 | + 27 |
| Saline | Phenylalanine | 11 420 ± 563 | + 4 |
| Phenylalanine | Saline | 15 030 ± 579 | + 37 |

* Compared to polypeptide synthesis by 40S and 60S subunits obtained from saline-treated animals.

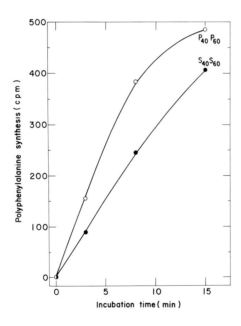

Fig. 9. Influence of phenylalanine loading on polypeptide elongation by ribosomal subunits from infant rat cerebral
cortex. Ribosomal subunits were prepared from cerebral cortices of infant rats given an intraperitoneal injection of
3.0% L-phenylalanine (2 mg/g body wt.) in 0.45% NaCl, or an equivalent volume of 0.9% NaCl, 1 h earlier. The
incubation mixture (50 μl) contained $0.02 A_{260}$ units of 40S subunits, $0.05 A_{260}$ units of 60S subunits, 100 mM KCl,
20 mM Tris–HCl, pH 7.5, 1.0 mM GTP, 2.1 mM phosphoenol pyruvate, 0.3 IU of pyruvate kinase, 1 mM dithiothreitol, 10 mM MgCl, $0.2 A_{260}$ units of poly(U), 10 pmoles of [3H]PhetRNA and saturating levels of eukaryotic
elongation factors, EF-1 and EF-2. The reaction mixtures were incubated at 37°C, and the reaction was terminated by
the addition of 1 ml of cold 10% trichoroacetic acid. The precipitates of polyphenylalanine were then processed for
measurement of radioactivity by liquid scintillation spectrometry (Merrick, 1979). $P_{40}$, $P_{60}$, ribosomal subunits from
phenylalanine-treated rats. $S_{40}$, $S_{60}$, ribosomal subunits from saline-treated animals.

208

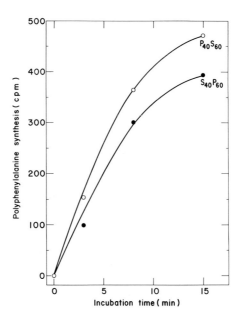

Fig. 10. Localization of phenylalanine-induced alterations in polypeptide elongation in 40S ribosomal subunits from infant rat cerebral cortex. Treatment of animals and conditions of incubation in the elongation assay system were the same as described in the legend to Fig. 9.

These experiments suggested that some phase of the translational process in brain protein synthesis was accelerated in hyperphenylalaninemic infant rats. The possibility of phenylalanine-induced enhancement of initiation mechanisms seemed unlikely in view of the finding that polypeptide synthesis by cerebral polyribosomes from infant rats in the presence of endogenous messenger RNA was unaffected by phenylalanine loading (Roberts, 1977). Moreover, results from this and other laboratories had previously indicated that initiation mechanisms in brain protein synthesis may be depressed in experimental hyperphenylalaninemia (Taub and Johnson, 1975; Roberts and Morelos, 1976; Hughes and Johnson, 1978a,b). In view of these various findings, investigations were undertaken of the possible effects of phenylalanine loading on the elongation process of brain protein synthesis. In these more recent experiments, highly purified preparations of ribosomal subunits from control and hyperphenylalaninemic infant rats were incubated in an elongation system containing poly(U), [$^3$H]phenylalanyl-tRNA and purified eukaryotic elongation factors (L. Holbrook and S. Roberts, unpublished observations). Under these conditions, polyphenylalanine synthesis appeared to be significantly enhanced by prior phenylalanine loading (Fig. 9). Moreover, this increase in elongation mechanisms was localized in the cerebral 40S subunit (Fig. 10). The tentative conclusion that can be drawn from these preliminary observations is that phenylalanine loading, by speeding up polypeptide elongation on cerebral ribosomes, may result in the formation of incomplete proteins incapable of serving normal brain functions. Additional work is required to substantiate these findings, particularly in view of earlier observations which suggested that phenylalanine loading inhibited polypeptide elongation by isolated mouse brain polyribosomes incubated with a crude preparation of soluble protein synthesis factors (Hughes and Johnson, 1978b). The limitations of such experiments have been described above.

These results do not, in themselves, provide definitive evidence that the phenylalanine-induced decrease in phosphorylation of the cerebral S6 ribosomal protein is solely or partially responsible for the defects in protein synthesis observed in hyperphenylalaninemic animals or phenylketonuric human patients. Thus, phenylalanine loading, by inhibiting the activity of brain cAMP-dependent protein kinases, may result in other metabolic defects which directly or indirectly depress protein synthesis. Moreover, the alterations in phosphorylation of the cerebral S6 ribosomal protein observed under these conditions may be accompanied by other changes in the structure and function of the 40S ribosomal subunits. In efforts to resolve these problems, experiments are underway in our laboratory in which polypeptide elongation will be assessed in purified systems with the use of cerebral 40S ribosomal subunits containing the S6 protein in various states of phosphorylation induced in cellular preparations with cAMP and other effectors, as well as in reconstituted ribosome-protein kinase systems. Comparable experiments are also underway to study the influence of variations in cerebral ribosomal protein phosphorylations in hyperphenylalaninemia and the other conditions outlined above on sequential steps in the initiation of brain protein synthesis. It is anticipated that these investigations may help to elucidate basic biochemical processes which underlie normal and abnormal neural activity in the central nervous system, as well as contribute to knowledge of the role of ribosomal protein phosphorylation in eukaroytic protein synthesis.

## ACKNOWLEDGEMENT

These investigations were supported by a research grant from the National Institutes of Health, U.S. Public Health Service (NS-13295). The bibliographic and editorial assistance of Jona Huefe is gratefully acknowledged.

## REFERENCES

Ashby, C.D. and Roberts, S. (1975) Phosphorylation of ribosomal proteins in rat cerebral cortex in vitro. *J. biol. Chem.*, 250: 2546–2555.

Bogucki, B. and Roberts, S. (1979) Influence of elevated levels of phenylalanine on amino acid and protein metabolism in rat cerebral cortex in vitro. *Fed. Proc.*, 38: 947 (abstr. 3792).

Cohen, P. (Ed.) (1980) *Molecular Aspects of Cellular Regulation*, Vol. 1, Protein Phosphorylation in Regulation, Elsevier/North-Holland, Amsterdam.

Daly, J. (1977) *Cyclic Nucleotides in the Nervous System*, Plenum Press, New York, London.

Francis, T.A. (1980) *Phosphorylation of Ribosomal Proteins in Isolated Ribosome-Protein Kinase Systems from Rat Cerebral Cortex*. Ph.D. Dissertation, University of California, Los Angeles, CA.

Francis, T.A. and Roberts, S. (1978) Ribosomal protein phosphorylation in rat cerebral 40S subunits catalyzed by protein kinase catalytic subunit. *Fed. Proc.*, 37: 1406 (abstr. 753).

Francis, T.A. and Roberts, S. (1980) Ribosomal protein phosphorylation catalyzed by protein kinase catalytic subunit from rat cerebral cortex in vitro. *Fed. Proc.*, 39: 1743 (abstr. 737).

Gaull, G.E., Tallan, H.H., Lajtha, A. and Rassin, D.K. (1975) Pathogenesis of brain dysfunction in inborn errors of amino acid metabolism. In *Biology of Brain Dysfunction*, G.E. Gaull (Ed.), Plenum Press, New York, London.

Genot, A., Reboud, J.P., Cenatiempo, Y. and Cozzone, A.J. (1978) Endogenous phosphorylation of ribosomal proteins from membrane-free rat liver polysomes. *FEBS Lett.*, 86: 103–107.

Grankowski, N. and Gasior, E. (1975) An in vivo and in vitro phosphorylation of yeast ribosomal proteins. *Acta biochem. pol.*, 22: 45–56.

Gressner, A.M. and Wool, I.G. (1974a) The phosphorylation of liver ribosomal proteins in vivo. Evidence that only a single small subunit protein (S6) is phosphorylated. *J. biol. Chem.*, 249: 6917–6925.

Gressner, A.M. and Wool, I.G. (1974b) The stimulation of the phosporylation of ribosomal protein S6 by cycloheximide and puromycin. *Biochem. biophys. Res. Commun.*, 60: 1482–1489.

Gressner, A.M. and Wool, I.G. (1976) Effect of experimental diabetes and insulin on phosphorylation of rat liver ribosomal protein S6. *Nature (Lond.)*, 259: 148–150.

Hofmann, F., Bechtel, P.J. and Krebs, E.G. (1977) Concentrations of cyclic AMP-dependent protein kinase subunits in various tissues. *J. biol. Chem.*, 252: 1441–1447.

210

Hughes, J.V. and Johnson, T.C. (1976) The effects of phenylalanine on amino acid metabolism and protein synthesis in brain cells in vitro. *J. Neurochem.*, 26: 1105–1113.

Hughes, J.V. and Johnson, T.C. (1977a) Hyperphenylalaninemia: effect on brain polyribosomes can be partially reversed by other amino acids. *Science*, 195: 402–404.

Hughes, J.V. and Johnson, T.C. (1977b) The effects of hyperphenylalaninaemia on the concentrations of aminoacyl-transfer ribonucleic acid in vivo. A mechanism for the inhibition of neural protein synthesis by phenylalanine. *Biochem. J.*, 162: 527–537.

Hughes, J.V. and Johnson, T.C. (1978a) Abnormal amino acid metabolism and brain protein synthesis during neural development. *Neurochem. Res.*, 3: 381–399.

Hughes, J.V. and Johnson, T.C. (1978b) Experimentally induced and natural recovery from the effects of phenylalanine on brain protein synthesis. *Biochem. biophys. Acta*, 517: 473–485.

Issinger, O.-G. (1977) Phosphorylation of acidic ribosomal proteins from rabbit reticulocytes by a ribosome-associated casein kinase. *Biochim. biophys. Acta*, 477: 185–189.

Issinger, O.-G., Beier, H., Speichermann, N., Flokerzi, V. and Hofmann, F. (1980) Comparison of phosphorylation of ribosomal proteins from HeLa and Krebs II ascites-tumour cells by cyclic AMP-dependent and cyclic GMP-dependent protein kinases. *Biochem. J.*, 185: 89–99.

Kramer, G., Henderson, A.B., Pinphanichakarn, P., Wallis, M.H. and Hardesty, B. (1977) Partial reaction of peptide initiation inhibited by phosphorylation of either initiation factor eIF-2 or 40S ribosomal proteins. *Proc. nat. Acad. Sci (Wash.)*, 74: 1445–1449.

Krystosek, A., Bitte, L.F., Cawthon, M.L. and Kabat, D. (1974) Phosphorylation of ribosomal proteins in eukaryotes. In *Ribosomes*, M. Nomura, A. Tissières and P. Lengyel (Eds.), Cold Spring Harbor Laboratory, pp. 855–870.

Kudlicki, W., Szyszka, R., Palén, E. and Gasior, E. (1980) Evidence for a highly specific protein kinase phosphorylating two strongly acidic proteins of yeast 60S ribosomal subunit. *Biochim. biophys. Acta*, 633: 376–385.

Lastick, S.M. and McConkey, E.H. (1981) HeLa ribosomal protein S6: insulin and dibutyryl cyclic AMP affect different phosphopeptides. *J. biol. Chem.*, 256: 583–585.

Leader, D.P. (1980) The control of phosphorylation of ribosomal proteins. In *Molecular Aspects of Cellular Regulation*. Vol. 1, P. Cohen (Ed.), Elsevier/North-Holland, Amsterdam, pp. 203–233.

Leader, D.P. and Coia, A.A. (1978) The phosphorylation of ribosomal protein S6 on the monoribosomes and polyribosomes of baby hamster kidney fibroblasts. *FEBS Lett.*, 90: 270–274.

Martini, O.H.W. and Kruppa, J. (1979) Ribosomal phosphoproteins of mouse myeloma cells. Changes in the degree of phosphorylation induced by hypertonic initiation block. *Eur. J. Biochem.*, 95: 349–358.

Merrick, W.C. (1979) Assays for eukaryotic protein synthesis. *Meth. Enzymol.*, 60: 108–123.

Moldave, K. and Grossman, L. (Eds.) (1979) *Methods in Enzymology*, Vol. 60, Nucleic Acids and Protein Synthesis, Academic Press, New York, San Francisco, London.

Möller, W., Slobin, L.I., Amons, R. and Richter, D. (1975) Isolation and characterization of two acidic proteins of 60S ribosomes from Artemia salina cysts. *Proc. nat. Acad. Sci. (Wash.)*, 72: 4744–4748.

Palmer, W.K., McPherson, J.M. and Walsh, D.A. (1980) Critical controls in the evaluation of cAMP-dependent protein kinase activity ratios as indices of hormonal action. *J. biol. Chem.*, 255: 2663–2666.

Roberts, S. (1968) Influence of elevated circulating levels of amino acids on cerebral concentrations and utilization of amino acids. In *Progress in Brain Research*, Vol., 29, A. Lajtha and D.H. Ford (Eds.), Elsevier, Amsterdam, pp. 235–243.

Roberts, S. (1977) Translational control of brain protein synthesis. In *Mechanisms, Regulation and Special Functions of Protein Synthesis in the Brain*, S. Roberts, A. Lajtha and W.H. Gispen (Eds.), Elsevier/North-Holland, Amsterdam, New York, pp. 3–20.

Roberts, S. and Ashby, C.D. (1978) Ribosomal protein phosphorylation in rat cerebral cortex in vitro. Influence of cylcic adenosine 3′:5′-monophosphate. *J. biol. Chem.*, 253: 288–296.

Roberts, S. and Morelos, B.S. (1976) Role of ribonuclease action in phenylalanine-induced disaggregation of rat cerebral polyribosomes. *J. Neurochem.*, 26: 387–400.

Roberts, S. and Morelos, B.S. (1979) Phosphorylation of multiple proteins of both ribosomal subunits in rat cerebral cortex in vivo. Effect of adenosine 3′:5′-cyclic monophosphate. *Biochem. J.*, 184: 233–244.

Roberts, S. and Morelos, B.S. (1980) Cerebral ribosomal protein phosphorylation in experimental hyperphenylalaninaemia. *Biochem. J.*, 190: 405–419.

Roberts, S. and Morelos, B.S. (1982) Inhibition of cerebral protein kinase activity and cyclic AMP-dependent ribosomal-protein phosphorylation in experimental hyperphenylalaninemia. *Biochem. J.*, 202: 343–351.

Roberts, S., Lajtha, A. and Gispen, W.H. (Eds.) (1977) *Mechanisms, Regulation and Special Functions of Protein Synthesis in the Brain*, Elsevier/North-Holland, Amsterdam, New York.

Rosenberg, L.E. and Scriver, C.R. (1980) Disorders of amino acid metabolism. In *Metabolic Control and Disease*,

8th Edn., P.K. Bondy and L.E. Rosenberg (Eds.), W.B. Saunders, Philadelphia, London, Toronto, pp. 583–776.

Rubin, C.S., Rangel-Aldao, R., Sackar, D., Erlichman, J. and Fleischer, N. (1979) Characterization and comparison of membrane-associated and cytosolic cAMP-dependent protein kinases. Physicochemical and immunological studies on bovine cerebral cortex protein kinases. *J. biol. Chem.*, 254: 3797–3805.

Scriver, C.R. and Rosenberg, L.E. (1973) *Amino Acid Metabolism and its Disorders*, W.B. Saunders, Philadelphia, London, Toronto.

Sherton, C.C. and Wool, I.G. (1972) Determination of the number of proteins in liver ribosomes and ribosomal subunits by two-dimensional polyacrylamide gel electrophoresis. *J. biol. Chem.*, 247: 4460–4467.

Sherton, C.C. and Wool, I.G. (1974) A comparison of the proteins of rat skeletal muscle and liver ribosomes by two-dimensional polyacrylaminde gel electrophoresis. Observations on the partition of proteins between ribosomal subunits and a description of two acidic proteins in the large subunit. *J. biol. Chem.*, 249: 2258–2267.

Siegel, F.L., Aoki, K. and Colwell, R.E. (1971) Polyribosome disaggregation and cell-free protein synthesis in preparations from cerebral cortex of hyperphenylalaninemic rats. *J. Neurochem.*, 18: 537–547.

Taub, F. and Johnson, T.C. (1975) The mechanism of polyribosome disaggregation in the brain tissue by phenylalanine. *Biochem. J.*, 151: 173–180.

Terao, K. and Ogata, K. (1979a) Proteins of small subunits of rat liver ribosomes that interact with poly(U). II. Cross-links between poly(U) and ribosomal proteins in 40S subunits induced by UV irradiation. *J. Biochem.*, 86: 605–617.

Terao, K. and Ogata, K. (1979b) Proteins of small subunits of rat liver ribosomes that interact with poly(U). I. Effects of preincubation of poly(U) with 40S subunits on the interactions of 40S subunit proteins with aurintricarboxylic acid with $NN'$-$p$-phenylenedimaleimide. *J. Biochem.*, 86: 597–603.

Thomas, G., Siegmann, M., Kubler, A.-M., Gordon, J. and Jimenez de Asua, L. (1980) Regulation of 40S ribosomal protein S6 phosphorylation in Swiss mouse 3T3 cells. *Cell*, 19: 1015–1023.

Todokoro, K., Ulbrich, N., Chan, Y.-L. and Wool, I.G. (1981) Characterization of the binding of rat liver ribosomal proteins L6, L8, L19, S9, and S13 to 5.8 S ribosomal ribonucleic acid. *J. biol. Chem.*, 256: 7202–7212.

Traugh, J.A. (1981) Regulation of protein synthesis by phosphorylation. In *Biochemical Actions of Hormones*, Vol. 8, G. Litwack (Ed.), Academic Press, New York, London, Toronto, Sydney, San Francisco, pp. 167–208.

Traugh, J.A. and Porter, G.G. (1976) A comparison of ribosomal proteins from rabbit reticulocytes phosphorylated in situ and in vitro. *Biochemistry*, 15: 610–616.

Treloar, M.A., Treloar, M.W. and Kisilevsky, R. (1977) Ethionine and the phosphorylation of ribosomal protein S6. *J. biol. Chem.*, 252: 6217–6221.

Ulbrich, N. and Wool, I.G. (1978) Identification by affinity chromatography of the eukaryotic ribosomal proteins that bind to 5S ribosomal ribonucleic acid. *J. biol. Chem.*, 253: 9049–9052.

Ulbrich, N., Wool, I.G., Ackerman, E. and Sigler, P.B. (1980) The identification by affinity chromatography of the rat liver ribosomal proteins that bind to elongator and initiation transfer ribonucleic acids. *J. biol. Chem.*, 255: 7010–7016.

Ventimiglia, F.A. and Wool, I.G. (1974) A kinase that transfers the $\gamma$-phosphoryl group of GTP to proteins of eukaryotic 40S ribosomal subunits. *Proc. nat. Acad. Sci. (Wash.)*, 71: 350–354.

Von Hungen, K. and Roberts, S. (1974) Neurotransmitter-sensitive adenylate cyclase systems in the brain. In *Reviews of Neuroscience*, Vol. 1, S. Ehrenpreis and I.J. Kopin (Eds.), Raven Press, New York, pp. 231–281.

Weller, M. (1979) *Protein Phosphorylation*, Pion, London.

Westermann, P., Heuman, W., Bommer, U.-A., Bielka, H., Nygard, O. and Hultin, T. (1979) Crosslinking of initiation factor eIF-2 to proteins of the small subunit of rat liver ribosomes. *FEBS Lett.*, 97: 101–104.

Wettenhall, R.E.H. and Howlett, G.J. (1979) Phosphorylation of a specific ribosomal protein during stimulation of thymocytes by concanavalin A and prostaglandin $E_1$. *J. biol. Chem.*, 254: 9317–9323.

Wicks, W.D. (1974) Regulation of protein synthesis by cyclic AMP. In *Advances in Cyclic Nucleotide Research*, Vol. 4, P. Greengard and G.A. Robison (Eds.), Raven Press, New York, pp. 335–438.

Wool, I.G. (1979) The structure and function of eukaryotic ribosomes. *Annu. Rev. Biochem.*, 48: 719–754.

Wool, I.G. and Stöffler, G. (1974) Structure and function of eukaryotic ribosomes. In *Ribosomes*, M. Nomura, A. Tissières and P. Lengyel (Eds.), Cold Spring Harbor, pp. 417–460.

Zomzely, C.E., Roberts, S., Gruber, C.P. and Brown, D.M. (1968) Cerebral protein synthesis. II. Instability of cerebral messenger ribonucleic acid-ribosome complexes. *J. biol. Chem.*, 243: 5396–5409.

Zomzely-Neurath, C., York, C. and Moore, B.W. (1973) In vitro synthesis of two brain-specific proteins (S100 and 14-3-2) by polyribosomes from rat brain. *Arch. Biochem. Biophys.*, 155: 58–69.

# Phosphorylation in Relation to the Modulation of Brain Protein Synthesis by ACTH-Like Neuropeptides

P. SCHOTMAN, H. FRANKENA, L.H. SCHRAMA and P.M. EDWARDS

*Division of Molecular Neurobiology, Institute of Molecular Biology,*
*Laboratory of Physiological Chemistry, and Rudolf Magnus Institute for*
*Pharmacology, State University of Utrecht, Utrecht, The Netherlands*

## 1. INTRODUCTION

$NH_2$-terminal fragments of corticotrophin (ACTH) are involved in central nervous functioning by a direct interaction with subcortical structures (De Wied and Gispen, 1977; Dunn and Schotman, 1981). The biochemical effects of ACTH include changes in brain RNA and protein synthesis (Dunn and Schotman, 1981), in cyclic nucleotide levels, in the activity of a membrane-bound protein kinase and in the turnover of polyphosphoinositides (Wiegant et al., 1981). In order to explain the diverse actions of ACTH on various peripheral target organs, Schwyzer (1980) has proposed a model in which different parts of the peptide molecule are responsible for specific physiological functions, e.g., receptor binding, $Mg^{2+}$ accumulation and steroidogenesis. The various neurotropic actions of ACTH on behavioural and neurochemical parameters could similarly be assigned to specific sequences. The relatively large peptides $ACTH_{1-24}$ and $ACTH_{5-18}$ display the full range of activities, whereas smaller fragments only show a proportion of these. For instance, $ACTH_{4-10}$ alters brain protein synthesis and behaviour in certain avoidance and reward-motivated tests (Dunn and Schotman, 1981; De Wied and Gispen, 1977), but does not cause the changes in membrane phosphorylation or the grooming activity associated with $ACTH_{1-24}$ (Gispen and De Wied, 1980). In peripheral target cells most, but not all, actions of ACTH are mediated by a cAMP increase which differs from the classical second messenger mechanism (Sutherland, 1972) in that calcium ions are required for the hormone/receptor-adenylate cyclase coupling (Saez et al., 1981). In the nervous system, many of the changes in metabolic processes evoked by ACTH have been shown to be independent of cAMP (Wiegant et al., 1981).

## 2. MODULATION OF PROTEIN SYNTHESIS

The changes in brain protein synthesis observed in the brain in vivo and in brain slices and pineal glands in vitro have recently been shown to occur in a cell-free preparation of brain tissue (Schotman et al., 1980; Schotman and Allaart, 1981). Fig. 1A shows that, under certain conditions (high $Mg^{2+}$ and $K^+$ concentrations), $ACTH_{1-24}$ ($10^{-8}$ M) prevented the rapid decay of the protein synthesis seen in control incubations. In the absence of ACTH, the protein

---

Correspondence and reprint requests to: Dr. P. Schotman, Institute of Molecular Biology, University of Utrecht, Padualaan 8, 3508 TB Utrecht, The Netherlands.

214

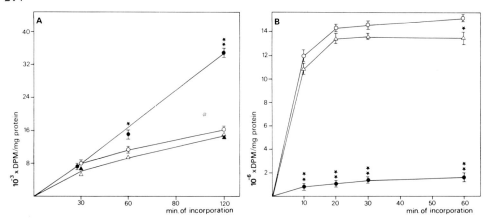

Fig. 1.A: Effects of $ACTH_{1-24}$ ($10^{-8}$ M) on leucine incorporation into proteins. A post-mitochondrial supernatant fraction $S_{20}$ (10 min, $20\,000 \times g$) of brain was incubated with L-[U-$^{14}$C]leucine (340 mCi/mmole) in the presence of 12 mM $Mg^{2+}$ and 200 mM $K^+$ (Schotman and Allaart, 1981) and with (●) or without (○) $ACTH_{1-24}$ ($10^{-8}$ M) for the times indicated. The effect of aurintricarboxylic acid (ATA), an inhibitor of initiation, at 50μM, is shown in the presence (▲) or absence (△) of $ACTH_{1-24}$ ($10^{-8}$ M). The symbols represent mean ± S.E.M. of three incubations. *$2P$ < 0.05; **$2P$ < 0.01, Student's $t$ test. Taken from Schotman and Allaart (1981). B: Effects of $ACTH_{11-24}$ ($10^{-4}$ M) on leucine incorporation into proteins. An $S_{20}$ (see A) was incubated with L-[4,5-$^3$H]leucine (131 Ci/mmole) in the presence of 4 mM $Mg^{2+}$ and 100 mM $K^+$ and with (●) or without (○) $ACTH_{11-24}$ ($10^{-4}$ M) for the times indicated (Schrama et al., in preparation). The effect of edeine, an inhibitor of initiation, at $10^{-6}$ M is shown in the absence (△) of $ACTH_{11-24}$ ($10^{-4}$ M). In the presence of ACTH, edeine had no effect (data not shown). Symbols represent mean ± S.E.M. of three incubations. *$2P$ < 0.05; **$2P$ < 0.05, Student's $t$ test.

synthesis observed was almost entirely the result of elongation of peptide chains, as is shown by the fact that aurintricarboxylic acid (ATA, an inhibitor of chain initiation; Safer and Anderson, 1978) had negligible effect. However, addition of $ACTH_{1-24}$ ($10^{-8}$ M) doubled the amount of labelled protein formed over 2 h and this effect was abolished by ATA. These data suggest that the presence of ACTH resulted in re-initiation of peptide chain synthesis amounting to a mean of once for each messenger (Fig. 1A). The influence of $ACTH_{1-24}$ on the cell-free system showed a biphasic pattern. Low concentrations stimulated protein synthesis as described above; high concentrations ($10^{-4}$ M) inhibited. The stimulatory effect of $ACTH_{1-24}$ could also be brought about by the N-terminal sequence $ACTH_{4-10}$ (Schotman and Allaart, 1981). The inhibitory action of high concentrations of $ACTH_{1-24}$ could be elicited by peptide sequences (5–18) and (11–24) closer to the C terminal of the molecule (Fig. 1B, shown for (11–24)). The inhibitory effect of $ACTH_{11-24}$ was concentration-dependent between $10^{-7}$ and $10^{-4}$ M and at the latter concentration, 80% inhibition was attained. The stimulation caused by low concentrations of $ACTH_{1-24}$ was not seen at any concentration of $ACTH_{11-24}$. The system used in the experiments reported in Fig. 1A was modified (the significant changes were lower $Mg^{2+}$ and $K^+$ concentrations) to give the higher rate (10–15-fold) of protein synthesis shown in Fig. 1B. However, the contribution from initiation of new peptide chains remained low as is shown by the small effect of edeine, another inhibitor of initiation (Safer and Anderson, 1978).

The inhibitory effect of $ACTH_{11-24}$ in this system, therefore, must be explained in terms of an interference with the elongation of pre-existing peptide chains. The initiation of new peptide chains has been proposed as the main regulatory site for translation of mRNA into proteins. Nevertheless, there are several examples of regulation of the elongation rate by physiological stimuli (Roper and Wicks, 1978; Nielsen and McConkey, 1980) and of a correlation between

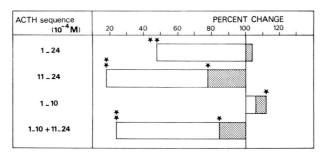

Fig. 2. Effect of different ACTH sequences at $10^{-4}$ M on leucine incorporation at different $Mg^{2+}$ concentrations. The experimental conditions were as described in the legend to Fig. 1B, except that open bars represent the data at 4 mM and shaded bars at 12 mM $Mg^{2+}$. The blocks represent the mean incorporation at four time points in three separate incubations. Analysis of variance was used to determine the significance of peptide effects. *$P < 0.05$; **$P < 0.01$.

physiological changes in protein synthesis and differences in elongation rate, for example during the development of the nervous system (Campagnoni and Harris, 1977) and after hypophysectomy (Schotman et al., 1980). The effect of the ACTH sequences (5–18) and (11–24) on elongation rates possibly results from an interaction with regulatory sites that bind spermine and $Mg^{2+}$ (Schrama and Schotman, 1981). Structure–activity studies have indicated that lysine residues in the peptides are essential for this action (Schrama et al., in preparation).

The critical role of $Mg^{2+}$ in ACTH regulation of protein synthesis is also evident in the data shown in Fig. 2. At high $Mg^{2+}$ concentrations (10–12 mM) peptide fragments ($10^{-4}$ M) of ACTH showed divergent effects, viz. $ACTH_{1-10}$ caused a 12% increase and $ACTH_{11-24}$ a 20% decrease. At 4 mM $Mg^{2+}$, $ACTH_{11-24}$ inhibited protein synthesis by 83%, whereas $ACTH_{1-10}$ was inactive. The interaction between $Mg^{2+}$ ions and the peptide sequence (11–24) in our brain-derived system is particularly interesting in view of the effect of the same portion of the ACTH molecule on $Mg^{2+}$ accumulation in peripheral target organs (Schwyzer, 1980).

In summary, ACTH-like peptides alter protein synthesis in a cell-free system derived from brain in a bimodal fashion: (i) the N-terminal part of the molecule is responsible for a stimulation of re-initiation of mRNA translation occurring at low peptide ($< 10^{-8}$ M) and high $Mg^{2+}$ (12 mM) and $K^+$ (200 mM) concentrations; (ii) a portion closer to the C terminal, containing several basic amino acid residues, is responsible for the inhibition of chain elongation at high peptide ($> 10^{-7}$ M) and low $Mg^{2+}$ (4 mM) concentrations. These actions might explain similar bimodal effects of ACTH on behavioural parameters (De Wied and Gispen, 1977) and on in vivo brain protein synthesis (Schotman et al., 1976).

Studies on the effect of ACTH on protein synthesis in intact pineal glands in vitro indicated an important role for the release of endogenous transmitters (Schotman et al., 1981). In the cell-free system derived from brain, it is highly unlikely that the observed effects of ACTH on protein synthesis are mediated by release of endogenous transmitters since careful examination of the preparation by electron microscopy revealed no intact synaptosomal structures (Fig. 3). The cell-free preparation contains considerable quantities of membrane structures (Fig. 3). Some of this material can be identified as deriving from the endoplasmic reticulum but small fragments of plasma membrane are also likely to be present. Therefore, membrane-mediated mechanisms of action of the peptides cannot be excluded. However, it is known that certain peptide hormone receptor complexes are internalised (Goldfine, 1978) and that ACTH itself can penetrate membranes (Schwyzer, 1980). A direct effect of the ACTH-like peptides on the protein machinery is therefore theoretically possible.

Fig. 3. The supernate of a centrifugation at 20 000 × g for 10 min (S$_{20}$) was centrifuged at 160 000 × g for 60 min. Slices of the resulting pellet were fixed and stained in glutaraldehyde and stained with uranyl acetate using standard procedures. No structures resembling intact synaptosome myelin fragments were visible. The electron micrograph shown is at a magnification of 1:33 000. The predominant organelles present are the ribosomes (black dots). The numerous vesicular structures of various size may derive from the plasma membrane and/or transmitter-containing vesicles.

Fig. 4. One- and two-dimensional separation of proteins and phosphoproteins in the post-mitochondrial supernatant (S$_{20}$) fraction of brain. The post-mitochondrial supernatant fraction prepared from rat brain stem was incubated for 15 sec in the presence of 12 mM Mg$^{2+}$, 200 mM K$^+$, $10^{-4}$ M GTP and 3–8 $\mu$Ci [$\gamma$-$^{32}$P]ATP (3000 Ci/mmole). (a) The proteins were separated by SDS–polyacrylamide gel electrophoresis. A mixture of standard proteins was run alongside the brain proteins; the molecular weight of each standard protein is indicated on the left of the figure at its respective position in the gel. The three tracks on the left of the figure were stained with fast green to show the position of protein. The three tracks on the right show the pattern obtained after autoradiography of the $^{32}$P-labelled phosphoproteins. (b, c) Photographs and densitometric scans of autoradiograms of $^{32}$P-labelled phosphoproteins in S$_{20}$ incubated as described for (a) in the presence and absence of cyclic nucleotides at the concentrations shown. The optical density scans of the control tracks (solid line in (b)) and the cAMP and cGMP tracks (shaded area in (b)) are shown. (d, e) Autoradiograms of $^{32}$P-labelled phosphoproteins separated in the first dimension according to isoelectric point (IEP) and in the second dimension according to molecular weight (MW). Incubations were carried out in the absence (d) or presence (e) of cAMP ($10^{-5}$ M). (f) Diagram of 7 phosphoproteins that can be clearly identified after the two-dimensional separation shown in (d) and (e). 1, 75 K (IEP 4.2); 2, 73 K (IEP 5.8–7.0); 3, 58 K (IEP 5.4–6.8); 4, 58 K (IEP 4.8–5.1); 5, 54 K (IEP 4.7); 6, 50 K (IEP 4.7); 7, 47 K (IEP 4.8). *2P 0.01, Student's $t$ test, $n = 3$. Taken from Van Dijk et al. (1981).

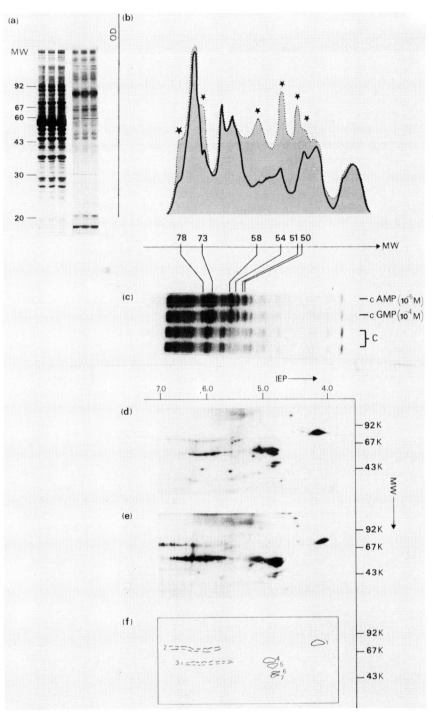

## 3. MODULATION OF PHOSPHORYLATION

Studies on the mechanism of action of ACTH on brain membrane function have demonstrated the involvement of a protein kinase that phosphorylates the substrate protein B-50 (Zwiers et al., 1976; Wiegant et al., 1981). The latter protein plays a role in the turnover of membrane (poly)phosphoinositides (Jolles et al., 1980), which in turn can mediate changes in $Ca^{2+}$ fluxes (Michell, 1979). The ACTH-sensitive protein phosphorylation system in brain membranes is insensitive to cAMP (Wiegant et al., 1981), but effects of ACTH on cAMP-dependent phosphorylation of regulatory proteins have also been described in peripheral target tissues (Saez et al., 1981; Boyd and Gorban, 1980).

The action of ACTH-like peptides on protein synthesis may also be mediated by protein phosphorylation in an analogous fashion. Phosphorylation of proteins associated with the ribosomal system has been implicated in the regulation of the rate of protein synthesis in many tissues (see review by Traugh, 1980). In the central nervous system, phosphorylation of several ribosomal proteins has been demonstrated in rat cerebral cortex in vitro (Ashby and Roberts, 1975) and in vivo (Roberts and Morelos, 1979). Some of these proteins were affected by cAMP (Roberts and Morelos, 1979). We report here on studies of phosphorylation of proteins in the same post-mitochondrial supernatant fraction as was used to study ACTH modulation of protein synthesis. This has the advantage that one can assume that the regulatory principles are present. A serious disadvantage, however, is that this preparation contains not only ribosomal phosphoproteins but also all the soluble phosphoproteins and a considerable quantity of membrane-bound material (Fig. 3). The constituent proteins of the post-mitochondrial supernatant fraction were labelled by incubation with $[\gamma\text{-}^{32}P]ATP$ and separated by SDS–polyacrylamide gel electrophoresis. Fig. 4a shows the protein profile obtained after fast green staining, together with the position of six molecular weight markers to indicate approximate molecular weights. The corresponding autoradiograms (Fig. 4a, c) revealed the presence of many phosphoproteins. With a few exceptions (e.g., the 54 K band), the labelled phosphoprotein bands did not coincide with bands stained with fast green. Hence, almost all phosphoproteins are minor protein components in the post-mitochondrial supernatant fraction from rat brain. The molecular weight and relatively high concentration of protein in the 54 K band suggests that it contains the phosphorylated subunits of tubulin (Weller, 1979; Zisapel et al., 1980).

## 4. CHARACTERISTICS OF PROTEIN PHOSPHORYLATION IN POST-MITOCHONDRIAL SUPERNATE

### 4.1. *Sensitivity to cyclic nucleotides*

Both cAMP and cGMP enhanced phosphorylation of six phosphoprotein bands (50, 51, 54, 58, 73 and 78 K) (Fig. 4b, c). However, the system was 10 times more sensitive to cAMP than to cGMP (10 $\mu$M and 100 $\mu$M nucleotide, respectively, gave equivalent stimulation). This is consistent with the results of others (Miyamoto et al., 1969; Tao et al., 1970) showing that the effect of 0.1–10 $\mu$M cAMP on protein kinases in cell-free preparations derived from brain and reticulocytes could be reproduced by cGMP but only at 10–100-fold higher concentrations. We further characterised the phosphoproteins present in the post-mitochondrial supernate by separating proteins by isoelectric focussing prior to SDS–PAGE in the second dimension (Fig. 4e; Van Dijk et al., 1981). The stimulation of phosphorylation by cAMP was evident in four regions (compare Fig. 4e with 4d) corresponding to the proteins identified in Fig. 4f: (2) 73 K, pI 5.8–7.0; (3) 58 K, pI 5.4–6.8; (4) 54 K, pI 4.7; (5) 50 K, pI 4.7. Surprisingly, phosphorylation of the 34 K phosphoprotein band was not altered by cAMP although this protein seems likely to be the S6 ribosomal protein, which has been shown to be sensitive to cAMP in many tissues including the brain (Hunt, 1980; Traugh, 1980; Jagus et al., 1981; Roberts and Morelos, 1979). The effects of cyclic nucleotides were essentially the same when GTP was omitted from the incubation medium (data not shown). This is in marked contrast to the effects of GTP on basal phosphorylation and on the response to ACTH, as described below.

## 4.2. Sensitivity to GTP

The incubation medium used for measuring protein synthesis in the post-mitochondrial supernate contained GTP, which is essential at several steps in protein synthesis (Safer and Anderson, 1978). We therefore investigated the effect of GTP on the phosphorylation of proteins and found the system highly sensitive to GTP concentration. GTP could act in a number of ways. (1) It could act by modulation of kinase and/or phosphatase enzymes. (2) It could compete with labelled ATP for kinases utilising both nucleotides. (3) It could alter the relative amounts of labelled GTP and ATP in the system. The enzyme nucleotide diphosphokinase catalyses the exchange of the $\gamma$-phosphate group between adenosine and other nucleotides (ATP + NDP $\rightleftharpoons$ NTP + ADP) (Wemmer, 1979). Thus added GTP, in combination with endogenous ADP can give rise to ATP formation. Addition of GTP inevitably adds GDP to the system since not only is GDP a contaminant of commercially available GTP preparations, but also GTP will be hydrolysed by a number of enzymes. The resulting GDP will be a substrate for the exchange reaction using $[\gamma\text{-}^{32}P]ATP$ and giving rise to $[\gamma\text{-}^{32}P]GTP$. Addition of unlabelled GTP ($10^{-4}$ M) decreased the incorporation of $^{32}P$ from $[\gamma\text{-}^{32}P]ATP$ into specific phosphoprotein bands at 24, 34, 38, 40, 50, 58 and 64 K (Fig. 5a). One explanation for this observation might be the generation of unlabelled ATP as explained above. However, this is not tenable since the phosphorylation of other protein bands (17, 20, 47, 67 and 75 K) was increased by GTP, whereas addition of unlabelled ATP resulted in uniform reduction of $^{32}P$ incorporation into all bands (Van Dijk et al., 1981). The possibility that nucleotide diphosphokinase enzyme activity results in the generation of $[\gamma\text{-}^{32}P]GTP$ from $[\gamma\text{-}^{32}P]ATP$ and GDP derived from unlabelled GTP is discussed in section 4.4. Selective decrease in certain phosphoprotein bands by addition of unlabelled GTP may be indicative of a kinase which can utilise GTP in place of the $[^{32}P]ATP$ as a substrate. The so-called casein kinase II or phosvitin kinase, for example, can use either nucleotide in phosphorylation reactions (Weller, 1979). However, this still does not explain the observed increase in $^{32}P$ incorporation into five protein bands. Regulatory effects of GTP, independent of its role as a potential kinase substrate, could explain both stimulatory and inhibitory actions on phosphoprotein labelling. Such a system, involving GTP in both activation and inhibition, has been described for hormonal regulation of adenylate cyclase activity (Londos et al., 1981). In relation to protein phosphorylation, certain protein kinases (Wiegant et al., 1978; Gross et al., 1981) and phosphoprotein phosphatases (England, 1980; Traugh, 1980) have been shown to be regulated by nucleotides (ATP and GTP).

The $[\gamma\text{-}^{32}P]ATP$-labelling method indicates the turnover of the phosphate moiety of phosphoproteins, rather than net phosphorylation. Therefore, a single effect on phosphatase enzymes could produce opposite effects on incorporation of label into individual phosphoproteins depending on whether kinase activity or kinase substrate (dephosphorylated protein) was the limiting factor in the phosphorylation process. Furthermore, in most systems there is a competition between a number of substrates for phosphatase activity, so a decrease in the affinity of the phosphoprotein phosphatase for one substrate, such as has been shown to result

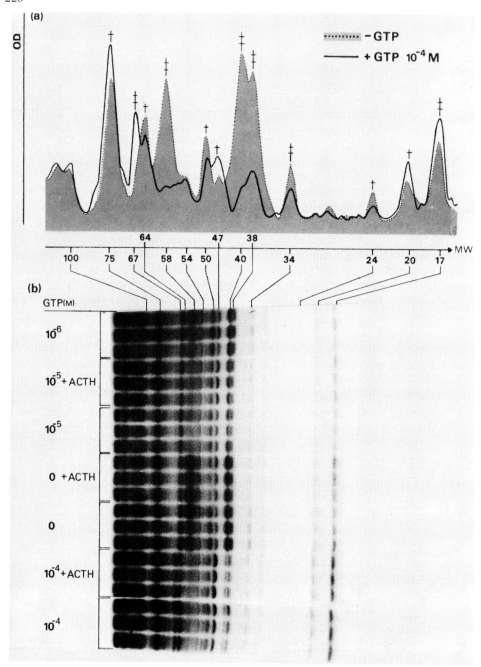

Fig. 5. Incubations were carried out as described in Fig. 4 except that the GTP concentration was varied from 0 to $10^{-4}$ M. Autoradiograms obtained after incubation in the presence or absence of $ACTH_{1-24}$ ($10^{-4}$ M) at the GTP concentrations indicated are shown in (b). Densitometric scans of the autoradiograms obtained in the presence (solid line) or absence (shaded area) of GTP ($10^{-4}$ M) are shown in (a). $^{+}2P < 0.05$; $\ddagger 2P < 0.01$, Student's $t$ test, $n = 3$. Taken from Van Dijk et al., (1981).

from GTP binding to the initiation factor eIF-2 (Jagus et al., 1981), will result in increased dephosphorylation of another substrate.

### 4.3. *Sensitivity to ACTH and its modulation by GTP*

ACTH$_{1-24}$ ($10^{-4}$ M) altered the phosphorylation of eight proteins (Figs. 5b and 6) all of which were also modulated by GTP. The phosphorylation of seven of these proteins (molecular weights 24, 34, 38, 50, 64, 67 and 75 K) is decreased by ACTH$_{1-24}$ and of one is increased (47 K). The sensitivity of ACTH varied with the GTP concentration (Fig. 6) in the incubation medium. The GTP concentration that gave the maximum ACTH effects was not the same for all phosphoproteins, but was in most cases the GTP concentration that gave the highest

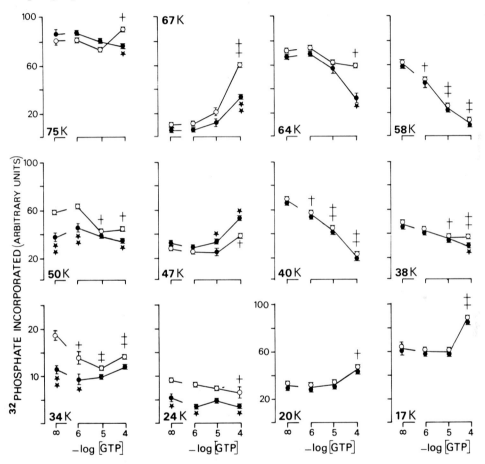

Fig. 6. GTP-sensitive phosphorylation and the effect of ACTH$_{1-24}$ ($10^{-4}$ M). The phosphorylation of 12 GTP-sensitive phosphoprotein bands was quantified by densitometric scanning of the autoradiogram shown in Fig. 5b. The labelling of the phosphoproteins was quantified by taking peak height in mm above background. The 24 K phosphoband was quantified from an autoradiogram exposed to the radioactive gel about 10 times longer than was necessary for the other bands. Open circles indicate the mean ± S.E.M. from incubations without ACTH, closed circles from incubations in the presence of ACTH$_{1-24}$ ($10^{-4}$ M). In the absence of ACTH, $^{+}2P < 0.05$; $^{‡}2P < 0.01$ indicates significance of difference (Student's $t$ test) from value with no GTP present ($\infty$). The effect of ACTH was measured by comparison with the control at each GTP concentration; $^{*}2P < 0.05$; $^{**}2P < 0.01$, Student's $t$ test, $n = 3$. Taken from Van Dijk et al. (1981).

222

phosphorylation of that protein in the absence of ACTH. There are other examples where sensitivity to hormones is highest when the basal activity is maximal (Zatz, 1978). Such a correlation has been observed for ACTH in the stimulation of protein synthesis in pineal glands (Schotman et al., 1981) and in cell-free systems (Schotman et al., 1980). However, the coincidence of GTP concentration at which basal phosphorylation is maximal with that at which sensitivity to ACTH is greatest may suggest a convergent pathway for the action of the two agents. Such a convergence has been proposed for the effect of ACTH and GTP on adenyl cyclase activity in the fat cell (Londos et al., 1981).

### 4.4. *Influence of phosphate donor*

In an attempt to elucidate the role of nucleotides in modulating ACTH effects on phosphorylation, we investigated the effect of replacing $[\gamma\text{-}^{32}P]ATP$ with $[\gamma\text{-}^{32}P]GTP$ as the phosphate donor. A completely different spectrum of $^{32}P$-labelled proteins was seen (Fig. 7). Three new phosphoprotein bands appeared at 28, 36 and 96 K, suggesting that the responsible protein kinase(s) are completely dependent on GTP as phosphate donor.

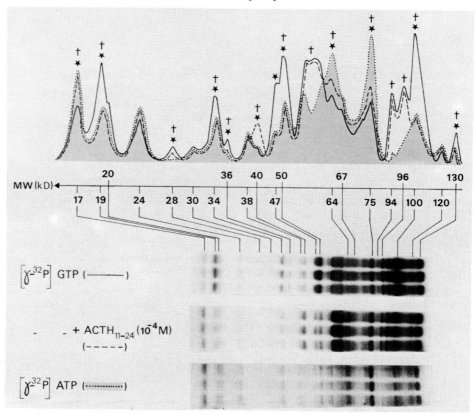

Fig. 7. Phosphate labelling of proteins with $[\gamma\text{-}^{32}P]GTP$ and $[\gamma\text{-}^{32}P]ATP$. Incubations were carried out in the presence of either $[\gamma\text{-}^{32}P]GTP$ in the presence (–––) or absence (——) of ACTH$_{11-24}$ ($10^{-4}$ M) or $[\gamma\text{-}^{32}P]ATP$ in the presence of GTP ($10^{-4}$ M) (shaded area). The experimental conditions and preparations of autoradiograms and scans were as described in Figs. 3 and 5. Significant differences in labelling in the presence of $[\gamma\text{-}^{32}P]GTP$ as compared with that in the presence of $[\gamma\text{-}^{32}P]ATP$ are indicated by $^+2P < 0.05$, Student's $t$ test ($n = 3$). Labelling in the presence of ACTH$_{11-24}$ and $[\gamma\text{-}^{32}P]GTP$ has been compared to that in the presence of $[\gamma\text{-}^{32}P]GTP$ alone; $^*2P < 0.01$, Student's $t$ test ($n = 3$).

A protein kinase that transfers the $\gamma$-phosphoryl group of GTP to protein components of eukaryotic 40S and 60S ribosomal subunits has been described (Ventimiglia and Wool, 1974; Leader, 1980). This enzyme is found both in the cytosol and associated with ribosomal particles; the phosphorylation of 60S ribosomal subunit proteins may be linked to the GTPase activity involved in peptide chain elongation (Leader, 1980).

In addition to the appearance of three new phosphoprotein bands when $[\gamma\text{-}^{32}P]GTP$ was used as a phosphate donor, marked alterations of relative labelling of other bands were seen (Fig. 7). The labelling of phosphoprotein bands at 19, 34, 50, 54–58, 94, 100 and 130 K was increased and that of the bands at 17, 64 and 75 K was decreased. Addition of unlabelled GTP ($10^{-4}$ M) did not alter the relative labelling of the protein bands as was seen when $[\gamma\text{-}^{32}P]ATP$ was the precursor (cf. section 4.2 and Figs. 5 and 6). In the presence of $[\gamma\text{-}^{32}P]GTP$, unlabelled GTP caused an overall decrease in labelling (data not shown). This is simply a consequence of the decreased specific activity of the $[\gamma\text{-}^{32}P]GTP$ in the incubation. The failure of GTP to alter the relative labelling of phosphoprotein bands from $[\gamma\text{-}^{32}P]GTP$ provides evidence that the effect of GTP on the labelling from $[\gamma\text{-}^{32}P]ATP$ is more likely to be related to generation of an alternative substrate ($[\gamma\text{-}^{32}P]GTP$) than to regulation of some enzyme activity. In the latter case, regulation might be predicted to modify labelling from both $[\gamma\text{-}^{32}P]ATP$ and $[\gamma\text{-}^{32}P]GTP$. In the former case, GTP can only affect labelling from $[\gamma\text{-}^{32}P]ATP$. Such a change in available phosphate donor would cause a shift in the contribution made by casein kinase I (which has an absolute requirement for ATP) and casein kinase II (which can utilise GTP or ATP) (Hathaway and Traugh, 1979). Since these kinases probably have differing affinities for various endogenous substrates, addition of GTP would lead, via generation of GDP and hence labelled GTP, to a decreased labelling of protein substrates of casein kinase I and an increase labelling of substrates of kinase II. This hypothesis is compatible with our finding that changes induced by GTP are different from those induced by cAMP (Fig. 4), since both enzymes are cyclic nucleotide-independent (Traugh, 1980).

The enzyme nucleotide diphosphokinase (NDPK) (Weller, 1979), which is very active in the cytosol, will play an important role in determining the relative amounts of labelled GTP and ATP available for phosphorylation. For example, after 1 min of incubation with $[\gamma\text{-}^{32}P]ATP$, it has been found that only 30–40% of the initial label remained in ATP, whereas 20% was recovered in GTP (Ernst et al., 1979). A similar exchange might be predicted to occur in the reverse direction when $[\gamma\text{-}^{32}P]GTP$ is used as precursor. Thus, some of the effects of adding unlabelled GTP to the $[\gamma\text{-}^{32}P]ATP$-labelling system (or unlabelled ATP to the $[\gamma\text{-}^{32}P]GTP$ system, data not shown) may be related to the generation, via diphosphonucleotide formation of $\gamma$-$^{32}P$-labelled alternative triphosphonucleotide.

With $[\gamma\text{-}^{32}P]GTP$ as substrate (Fig. 7), addition of $ACTH_{11-24}$ resulted in a decrease in labelling of eight protein bands (19, 28, 34, 36, 47, 50, 100 and 130 K) and an increase in four bands (17, 40, 64 and 75 K). Only for the 34 and 50 K have similar changes been observed with $[\gamma\text{-}^{32}P]ATP$ as precursor and this only in the absence of GTP (Fig. 6).

With few exceptions (40, 94 and 96 K bands and poorly separated proteins in the 55–60 K region), the effect of ACTH was to alter the profile seen with $[\gamma\text{-}^{32}P]GTP$ towards that seen with $[\gamma\text{-}^{32}P]ATP$ as the precursor in the presence of unlabelled GTP. We cannot, at present, give any explanation for this intriguing situation.

### 4.5. ACTH effect is cAMP-independent

In the adrenal cortex, the majority of observed effects of ACTH result from an initial stimulation of adenylate cyclase activity (Boyd and Gorban, 1980). Cyclic nucleotide concentrations in the brain are also modulated by ACTH (Wiegant et al., 1979). Regulation of protein synthesis by cyclic nucleotides has been shown for many systems (Wicks, 1974) including the pineal gland (Schotman et al., 1981) and a cell-free system derived from brain stem (Schotman et al., 1980).

However, ACTH effects on protein phosphorylation in the brain post-mitochondrial supernate cannot be mediated by cAMP since cAMP increased the phospholabelling of a completely different selection of protein bands (Figs. 4 and 5). The response to cGMP is similar to that to cAMP. A cyclic nucleotide-independent pathway is likewise implicated in the ACTH-induced changes in phosphorylation of membrane proteins (Wiegant et al., 1981; Saez et al., 1981). Only one protein (50 K) was sensitive to both ACTH and cAMP. Phospholabelling of this protein was increased by cAMP and decreased by ACTH. The molecular weight of this band is similar to that (54 K) reported for the regulatory subunit of the cAMP-dependent protein kinase II ($R_{II}$). This subunit is phosphorylated (Weller, 1979) by the catalytic subunit both in the holoenzyme state and in the free state. cAMP does not stimulate the auto-phosphorylation of the holoenzyme but may stimulate a catalytic phosphorylation of free $R_{II}$ (Rangal-Aldao and Rosen, 1976). This action of the catalytic subunit on $R_{II}$ may have different characteristics from that on other protein substrates. This could explain why ACTH affects the phosphorylation of $R_{II}$ but not other cAMP-dependent protein bands. A parallel may be drawn with the effects of ACTH on the auto-phosphorylation of the protein B-50 kinase complex in membranes (Zwiers et al., this volume).

The link between effects on protein phosphorylation and protein synthesis may, however, involve cAMP. We cannot exclude the possibility that a modulation of adenylate cyclase activity results from the observed changes in phosphoprotein turnover. In this respect it is interesting to note the recent observations by Wiegant et al. (this volume), that the actions of ACTH on brain membrane protein phosphorylation involve protein kinases, probably via $Ca^{2+}$- and GTP-sensitive mechanisms. Similar mechanisms are involved in the effect of ACTH on adrenal cortical cells, where adenylate cyclase is stimulated (Saez et al., 1981).

## 5. PEPTIDE STRUCTURES REQUIRED FOR PHOSPHOPROTEIN REGULATION. COMPARISON WITH PROTEIN SYNTHESIS

Structure–activity studies demonstrated that most of the effects of $ACTH_{1-24}$ on phosphorylation could also be elicited by the sequence $ACTH_{11-24}$. This suggested that the phosphoprotein effects were more likely to be related to the actions of ACTH on peptide chain elongation (Fig. 1B) than to effects on initiation (Fig. 1A). Only one protein band (24 K) was sensitive to $ACTH_{1-24}$, but not to $ACTH_{11-24}$, and this protein was insensitive to the peptide-chain initiation stimulator, $ACTH_{1-10}$. Caution must be exercised in making correlations between the phosphorylation and protein synthesis data, since the time scales of the experiments are very different (15 sec incubations in the former studies and 10–60 min incubations in the latter). In reticulocyte systems, initiation of new peptide chains decays very rapidly during incubation without hemin (Jagus et al., 1981). Inactivation of the initiation processes can be prevented in systems derived from reticulocytes and other cells (Ochoa and de Haro, 1979) by addition of hemin. We have been unable to preserve initiation of peptide chain formation in our brain-derived preparation but we cannot exclude the possibility that initiation was occurring during the first 15 sec of incubation, the period corresponding to the phosphorylation period. Therefore, the possible role of proteins phosphorylated in our preparation in peptide-chain initiation can only be tentatively surmised from the known role of similar proteins in other systems. Irrespective of possible undetected effects of ACTH on initiation, peptide chain elongation was clearly inhibited by $ACTH_{11-24}$ and this effect may be related to some of the observed rapid effects of this peptide on protein phosphorylation. Our data on the peptide- and $Mg^{2+}$-concentration dependency of the two systems tend to support this view.

## 6. MAGNESIUM DEPENDENCY

Both protein synthesis and phosphorylation were highly sensitive to the Mg concentration in the absence of ACTH (Fig. 8, +GTP). The effects of magnesium on protein phosphorylation cannot be related to formation of Mg–ATP or Mg–GTP, the preferred substrates of protein kinases (Weller, 1979), since the magnesium concentrations studied are an order of magnitude higher than those required to saturate the nucleotides. The biphasic relationship between magnesium concentration and protein synthesis was not matched in the phosphorylation of any single protein, suggesting that a simple correlation does not exist. The same is true for the effect of ACTH on magnesium dependency. The presence of ACTH ($10^{-4}$ M) dramatically altered the sensitivity of protein synthesis to magnesium and vice versa. The effect of ACTH was greatest at the magnesium concentration that also gave the highest basal activity. The frequency of coincidence of these two maxima has already been commented on above (section 4.3). Magnesium also markedly altered the effect of ACTH on protein phosphorylation. Fig. 8 (+GTP) shows the relationship between magnesium concentration and phospholabelling in

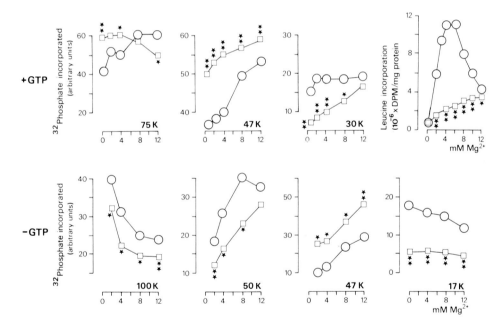

Fig. 8. Magnesium dependency of protein synthesis and phosphorylation of selected proteins. The phosphorylation at 100 mM $K^+$ of six phosphoprotein bands sensitive to $ACTH_{11-24}$ is compared to the $Mg^{2+}$ dependency of leucine incorporation (see Fig. 2) between 0.75 and 12 mM magnesium and the effect of $ACTH_{11-24}$ on both parameters is shown. The selection of the phosphoprotein bands was made according to their sensitivity to $ACTH_{11-24}$ at 4 mM $Mg^{2+}$ and 100 mM $K^+$ (optimum for protein synthesis), in the presence (+GTP) or absence (−GTP) of GTP ($10^{-4}$ M) in the incubation mixture. Incubations were performed as described for Figs. 3 and 5, in the absence (o) or presence (□) of $ACTH_{11-24}$ ($10^{-4}$ M). *$2P < 0.05$; **$2P < 0.01$, Student's $t$ test ($n = 3$). Taken from Schrama et al., 1982.

the three protein bands that showed the greatest modulation of ACTH effects by the cation.

Increasing $Mg^{2+}$ concentration reduced (47 K, 30 K) or even inverted (75 K) the effect of ACTH on protein phosphorylation. Once again, the absence of directly comparable effects on a single protein band and on protein synthesis proscribe any simple correlations. In view of the marked effect of GTP on protein phosphorylation and sensitivity to ACTH, we also checked $Mg^{2+}$ dependency of these parameters in the absence of GTP. With the exception of the 47 K protein band, which behaved similarly under the two conditions, different phosphoproteins were sensitive to ACTH in the absence of GTP, as has already been discussed (section 4.3). Four protein bands, 100, 50, 47 and 17 K (the same protein bands as were sensitive to ACTH when $[\gamma-^{32}P]GTP$ was the precursor; Fig. 7) were sensitive to ACTH and these bands differed from each other in their response to changing magnesium concentration. Unlike the situation in the presence of GTP, magnesium had no marked effects on the sensitivity to ACTH. The complexity of the effects of magnesium on $^{32}P$ labelling of phosphoproteins may result from a combination of effects on various kinases and/or phosphatases, but could also result from modulation of a single enzyme. For instance a protease-activated kinase (also known as kinase C and calcium/lipid-dependent protein kinase), which is very active in brain (Takai et al., 1977) shows different magnesium optima for different exogenous substrates (Takai et al., 1977). Phosphatase enzymes may also be involved, since, as was discussed in section 4.2, modulation of a single enzyme may result in diverse effects in different substrates. Two magnesium-sensitive phosphatases have been described in the literature: the myosin light chain phosphatase (Adelstein et al., 1981) and the pyruvate dehydrogenase phosphatase (England, 1980). We cannot currently distinguish between phosphatase and kinase effects in our system.

## 7. CONCENTRATION OF ACTH

If the effects of ACTH on protein synthesis and phosphorylation are related, one would predict similar concentration–effect relationships. We chose for our phosphorylation studies to use conditions (4mM $Mg^{2+}$, $10^{-4}$ M GTP), which gave the maximal sensitivity to $ACTH_{11-24}$ in the protein synthesis assay (Fig. 2). The effect of peptide concentration on protein synthesis and protein phosphorylation are shown in Fig. 9. Three protein bands (75 K, 47 K and 30 K) showed changes in $^{32}P$ labelling related to ACTH concentration.

Phospholabelling of the 75 K band was stimulated by ACTH, but only at low ($< 10^{-6}$ M) concentrations of the peptide. High concentrations ($> 10^{-5}$ M) of ACTH were required to cause the observed decrease in labelling of the 30 K band. The most interesting pattern was that of the 47 K protein band, which was less phosphorylated at low ACTH concentrations ($10^{-10}$–$10^{-8}$ M) and more phosphorylated at high concentrations ($> 10^{-5}$ M). This is not unlike the biphasic change in protein synthesis, which is stimulated at $10^{-8}$ M and inhibited at $> 10^{-7}$ M.

## 8. SENSITIVITY TO HEMIN

Hemin is a regulator of protein synthesis which shows a biphasic action on a cell-free system from reticulocytes (Hunt, 1980). Its mode of action is believed to be via prevention of the activation of a kinase enzyme, the hemin-controlled repressor (HCR), that in turn phosphorylates and inactivates the eIF-$2\alpha$ initiation factor (see review by Traugh, 1980). In view of this

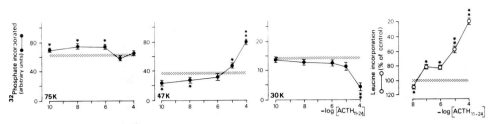
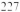

Fig. 9. Concentration dependency of the effects of $ACTH_{11-24}$ on protein synthesis and phosphorylation. The effects of $ACTH_{11-24}$ on the phosphorylation of 3 phosphobands in the presence of 4 mM $Mg^{2+}$, 100 mM $K^+$ and $10^{-4}$ M GTP (see Fig. 8) are compared to the effects of $ACTH_{11-24}$ on leucine incoporation under these conditions. Incubations were performed as described for Figs. 3 and 5, in the presence of varying concentrations of $ACTH_{11-24}$. The shaded bars represent the means ± S.E.M. of values obtained in the absence of ACTH. *$2P < 0.05$; **$2P < 0.01$, Student's $t$ test ($n = 3$). Taken from Schrama et al., 1982.

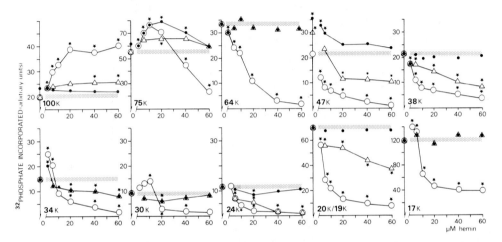

Fig. 10. Sensitivity to hemin of the phosphorylation of ten phosphoprotein bands at 4 mM $Mg^{2+}$, 100 mM $K^+$ and $10^{-4}$ M GTP (o) and the effects of the presence of $ACTH_{11-24}$ at $10^{-4}$ M (●) or at $10^{-5}$ M (△). The hemin concentrations were 0, 2, 5, 10, 20, 40 and 60 $\mu$M. The methods were as described in Figs. 3 and 5. *$2P < 0.05$, Student's $t$ test ($n = 3$), significantly different from controls, without hemin (shaded bars).

link between protein phosphorylation and protein synthesis, we studied the effects of hemin in our system. As is shown in Fig. 10, low concentrations of hemin affected the phosphorylation of a large number of protein bands. The direction and concentration dependence of the changes were different for individual proteins. $ACTH_{11-24}$ had very large effects on protein phosphorylation in the presence of hemin in all the protein bands. The effect of hemin was reduced or totally abolished even in protein bands (64 K, 38 K, 34 K, 30 K, 24 K, 20 K, 17 K) where ACTH had no effect on phosphorylation in the absence of hemin under the incubation conditions used. Nevertheless, all these phosphoprotein bands have been mentioned as being sensitive to ACTH, either at low GTP ($< 10^{-6}$ M) and high $Mg^{2+}$ (Fig. 5) or with [$\gamma$-$^{32}$P]GTP as precursor (Fig. 7). The effect of ACTH varied to different extents with the hemin concentration indicating that it was not due to a direct interaction between the two agents. Furthermore, the effect of ACTH is often most marked at the highest hemin concentrations, which argues against competition at a single site.

The parallel shift in the hemin concentration curve of the phosphorylation of the 47 K band caused by the presence of ACTH suggests a non-competitive interaction between hemin and ACTH. Close correlation between the two agents is also suggested by the fact that in the case of four protein bands (75, 34, 30 and 17 K) hemin had a biphasic action and ACTH inhibited both the stimulatory and inhibitory phases. The effect of ACTH was concentration-dependent. With one exception (30 K) all the bands sensitive to hemin are also sensitive to GTP. We cannot unequivocally identify the hemin-controlled repressor (MW 100 K or 77 K, pI 6.0) or its substrate, eIF-2$\alpha$ (MW 34 K, pI 5.0), which would show a decrease in phosphorylation in the presence of hemin (Traugh, 1980; Hunt, 1980). From the evidence of (i) molecular weight, (ii) increased phospholabelling by hemin under conditions where protein synthesis is inhibited and (iii) sensitivity to GTP (data for GTP effect not shown), our protein bands 75 K and 100 K are possible candidates for HCR and our protein bands at 38 K and 34 K for e IF-2$\alpha$.

Although hemin is considered to act as a specific regulator of cell-free protein synthesis, a more general interaction with protein phosphorylation is indicated by the variety of kinase enzymes sensitive to hemin (Hirsch and Martelo, 1976; Traugh, 1980). However, most reports on the role of protein phosphorylation in the regulation of protein synthesis by hemin have only considered the inhibitory effects of hemin on the phosphorylation of the hemin-controlled repressor and its substrate, eIF-2$\alpha$ (Traugh, 1980). The relatively non-specific inhibition of protein phosphorylation by hemin which we, and others, have shown, suggests that a more stringent criterion is required to indicate a connection between the two systems. The biphasic effect of hemin on the phosphorylation of a small number of protein bands (Fig. 10) may be a phenomenon related to regulation of protein synthesis since a similar biphasic effect of hemin on protein synthesis has been reported (Tahara et al., 1978).

## 9. PHOSPHOPROTEINS SENSITIVE TO ACTH

We are unable, as yet, to identify unequivocally any of the phosphoproteins that are regulated by ACTH. Although a great deal of work has been done on the characterisation of soluble protein kinases acting on exogenous substrates (Weller, 1979), much less is known of their endogenous substrates. In brain membrane preparations, several phosphoprotein bands have been reported to be sensitive to ACTH-like peptides; two proteins (50 and 52 K) are sensitive to enkephalin (Bär et al., 1980); protein B-50 (48 K, pI 4.5) to ACTH$_{1-24}$ (Zwiers et al., 1976) and two proteins (17 and 20 K) to ACTH$_{1-24}$ (Zwiers et al., 1976, 1978) and endorphins (Ehrlich et al., 1980). Behavioural treatments that may be related to peptide effects have also been shown to alter the extent of phosphorylation of the $\alpha$-subunit of pyruvate dehydrogenase (MW 41 K) (Morgan and Routtenberg, 1980; Ehrlich et al., 1980). Only the B-50 protein is an exclusively membrane protein; pyruvate dehydrogenase is a mitochondrial protein. In the adrenal cortex, ACTH increases the phosphorylation of a 16 K protein and a 150 K cytosolic protein (Podesta et al., 1979). As discussed in section 2, our post-mitochondrial supernate contains membrane fragments, so we might expect to detect the ACTH-sensitive proteins previously described in membrane fragments. Changes in phospholabelling of proteins in the appropriate molecular weight ranges (our proteins 17 K, 20 K, 40 K, 47 K and 50 K) are observed in the post-mitochondrial supernate, but we have no firmer evidence for the identity of these proteins.

## 10. RELATIONSHIP BETWEEN PHOSPHOPROTEINS AND PROTEIN SYNTHESIS

Many of the proteins in the protein synthetic system are phosphoproteins but, with the possible exceptions of the hemin-controlled repressor (HCR) and eIF-2$\alpha$, the relationship between phosphoproteins and protein synthesis rate is far from clear. cAMP, insulin and many other factors can modulate both protein phosphorylation and protein synthesis but the connection between these two effects has not been unequivocally established (Safer and Anderson, 1978; Leader, 1980; Hunt, 1980; Traugh, 1980). The phosphoproteins that have molecular weights comparable to the ACTH-sensitive bands in our system are included in Table I. Most of the studies on the role of phosphoproteins in protein synthesis have focussed on peptide chain initiation (Ochoa and de Haro, 1979; Hunt, 1980; Traugh, 1980; Jagus et al., 1981).

Correlations between effects on elongation (such as we see with ACTH$_{11-24}$, Fig. 1B) and phosphorylation have been reported for the S6 ribosomal protein and tRNA synthetases (Leader, 1980; Traugh, 1980; Cohen, 1980). The extent of phosphorylation of the proteins involved in protein synthesis is regulated by protein kinases and phosphoprotein phosphatases. Several of these enzymes are also present in ribosomal fractions (Traugh, 1980). Modulation of both enzyme systems is known to occur (Traugh, 1980; Grankowski et al., 1980). The possible importance of these and other enzymes in the observed effects of ACTH on phosphoprotein labelling is discussed below.

## 11. ENZYMES

The ACTH-induced changes in the incorporation of labelled phosphate into phosphoproteins could be the result of an interaction with three types of enzyme systems: protein kinases, phosphoprotein phosphatases and enzymes involved in the availability of the nucleotide triphosphate precursor (ATPases, GTPases and nucleotide diphosphokinase).

### 11.1. *Protein kinases*

The effect of ACTH cannot be related to a simple effect on any single kinase enzyme, since such an action could not explain its divergent effects on different protein substrates. One would have to propose a combination of effects, which may indeed be the case. Many kinases, both dependent and independent of cyclic nucleotides, can phosphorylate proteins in the protein synthetic apparatus (Leader, 1980; Hunt, 1980; Ochoa and de Haro, 1979; Traugh, 1980). These enzymes are indicated in Table I alongside their reported protein substrates. It is clear that ACTH-induced changes in phospholabelling in our system are not mediated by cyclic nucleotides. However, an effect on the cAMP-dependent protein kinase cannot be excluded since, as was discussed in section 4.5, an interaction with the auto-phosphorylation of kinase II is suggested from the characteristics of our phosphoprotein band 50 K. Moreover, several proteins may be phosphorylated by both cAMP-dependent and -independent enzymes. The relative affinities of cAMP-independent casein kinases I and II for ATP and GTP differ (Weller, 1979; Traugh, 1980). This undoubtedly has some influence on the spectrum of protein phosphorylated under the different conditions ([$\gamma$-$^{32}$P]ATP, [$\gamma$-$^{32}$P]-ATP + GTP, [$\gamma$-$^{32}$P]GTP and [$\gamma$-$^{32}$P]GTP + ATP) we have studied. However, no simple explanation of the effect of altering the triphosphonucleotide in the medium nor the effects of ACTH can be put forward on this basis. It is tempting to propose that the protease-activated kinase II, probably

TABLE I

| Phosphoprotein bands of post-mitochondrial supernate | | | | | | | Phosphoproteins from literature | | |
|---|---|---|---|---|---|---|---|---|---|
| MW/pI | ACTH (11–24)[a] | cAMP cGMP[b] | Phosphate donor[c] | GTP[d] (10⁻⁴ M) | Hemine[e] | MW/pI | Phospho-proteins[f] | | Protein kinases (phosphate donor)[g] |
| 130 | − | o | + | ? | o | 150 | eIF-5, GTP-ase | | CKII (GTP/ATP) |
|  |  |  |  |  |  | 130 | eIF-3 | | CKII (GTP/ATP) |
| 100 | − | o | + | ? | + | 96/5.6 | HCR | | HCR (ATP) |
| 96 | o | ? | + | o | o |  |  |  |  |
| 94 | o | ? | + | o | o |  |  |  |  |
| 78 | o | + | + | ? | o |  |  |  |  |
| 75/4.2 | +/−[i] | o | − | + | +/−[h] | 80 | HCR | | HCR (ATP) |
|  |  |  |  |  |  | 80 | eIF-4B, CAPbinding kinase C | | CKI (ATP) |
|  |  |  |  |  |  | 75/5.6 |  | | C (ATP) |
| 73/5.8–7.0 | o | + | o | o | o | 69 | eIF-3 | | CKII (GTP/ATP) |
| 67 | − | o | o | + | o | 67 | DAI | | DAI (ATP) |
| 64 | − | o | o | + | − | 64 |  | |  |
| 58/5.8–6.8 | o | + | + | − | o |  |  |  |  |
| 4.8–5.1 |  |  |  |  |  |  |  |  |  |
| 54/5.7 | o | + | o | o | o | 54 | RII | | CII (ATP) |
| 51 | o | + | o | o | o |  |  |  |  |
| 50/4.7 | − | + | − | + | o | 50/5.4 | eIF-2β | | CKII (GTP/ATP) |
| 47/4.8 | +/−[h,i] | o | o | + | − |  |  | | PAKII (ATP), C (ATP) |
| 40 | − | o | − | − | o | 48 | B-50 | | C (ATP) |
| 38 | − | o | o | − | − | 38 | eIF-2α | | HCR (ATP), DAI (ATP) |
|  |  |  |  |  |  | 37 | CKI | | CKI (ATP), |
| 36 | − | o | + | o | o | 35 | eIF-3 | | CKII (GTP/ATP) |
| 34 | − | o | + | − | +/−[h] | 34 | S₆ | | A (ATP), G (GTP), CKII (GTP/ATP), PAKII (ATP) |

| | | | | | | | |
|---|---|---|---|---|---|---|---|
| 30 | − | o | − | | | +/−[h] | |
| 28 | − | o | + | | | o | |
| 24 | − | o | + | − | 24 | − | inhibitor A | CKII (GTP/ATP) |
| 24 | − | o | − | | 24 | − | CKII | CKII (GTP/ATP) |
| 20 | o | o | o | − | | | | |
| 19 | − | o | + | − | 17 | +/−[h] | S$_{10}$ | PKI (ATP) |
| 17 | − | o | + | | 14–30/4.5 | | L12, GTP-ase | AI (ATP), PAKI (ATP) |
| | | | | | | | L12 | |

[a] This includes any ACTH effect, independent of the experimental conditions (Figs. 6, 7, 8, 9).

[b] Data from Fig. 4.

[c] The phosphorylation with $[\gamma\text{-}^{32}P]$GTP is compared to that with $[\gamma\text{-}^{32}P]$ATP and $10^{-4}$ M GTP (Fig. 7).

[d] The phosphorylation with $[\gamma\text{-}^{32}P]$ATP and $10^{-4}$ M GTP present is compared to that in the absence of GTP (Fig. 5).

[e] The influence of hemin over a range of concentrations with $[\gamma\text{-}^{32}P]$ATP (Fig. 10).

[f] eIF indicates eukaryotic initiation factor, RII the regulatory subunit of cAMP-dependent protein kinase II. B-50 (see Aloyo et al., this volume); S$_6$, S$_{10}$ proteins of the 40S ribosomal subunit; L12, L12′ proteins of the 60S ribosomal subunit.

[g] A, cAMP-dependent protein kinase; G, cGMP-dependent protein kinase; CKI, casein kinase I; CKII, casein kinase II; PAKI, protease-activated kinase I; PAKII, protease-activated kinase II; C, lipid-activated kinase C; HCR, hemin-controlled regulator; DAI, double-stranded RNA-activated inhibitor.

[h] Biphasic response dependent on the concentration.

[i] An increase or decrease dependent on the experimental condition. +, increase; −, decrease; o, no effect.

the same as kinase C (Takai et al., 1979; Traugh, 1980), may be involved in some of the effects of ACTH in view of the suggestion that it is identical to the ACTH-sensitive B-50 kinase enzyme (Aloyo et al., this volume) and the complex effects of magnesium on both this enzyme and ACTH effects in our system (see section 6).

## 11.2. *Phosphoprotein phosphatases*

Phosphoprotein phosphatases have been less extensively investigated than protein kinase enzymes but there is some evidence that they may play an important role in the phosphorylation of proteins involved in the protein synthetic apparatus. All the phosphoproteins shown in Table I are substrates for phosphoprotein phosphatases. Aminoacyl tRNA synthetases are also phosphoproteins and their enzyme activity differs with degree of phosphorylation (Traugh, 1980). Regulation of protein synthesis by an effect on peptide chain elongation rate has been reported to correlate with effects on aminoacyl tRNA synthetase phosphatases. Mediation by phosphoprotein phosphatases of hormonal effects on protein phosphorylation has also been suggested for the effect of insulin on pyruvate dehydrogenase (Kiechle et al., 1981). In addition to several specific phosphatases that have been described, there is a phosphoprotein phosphatase with broad substrate specificity. The activity of this phosphatase is regulated by an inhibitory subunit of the enzyme itself, by unidentified heat-stable inhibitory factors (such as has been found in muscle) and by various low molecular weight factors including ATP and GTP. The rate of dephosphorylation of individual proteins is also regulated independently of effects on the absolute activity of the enzyme itself (so-called substrate-directed regulation; England, 1980). The possibility of seeing different effects on different proteins is further increased because we measured phosphoprotein labelling not net phosphorylation of proteins in our system (section 4.2).

The effect of insulin on pyruvate dehydrogenase phosphatase depends on the release of a small molecular weight mediator, indicating an additional step in the mechanism of action of the hormone (Kiechle et al., 1981). A small molecular weight component, known as the phosphorylation inhibiting peptide, is also implicated in the regulation of the phosphorylation of protein B-50 by ACTH (Zwiers et al., 1980).

## 11.3. *Enzymes involved in trinucleotide metabolism*

The post-mitochondrial supernate is predicted to contain many enzymes that can hydrolyse added trinucleotides and the nucleotide diphosphate kinase that catalyses the transfer of the $\gamma$-phosphate group of ATP to other diphosphonucleotides (Weller, 1979). The combined activity of these enzymes can alter the relative concentrations and specific activities of $[\gamma\text{-}^{32}P]ATP$ and $[\gamma\text{-}^{32}P]\text{-}GTP$ present in the incubation mixture.

The protein kinases have different relative affinities for the two nucleotides so a shift in the contribution of various kinases to the phosphorylation observed would be predicted to result from changes in ATP and GTP. It is difficult to predict precisely how changes in the nucleotides would alter the spectrum of proteins labelled. However, an effect of ACTH on the enzymes of trinucleotide metabolism would be expected to produce a complex pattern of changes that show certain of the characteristics we have observed (dependence on GTP concentration and on the labelled precursor used). As has been mentioned in section 11.2, changes in trinucleotide levels can modulate the activity of certain phosphoprotein phosphatases.

In this chapter, we have shown the abundancy of possible regulatory mechanisms whereby ACTH-like peptides may modulate protein synthesis via phosphorylation. The extent to which observed influences of these peptides on phosphorylation are related to the known effects on protein synthesis remains to be demonstrated. In this respect, this uncertainty reflects a more general lack of knowledge about the role of phosphorylation in the regulation of protein synthesis. Other approaches, such as in vivo/in vitro studies may be required to help solve the problem. Studies directed at specific enzyme systems may also be helpful, although the information on endogenous protein substrates is, currently, limited.

## 12. SUMMARY

ACTH peptides affect protein synthesis by actions on initiation and elongation of peptide chains. They also have complex effects on protein phosphorylation. We have attempted to elucidate the relationship between these two effects by (i) using the same cell-free system for studying both processes, (ii) investigating the effects of agents (magnesium, phosphonucleotides and hemin) that alter both processes, (iii) comparing the peptide structure and concentration required for modulation of both processes, and (iv) by comparison of the observed effects of ACTH peptides on phosphorylation with known or proposed factors in protein synthesis regulation. We have also considered the possible mechanisms involved in the observed changes in phosphoprotein labelling.

## ACKNOWLEDGEMENTS

We gratefully acknowledge valuable discussions with Professor H.O. Voorma and Drs. R. Benne and H. Zwiers and the technical assistance of Lia Claessens and Ed Kluis. Part of the data have been collected by Dr. A.M.A. Van Dijk. Electron microscopy was performed by Thea Horsten, Department of Molecular Cell Biology, Ultrastructural Research Unit.

This research was supported by grant 13-31-43 from the Netherlands Organization for the Advancement of Pure Research.

## REFERENCES

Adelstein, R.S., Pato, M.D. and Conti, M.A. (1981) The role of phosphorylation in regulating contractile proteins. *Adv. cycl. Nucl. Res.*, 14: 361–373.

Ashby, C.D. and Roberts, S. (1975) Phosphorylation of ribosomal proteins in rat cerebral cortex in vitro. *J. biol. Chem.*, 250: 2546–2555.

Bär, P.R., Schotman, P. and Gispen, W.H. (1980) Enkephalins affect hippocampal membrane phosphorylation. *Eur. J. Pharmacol.*, 65: 165–174.

Boyd, G.S. and Gorban, A.M.S. (1980) Protein phosphorylation and steroidogenesis. In *Recently Discovered Systems of Enzyme Regulation by Reversible Phosphorylation*, P. Cohen (Ed.), Elsevier/North-Holland Biomedical Press, Amsterdam, pp. 95–134.

Campagnoni, A.T. and Harris, J.R. (1977) In vitro protein synthesis on free polyribosomes isolated from the developing mouse brain. *J. Neurochem.*, 28: 589–596.

Cohen, P. (Ed.) (1980) *Recently Discovered Systems of Enzyme Regulation by Reversible Phosphorylation*, Elsevier/North-Holland Biomedical Press, Amsterdam.

De Wied, D. and Gispen, W.H. (1977) Behavioral effects of peptides. In *Peptides in Neurobiology*, H. Gainer (Ed.), Plenum Press, New York, pp. 397–448.

Dunn, A.J. and Schotman, P. (1981) Effects of ACTH and related peptides on cerebral RNA and protein synthesis. *Pharmacol. Ther.*, 12: 353–372.

Ehrlich, Y.H., Davis, L.G., Keen, P. and Brunngraber, E.G. (1980) Endorphin-regulated protein phosphorylation in brain membranes. *Life Sci.*, 26: 1765–1772.

England, P.J. (1980) Regulation by phosphorylation and dephosphorylation. In *The Enzymology of Posttranslational*

234

*Modification of Proteins,* Vol. 1, R.B. Freedman and H.C. Hawkins (Eds.), Academic Press, New York, pp. 292–344.

Ernst, V., Levin, D.H. and London, I.M. (1979) In situ phosphorylation of the $\alpha$-subunit of eukaryotic initiation factor 2 in reticulocyte lysates inhibited by heme deficiency, double stranded RNA, oxidized glutathione, or the heme regulated protein kinase. *Proc. nat. Acad. Sci. (Wash.),* 76: 2118–2122.

Gispen, W.H. and de Wied, D. (1980) ACTH as neuromodulator: Behavioral and neurochemical aspect. In *Neurochemistry and Clinical Neurology,* L. Battiolin, G. Haskin and A. Lajtha (Eds.), Alan R. Liss, New York, pp. 251–263.

Goldfine, I.D. (1978) Insulin receptors and the site of action of insulin. *Life Sci.,* 23: 2639–2648.

Grankowski, N., Lehmusvirta, D., Kramer, G. and Hardesty, B. (1980) Partial purification and characterization of reticulocyte phosphatase with activity for phosphorylated initiation factor 2. *J. biol. Chem.,* 255: 310–318.

Gross, M., Watt-Morse, P. and Kaplansky, D.A. (1981) Characterization of a rabbit reticulocyte supernatant factor that reverses the translational inhibition of heme deficiency. *Biochim. biophys. Acta,* 654: 219–226.

Hathaway, G.M. and Traugh, J.A. (1979) Cyclic nucleotide-independent protein kinases from rabbit reticulocytes: Purification of casein kinase. *J. biol. Chem.,* 254: 762–768.

Hirsch, J.D. and Martelo, O.J. (1976) Inhibition of rabbit reticulocyte protein kinase by hemin. *Biochem. biophys. Res. Commun.,* 71: 926–932.

Hunt, T. (1980) Phosphorylation and control of protein synthesis in reticulocytes. In *Recently Discovered Systems of Enzyme Regulation by Reversible Phosphorylation,* P. Cohen (Ed.), Elsevier/North-Holland Biomedical Press., Amsterdam, pp. 175–202.

Jagus, R., Anderson, W.F. and Safer, B. (1981) The regulation of initiation of mammalian protein synthesis. *Progr. nucl. Acid. Res. mol. Biol.,* 25: 127–185.

Jolles, J., Zwiers, H., van Dongen, C., Schotman, P., Wirtz, K.W.A. and Gispen, W.H. (1980) Modulation of brain polyphosphoinositide metabolism by ACTH-sensitive protein phosphorylation. *Nature (Lond.),* 286: 623–625.

Kiechle, F., Jaralt, L., Kotagal, N. and Popp, D.A. (1981) Partial purification from rat adipose plasma membranes of a chemical mediator which stimulates the action of insulin on pyruvate dehydrogenase. *J. biol. Chem.,* 256: 2945–2951.

Leader, D.P. (1980) The control of phosphorylation of ribosomal proteins. In *Recently Discovered Systems of Enzyme Regulation by Reversible Phosphorylation,* P. Cohen (Ed.), Elsevier/North-Holland Biomedical Press, Amsterdam, pp. 203–234.

Londos, C., Cooper, D.M.F. and Rodbell, M. (1981) Receptor-mediated stimulation and inhibition of adenylate cyclases: The fat cell as a model system. *Adv. cycl. Nucl. Res.,* 14: 163–171.

Michell, R.H. (1979) Inositol phospholipids in membrane function. *Trends biochem. Sci.,* 4: 128–131.

Miyamoto, E., Kuo, J.F. and Greengard, P. (1969) Cyclic nucleotide dependent protein kinases. *J. biol. Chem.,* 244: 6395–6402.

Morgan, D.G. and Routtenberg, A. (1980) Evidence that a 41,000 dalton brain phosphoprotein is pyruvate dehydrogenase. *Biochem. biophys. Res. Commun.,* 95: 559–576.

Nielsen, P.J. and McConkey, E.H. (1980) Evidence for control of protein synthesis in Hela cells, via the elongation rate. *Cell. Physiol.,* 104: 269–281.

Ochoa, S. and de Haro, C. (1979) Regulation of protein synthesis in eukaryotes. *Annu. Rev. Biochem.,* 48: 549–580.

Podesta, E.J., Milani, A., Steffen, H. and Neher, R. (1979) Adrenocorticotropin (ACTH) induced phosphorylation of a cytoplasmic protein in intact isolated adrenocortical cells. *Proc. nat. Acad. Sci. (Wash.),* 76: 5187–5191.

Rangal-Aldao, R. and Rosen, O.M. (1976) Mechanism of selfphosphorylation of adenosine 3',5'-monophosphate-dependent protein kinase from bovine cardiac muscle. *J. biol. Chem.,* 251: 7526–7529.

Roberts, S. and Morelos, B.S. (1979) Phosphorylation of multiple proteins of both ribosomal subunits in rat cerebral cortex in vivo. Effect ot adenosine 3',5'-cyclic monophosphate. *Biochem. J.,* 184: 233–244.

Roper, M.P. and Wicks, W.D. (1978) Evidence for the acceleration of the rate of elongation of tyrosine aminotransferase nascent chains by dibutyryl cyclic AMP. *Proc. nat. Acad. Sci. (Wash.),* 75: 140–144.

Saez, J.H., Morera, A.M. and Dazord, A. (1981) Mediation of the effects of ACTH on adrenal cells. *Adv. cycl. Nucl. Res.,* 14: 563–579.

Safer, B. and Anderson, W.F. (1978) The molecular mechanism of hemoglobin syntheis and its regulation in the reticulocyte. *CRC crit. Rev. Biochem.,* 5: 261–290.

Schotman, P. and Allaart, J. (1981) Biphasic modulation by ACTH-like peptides of protein synthesis in a cell-free system from rat brain. *J. Neurochem.,* 37: 1349–1352.

Schotman, P., Reith, M.E.A., van Wimersma Greidanus, Tj.B., Gispen, W.H. and de Wied, D. (1976) Hypothalamic and pituitary peptide hormones and the central nervous system: with special references to the neurochemical effects of ACTH. In *Molecular and Functional Neurobiology,* W.H. Gispen (Ed.), Elsevier, Amsterdam, pp. 309–344.

Schotman, P., Van Heuven-Nolsen, D. and Gispen, W.H. (1980) Protein synthesis in a cell-free system from rat brain sensitive to ACTH-like peptides. *J. Neurochem.*, 34: 1661–1670.

Schotman, P., Allaart, J. and Gispen, W.H. (1981) Pineal protein synthesis highly sensitive to ACTH-like neuropeptides. *Brain Res.*, 219: 121–135.

Schrama, L.H. and Schotman, P. (1981) Interaction of corticotropin (ACTH) 11–24 with $Mg^{2+}$ spermine sites involved in cell-free brain protein synthesis. *Abstr. 8th Meeting Int. Soc. Neurochem.*, p. 221.

Schwyzer, R. (1980) Organisation and transduction of peptide information. *Trends phys. Sci.*, 3, 327–331.

Sutherland, E.W. (1972) Studies on the mechanism of hormone action. *Science*, 177: 401–408.

Tahara, S.M., Traugh, J.A., Sharp, S.B., Lundak, T.S., Safer, B. and Merrick, W.C. (1978) Effect of hemin on site-specific phosphorylation of eukaryotic initiation factor 2. *Proc. nat. Acad. Sci. (Wash.)*, 75: 787–793.

Takai, Y., Kishimoto, A., Inoue, M. and Nishizuka, Y. (1977) Studies on a cyclic nucleotide-independent protein kinase and its proenzyme in mammalian tissues. *J. biol. Chem.*, 252: 7603–7609.

Takai, Y., Kishimoto, A., Iwasa, Y., Kawahara, Y., Mori, T. and Nishizuka, Y. (1979) Calcium-dependent activation of a multifunctional protein kinase by membrane phospholipids. *J. biol. Chem.*, 254: 3692–3695.

Tao, M., Salas, M.L. and Lipmann, F. (1970) Mechanism of activation by adenosine 3′,5′-cyclic monophosphate of a protein phosphokinase from rabbit reticulocytes. *Proc. nat. Acad. Sci. (Wash.)*, 67: 403–414.

Traugh, J.A. (1980) Regulation of protein synthesis. *Biochem. Action Horm.*, 8: 167–208.

Van Dijk, A.M.A., Benitez-King, G., Schotman, P. and Gispen, W.H. (1981) Phosphorylation of proteins in a post-mitochondrial supernatant from rat brain stem affected by $ACTH_{1-24}$ and cyclic nucleotides. *Neurochem. Res.*, 6: 847–860.

Ventimiglia, F.A. and Wool, I.G. (1974) A kinase that transfers the $\gamma$-phosphoryl group of GTP to proteins of eukaryotic 40S ribosomal subunits. *Proc. nat. Acad. Sci. (Wash.)*, 71: 350–351.

Weller, M. (1979) *Protein Phosphorylation. The nature, Function, and Metabolism of Proteins, which Contain Covalently Bound Phosphorus.* PION, London, pp. 1–557.

Wicks, W.D. (1974) Regulation of protein synthesis by cyclic AMP. *Adv. cycl. Nucl. Res.*, 4: 335–337.

Wiegant, V.M., Zwiers, H., Schotman, P. and Gispen, W.H. (1978) Endogenous phosphorylation of rat brain synaptosomal plasma membranes in vitro: Some methodological aspects. *Neurochem. Res.*, 3: 443–453.

Wiegant, V.M., Dunn, A.J., Schotman, P. and Gispen, W.H. (1979) ACTH-like neurotropic peptides: Possible regulation of rat brain cyclic AMP. *Brain Res.*, 168: 565–584.

Wiegant, V.M., Zwiers, H. and Gispen, W.H. (1981) Neuropeptides and brain cyclic AMP and phosphoproteins. *Pharmacol. Ther.*, 12: 463–490.

Zatz, M. (1978) Sensitivity and cyclic nucleotides in the rat pineal gland. *J. neural Transm.*, Suppl., 13: 175–201.

Zisapel, N., Levi, M. and Gozes, I. (1980) Tubulin, an integral protein of mammalian synaptic vesicles membrane. *J. Neurochem.*, 34: 26–32.

Zwiers, H., Veldhuis, D., Schotman, P. and Gispen, W.H. (1976) ACTH, cyclic nucleotides and brain protein phosphorylation in vitro. *Neurochem. Res.*, 1: 669–677.

Zwiers, H., Wiegant, V.M., Schotman, P. and Gispen, W.H. (1978) ACTH-induced initiation of endogenous rat brain protein phosphorylation in vitro: structure–activity. *Neurochem. Res.*, 3: 455–463.

Zwiers, H., Verhoef, J., Schotman, P. and Gispen, W.H. (1980) A new phosphorylation-inhibiting peptide (PIP) with behavioral activity from rat brain membranes. *FEBS Lett.*, 112: 168–172.

# Role of Calmodulin in Brain Function

WAI YIU CHEUNG

*Departments of Biochemistry, St. Jude Children's Research Hospital and
University of Tennessee Center for the Health Sciences,
Memphis, TN 38101, U.S.A.*

## INTRODUCTION

Brain is a complex organ. Its main function, the processing and storage of information, requires rapid integration of incoming and outgoing signals. The transmission of these signals depends on the generation of action potential and the release of transmitters — both intimately involving $Ca^{2+}$. The importance of $Ca^{2+}$ in cellular functions has been appreciated for more than three decades, but its mode of action at the molecular level is only beginning to be unraveled as a result of research on calcium-binding proteins, calmodulin in particular.

This chapter reviews the salient features of calmodulin and some of the recent findings on its role in cellular processes of the brain. Only selected references are cited; a more comprehensive list is available in other reviews (Cheung, 1980a,b; Klee et al., 1980; Means and Dedman, 1980; Brostrom and Wolff, 1981).

## GENERAL PROPERTIES OF CALMODULIN

Originally discovered as an activator of cyclic nucleotide phosphodiesterase (Cheung, 1981), calmodulin is a $Ca^{2+}$-modulated protein found in all eukaryotes that have been examined. Its functional status as a protein is unique: it has no intrinsic enzyme activities, but has the ability to regulate the activity of many enzymes. Table I lists the enzymes that clearly depend on calmodulin for activity. Increasing evidence now indicates that calmodulin serves as a major, if not the principal, mediator of $Ca^{2+}$ actions.

Calmodulin is a single polypeptide with 148 amino acids (see Fig. 1) and a molecular weight of 16 700. Some 30 % of its amino acids consist of aspartate or glutamate, which accounts for the low isoelectric point (4.3). It contains no cysteine, hydroxyproline or tryptophan, but does contain a trimethylated lysine at position 115. Calmodulin isolated from certain sources contains no trimethylated lysine and appears to be equally active, at least in activating bovine brain phosphodiesterase. The lack of cysteine and hydroxyproline would allow calmodulin to have a flexible tertiary structure, a desirable feature for a multifunctional protein that interacts with many different receptor proteins (Cheung, 1980a). The high ratio of phenylalanine (eight residues) to tyrosine (two residues) in calmodulin results in an unusual ultraviolet absorption spectrum with five peaks — at 253, 259, 265, 269 and 272 nm and a shoulder at 282 nm.

One striking characteristic of calmodulin is its tendency to retain biologic activity after exposure to heat (99° C), urea (8 M), acidic pH and detergents. Another is its lack of both tissue

## TABLE I

### CALMODULIN-REGULATED ENZYMES

| Enzyme | Reference |
| --- | --- |
| Cyclic nucleotide phosphodiesterase | Cheung, 1980a,b |
| Adenylate cyclase | Brostrom et al., 1975; Cheung et al., 1975a |
| Guanylate cyclase | Nagao et al., 1979 |
| $Ca^{2+}$-ATPase | Gopinath and Vincenzi, 1977; Jarrett and Penniston, 1977 |
| Myosin light chain kinase | Dabrowska and Hartshorne, 1978; Yagi et al., 1978 |
| Phosphorylase $b$ kinase | Cohen et al., 1978 |
| Glycogen synthetase kinase | Payne and Soderling, 1980 |
| $Ca^{2+}$-dependent protein kinase | Schulman and Greengard, 1978 |
| NAD kinase | Anderson and Cormier, 1978 |

The table lists enzymes with activities that are clearly dependent on calmodulin. Although $Ca^{2+}$-dependent protein kinase(s) has been reported in numerous tissues, the enzyme has not been characterized vigourously.

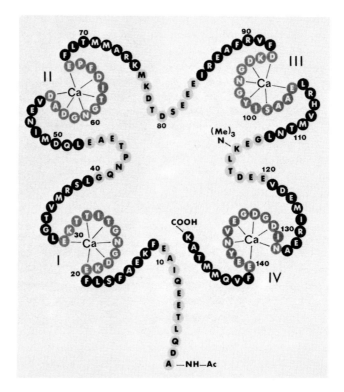

Fig. 1. Amino acid sequence of bovine brain calmodulin as determined by Watterson et al. (1980). The scheme depicts the four putative $Ca^{2+}$-binding domains consisting of a twelve-residue loop (gray circles) flanked on each side by an eight-residue helix (dark circles) based on the E-F hand model of Kretsinger and Barry (1975). The predicted $Ca^{2+}$-binding residues are indicated by the solid lines in each loop. The amino acids are designed by the one-letter abbreviations: A, alanine; D, aspartic acid; E, glutamic acid; F, phenylalanine; G, glycine; H, histidine; I, isoleucine; K, lysine; L, leucine; M, methionine; N, asparagine; P, proline; Q, glutamine; R, arginine; S, serine; T, threonine; V, valine; Y, tyrosine.

and species specificity. A third is that calmodulin from a variety of sources possesses many similar physicochemical properties. In fact, calmodulin isolated from several mammalian tissues have identical tryptic peptide maps and essentially identical amino acid sequences. More than 70 % of the amino acid sequence in calmodulin appear homologous with that of troponin $c$, even though the two proteins are functionally distinct. Bovine brain calmodulin can be substituted effectively for troponin $c$ in the activation of muscle actomyosin ATPase (Amphlett et al., 1976); whereas attempts to substitute troponin $c$ for calmodulin have invariably failed. From the crystal structure of parvalbumin and the similarity of its amino acid sequence to that of troponin $c$, Kretsinger and Barry (1975) predicted the three-dimensional structure of rabbit skeletal muscle troponin $c$ and identified the putative $Ca^{2+}$-binding residues in each domain. The corresponding residues in calmodulin are indicated in Fig. 1, which emphasizes the four $Ca^{2+}$-binding domains. Each domain comprises a 12-residue $Ca^{2+}$-binding loop, flanked on each side by an 8-residue helix. The four domains appear homologous; hence the protein may have evolved through repeated duplication of a gene coding for a peptide consisting of one $Ca^{2+}$-binding domain. The affinities of $Ca^{2+}$-binding have not been agreed upon, but most investigators distinguish two classes of binding sites, one with a $K_d$ of approximately $10^{-6}$ M and another of approximately $10^{-5}$ M. $Mn^{2+}$ substitutes for $Ca^{2+}$, with a $K_d$ of approximately $10^{-5}$ M. $Mg^{2+}$ binds to calmodulin, but the resulting complex is not biologically active. $Tb^{3+}$ also substitutes effectively for $Ca^{2+}$ in many situations, including the activation of phosphodiesterase (Tallant et al., 1980).

Attempts have been made to clarify the structure–function relationships of calmodulin. Modification of the single histidine or both tyrosines did not affect the protein's biological activity, whereas derivatization of methionine, lysine, arginine or carboxy groups impaired its activity to various extents. When controlled tryptic digestion was used to yield peptides of different sizes, peptide 1 (residues 1 through 77) and peptide 2 (residues 78 through 148) showed no biologic activity, although peptide 2 retained the ability to undergo conformational change and to form a complex with troponin I in the presence of $Ca^{2+}$. Peptide 3 (residues 1 through 106) was 1/200th as active as the native protein, but removal of a 16-residue fragment (residue 91 through 106) abolished the remaining activity (Walsh et al., 1977). These results suggest that the biologic activity of calmodulin depends heavily on the integrity of the entire molecule. Conceivably, the role of calmodulin in cellular function is of such basic importance that a mutation resulting in a gross change of the primary structure of the molecule would be lethal to the cell.

TABLE II

PHYSICAL AND CHEMICAL PROPERTIES OF BOVINE BRAIN CALMODULIN

| Determination | Value |
|---|---|
| $M_r$ (molecular weight) | 16 700 |
| $f : f_0$ (frictional ratio) | 1.20 |
| pI (isoelectric point) | 4.3 |
| $K_d$ ($Ca^{2+}$ binding) | $3.5 \times 10^{-6}$–$1.8 \times 10^{-5}$ M |
| $S_{20,w}$ (sedimentation coefficient) | 1.85 S |
| $\bar{v}$ (partial specific value) | 0.72 cm$^3$/g |
| $D$ (diffusion coefficient) | $1.09 \times 10^{-6}$ cm$^2$/S |
| Stokes radius | 20.9 Å |
| $E_{276}^{1\%}$ | 1.8 |
| Amino acids | 148 |

Calmodulin undergoes a conformational change upon binding $Ca^{2+}$, and exposes a hydrophobic domain that may serve as an interface for its receptor proteins (LaPorte et al., 1980). Trifluoperazine, an antipsychotic drug, binds calmodulin with a $K_d$ of $10^{-6}$ M, presumably to the hydrophobic domain, and suppresses its activity by blocking the formation of a calmodulin-receptor complex. The inhibition is reversed when the drug is removed. The high affinity of calmodulin for trifluoperazine has been cleverly exploited to devise a specific affinity column (Charbonneau and Cormier, 1979; Jamieson and Vanaman, 1979) for isolating the protein from various tissues.

Calmodulin has been extensively characterized, and some of its physicochemical properties are summarized in Table II.

## MECHANISM OF CALMODULIN ACTION

The mechanism by which calmodulin activates an enzyme has been studied most extensively with phosphodiesterase (for review, see Cheung, 1980a; Klee et al., 1980). As depicted in the equations below, neither $Ca^{2+}$ nor calmodulin (CaM) alone is active.

$$4\ Ca^{2+} + CaM_{(inactive)} \qquad CaM^* \cdot Ca^{2+}_{4\ (active)} \qquad (1)$$

$$E_{(less\ active)} + CaM^* + Ca^{2+}_4 \qquad E^* \cdot CaM^* \cdot Ca^{2+}_{4\ (activated)} \qquad (2)$$

$Ca^{2+}$ binds to calmodulin sequentially (Kilhoffer et al., 1980; Tallant et al., 1980), but the exact order has not been established. The binding of $Ca^{2+}$ induces a conformational change in calmodulin, which then interacts with the apoenzyme (E) to form a ternary complex, the active holoenzyme. (The asterisks (*) in the above equations indicate a new conformation.) This process is reversible; under physiologic conditions, the direction of the reaction is likely controlled by intracellular concentration of $Ca^{2+}$. An increase of $Ca^{2+}$ favors the formation of the active holoenzyme, and a decrease favors its dissociation to the apoenzyme. Adenylate cyclase (Lynch et al., 1976), $Ca^{2+}$-ATPase (Lynch and Cheung, 1979), myosin light chain kinase (Hathaway et al., 1981) and NAD kinase (Jarrett et al., 1980) appear to be regulated similarly. In the case of phosphodiesterase and myosin light chain kinase, the active form of calmodulin contains $4\ Ca^{2+}$ (Huang et al., 1981; Blumenthal and Stull, 1980). Whether calmodulin binds the maximum number of bound $Ca^{2+}$ before interacting with other enzymes is not known.

Certain exceptions to the mechanism depicted above should be noted. Calmodulin is tightly bound to phosphorylase kinase and is not dissociated upon removal of the $Ca^{2+}$; moreover, a second molecule of calmodulin further activates phosphorylase kinase activity (Cohen et al., 1978).

## IMMUNOCYTOCHEMICAL LOCALIZATION OF CALMODULIN IN BRAIN

In mammalian cells, calmodulin is associated with the cytosol and the particulate fractions. In bovine brain cortex, some 60% of the total calmodulin is associated with particulate fractions (Table III).

Using immunocytochemical techniques, Wood et al. (1980a,b) localized calmodulin in mouse and rat basal ganglia, cerebellum and cerebral cortex. In basal ganglia, anticalmodulin

TABLE III

SUBCELLULAR DISTRIBUTION OF CALMODULIN IN BOVINE BRAIN CORTEX

| Fraction | Distribution (%) |
|---|---|
| Homogenate | 100 |
| 100 000 × $g$ supernatant | 41 |
| Nuclear | 1 |
| Mitochondrial | 36 |
| Microsome | 25 |

The amount of calmodulin in the homogenate of bovine brain cortex is taken as 100%; the activities in other fractions are expressed as percentage of the total (from Cheung et al., 1975).

was found in the soma, but not the nucleus, and within processes emanating from these cells. Labeled punctates which appeared to be cell processes cut longitudinally were dispersed throughout the neutrophile. The islands of white matter that contained bundles of myelinated axons did not show detectable reaction product.

In the cerebellum, all identifiable neurons — including Purkinje cells, basket and stellate cells, granule and Golgi II cells, and neurons of the deep cerebellar nuclei — contained reaction product. In Purkinje cells, in which dendrites could be clearly identified, the reaction product is evident (Wood et al., 1980a,b).

With the electron microscope, reaction product was evident in the soma and their processes. The staining within the soma was distributed among various organelles, especially on their membranes facing the cytoplasm, and was invariably heavier at the cell periphery than in the perinuclear region. Oligodendroglia astrocytes, or myelinated axons, were not stained. Many cell processes, cut in longitudinal or cross-sections, contained label. Many were postsynaptic to unlabeled presynaptic terminals, and thus appeared to be dendrites, although the possibility that some of the smaller profiles were unmyelinated axons could not be ruled out. In areas where the postsynaptic densities (PSD) were localized, the staining was heavy, even though in some fields a few PSDs were not labeled, perhaps because antibodies had not penetrated to these sites (Fig. 2). Calmodulin has been found to be a component of isolated PSDs (Grab et al., 1979).

Anticalmodulin also labeled the microtubules and the outer membranes of mitochondria. In heavily labeled dendrites, the antibodies obscured the details of stained elements, whereas in lightly labeled ones, they clearly decorated the microtubules. The staining pattern of mitochondria was erratic, being usually found at the outer membrane facing an area of heavy staining. Label was also associated with various cellular organelles, including free ribosomes and polysomes. Similar labeling patterns were observed in cerebellum (Lin et al., 1980).

## CALMODULIN AND CYCLIC NUCLEOTIDE METABOLISM

Most mammalian tissues contain multiple forms of phosphodiesterase. A particulate form that is sensitive to hormones has a low $K_m$ for cAMP. A second form is stimulated by cGMP and catalyzes the hydrolysis of cAMP and cGMP with comparable efficiency. A third form requires $Ca^{2+} \cdot$ calmodulin for activity. The activity of the different forms varies with the

242

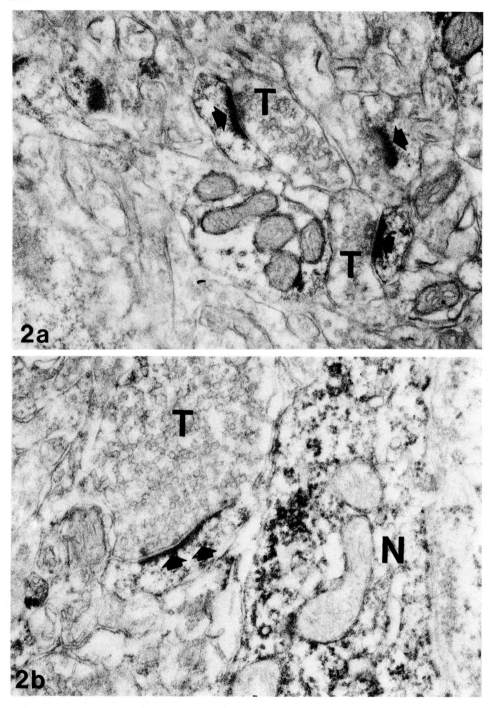

Fig. 2. Immunocytochemical localization of calmodulin in caudate-putamen of mouse. Two examples of fields showing anticalmodulin labeling of the postsynaptical densities (PSD, short arrows). T, presynaptic terminal; N, neuron. The neuron contains label deposited on cellular organelles, including certain parts of the outer mitochondrial membrane. (a) × 59 000; (b) × 61 700 (from Wood et al., 1980b).

tissue of origin. In the brain, the $Ca^{2+}$-dependent form accounts for a majority of phosphodiesterase activity (for a review, see Lin and Cheung, 1980).

The $Ca^{2+}$-dependent phosphodiesterase from bovine brain (Sharma et al., 1980) and heart (LaPorte et al., 1979) has been purified to apparent homogeneity. The enzyme consists of two identical subunits and has a molecular weight of 59 000. In the presence of $Ca^{2+}$, each catalytic subunit binds one molecule of calmodulin. Calmodulin increases the $V_{max}$ of the enzyme without affecting its apparent $K_m$ for the substrate. The enzyme displays normal Michaelis–Menton kinetics. $Ca^{2+}$-dependent phosphodiesterase can be activated by a brief treatment with trypsin or other endoproteases. Activation of phosphodiesterase by calmodulin proceeds stoichiometrically and reversibly. Activation by protease reduces the molecular weight of phosphodiesterase, so that the enzyme is unable to interact with and respond to calmodulin. Stimulation by either agent produces an activated enzyme with comparable final activities (Lin and Cheung, 1980). Stimulation of phosphodiesterase by protease is probably not relevant physiologically.

Brain adenylate cyclase is also stimulated by $Ca^{2+}$ through calmodulin. The enzyme is present in all regions of the brain that have been examined. Calmodulin-activatable adenylate cyclase may not be unique to brain; a similar enzyme has been found in pancreas and adrenal medulla (Cheung and Storm, 1982).

The observation that calmodulin stimulates the activities of both adenylate cyclase and phosphodiesterase should not necessarily be taken to imply concurrent stimulation. To the contrary, at micromolar concentrations of substrate, the $Ca^{2+}$-dependent phosphodiesterase catalyzes the hydrolysis of cGMP faster than cAMP, and the $Ca^{2+}$ flux may result in an increase of cAMP and a decrease of cGMP. Moreover, Piascik et al. (1980) noted that adenylate cyclase and phosphodiesterase differ in their sensitivity to $Ca^{2+}$. Brain adenylate cyclase is activated by low concentrations of $Ca^{2+}$ (0.03 $\mu$M) and at a concentration of $Ca^{2+}$ (0.3 $\mu$M) that activates phosphodiesterase, adenylate cyclase is already inhibited. The influx of $Ca^{2+}$ across the plasma membrane into the cell may cause sequential activation of adenylate cyclase and phosphodiesterase, resulting in a transient accumulation of cAMP (see Fig. 3).

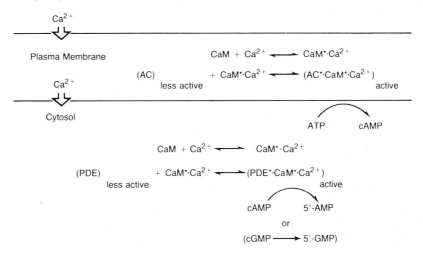

Fig. 3. Speculative scheme for the sequential activation of brain adenylate cyclase and phosphodiesterase by a cellular flux of $Ca^{2+}$. CaM, calmodulin; AC, adenylate cyclase; PDE, phosphodiesterase; the asterisk (*) indicates an active conformation (modified from Cheung et al., 1978).

An alternative mechanism has been suggested by Gnegy et al. (1977) who observed that a purified cAMP-dependent protein kinase in the presence of cAMP and ATP stimulated the release of calmodulin from a particulate to a soluble fraction of rat brain and adrenal medulla. The implication here is that the release of calmodulin would stimulate $Ca^{2+}$-dependent phosphodiesterase in the cytosol and thus facilitate the hydrolysis of cAMP towards the basal level, an example of feedback control. This notion appears attractive but is difficult to reconcile with the general finding that the concentration of calmodulin in cytosol is considerably higher than that of phosphodiesterase. It is more likely that the cellular concentration of $Ca^{2+}$ rather than that of calmodulin is rate-limiting for phosphodiesterase activity.

A further aspect of cAMP metabolism in the brain being investigated by Gnegy and her coworkers is the possibility that the sensitivity of striatal adenylate cyclase to dopamine is related to the membrane level of calmodulin. They found that the high level of calmodulin afforded supersensitivity whereas low levels afforded subsensitivity to the neurohormone, and that the calmodulin content in the striatal membrane changed in response to chronically altered dopaminergic activity. Calmodulin levels were elevated in striatal membranes in rats treated chronically with cataleptogenic antipsychotic drugs to decrease dopamine levels. These animals exhibited behavioral supersensitivity to apomorphone and the striatal adenylate cyclase had an increased affinity for dopamine. These results suggest that calmodulin may have a role in dopamine receptor function (Gnegy et al., 1980).

The regulation of brain adenylate cyclase by calmodulin may be even more complex. Partially purified adenylate cyclase from bovine brain cortex could be fractionated into two distinct fractions on a calmodulin–Sepharose affinity column. A minor fraction accounting for 20 % of the activity was stimulated by calmodulin. The predominant form, accounting for the remaining activity, was insensitive to calmodulin, but was made responsive to calmodulin by the addtition of a guanyl nucleotide-binding protein isolated from brain extract (Toscano et al., 1979). The significance of this finding remains to be clarified.

## CALMODULIN AND NEUROTRANSMISSION

$Ca^{2+}$ participates in the biosynthesis and release of neurotransmitters and the phosphorylation of certain specific proteins upon depolarization of the postsynaptic terminal. Tyrosine hydroxylase and tryptophan hydroxylase are key enzymes in the biosynthesis of catecholamines and serotonin, respectively. Yamauchi and Fujisawa (1979, 1980) demonstrated that both of these enzymes are activated by a calmodulin-dependent protein kinase.

When neurons are stimulated, their vesicles fuse with the presynaptic plasma membrane, and release their contents into the synaptic cleft, a process dependent on $Ca^{2+}$. DeLorenzo et al. (1979) showed that the release of neurotransmitters from the synaptic vesicles is closely linked to calmodulin-dependent phosphorylation of certain synaptic membrane proteins. Neurotransmitters released into the synaptic cleft bind to specific receptors on the postsynaptic membrane, resulting in an influx of $Ca^{2+}$ or an increased concentration of cAMP in the postsynaptic terminus. As already discussed, both the biosynthesis and degradation of cAMP in brain are regulated by $Ca^{2+}$ through the mediation of calmodulin. A $Ca^{2+}$-ATPase, the biochemical expression of the $Ca^{2+}$ pump, requires calmodulin for activity, and has been found in certain synaptic membranes (Sobue et al., 1979). Ueda and Greengard (1977) showed that a specific protein, protein I, located on the postsynaptic membrane and the surface of synaptic vesicles, is phosphorylated by a calmodulin-dependent or a cAMP-dependent protein kinase, although the sites of phosphorylation are distinct (Huttner et al., 1981). It appears that the entire process of neurotransmission from the biosynthesis of transmitters to the stimulation of the postsynaptic terminal is controlled by $Ca^+$ and that some of the underlying reactions, including the regulation of the neuronal level of $Ca^{2+}$, are mediated by calmodulin.

Why does calmodulin not contain tryptophan (precursor of serotonin) and only two tyrosines (precursor of dopamine and norepinephrine)? The level of calmodulin in brain is remarkably high, reaching several hundred milligrams per kilogram of tissue. If calmodulin were to contain the usual level of tryptophan and tyrosine as the average protein and to turnover at a half-life of about 20 h as in certain cultured cells (Chafouleas et al., 1981), there would be a continuous abundant supply of these amino acids, a condition that might lead to an excessive synthesis of neurotransmitters. As it stands, calmodulin metabolism in the brain does not affect the synthesis of neurotransmitters. Admittedly, this line of argument is teleologic.

## CALMODULIN AND CELLULAR SUPERSTRUCTURE

Welsh et al (1978), using indirect immunofluorescence techniques, demonstrated that anticalmodulin decorates the mitotic spindle of dividing cells. The fluorescence appeared most intense at the poles of the spindle where the mitotic apparatus was undergoing depolymerization. Colcemid and $N_2O$, agents that disrupt microtubule structure, also altered the distribution of fluorescence (Welsh et al., 1979). In vitro experiments with purified tubulin suggested that calmodulin accelerates the $Ca^{2+}$-dependent depolymerization of microtubules (Marcum et al., 1978). In this experiment, the concentration of calmodulin was stoichiometric with tubulin, and the effect was not specific, as troponin $c$ was more effective. The physiological relevance of this calmodulin effect remains to be shown.

Burke and DeLorenzo (1981) recently found a calmodulin-dependent protein kinase in brain that catalyzes the phosphorylation of tubulin, resulting in marked changes in its physicochemical properties and a temperature-dependent formation of non-random, insoluble "filamentous-like" structures that are distinct from microtubules (see DeLorenzo, this volume).

Calmodulin-dependent protein kinase also catalyzes the phosphorylation of numerous other proteins, with molecular weights ranging from 10 000 to 200 000 (DeLorenzo et al., 1981). The functions of these proteins have not been clarified.

## CALMODULIN-BINDING PROTEINS

A number of calmodulin-binding proteins with unknown biological functions have been described, and they may be additional calmodulin-regulated enzymes (for review, see Wang et al., 1980). One of these, with a molecular weight of 80 000, is present in high concentrations in the brain, especially in the putamen and caudate nucleus (Wallace et al., 1980). Now called calcineurin, the protein consists of two subunits with molecular weights of 60 000 and 16 500. The large subunit interacts with calmodulin, and the small subunit binds $4 Ca^{2+}$ with a $K_d$ of $10^{-6} M$ (Klee et al., 1979). Table IV shows that its levels in non-nervous tissues are much lower or insignificant. Using immunocytochemical techniques, Wood et al. (1980a,b) localized calcineurin at the postsynaptic densities and dendritic microtubules in the basal ganglia of mouse brain (Fig. 4), locations in which calmodulin is also found. These results suggest that the two proteins may be important in certain postsynaptic functions.

In a preliminary attempt to probe the function of calcineurin, we studied its concentration in developing rat brain. The level of calcineurin increased sharply between days 15 and 21 after

TABLE IV

THE LEVEL OF CALCINEURIN IN VARIOUS BOVINE TISSUES

| Tissue | Calcineurin (mg protein/kg tissue) |
|---|---|
| Adrenal | 3.3 ± 0.2 |
| Cerebellum | 29.4 ± 12.0 |
| Cerebrum | |
|     Grey matter | 36.0 ± 5.0 |
|     White matter | 15.9 ± 2.5 |
|     Caudate nucleus | 62.9 ± 10.9 |
|     Hippocampus | 36.4 ± 7.3 |
|     Hypothalamus | 31.3 ± 19.7 |
|     Putamen | 84.8 ± 20.0 |
|     Thalamus | 19.8 ± 7.0 |
| Heart | 0.7 ± 0.3 |
| Kidney | |
|     Cortex | 2.3 ± 0.7 |
|     Medulla | 3.4 ± 1.8 |
| Liver | 1.8 ± 0.5 |
| Lung | 3.2 ± 1.9 |
| Medulla oblongata | 2.5 ± 1.5 |
| Olfactory bulb | 17.2 ± 11.8 |
| Pons | 6.3 ± 3.9 |
| Skeletal muscle | 1.9 ± 0.6 |
| Spleen | 1.8 ± 0.6 |
| Testis | 3.1 ± 0.9 |
| Tongue | 2.8 ± 0.9 |
| Thyroid | 2.1 ± 1.5 |

An appropriate volume of a $100\,000\,g$ supernatant fluid from each tissue extract was assayed for calcineurin as determined by radioimmunoassay. The data represent the mean ± S.D. of four determinations on tissues from two animals; each assay was done in duplicate (from Wallace et al., 1980).

birth, a period corresponding to synaptogenesis (Tallant and Cheung, 1982). The exact role of calcineurin in synaptic function remains uncertain.

## CALMODULIN-DIRECTED SPECIFICITY

The versatility of calmodulin raises the question of how it acts specifically at the molecular level. Conceivably, different cells possess receptors that differ in structure and quantity, as well as in affinities, for calmodulin. In a given cell, which may contain multiple calmodulin-regulated enzymes, an increase of intracellular $Ca^{2+}$ could stimulate all these enzymes concurrently, or only a certain type(s). The latter possibility is much more likely, since the enzymes reside in different cellular compartments and are not equally accessible to $Ca^{2+}$ or to calmodulin. Moreover, their sensitivity to $Ca^{2+}$ differs: a concentration of $Ca^{2+}$ that activates one enzyme does not necessarily activate another, as may be the case of brain adenylate cyclase and $Ca^{2+}$-dependent phosphodiesterase (Piascik et al., 1980). Relevant to this point is the relative affinity of receptors for calmodulin. A receptor with a higher affinity for calmodulin is more likely to respond first to the cellular flux of $Ca^{2+}$. In addition, the apparent affinity of an

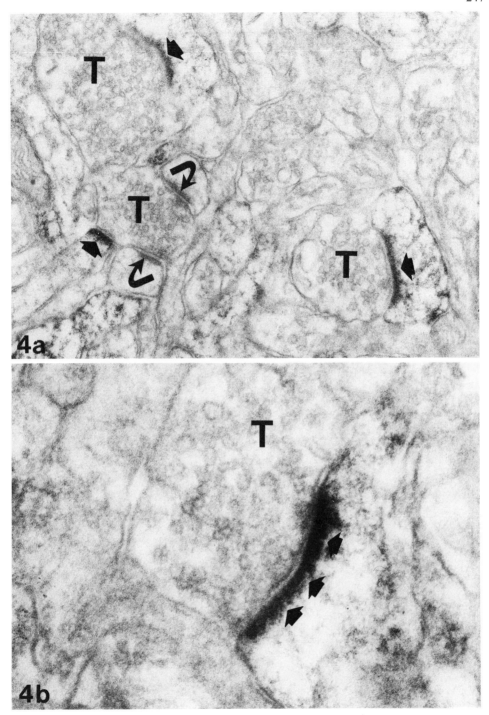

Fig. 4. Immunocytochemical localization of calcineurin in caudate-putamen of mouse. Two examples of fields showing anticalcineurin labeling of the postsynaptic densities. Curved arrows (a) contrast the lightly labeled with the heavily labeled PSD. T, presynaptic terminal. (a) × 58 500; (b) × 58 650 (from Word et al., 1980).

248

enzyme for calmodulin may be altered by certain cellular constituents; the change in affinity, though subtle, may alter the direction of one cellular activity in favor of another.

$Ca^{2+}$-stimulated phosphodiesterase activity is inhibited by calcineurin, presumably because it competes effectively with the enzyme for calmodulin. We showed recently that phosphodiesterase, in the presence of its substrate cAMP, increases its affinity for calmodulin, making it more refractory to inhibition by calcineurin (Cheung et al., 1981). Fig. 5 shows the effect of cAMP on the inhibition of phosphodiesterase (E) by calcineurin (I). In the middle curve, phosphodiesterase and calmodulin (A) were mixed briefly and then I was added. After various times of preincubation, an aliquot of the reaction mixture was removed to assay for phosphodiesterase activity. Phosphodiesterase activity decreased with preincubation time, indicating that calcineurin inhibited the enzyme. The holoenzyme of phosphodiesterase is an enzyme·calmodulin complex (abbreviated E·A for the sake of simplicity), which is in equilibrium with its components (E·A ⟶ E + A). During preincubation, I competed with E for A to form E·I, resulting in the time-dependent decrease of phosphodiesterase. In the second set of experiments (upper curve), E and A were mixed briefly in the presence of cAMP before I was added. There was a slight but detectable decrease of phosphodiesterase activity as a function of preincubation time, but the reduction was much less than that observed in the middle curve. In the presence of cAMP, phosphodiesterase activity apparently becomes more refractory to the inhibition by calcineurin. cAMP may increase the affinity of E for A or decrease that of I for A; in either case, more E is preserved in the form of E·A. In the lower curve, the calcineurin and calmodulin were preincubated in the presence of cAMP for various

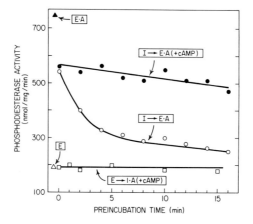

Fig. 5. Effect of cAMP on the inhibition of phosphodiesterase by calcineurin. The preincubation mixture contained 40 mM Tris–HCl (pH 8.0), 5 mM $MgCl_2$, 250 $\mu$M $CaCl_2$ and other components, as indicated for each curve. Middle curve ( O – – – O ): other components: E (0.13 unit) and A (100 pmoles) in a volume of 1.7 ml. The mixture was preincubated for 2 min at 30°C and I (240 pmoles) was then added; at indicated times, aliquots were removed and assayed immediately for phosphodiesterase activity. Upper curve ( ●——● ): the composition of the preincubation was the same as the middle curve except that it contained 2.5 mM cAMP. Immediately after the addition of cAMP, I was added to the preincubation mixture, and at indicated times, one aliquot (a) was collected in a tube kept at 100°C to terminate the reaction, and another aliquot (b) was transferred to a tube kept at 30°C for a further 5-min incubation. The amount of cAMP hydrolyzed in (a) gave the amount of cAMP hydrolyzed during the preincubation period; the algebraic difference between (b) and (a) gave the amount of cAMP hydrolyzed during the 5-min incubation. Lower curve ( □ – – – □ ): other components were A (100 pmoles), I (240 pmoles) and 2.5 mM cAMP. At indicated times, an aliquot was transferred to a tube containing E (5 milliunits), incubated for 5 min and the amount of cAMP hydrolyzed was determined. E(Δ)), basal phosphodiesterase or apoenzyme activity; E·A (▲) stimulated phosphodiesterase or holoenzyme activity (from Cheung et al., 1981).

times before E was added to start the phosphodiesterase assay. The enzyme activity at all preincubation times was comparable to the basal level, suggesting that cAMP did not decrease the affinity of I for A; a reduction in the I·A complex would have allowed the formation of more E·A complex (i.e., an apparent increase of phosphodiesterase activity with preincubation). Collectively, these results indicate that cAMP renders phosphodiesterase more refractory to inhibition by calcineurin by increasing the affinity of the enzyme for calmodulin.

To obtain a rough estimate of the relative rates of dissociation of E·A complex to E + A in the presence or absence of cAMP, we determined the initial slopes of the upper and middle curves as indications of the rates of dissociation of the E·A complex. Assuming that the formation of I·A complex was not the rate-limiting step, we estimated that the rate of dissociation of the E·A complex was approximately 14 times faster in the absence than in the presence of cAMP. Since cAMP did not appear to diminish the affinity of I for A (lower curve), the data suggest that cAMP enhanced the affinity of E for A 14-fold. In a separate experiment, using equilibrium dialysis, we found that neither I, A nor a mixture of I·A bound any cAMP.

When cAMP was present in the preincubation mixture (upper curve of Fig. 5), 5'-AMP was formed, raising the possibility that 5'-AMP affected the affinity of A for E or I. This was excluded by another experiment in which 5'-AMP was added to the preincubation mixture in place of cAMP [i.e., I → E·A (+ 5'-AMP)]. Phosphodiesterase activity decreased with preincubation time in a manner similar to the experiment containing no cAMP. In another experiment, E was added to the preincubation mixture containing I·A and 5'-AMP [i.e., E → I·A (+ 5'-AMP)]; in this instance, phosphodiesterase activity was comparable to the basal level, suggesting that 5'-AMP did not alter the affinity of A for E of for I.

The finding that cAMP enhances the affinity of phosphodiesterase for calmodulin may have implications in vivo. Indeed, the alteration of selectivity of calmodulin by cAMP in favor of its own hydrolysis might represent one example of calmodulin-directed specificity (Fig. 6), a phenomenon that could have a wider physiological relevance. "I" does not necessarily have to be calcineurin; it may represent any other calmodulin-regulated enzyme. Hence, the conclusion reached above remains valid as long as cAMP does not affect the affinity of I for calmodulin. Indeed, the scheme may apply theoretically to other pairs of calmodulin-governed systems if we replace cAMP with an effector that changes the affinity of calmodulin for only one of the two receptor proteins. Although attractive, this notion is supported by preliminary evidence only. It would be important to determine whether such a mechanism indeed operates in vivo and whether a similar mechanism applies to other calmodulin-regulated enzymes.

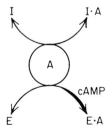

Fig. 6. A scheme showing the competition of phosphodiesterase (E) and calcineurin (I) for calmodulin (A). In the presence of cAMP, the affinity of E for A is increased, with I becoming less able to compete for A; the formation of the E·A complex is favored over that of I·A. Thus, an increase of cAMP tends to favor its own hydrolysis. Although I represents calcineurin, it may be any other calmodulin-regulated enzyme, and the scheme is valid as long as cAMP does not affect the affinity of I for calmodulin. The scheme may prove to be a general one; I and E could be any other sets of calmodulin-regulated systems provided that cAMP is replaced with an appropriate effector that selectively affects the affinity of calmodulin for one of the calmodulin receptors (from Cheung et al., 1981).

## CALMODULIN AS AN INTEGRATOR OF CELLULAR MESSENGERS

Brain is one of the most active tissues in cAMP metabolism, and the important role of cAMP in neuronal function has been extensively reviewed. The close relationship between cAMP and $Ca^{2+}$ is perhaps best illustrated by reactions in the brain. $Ca^{2+}$ controls both the synthesis and degradation of cAMP, which activates the cAMP-dependent protein kinase. $Ca^{2+}$ regulates a separate protein kinase that is calmodulin-dependent. The two kinases catalyze the phosphorylation of the same or different proteins or the same protein at distinct sites. cAMP may

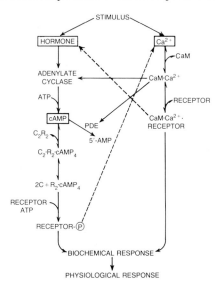

Fig. 7. Integration of cellular regulators by calmodulin. Stimulation of a cell leads to the release of hormones or $Ca^{2+}$ or both. Catecholamines and certain peptide hormones activate adenylate cyclase and cause an increase of intracellular cAMP. Upon binding cAMP, the regulatory subunit (R) of protein kinase ($C_2R_2$) is dissociated from the catalytic subunit (C), which becomes active, and catalyzes the phosphorylation of an effector protein. Phosphorylation of a protein either stimulates or inhibits its biological activity; the phosphorylated protein serves as an effector or a modulator of a cellular process. The influx of $Ca^{2+}$ or the release of $Ca^{2+}$ from the cell membrane or sarcoplasmic reticulum activates calmodulin, which forms a complex with a receptor protein to initiate a biochemical or physiological response. CaM·$Ca^{2+}$·receptor presents the active form of adenylate cyclase, phosphodiesterase or any of the calmodulin-regulated enzymes. Calmodulin regulates the metabolism of cAMP, which in turn affects the availability of $Ca^{2+}$. Thus, the function and metabolism of these cellular regulators are interrelated, and calmodulin integrates them on a molecular basis. The dashed lines denote relationships that have yet to be clearly established on a molecular basis.

regulate the metabolism of $Ca^{2+}$ as well as the cellular distribution of calmodulin. Fig. 7 illustrates the integration of the two cellular messengers. In view of the number of enzymes regulated by calmodulin, including several protein kinases, the involvement of $Ca^{2+}$ and cAMP are interconnected, it is perhaps more appropriate to refer to them simply as cellular messengers or regulators rather than second messengers.

## CONCLUSIONS

The importance of calmodulin in brain function is unlikely to be limited to the processes described in the text. Some of the enzymes listed in Table I that have not been discussed in the text may well prove to be important. Although the central role of $Ca^{2+}$ in neural physiology has been studied extensively, much remains to be learned. Not only is it important to identify cellular reactions that are calmodulin-dependent, but one must also establish those that are not. As other $Ca^{2+}$ receptors are found, a much better understanding of the role of $Ca^{2+}$ in the central nervous system will begin to emerge.

## NOTE ADDED IN PROOF

Recent experiments from our laboratory indicate that calcineurin is a calmodulin-dependent protein phosphatase. Biochem. Biophys. Res. Commun. (in press) Yang, S.-D., Tallant, E.A. and Cheung, W.Y. (1982).

## ACKNOWLEDGEMENTS

The work in my laboratory has been supported by grants NS 08059 and GM 28178 from the United Public Health Service and by ALSAC.
I thank John Gilbert for editorial assistance and Pat Nicholas for typing the manuscript.

### REFERENCES

Amphlett, G.W., Vanaman, T.C. and Perry, S.V. (1976) Effect of the troponin $c$-like protein from bovine brain (brain modulator protein) on the $Mg^{2+}$-stimulated ATPase of skeletal muscle actomyosin. *FEBS Lett.*, 72: 163–168.

Anderson, J.M. and Cormier, M.J. (1978) Calcium-dependent regulator of NAD kinase in higher plants. *Biochem. biophys. Res. Commun.*, 84: 595–602.

Blumenthal, D.K. and Stull, J.T. (1980) Activation of skeletal muscle myosin light chain kinase by calcium and calmodulin. *Biochemistry*, 19: 5608–5614.

Brostrom, C.O. and Wolff, D.J. (1981) Properties and functions of calmodulin. *Biochem. Pharmacol.*, 30: 1395–1405.

Brostrom, C.O., Huang, Y.-C., Breckenridge, B.McL. and Wolff, D.J. (1975) Identification of a calcium-binding protein as a calcium-dependent regulator of brain adenylate cyclase. *Proc. nat. Acad. Sci. (Wash.)*, 72: 64–68.

Burke, B.E. and DeLorenzo, R.J. (1981) $Ca^{2+}$- and calmodulin-stimulated endogenous phosphorylation of neurotubulin. *Proc. nat. Acad. Sci. (Wash.)*, 78: 991–995.

Chafouleas, J.G., Pardue, R., Brinkley, B.R., Dedman, J.R. and Means, A.R. (1981) Regulation of intracellular levels of calmodulin and tubulin in normal and transformed cells. *Proc. nat. Acad. Sci. (Wash.)*, 78: 996–1000.

Charbonneau, H. and Cormier, M.J. (1979) Purification of plant calmodulin by fluphenazine-sepharose affinity chromatography. *Biochem. biophys. Res. Commun.*, 90: 1039–1047.

Cheung, W.Y. (1980a) Calmodulin plays a pivotal role in cellular regulation. *Science*, 207: 19–27.

Cheung, W.Y. (Ed.) (1980b) *Calcium and Cell Function*, Vol. 1, Calmodulin, Academic Press, New York.

Cheung, W.Y. (1981) Discovery and recognition of calmodulin: A personal account. *J. cycl. Nucl. Res.*, 7: 71–84.

Cheung, W.Y. and Storm, D. (1982) Calmodulin regulation of cyclic AMP metabolism. *Handbook exp. Pharmacol.*, 58: 301–323.

Cheung, W.Y., Bradham, L.S., Lynch, T.J., Lin, Y.M. and Tallant, E.A. (1975a) Protein activator of cyclic 3′:5′-nucleotide phosphodiesterase of bovine on rat brain also activates its adenylate cyclase. *Biochem. biophys. Res. Commun.*, 66: 1055–1062.

Cheung, W.Y., Lin, Y.M. and Liu, Y.P. (1975b) Regulation of bovine brain cyclic 3′,5′-nucleotide phosphodiesterase by its protein activator. In *Cyclic Nucleotides in Diseases*, B. Weiss (Ed.), University Park Press, pp. 321–350.

Cheung, W.Y., Lynch, T.J. and Wallace, R.W. (1978) An endogenous $Ca^{2+}$-dependent activator protein of brain adenylate cyclase and cyclic nucleotide phosphodiesterase. Adv. cyclic Nucleot. Res., 9: 233–251.

Cheung, W.Y., Lynch, T.J., Wallace, R.W. and Tallant, E.A. (1981) cAMP renders $Ca^{2+}$-dependent phosphodiesterase refractory to inhibition by a calmodulin-binding protein (calcineurin). *J. biol. Chem.*, 256: 4439–4443.

Cohen, P., Burchell, A., Foulkes, J.G., Cohen, T.W., Vanaman, T.C. and Nairn, A.L. (1978) Identification of the $Ca^{2+}$-dependent modulator protein as the fourth subunit of rabbit skeletal muscle phosphorylase kinase. *FEBS Lett.*, 92: 287–293.

Dabrowska, R. and Hartshorne, D.J. (1978) A $Ca^{2+}$- and modulator-dependent myosin light chain kinase from non-muscle cells. *Biochem. biophys. Res. Commun.*, 85: 1352–1359.

DeLorenzo, R.J., Freedman, S.D., Yobe, W.B. and Maurer, S.C. (1979) Stimulation of $Ca^{2+}$-dependent neurotransmitter release and presynaptic nerve-terminal protein phosphorylation by calmodulin and a calmodulin-like protein isolated from synaptic vesicles. *Proc. nat. Acad. Sci. (Wash.)*, 76: 1838–1842.

DeLorenzo, R.J., Burdette, S. and Holderness, J. (1981) Benzodiazepine inhibition of the calcium-calmodulin protein kinase in brain membrane. *Science*, 213: 546–549.

Gnegy, M.E., Lucchelli, A. and Costa, E. (1977) Correlation between drug-induced supersensitivity of dopamine-dependent striatal mechanisms and the increase in striatal content of the $Ca^{2+}$-regulated protein activaotr of cAMP phosphodiesterase. *Arch. Pharmacol.*, 301: 121–127.

Gnegy, M.E., Lau, Y.S. and Treisman, G. (1980) Role of calmodulin in states of altered catecholamine sensitivity. *Ann. N.Y. Acad. Sci.*, 356: 304–318.

Gopinath, R.M. and Vincenzi, F.F. (1977) Phosphodiesterase protein activator mimics red blood cell cytoplasmic activator of $(Ca^{2+}–Mg^{2+})$ATPase. *Biochem. biophys. Res. Commun.*, 77: 1203–1209.

Grab, D.J., Berzins, K., Cohen, R.S. and Siekevitz, P. (1979) Presence of calmodulin in postsynaptic densities isolated from canine cerebral cortex. *J. biol. Chem.*, 254: 8690–8696.

Hathaway, D.R., Adelstein, R.S. and Klee, C.B. (1981) Interaction of calmodulin with myosin light chain kinase and cAMP-dependent protein kinase in bovine brain. *J. biol. Chem.*, 256: 8183–8189.

Huang, C.Y., Chan, V., Chock, P.B., Wang, J.H. and Sharma, R.K. (1981) Mechanism of activation of cyclic nucleotide phosphodiesterase: Requirement of the binding of four $Ca^{2+}$ to calmodulin for activation. *Proc. nat. Acad. Sci. (Wash.)*, 78: 871–874.

Huttner, W.B., DeGennaro, L.J. and Greengard, P. (1981) Differential phosphorylation of multiple sites in purified protein I by cyclic AMP-dependent and calcium-dependent protein kinase. *J. biol. Chem.*, 256: 1482–1488.

Jamieson, G.A. and Vanaman, T.C. (1979) Calcium-dependent affinity chromatography of calmodulin on an immobilized phenothiazine. *Biochem. biophys. Res. Commun.*, 90: 1048–1056.

Jarrett, H.W. and Penniston, J.T. (1977) Partial purification of the $Ca^{2+}–Mg^{2+}$ ATPase activator from human erythrocytes: Its similarity to the activator of $3':5'$-cyclic nucleotide phosphodiesterase. *Biochem. biophys. Res. Commun.*, 77: 1210–1216.

Jarrett, H.W., Charbonneau, H., Anderson, J.M., McCann, R.O. and Cormier, M.J. (1980) Plant calmodulin and the regulation of NAD kinase. *Ann. N.Y. Acad. Sci.*, 356: 119–129.

Kilhoffer, M.-C., Gerara, D. and Demaille, J.G. (1980) Terbium binding to octopus calmodulin provides the complete sequence of ion binding. *FEBS Lett.*, 120: 99–103.

Klee, C.B., Crouch, T.H. and Krinks, M.M. (1979) Calcineurin: A calcium- and calmodulin-binding protein of the nervous system. *Proc. nat. Acad. Sci. (Wash.)*, 76: 6270–6273.

Klee, C.B., Crouch, T.H. and Richman, P. (1980) Calmodulin. *Annu. Rev. Biochem.*, 49: 489–515.

Kretsinger, R.H. and Barry, C.D. (1975) The predicted structure of the calcium-binding component of troponin. *Biochim. biophys. Acta*, 405: 40–52.

LaPorte, D.C., Toscano, W.A. and Storm, D.R. (1979) Cross-linking of iodine-125-labeled calmodulin to the $Ca^{2+}$-sensitive phosphodiesterase purified from bovine heart. *Biochemistry*, 18: 2820–2825.

LaPorte, D.C., Wierman, B.M. and Storm, D.R. (1980) Calcium-induced exposure of a hydrophobic surface on calmodulin. *Biochemistry*, 19: 3814–3819.

Lin, Y.M. and Cheung, W.Y. (1980) $Ca^{2+}$-dependent cyclic nucleotide phosphodiesterase. In *Calcium and Cell Function*, Vol. 1, Calmodulin, W.Y. Cheung (Ed.), Academic Press, New York, pp. 79–100.

Lin, C.T., Dedman, J.R., Brinkley, B.R. and Means, A.R. (1980) Localization of calmodulin in rat cerebellum by immunoelectron microscopy. *J. Cell Biol.*, 85: 473–480.

Lynch, T.J. and Cheung, W.Y. (1979) Human erythrocyte $Ca^{2+}–Mg^{2+}$-ATPase: Mechanism of stimulation by $Ca^{2+}$. *Arch. Biochem. Biophys.*, 194: 165–170.

Lynch, T.J., Tallant, E.A. and Cheung, W.Y. (1976) $Ca^{2+}$-dependent formation of brain adenylate cyclase-protein activator complex. *Biochem. biophys. Res. Commun.*, 68: 616–625.

Marcum, J.M., Dedman, J.R., Brinkley, B.R. and Means, A.R. (1978) Control of microtubule assembly–disassembly by calcium-dependent regulator protein. *Proc. nat. Acad. Sci. (Wash.)*, 75: 3771–3775.

Means, A.R. and Dedman, J.R. (1980) Calmodulin — an intracellular calcium receptor. *Nature (Lond.)*, 285: 73–77.

Nagao, S., Suzuki, Y. and Watanabe, Y. (1979) Activation by a calcium-binding protein of guanylate cyclase in

*Tetrahymena pyriformis. Biochem. biophys. Res. Commun.*, 90: 261–268.

Payne, M.E. and Soderling, T.R. (1980) Calmodulin-dependent glycogen synthase kinase. *J. biol. Chem.*, 255: 8054–8056.

Piascik, M.T., Wisler, P.L., Johnson, C.L. and Potter, J.D. (1980) $Ca^{2+}$-dependent regulation of guinea pig brain adenylate cyclase. *J. biol. Chem.*, 255: 4176–4181.

Schulman, H. and Greengard, P. (1978) $Ca^{2+}$-dependent protein phosphorylation system in membranes from various tissues and its activation by "calcium-dependent regulator". *Proc. nat. Acad. Sci. (Wash.)*, 75: 5432–5436.

Sharma, R.K., Wang, T.H., Wirch, E. and Wang, J.H. (1980) Purification and properties of bovine brain calmodulin-dependent cyclic nucleotide phosphodiesterase. *J. biol. Chem.*, 255: 5916–5923.

Sobue, K., Ichida, S., Yoshida, H., Yamazaki, R. and Kakiuchi, S. (1979) Occurrence of a $Ca^{2+}$- and modulator protein-activatable ATPase in the synaptic plasma membranes of brain. *FEBS Lett.*, 99: 199–202.

Tallant, E.A. and Cheung, W.Y. (1982) Calcineurin increases during synaptogenesis. Fed. Proc., 41: 1213 (Abstract).

Tallant, E.A., Wallace, R.W., Dockter, M.E. and Cheung, W.Y. (1980) Activation of calmodulin by terbium ($Tb^{3+}$) and its use as a fluorescence probe. *Ann. N.Y. Acad. Sci.*, 356: 436.

Toscano, W.A., Westcott, K.R., LaPorte, D.C. and Storm, D.R. (1979) Evidence for a dissociable subunit required for calmodulin stimulation of brain adenylate cyclase. *Proc. nat. Acad. Sci. (Wash.)*, 76: 5582–5586.

Ueda, T. and Greengard, P. (1977) Adenosine $3':5'$-monophosphate-regulated phosphoprotein system of neuronal membranes. *J. biol. Chem.*, 252: 5155–5163.

Wallace, R.W., Tallant, E.A. and Cheung, W.Y. (1980) High levels of a heat-labile calmodulin-binding protein ($CaM$-$BP_{80}$) in bovine neostriatum. *Biochemistry*, 19: 1831–1837.

Walsh, M., Steven, F.C., Kuznicki, J. and Drabikowski, W. (1977) Characterization of tryptic fragments obtained from bovine brain modulator of cyclic nucleotide phosphodiesterase. *J. biol. Chem.*, 252: 7440–7443.

Wang, J.H., Sharma, R.K. and Tam, S.W. (1980) Calmodulin-binding proteins. In *Calcium and Cell Function*, Vol. 1, Calmodulin, W.Y. Cheung (Ed.), Academic Press, New York, pp. 305–328.

Watterson, D.M., Sharief, F. and Vanaman, T.C. (1980) The complete amino acid sequence of $Ca^{2+}$-dependent modulator protein (calmodulin) of bovine brain. *J. biol. Chem.*, 255: 462–475.

Welsh, M.J., Dedman, J.R., Brinkley, B.R. and Means, A.R. (1978) Calcium-dependent regulator protein: Localization in mitotic apparatus of eukaryotic cells. *Proc. nat. Acad. Sci. (Wash.)*, 75: 1867–1871.

Welsh, M.J., Dedman, J.R., Brinkley, B.R. and Means, A.R. (1979) Tubulin and calmodulin: Effects of microtubules and microfilament inhibitors on localization in the mitotic apparatus. *J. Cell Biol.*, 81: 624–634.

Wood, J.G., Wallace, R.W. and Cheung, W.Y. (1980a) Immunocytochemical studies of the localization of calmodulin and $CaM$-$BP_{80}$ in brain. In *Calcium and Cell Function*, Vol. 1, Calmodulin, W.Y. Cheung (Ed.), Academic Press, pp. 291–304.

Wood, J.G., Wallace, R.W., Whitaker, J.N. and Cheung, W.Y. (1980b) Immunocytochemical localization of calmodulin and a heat-labile calmodulin-binding protein in basal ganglia of mouse brain. *J. Cell Biol.*, 84: 66–76.

Yagi, K., Yazawa, M., Kakiuchi, S., Ohshima, M. and Uenishi, K. (1978) Identification of an activator protein for myosin light chain kinase as the $Ca^{2+}$-dependent modulator protein. *J. biol. Chem.*, 253: 1388–1340.

Yamauchi, T. and Fujisawa, H. (1979) Activation of tryptophan-5-monooxygenase by calcium-dependent regulator protein. *Biochem. biophys. Res. Commun.*, 90: 28–35.

Yamauchi, T. and Fujisawa, H. (1980) Involvement of calmodulin in the $Ca^{2+}$-dependent activation of rat brainstem tyrosine-3-monooxygenase. *Biochem. int.*, 1: 98–104.

# Ca²⁺-Calmodulin Tubulin Kinase System and its Role in Mediating the Ca²⁺ Signal in Brain

ROBERT J. DELORENZO, BASILIO GONZALEZ,
JAMES GOLDENRING, ALLEN BOWLING and RONALD JACOBSON

*Department of Neurology, Yale Medical School, 333 Cedar Street,*
*New Haven, CT 06510, U.S.A.*

## INTRODUCTION

$Ca^{2+}$ plays a major role in the function of nervous tissue (Rubin, 1972; Rasmussen and Goodman, 1977). One of the most widely recognized roles of $Ca^{2+}$ in synaptic function is its action in neurotransmission. Early studies showed that the release of neurotransmitter substances by vertebrate neuromuscular juctions was dependent upon the $Ca^{2+}$ ion concentration in the media (Rubin 1972; Del Castillo and Stark, 1952). Elegant studies at the synaptic level most convincingly demonstrated that the effects of $Ca^{2+}$ on neurotransmission were not secondary to effects of $Ca^{2+}$ on the presynaptic action potential, but were directly dependent upon the entry of $Ca^{2+}$ into the nerve terminal (Katz and Miledi, 1969, 1970; Miledi and Slater, 1966; Miledi, 1973). The role of $Ca^{2+}$ in stimulus–secretion coupling has also been demonstrated in a variety of secretory processes in several tissues (Douglas, 1968). Thus, the role of $Ca^{2+}$ in synaptic function is well established. One of the major questions in neuroscience research at the present time is what is the molecular mechanism mediating the effects of $Ca^{2+}$ on synaptic activity.

Research in this laboratory over the last 10 years has been directed at providing a molecular approach to studying the biochemistry of the $Ca^{2+}$ signal in neurotransmitter release and synaptic modulation. In vitro and in vivo preparations were developed and employed to study the effects of $Ca^{2+}$ on neurotransmitter release (DeLorenzo and Freedman, 1977a,b, 1978; DeLorenzo et al., 1979; DeLorenzo, 1980a), synaptic protein phosphorylation (Burke and DeLorenzo, 1981a–c; DeLorenzo, 1976, 1977, 1980a,b, 1981d; DeLorenzo et al., 1977, 1981; DeLorenzo and Glaser, 1976), and synaptic vesicle and synaptic membrane interactions (DeLorenzo, 1980a, 1981a–c). These results provided a molecular approach to studying the $Ca^{2+}$ signal and suggested that $Ca^{2+}$ kinase activity may be involved in mediating the effects of $Ca^{2+}$ and several neuroleptic drugs at the synapse.

Calmodulin is a major $Ca^{2+}$ receptor protein in brain and other tissues and has been shown to modulate the effects of $Ca^{2+}$ on several important enzyme systems (Cheung, 1980; Klee et al., 1980). Thus, we extended the work on the $Ca^{2+}$ signal in this laboratory to investigate the role of calmodulin in synaptic function and neurotransmitter release. Our results have demonstrated that calmodulin can be isolated from the synaptic nerve terminal (DeLorenzo, 1980a) and regulates the effects of $Ca^{2+}$ on synaptic protein phosphorylation, neurotransmitter release, and synaptic vesicle–synaptic membrane interactions in several experimental systems (DeLorenzo, 1980a; 1981a–e). In addition, synaptic tubulin has been shown to be a major substrate for the $Ca^{2+}$-calmodulin protein kinase system and the phosphorylation of this major

256

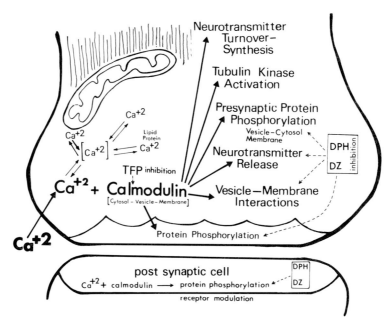

Fig. 1. Schematic model representing a summary of existing evidence supporting a role for the calmodulin hypothesis of neurotransmission (DeLorenzo 1980a, 1981b,c). Presynaptic and postsynaptic calmodulin serves as a $Ca^{2+}$ receptor activating several enzyme processes and synaptic events. The inhibition of calmodulin by trifluoperazine (TFP) is shown and the model indicates that this drug would be expected to affect all calmodulin-dependent processes. The $Ca^{2+}$ kinase inhibitors (phenytoin, DPH; diazepam, DZ) have been shown to inhibit not only kinase activity but vesicle–membrane interactions and neurotransmitter release, suggesting that synaptic protein phosphorylation may play a role in modulating these processes (from DeLorenzo, 1981c).

synaptic cytoskeletal protein may play a role in converting the $Ca^{2+}$ signal into a motor force at the synapse (Burke and DeLorenzo, 1981a–c). These studies provided an experimental framework to demonstrate that calmodulin, a major $Ca^{2+}$ receptor protein in brain, modulates many of the biochemical effects of $Ca^{2+}$ on synaptic preparations. From this evidence the calmodulin hypothesis of neuronal transmission was developed (DeLorenzo, 1980a,b; 1981a–c). This hypothesis (summarized in Fig. 1) states that as $Ca^{2+}$ enters the presynaptic nerve terminal, it binds to calmodulin and activates several $Ca^{2+}$-calmodulin-regulated processes that modulate synaptic and that $Ca^{2+}$ can also reach and regulate through calmodulin some of the postsynaptic effects of this cation.

The calmodulin hypothesis of neurotransmission suggests that $Ca^{2+}$ modulates the activity of many calmodulin–regulated processes at the synapse, including protein phosphorylation, neurotransmitter release, neurotransmitter turnover, vesicle–membrane interactions, and phosphorylation of synaptic tubulin (Fig. 1). Although this hypothesis provides a molecular synaptic receptor for $Ca^{2+}$ that can then activate several synaptic events, it is important to try and take the next step in providing a biochemical understanding of the action of $Ca^{2+}$ at the synapse and attempt to explain the dynamic functional aspects of the $Ca^{2+}$ signal in molecular terms.

In this presentation we will focus on the work from this laboratory that suggests that $Ca^{2+}$-calmodulin protein phosphorylation, especially the tubulin kinase system, provides an important mechanism for regulating synaptic activity. Tubulin has been identified as a major substrate for the calmodulin kinase system (Burke and DeLorenzo, 1981a–c) and this major cytoskeletal protein may provide an important insight into how $Ca^{2+}$ dynamically alters synaptic function. The phosphorylation of tubulin by the $Ca^{2+}$ kinase results in a marked allosteric alteration in the tubulin molecule resulting in the formation of very stable tubulin aggregates that form microfilaments (DeLorenzo, 1981b,c). Thus, $Ca^{2+}$ can produce marked changes in the physicochemical properties of tubulin through the action of the calmodulin tubulin kinase system. This system provides an attractive biochemical model for converting the $Ca^{2+}$ signal into molecular change. The evidence for the role of $Ca^{2+}$ kinases and specifically the tubulin kinase system in synaptic modulation will be discussed.

## $Ca^{2+}$-CALMODULIN–STIMULATED SYNAPTIC PROTEIN PHOSPHORYLATION AND NEUROTRANSMISSION

The evidence is accumulating to indicate that $Ca^{2+}$-calmodulin–regulated synaptic biochemical processes may regulate the effect of $Ca^{2+}$ on synaptic activity (DeLorenzo, 1980a; 1981a–c). Thus, it would be important to determine which calmodulin–regulated enzyme systems are involved in specific aspects of synaptic function. $Ca^{2+}$-stimulated endogenous protein phosphorylation was initially described in whole rat and human brain homogenates and synaptosome preparations (DeLorenzo, 1976; 1977; DeLorenzo et al., 1977; DeLorenzo and Glaser, 1976) and it was suggested that the effects of $Ca^{2+}$ on protein kinase activation might mediate the effects of $Ca^{2+}$ on neurotransmitter release and synaptic function. These results demonstrated that $Ca^{2+}$ stimulated the endogenous phosphorylation of many brain proteins, but partially proteins in the 10 000–20 000, 50 000–54 000, 60 000–64 000, and 150 000–300 000 molecular weight ranges. Two proteins with molecular weights of 52 000–54 000 and 60 000–64 000 dalton (proteins DPH-M and DPH-L, respectively) were of particular interest, since they were most dramatically stimulated by $Ca^{2+}$ and inhibited by phenytoin, an anticonvulsant that blocks several $Ca^{2+}$-dependent processes, including neurotransmitter release (DeLorenzo, 1980b). An hypothesis was developed from these findings, suggesting that $Ca^{2+}$-dependent protein phosphorylation (a new phosphorylation system distinct from cyclic AMP (cAMP) kinases) may regulate the effects of $Ca^{2+}$ on synaptic function and neurotransmitter release (DeLorenzo and Freedman, 1977a,b). The synaptic $Ca^{2+}$-dependent pattern of endogenous protein phosphorylation with proteins DPH-L and DPH-M as major bands has been confirmed by several laboratories in several isolated brain fractions (Ehrlich, 1978; Schulman and Greengard, 1978; Grab et al., 1980).

Calmodulin has been shown to mediate the activation of specific kinase systems in nonneuronal tissues (Adelstein et al., 1980; Cohen et al., 1980), crude brain membrane (Schulman and Greengard, 1978), and highly enriched synaptic preparations, including synaptic vesicle (DeLorenzo et al., 1979; DeLorenzo, 1980a), synaptic membrane (DeLorenzo, 1980a,b, 1981a–c), synaptic junction (DeLorenzo, 1980a), and postsynaptic density fractions (Grab et al., 1980; DeLorenzo, 1980a). Several distinct calmodulin kinases have been described in brain (Yamauchi and Fujisawa, 1980). Thus, $Ca^{2+}$-regulated protein kinase activity is a major enzyme system that may mediate the effects of calmodulin on synaptic function.

It was then demonstrated that the $Ca^{2+}$-calmodulin–dependent release of neurotransmiteer substances from synaptic vesicles was also dependent on $Mg^{2+}$ and ATP (DeLorenzo and Freedman, 1978; DeLorenzo et al., 1979; DeLorenzo, 1980b), suggesting that utilization of ATP by synaptic protein kinases may be involved in the release process. Experiments that

258

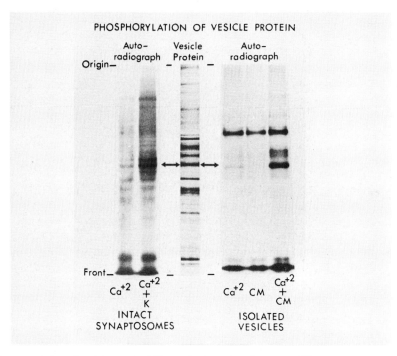

Fig. 2. Phosphorylation of vesicle protein. Effects of calmodulin (CM) and $Ca^{2+}$ on protein phosphorylation in isolated calmodulin-depleted synaptic vesicles (right) and of depolarization-dependent $Ca^{2+}$ uptake on protein phosphorylation of synaptic vesicles isolated from $^{32}$P-labeled intact synaptosomes (left) (DeLorenzo, 1980a). For experiments with isolated vesicles, $[\gamma\text{-}^{32}P]ATP$ was added to the reaction mixture and incubated for 1 min in the presence and/or absence of $Ca^{2+}$ (free $Ca^{2+}$, 10 $\mu$M) and CM (5 $\mu$g). For experiments with intact synaptosomes, synaptosomes were preincubated with $^{32}$P and then incubated with $Ca^{2+}$ (1 mM) or $Ca^{2+}$ (1 mM) plus $K^+$ (65 mM). Following incubation, synaptic vesicles were rapidly isolated from each incubated synaptosome reaction and analyzed for vesicle protein phosphorylation. Protein DPH-M is designated by arrows (from DeLorenzo, 1980a).

simultaneously studied $Ca^{2+}$-calmodulin–stimulated neurotransmitter release and protein phosphorylation in isolated vesicles and intact synaptosomes led to the hypothesis that $Ca^{2+}$-calmodulin–regulated synaptic protein phosphorylation, a distinct phosphorylation system from the cAMP protein kinases (Burke and DeLorenzo, 1981b; DeLorenzo, 1981a), may mediate the effects of $Ca^{2+}$ on neurotransmission (DeLorenzo, 1976, 1977, 1981a–c). The evidence supporting this hypothesis is summarized below.

Protein phosphorylation (Fig. 2) and neurotransmitter release calmodulin in depleted synaptic vesicles was shown to be (Table I) simultaneously stimulated by $Ca^{2+}$ and calmodulin (DeLorenzo et al., 1979; DeLorenzo, 1980b, 1981a). In addition it was shown that vesicle protein phosphorylation and neurotransmitter release had the same requirements for $Mg^{2+}$, ATP, $Ca^{2+}$, and calmodulin (DeLorenzo and Freedman, 1978; DeLorenzo, 1980a,b). Various incubation conditions such as pH and buffer solutions that produced maximal $Ca^{2+}$–stimulated release also gave maximal levels of phosphorylation (DeLorenzo and Freedman, 1978; DeLorenzo, 1981a). Phenytoin (DeLorenzo and Glaser, 1976; DeLorenzo et al., 1977; DeLorenzo, 1980b) and diazepam (Burdette and DeLorenzo, 1980; DeLorenzo et al., 1981) which specifically inhibit the vesicle $Ca^{2+}$-calmodulin kinase system were also shown to significantly inhibit neurotransmitter release (Table I) (DeLorenzo, 1981a,c,d). Trifluoperazine also simultaneously inhibited vesicle protein phosphorylation and neurotransmitter re-

TABLE I

EFFECTS OF CALMODULIN AND Ca$^{2+}$-CALMODULIN KINASE INHIBITORS ON Ca$^{2+}$-CALMODULIN-STIMULATED PROTEIN PHOSPHORYLATION AND NEUROTRANSMITTER RELEASE IN ISOLATED SYNAPTIC VESICLES

| Condition | Neurotransmitter release (%) | | Protein DPH-M phosphorylation (%) |
| --- | --- | --- | --- |
| | Acetylcholine | Norepinephrine | |
| Control | 34 | 38 | 21 |
| Ca$^{2+}$ | 41 | 44 | 25 |
| Calmodulin | 36 | 39 | 22 |
| Ca$^{2+}$ + calmodulin | 100 | 100 | 100 |
| Ca$^{2+}$ + calmodulin | | | |
| + trifluoperazine | 62 | 68 | 55 |
| + phenytoin | 69 | 72 | 49 |
| + diazepam | 61 | 63 | 47 |

Calmodulin depleted synaptic vesicles were isolated and studied for neurotransmitter release and protein DPH-M phosphorylation as described previously (DeLorenzo et al., 1979). The data give the means of ten determinations and are expressed as percentage of the maximally stimulated condition (100 %). The largest S.E.M. was 5.6. The effects of trifluoperazine (15 $\mu$M), phenytoin (80 $\mu$M), and diazepam (15 $\mu$M) were found to be statistically significant in comparison to maximally stimulated values. $P < 0.001$. (From DeLorenzo, 1981c.)

lease (DeLorenzo, 1981b,c) (Table I). Vesicles prepared under conditions that inactivated the labile Ca$^{2+}$-calmodulin kinase system, also showed no significant Ca$^{2+}$–calmodulin–stimulated release. Thus, in the isolated vesicle preparation, there is convincing evidence that protein phosphorylation and neurotransmitter release are simultaneously activated by Ca$^{2+}$ and calmodulin and that the release of neurotransmitter substances is directly dependent on the stimulation of vesicle protein phosphorylation. Several proteins are phosphorylated in the vesicle system, but proteins DPH-M and DPH-L (Fig. 2) were the most consistently observed phosphoproteins that showed the greatest Ca$^{2+}$-calmodulin–stimulated incorporation of [$^{32}$P]phosphate and the most significant inhibition by phenytoin.

In intact synaptosome preparations, depolarization of the synaptosome membrane in the presence of Ca$^{2+}$ stimulated the phosphorylation of an 80 000 dalton protein, designated protein I (Krueger et al., 1977). Depolarization-dependent Ca$^{2+}$ uptake was also shown to stimulate the phosphorylation of proteins DPH-L and DPH-M in intact synaptosomes (DeLorenzo et al., 1979; DeLorenzo, 1980a,b). Since synaptosome preparations are not pure, it was important to demonstrate that the depolarization-dependent increase in protein phosphorylation was actually occuring within the synaptosomes. Experiments were conducted to isolate synaptic vesicle, synaptic membrane, synaptic junction, and postsynaptic density fractions from $^{32}$P-labeled synaptosomes incubated under various conditions. These experiments demonstrated that depolarization-stimulated phosphorylation of proteins DPH-L and DPH-M was occurring in specific synaptosome fractions (DeLorenzo, 1980a).

It was also shown that depolarization-dependent Ca$^{2+}$ uptake simultaneously stimulated both protein phosphorylation and neurotransmitter release in intact synaptosome preparations (DeLorenzo et al., 1979; DeLorenzo, 1980a,b; 1981a,b) (Table II). The phosphorylation of proteins DPH-L, DPH-M, and several other proteins correlated with release in these studies. Furthermore, the level of phosphorylation of protein DPH-M in synaptic vesicle, synaptic junction, and postsynaptic density fractions from intact synaptosomes was shown to also correlate with neurotransmitter release (DeLorenzo, 1980a). Since the Ca$^{2+}$-stimulated levels

TABLE II

EFFECTS OF CALMODULIN AND $Ca^{2+}$-CALMODULIN KINASE INHIBITORS ON NEUROTRANSMITTER RELEASE AND PROTEIN PHOSPHORYLATION IN INTACT NERVE TERMINAL PREPARATIONS

| Condition | Neurotransmitter release (%) | | Protein phosphorylation (%) | |
|---|---|---|---|---|
| | Acetylcholine | Norepinephrine | Whole synaptosome | Synaptic vesicles |
| Control | 45 | 52 | 58 | 39 |
| $Ca^{2+}$ | 51 | 56 | 61 | 44 |
| $Ca^{2+}$, K | 100 | 100 | 100 | 100 |
| + trifluoperazine | 63 | 68 | 69 | 61 |
| + phenytoin | 68 | 70 | 68 | 67 |
| + diazepam | 64 | 59 | 72 | 67 |
| $Ca^{2+}$, A 23187 | 94 | 98 | 91 | 96 |
| + trifluoperazine | 69 | 73 | 72 | 76 |
| + phenytoin | 74 | 76 | 73 | 70 |
| + diazepam | 78 | 75 | 75 | 72 |

Intact synaptosomes were incubated under various conditions after preincubation with $^{32}P$ followed by quantitation of neurotransmitter release and protein DPH-L phosphorylation as described (DeLorenzo et al., 1979; DeLorenzo, 1980a). Concentrations of trifluoperazine, phenytoin, and diazepam were 15, 80 and 20 $\mu$M, respectively. The data give the means of eight determinations and are expressed as percentage of the maximally stimulated condition (100 %). The largest S.E.M. was 6.3. The effects of changes produced by all three drugs in comparison to the maximally stimulated condition was statistically significant. $P < 0.001$. (From DeLorenzo, 1981c.)

of phosphorylation of proteins DPH-L and DPH-M and several other proteins were shown to be dependent on calmodulin in vesicle (DeLorenzo et al., 1979), membrane (DeLorenzo, 1980a), and synaptic junction preparations (DeLorenzo, 1980a; Grab et al., 1980), it is reasonable to conclude that depolarization-dependent $Ca^{2+}$ uptake simultaneously stimulates $Ca^{2+}$-calmodulin-dependent protein phosphorylation and neurotransmitter release in intact synaptosome preparations.

Although work in this laboratory has shown that $Ca^{2+}$ entry into the nerve terminal simultaneously stimulates neurotransmitter release and protein phosphorylation, a more definitive correlation is needed to clearly implicate $Ca^{2+}$-calmodulin kinase activity in the process of neurotransmission. Our studies employing trifluoperazine, diazepam, and phenytoin demonstrated a more direct relationship between phosphorylation and release (Table II) (DeLorenzo, 1981b,c).

Trifluoperazine inhibited both synaptic protein phosphorylation and neurotransmitter release in intact synaptosome preparations (DeLorenzo, 1981b,c). The effect of trifluoperazine on protein phosphorylation was exactly the same as its effect on neurotransmitter release (described above). Trifluoperazine inhibited phosphorylation by both inhibiting depolarization-dependent $Ca^{2+}$ uptake induced by high $K^+$, and by directly inactivating the calmodulin kinase system, as seen in the presence of A 23187. Phenytoin and diazepam also inhibited the activation of calmodulin kinase activity in intact synaptosomes while simultaneously inhibiting neurotransmitter release (Table II). Thus, direct inactivation of calmodulin and the calmodulin kinase system inhibit the $Ca^{2+}$-dependent release process in intact synaptosomes. Combining the direct studies on the isolated vesicle system with the pharmacologic data obtained in the intact synaptosome preparation, it is reasonable to suggest that synaptic $Ca^{2+}$-calmodulin kinase activity may play an important role in mediating the effects of $Ca^{2+}$ on synaptic transmission.

# IDENTIFICATION OF TUBULIN AS A MAJOR SUBSTRATE FOR $Ca^{2+}$-CALMODU-LIN KINASE

To investigate the role of $Ca^{2+}$-calmodulin-stimulated protein phosphorylation in mediating synaptic function studies were initiated to determine the identity and possible function of two of the major synaptic phosphoproteins, proteins DPH-L and DPH-M. Although $Ca^{2+}$ was shown to stimulate the phosphorylation of many proteins in brain, two major phosphoproteins, designated proteins DPH-L and DPH-M, were of particular interest: $Ca^{2+}$-stimulated phosphorylation of these proteins was (1) inhibited by the anticonvulsant, phenytoin (DeLorenzo, 1977; DeLorenzo and Glaser, 1976; DeLorenzo et al., 1977), (2) dependent upon the $Ca^{2+}$-binding protein, calmodulin (DeLorenzo et al., 1979; DeLorenzo, 1980a,b, 1981a–c), (3) present in presynaptic nerve terminal preparations in association with synaptic vesicles, (4) shown to correlate with the $Ca^{2+}$-stimulated release of neurotransmitter substances in isolated synaptic vesicle and intact nerve terminal preparations (DeLorenzo et al., 1979; DeLorenzo, 1980a,b, 1981a), and (5) demonstrated to correlate with synaptic vesicle–synaptic membrane interactions (DeLorenzo, 1980a). In an attempt to determine the possible function or identity of proteins DPH-L and DPH-M, it was observed in our laboratory that these proteins had essentially the same molecular weight and comigrated with the $\alpha$ and $\beta$ subunits of tubulin on SDS–polyacrylamide gel electrophoresis (PAGE) (Burke and DeLorenzo, 1981a). Tubulin preparations have also been shown to contain endogenous protein kinase activity. These findings and the possible similarities between proteins DPH-L and DPH-M and the $\alpha$ and $\beta$ subunits of tubulin stimulated our interest in studying the effects of $Ca^{2+}$ and calmodulin on the endogenous phosphorylation of tubulin.

Tubulin is found in high concentrations in brain (Borisy and Taylor, 1967) and has been implicated in several physiological processes associated with nerve cell function, such as axonal transport, growth and differentiation, stimulus secretion coupling, electrical status of neuronal membranes, and structural and functional integrity of synaptic connections. $Ca^{2+}$ plays a major role in the regulation of tubulin and microtubular assembly and function. $Ca^{2+}$ also binds to neurotubulin, regulates ciliary and flagellar beating in several cell types, and may be involved in the organization of tubulin or tubulin-like proteins in the synaptic junctional complex. Given the significance of $Ca^{2+}$ in the function of the nervous system, it would be of great importance to understand the biochemical effects of $Ca^{2+}$ on tubulin. However, little is known about the molecular mechanism of the action of calcium on tubulin, or the extent to which the effects of calcium on tubulin might mediate the actions of $Ca^{2+}$ on cell function.

Results from this laboratory have shown that $Ca^{2+}$ stimulates the endogenous phosphorylation of neurotubulin isolated from rat brain and that a major part of bands DPH-L and DPH-M are $\alpha$- and $\beta$-tubulin (Burke and DeLorenzo, 1981a,b). The $Ca^{2+}$-stimulated phosphorylation of tubulin isolated by microtubule polymerization is dependent upon the presence of calmodulin and a tubulin-associated protein kinase system. A significant fraction of cytoplasmic calmodulin is associated with tubulin in the form of a $Ca^{2+}$-stimulated tubulin kinase complex, suggesting that the calmodulin-associated tubulin kinase system may modulate some of the effects of $Ca^{2+}$ on nerve cell function.

## $Ca^{2+}$-STIMULATED PHOSPHORYLATION OF TUBULIN

Previous results from this laboratory (Burke and DeLorenzo, 1981a,b) have shown that $Ca^{2+}$ stimulates the endogenous phosphorylation of tubulin in brain cytoplasm and synaptic

262

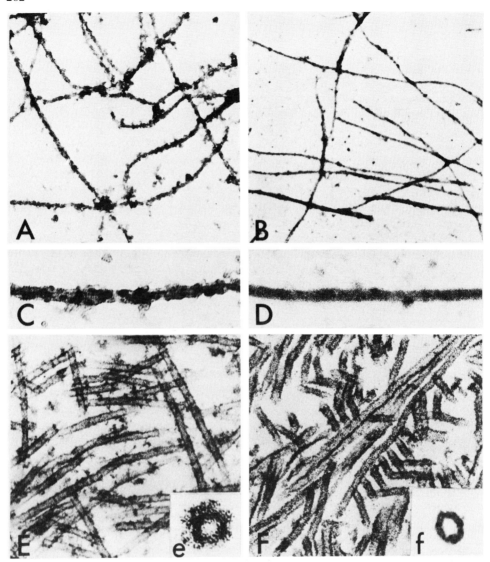

Fig. 3. Microtubules obtained from in vitro polymerization of rat brain tubulin (Shelanski et al., 1973). Briefly, rat brains from five animals were rapidly removed from the heads following decapitation and immediately homogenized at 4°C at a ratio of 1 g of brain to 1 ml of buffer (100 mM Pipes, 2 mM EGTA, 1 mM MgSO$_4$, 1 mM GTP, at pH 6.9). The homogenate was centrifuged at 100 000 × g for 1 h and the supernatant was mixed 1 : 1 with buffer containing 20% glycerol, incubated at 37°C for 30 min, and centrifuged at 100 000 × g at 25°C for 1 h, producing a crude microtubule pellet (tubulin A). The crude microtubule pellet was suspended in buffer (4°C) and put through four cycles of the microtubule assembly–disassembly scheme, producing a highly enriched preparation of tubulin, tubulin B. The resultant extracts (tubulin A extract) from each cycle of polymerization were combined and represented the material removal from tubulin A during the preparation of tubulin B. Negatively stained (A, B, × 16 600; C, D, × 116 200) and thin sections of embedded (E, F, × 50 000; e, f, × 207 500) specimens of microtubules from samples of tubulin A and tubulin B were prepared (Himes et al., 1977) and examined by electron microscopy. Negatively stained microtubules from tubulin A (A, C) appeared coated with an amorphous, granular material that was almost completely removed from the microtubules during multiple cycles of polymerization, producing tubulin B (B, D). The amorphous coating material associated with crude microtubules in tubulin A appeared as thin filamentous strands attached to the microtubules as seen in longitudinal (E) and transverse (e) sections of embedded specimens. Longitudinal (F) and transverse (f) sections of microtubules for tubulin B preparations revealed that most of this coating material had been removed. Adding the tubulin A extract back to the tubulin B preparation just prior to the final cycle of polymerization, produced the same coating material on the microtubules as seen in the tubulin A preparations. The electron micrographs shown are representative of studies from six separate preparations of microtubules.

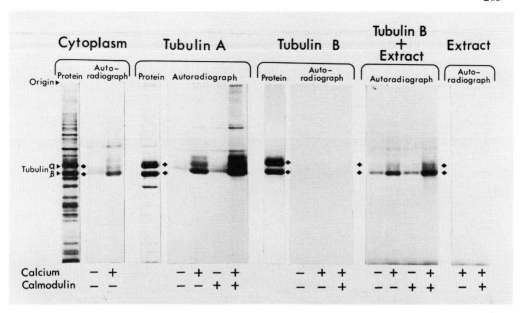

Fig. 4. Protein patterns and autoradiographs illustrating endogenous calcium- and calmodulin-stimulated phosphorylation of tubulin in preparations of brain cytoplasm, crude microtubules (tubulin A) and highly enriched microtubules (tubulin B). Brain cytoplasm, tubulin A, tubulin B, and tubulin A extract (extract) were obtained as described in Fig. 3. Immediately after preparation each fraction was dialyzed in less than 1 h in an Amicon multi-micro ultrafiltration system with a PM-10 membrane against an artificial intracellular medium (Iso-KCl medium plus EDTA, containing 160 mM KCl, 5 mM NaCl, 0.5 mM EDTA, and 10 mM Tris–maleate buffer, pH 6.9) to remove as much as possible of the GTP and magnesium that was introduced into the preparations during microtubule assembly (Fig. 3). The endogenous phosphorylation of tubulin in each fraction was investigated employing established procedures for studying calcium and calcium-stimulated (Burke and DeLorenzo, 1981a) protein phosphorylation in brain. Cytoplasm, tubulin A, and tubulin B (50 $\mu$g of protein) were incubated under standard conditions for 30 sec at 37°C in a 100 $\mu$l volume reaction mixture containing a final concentration of 10 $\mu$M [$\gamma$-$^{32}$P]ATP (5–10 Ci/mmole, from New England Nuclear), 4 mM MgCl$_2$, 100 mM KCl, 5 mM NaCl, 10 mM Tris–maleate, pH 6.5 in the presence or absence of 0.5 mM CaCl$_2$ and where indicated, calmodulin 10 $\mu$g and/or extract from tubulin A (20 $\mu$g). The reactions were indicated by the addition of calcium following a 2 min incubation at 4°C with [$\gamma$-$^{32}$P]ATP. The reactions were terminated by addition of 50 $\mu$l of "SDS stop solution" and a 40 $\mu$l sample of each reaction was analyzed by SDS–PAGE, protein staining, autoradiography, and quantitation of [$^{32}$P]phosphate incorporation (DeLorenzo, 1977). Quantitation of specific protein bands in each fraction was determined by densitometry of the protein pattern stained with fast green. [$^{32}$P]Phosphate incorporation into specific bands was shown to be linked to protein by phosphomonoester linkages and not to lipid or nucleic acids (DeLorenzo et al., 1979). The protein patterns and autoradiographs shown are representative of six separate experiments. Results similar to those shown for tubulin B were obtained when tubulin that was further enriched by phosphocellulose chromatography was substituted for tubulin B in the reaction mixtures. The positions of $\alpha$- and $\beta$-tubulin are indicated by arrows and the additions of calcium and/or calmodulin to the reaction mixtures are denoted by a plus. Activity of the calcium-stimulated endogenous tubulin kinase was decreased by prolonging the preparation time, especially delaying the time between removal of the brain and homogenization. Calmodulin was obtained from rat brain (DeLorenzo, 1980a). Calmodulin was isolated from tubulin A by heating the tubulin A preparation (95°C) for 8 min, cooling on ice, and centrifuging at 130 000 × g for 1 h. The resultant supernatant was then subjected to the standard isolation procedures for calmodulin by DEAE column chromatography and preparative gel electrophoreses.

nerve terminal preparations. The effects of Ca$^{2+}$ on the endogenous phosphorylation of tubulin are presented below.

Crude tubulin (tubulin A) and highly purified tubulin (tubulin B) were isolated from rat brain cytoplasm by microtubule assembly–disassembly (Fig. 3) and studied for endogenous Ca$^{2+}$-

TABLE III

DISTRIBUTION OF TOTAL PROTEIN, TUBULIN, CALMODULIN, AND CALCIUM-STIMULATED PHOSPHORYLATION OF TUBULIN IN EACH FRACTION OBTAINED FROM THE PREPARATION OF MICROTUBULES AND THE EFFECTS OF CALMODULIN AND TUBULIN A EXTRACT ON THIS CALCIUM-STIMULATED PROTEIN PHOSPHORYLATION

| | Total protein (%) | Tubulin (%) | Calmodulin (%) | Calcium-stimulated tubulin phosphorylation | |
| --- | --- | --- | --- | --- | --- |
| | | | | % | RSA |
| Cytoplasm | 100 | 100 | 100 | 100 | 1.00 |
| Supernatant | 87.7 ± 9.7 | 41.3 ± 6.3 | 90.7 ± 4.0 | 31.1 ± 7.4 | 0.35 |
| Tubulin A | 6.9 ± 2.1 | 53.6 ± 5.4 | 4.4 ± 2.1 | 22.4 ± 5.2 | 3.25 |
| + calmodulin | (7.8) | (53.6) | (104.4) | 44.2 ± 6.1 | 5.67 |
| Tubulin B | 3.7 ± 1.4 | 43.6 ± 7.1 | 0.0 | 0.0 | 0.00 |
| + calmodulin | (4.6) | (43.6) | (100) | 0.0 | 0.00 |
| + tubulin A extract | (6.8) | (51.0) | (2.7) | 9.1 ± 2.1 | 1.34 |
| + calmodulin and tubulin A extract | (7.7) | (51.0) | (102.7) | 29.3 ± 5.2 | 3.80 |
| Tubulin A extract | 3.1 ± 1.0 | 7.4 ± 1.6 | 2.7 ± 0.9 | 0.8 ± 0.3 | 0.26 |

Cytoplasm was prepared from rat brain homogenate (ten brains), incubated with microtubule polymerization buffer, and centrifuged as described in Fig. 3. The resultant supernatant was removed and the crude microtubule pellet (tubulin A) was suspended in buffer. Tubulin B and tubulin A extract were isolated from half of the tubulin A preparation by multiple cycles of assembly–disassembly (Fig. 3). Each fraction was dialyzed against Iso-KCl buffer (Fig. 4). Total protein, tubulin, calmodulin, and calcium-stimulated tubulin phosphorylation were determined for four separate preparations of cytoplasm and the mean values of each of these determinations are expressed as 100%, corresponding to mean absolute values of 51.3 mg, 3.54 mg, 0.46 mg, and $3.8 \times 10^5$ cpm, respectively. Total protein, tubulin, calmodulin, and phosphorylation for each cytoplasmic subfraction obtained during microtubule polymerization cycles are presented as the means ± S.E.M. of four separate preparations and are expressed as % starting cytoplasmic values. Relative specific activity (RSA) of calcium-stimulated tubulin phosphorylation for each fraction is expressed as the (mean % calcium-stimulated tubulin phosphorylation)/(mean % total protein). Highly purified calmodulin (Fig. 7) and/or tubulin A extract were added to tubulin A and B fractions in each of the four experiments to determine their effects on calcium-stimulated phosphorylation of tubulin and RSA of the fraction. The amount of calmodulin added to each fraction was equivalent to 100% of the calmodulin in the starting cytoplasm (0.9% total protein). The amount of tubulin A extract added to each fraction was equivalent to the percentage of this fraction in the starting cytoplasm (3.1%, total protein). The corrected calculated values of total protein, tubulin, and calmodulin in the combined fractions are shown in parentheses and represent the total amount in each mixture, taking into account the added protein. Since the amount of calmodulin and tubulin A extract added to the tubulin A and B preparations was constant, S.E.M. were omitted from these values for clarity. Calmodulin isolated from tubulin A and the tubulin kinase system (Fig. 7) produced qualitatively similar results to calmodulin isolated from whole brain. Protein was determined by the method of Lowry et al. (1951). For quantitation of tubulin and calmodulin in each fraction, samples were subjected to SDS–PAGE on slab gels (Fig. 2), which were stained and fixed in 0.5% Fast Green in 50% methanol–7% acetic acid for 1 h at 55°C, and then destained in 5% methanol–7% acetic acid for 1–2 h at 55°C; individual channels were scanned at 650 nm on a Transidyne RFT scanning densitometer (Transidyne General Co., Ann Arbor, MI) and peak areas corresponding to the positions of tubulin and calmodulin were measured with a Hewlett-Packard Model 3380A digital integrator (Hewlett-Packard, Avondale, PA) and expressed as % total protein in the scanned channel. Purified calmodulin and tubulin were used as protein markers. Calcium-stimulated protein phosphorylation was studied by incubating 50 $\mu$g of each franction in the presence or absence of calcium under standard conditions (Fig. 4). Incorporation of $[^{32}P][^{32}P]$phosphate into tubulin was determined by subjecting aliquots of each reaction mixture to SDS–PAGE and protein staining, by cutting out the protein staining bands corresponding to tubulin, and quantitating the radioactivity in each tubulin band by liquid scintillation counting. Radioactive bands comigrating with tubulin were shown to be due to incorporation of $[^{32}P]$phosphate into protein by phosphomonoester linkage as described previously. Calcium stimulation of $[^{32}P]$phosphate incorporation into tubulin is expressed as cpm/mg protein in comparison to the magnesium control condition. The calcium-stimulated phosphorylation of tubulin was significantly reduced by prolonging the length of subfractionation time, and thus the data shown were determined from four isolations that were performed in less than 5 h and immediately incubated under standard conditions.

dependent protein phosphorylation by our previously described procedures (Burke and DeLorenzo, 1981a). $Ca^{2+}$ caused a marked stimulation of endogenous incorporation of $[^{32}P]$ phosphate from $[\gamma\text{-}^{32}P]$-ATP into protein bands that comigrated on SDS–PAGE with the $\alpha$ and $\beta$ subunits of tubulin in both cytoplasmic and tubulin A preparations (Fig. 4, Table III). Tubulin A contained approximately 53.6 % of the tubulin and 22.4 % of the $Ca^{2+}$-stimulated phosphorylation of tubulin from the starting cytoplasm (Table III). The $\alpha$- and $\beta$-tubulins comprised 66.5 % of the total protein in the tubulin A preparation. The relative specific activity (RSA) of $Ca^{2+}$-stimulated phosphorylation of tubulin in the tubulin A preparation was increased 3.25-fold in comparison to the starting cytoplasm (Table III). To further demonstrate

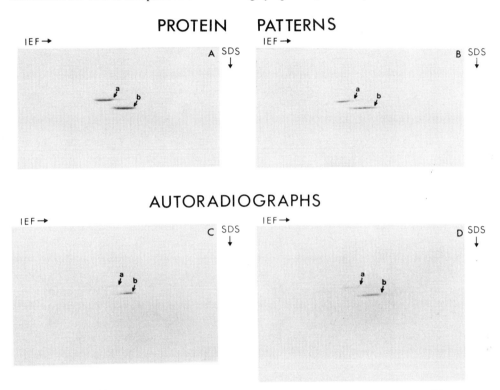

## PROTEIN    PATTERNS

## AUTORADIOGRAPHS

Fig. 5. Protein patterns of tubulin B (A) and the TK system (B) and autoradiographs of the $Ca^{2+}$-stimulated phosphorylation of tubulin A and the TK system (D) from two-dimensional gel electrophoresis. The isoelectric focusing (IEF) direction is from left to right with the basic isoelectric points to the left and acidic to the right. The direction of SDS–PAGE was from top to bottom as designated by arrows. The protein patterns were obtained by subjecting 8 $\mu$g of tubulin B (A) and 8 $\mu$g of the TK system prepared by DEAE column chromatography (B) to 2D gel electrophoresis and staining with Coomassie blue. The 2D gel system, utilizing isoelectric focusing followed by SDS gel electrophoresis, was performed as described by O'Farrell (1975) except for a minor modification of sample preparation due to the presence of SDS in our reaction mixtures. Protein samples were solubilized in our standard SDS stop solution mixture (1 % SDS) and samples for autoradiography were prepared by terminating the endogenous phosphorylation reactions after 20 sec with SDS stop solution as described in Fig. 4. All protein samples in the 1 % SDS stop solution were then mixed with 9 volumes of focusing buffer containing 9.5 M urea, 1.6 % (w/v) pH 5–7 ampholytes, 0.4 % (w/v) 3–10 ampholytes, 4 % (v/v) nonidet P-40, and 5 % (v/v) $\beta$-mercaptoethanol. Solubilization in this focusing buffer was performed at room temperature. Sample volume for the focusing gels was approximately 50 $\mu$l, containing 8 $\mu$g of sample protein. Dilution of the SDS concentration to 0.1 % with focusing buffer prior to isoelectric focusing prevented any artifacts due to SDS in the IEF direction, as determined by comparing these results to protein patterns of samples performed without the addition of SDS. Utilization of SDS in this system allowed us to study phosphorylation reactions that could be terminated at short time intervals with SDS.

266

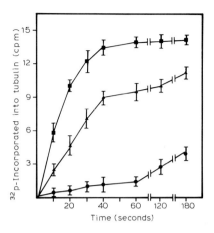

Fig. 6. Time course of calcium- and calmodulin-stimulated [$^{32}$P]phosphate incorporation into tubulin. Reactions were conducted under standard conditions with tubulin A and quantitated for [$^{32}$P]phosphate incorporation into tubulin as described (Fig. 4), except for variation in incubation time and with the following additions: 0.5 mM calcium (▲——▲); 0.5 mM calcium plus 10 $\mu$g calmodulin (■——■); and no additions (●——●). Data give the mean values ±S.E.M. for five determinations and are representative of six individual experiments. Calmodulin alone produced no change from the control conditions with no additions. Calmodulin isolated from whole rat brain was employed in the experiment shown, but calmodulin isolated from tubulin A and the tubulin kinase system (Fig. 8) produced identical results to those presented).

that the $^{32}$P-protein phosphate was incorporated into tubulin and not minor protein components comigrating with tubulin on SDS–PAGE, phosphorylated brain cytoplasm was subjected to two-dimensional (2D) gel electrophoresis. The majority of $Ca^{2+}$-stimulated [$^{32}$P]phosphate associated with tubulin staining in Fig. 4 was also found to comigrate with $\alpha$- and $\beta$-tubulin on 2D gels, as described in Fig. 5.

$Ca^{2+}$ stimulated both the initial rate and net level of phosphorylation of tubulin in these fractions, and reached half-maximal levels of [$^{32}$P]phosphate incorporation in less than 30 sec (Fig. 6). The free calcium concentration required to produce a half-maximal stimulation of tubulin phosphorylation in the tubulin A preparation was calculated to be 0.53 $\mu$M, using a $Ca^{2+}$–EGTA buffering system (Fig. 4). The activation of tubulin phosphorylation by $Ca^{2+}$ also required the presence of $Mg^{2+}$, as described for $Ca^{2+}$-stimulated phosphorylation of synaptosome and synaptic vesicle proteins (DeLorenzo et al., 1979; DeLorenzo, 1981a). The well described $Mg^{2+}$-dependent (Fig. 6) and cAMP-stimulated phosphorylation of tubulin (Jameson et al., 1980; Soifer, 1975) require much longer than $Ca^{2+}$-stimulated phosphorylation to reach half-maximal levels of phosphorylation, usually greater than 10–15 min. $Ca^{2+}$ also stimulated the phosphorylation of some of the other minor components in tubulin A preparations (Fig. 4), but the majority of $Ca^{2+}$-stimulated protein phosphorylation was associated with the $\alpha$ and $\beta$ subunits of tubulin under standard conditions. The majority of [$^{32}$P]phosphate radioactivity comigrating with tubulin was shown to be incorporated into tubulin protein by phosphomonoester linkage (Fig. 4).

The $Ca^{2+}$-stimulated endogenous phosphorylation of tubulin was lost when minor protein impurities were further removed from tubulin A preparations by multiple cycles of microtubule depolymerization and repolymerization, producing a highly enriched preparation of tubulin, tubulin B (Fig. 4, Table III). However, $Ca^{2+}$-stimulated endogenous phosphorylation of tubulin was restored to the tubulin B preparation when the protein impurities extracted from tubulin A were added back to tubulin B (Fig. 4, Table III). The tubulin A extract itself contained negligible amounts of endogenous $Ca^{2+}$-stimulated tubulin phosphorylation under standard conditions. Qualitatively identical results were obtained when tubulin that was further purified from tubulin B by phosphocellulose chromatography (Himes et al., 1977) was substituted for tubulin B in the phosphorylation reactions, demonstrating that highly purified tubulin can serve as a substrate for the $Ca^{2+}$-stimulated protein kinase system. These results indicate that the loss of $Ca^{2+}$-stimulated tubulin phosphorylation during further purification of tubulin was not the result of irreversible inactivation of the $Ca^{2+}$-dependent tubulin kinase system, but rather due to the removal from tubulin A of essential components of this phosphorylating system that could be added back to highly purified tubulin, restoring the endogenous $Ca^{2+}$-stimulated phosphorylation of tubulin.

The importance of microtubule-associated proteins in the function of tubulin has been suggested in several preparations and sources of tubulin. Examination of tubulin A and tubulin B preparations by electron microscopy of both negatively stained and thin sections specimens (Fig. 3) revealed that microtubules in tubulin A (Fig. 3A, C, E, e) were consistently coated with additional amorphous material. This coating material was almost totally removed from the microtubules during further cycles of purification, producing tubulin B (Fig. 3B, D, F, f). Addition of tubulin A extract back to tubulin B not only restored $Ca^{2+}$-stimulated phosphorylation of tubulin to this preparation (Fig. 4, Table III), but also produced the same coating appearance on the tubulin B microtubules as seen in the starting tubulin A, suggesting that some of these microtubule-associated materials might play a role in mediating the effects of $Ca^{2+}$ on the endogenous phosphorylation of tubulin. Electron microscopic examination has shown that filamentous (Himes et al., 1977) or amorphous coating material (Burns, 1978) are often attached to the walls of microtubules. More specifically, high molecular weight microtubule-associated proteins (MAPs) have been shown to produce filamentous coating on surfaces of microtubules assembled in vitro (Dentler et al., 1975) and to be distributed along the lengths of microtubules in situ (Connolly et al., 1978). Recently, highly enriched $MAO_2$ protein has been elegantly shown to produce a filamentous decoration of in vitro assembled brain microtubules (Kim et al., 1979). The possible presence of MAPs or other specific proteins in the tubulin kinase system is an important area for further investigation. Several minor high molecular weight components have been observed in the tubulin kinase system (Fig. 10), but more definitive studies are required to confirm the presence of MAPs in this $Ca^{2+}$-stimulated kinase system.

## CALMODULIN-STIMULATED $Ca^{2+}$-DEPENDENT PHOSPHORYLATION OF TUBULIN

The $Ca^{2+}$ receptor protein, calmodulin ($Ca^{2+}$-dependent regulator protein, CDR) or calmodulin-like proteins have been suggested to mediate many functions of calcium in neuronal and non-neuronal tissues (Cheung, 1980; Klee et al., 1980; DeLorenzo, 1980a). It would be important to determine if calmodulin is involved as a microtubule-associated protein in modulating the stimulatory effect of calcium on the phosphorylation of tubulin. To test this possibility, calmodulin was purified from bovine and rat brain by standard procedures (Fig. 7). The effects of this $Ca^{2+}$ receptor protein on $Ca^{2+}$-stimulated phosphorylation of tubulin were determined and are presented in Figs. 4 and 6 and Table III.

Calmodulin isolated from rat and bovine brain caused a significant increase in both the net level and initial rate of $Ca^{2+}$-stimulated [$^{32}P$]phosphate incorporation into tubulin (Fig. 6). The

268

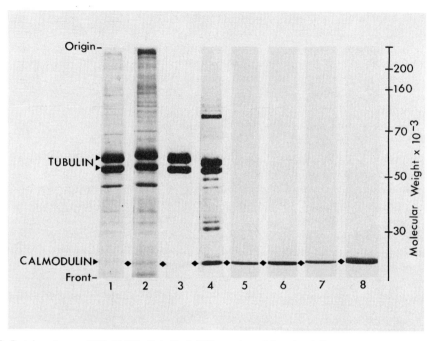

Fig. 7. Protein pattern on SDS–PAGE of tubulin A (250 $\mu$g, channel 1), calmodulin isolated from whole rat brain (15 $\mu$g, channel 2), calmodulin-like protein isolated from tubulin A (25 $\mu$g, channel 3) and the calmodulin tubulin kinase system fraction Fd (15 $\mu$g, channel 4), and a mixture of the protein samples in channels 2–4 (55 $\mu$g, channel 5). Tubulin A was isolated as described in Fig. 3. Highly purified calmodulin was isolated from rat brain as performed previously in the laboratory (DeLorenzo, 1980a). Calmodulin-like proteins (channels 3 and 4) were isolated from tubulin A and the tubulin kinase system by subjecting these protein fractions to the same isolation procedure employed to purify calmodulin from whole brain (heat treatment, DEAE column chromatography, and preparative non-SDS–PAGE). Protein samples were subjected to SDS–PAGE and stained with Coomassie blue (Fig. 4). The position of purified calmodulin is designated by arrows. For protein quantitation acrylamide gels were stained with Fast Green and quantitated by densitometry (Table III). Calmodulin comprised 0.21 % ± 0.05 of the total protein in tubulin A, expressed as the mean value of five isolation procedures ± S.E.M. Calmodulin proteins in the preparations of rat brain, tubulin A, and tubulin kinase system calmodulin (channels 2–4, respectively) were determined to comprise over 97 % of the total protein in each of these fractions. Calmodulin proteins isolated from tubulin A and the tubulin kinase system were shown to be immunologically identical (Fig. 8) and functionally identical to calmodulin isolated from whole brain.

concentration of calmodulin required to produce a half-maximal activation of the $Ca^{2+}$-stimulated phosphorylation of tubulin under standard conditions was about 1–3 $\mu$g. Calmodulin increased the RSA of $Ca^{2+}$-stimulated tubulin phosphorylation in tubulin A from 3.25 to 5.67 (Table III). Half-maximal stimulation of tubulin phosphorylation in the presence of calmodulin occurred at a free $Ca^{2+}$ concentration of approximately 0.41 $\mu$M (Fig. 4), which is consistent with the half-maximal concentrations of free $Ca^{2+}$ required to produce half-maximal activation of calmodulin-dependent phosphodiesterase (Klee et al., 1980).

Quantitation of the protein staining pattern of tubulin A (Fig. 7) revealed that approximately 0.21 % of the total protein in tubulin A comigrated as a single band with calmodulin from rat brain. This calmodulin-like protein was purified from tubulin A (Fig. 7) and shown to be a heat-stable protein that was immunologically identical to rat brain cytosol calmodulin (Fig. 8). Calmodulin isolated from tubulin A was also found to be functionally identical to calmodulin isolated from whole brain, since this microtubule-associated protein was shown in this

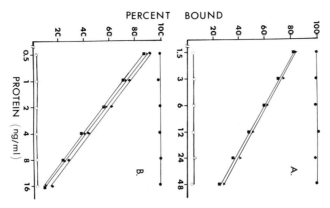

Fig. 8. Radioimmunoassays (RIA) for tubulin (A) and calmodulin (B) were developed using antisera from NZW (New Zealand White) female rabbits immunized with purified tubulin or calmodulin in complete Freund's adjuvant and boosted intravenously at 2-week intervals until suitable antisera were obtained. The assay method was modified from Hardin using a solid phase linked antigen in microtiter plates (Cooke Microtiter System). 100 $\mu$l of purified tubulin (A) or purified calmodulin (B) in PBS (0.05 M, pH 7.4) was absorbed to the microtiter plate wells by incubation for 18 h at 4°C. The wells were washed with PBS, incubated with PBS 0.3% gelatine for 2 h at 37°C, and washed again. 100 $\mu$l of anti-tubulin antisera (A) or anti-calmodulin antisera (B) were incubated in the wells for 24 h at 4°C with various concentrations of the proteins believed to be identical with the solid phase antigens in order to competitively inhibit the binding of antibody to the solid phase linked antigen. After washing the wells 100 $\mu$l of [$^{125}$I]Staphylococcal protein A (NEN, Pharmacia) was added to detect the amount of antibody bound to the solid phase antigen. Unbound [$^{125}$I]Staphylococcal protein A was then removed with three washes, and each well counted in a Beckman 4000 Gamma Counter. Maximum bound radioactivity (counts per minute) was determined for no added inhibitor protein ( ●——● , A and B), and the inhibition curve expressed as percentage of the maximum bound counts per minute. The assays were conducted in PBS 0.1% BSA, 0.2% azide to prevent nonspecific binding to the plastic wells. The assays were performed in triplicate and the largest standard error of the mean was ± 5%. The tubulin RIA (A) demonstrated a reaction of identity or parallel inhibition curves between tubulin isolated from a microtubulin preparation, tubulin B, ( ■——■ ) and tubulin isolated from the tubulin kinase system, fraction Fd ( ▲——▲ ). The calmodulin RIA (B) shows the reaction of identity between rat brain calmodulin ( ▲——▲ ), calmodulin from the Fd fraction ( ■——■ ), and calmodulin from crude tubulin A ( ◆——◆ ). Highly purified tubulin was obtained from tubulin A and Fd fractions by isolation of tubulin from each preparation by SDS–PAGE (Figs. 4 and 10), localization of tubulin on the gels by scanning at 265 nm with a Transidyne RFT scanning densitometer, and extraction of the tubulin from the gels according to the procedure developed by Matus et al., 1979. Tubulin isolated from these preparations was then dialyzed against 5000 × the volume of 10 mM Tris–maleate buffer, pH 7.0, for 24 h, concentrated in an Amicon UM 8 unit, and used for inhibition studies in the RIA. Highly purified calmodulin was isolated from rat brain cytosol and the proteins believed to be identical to calmodulin were isolated from tubulin A and Fd fractions as described in Fig. 10. Preimmune sera ( ○——○ ) served as control for blank values in both assays. Calmodulin in the tubulin assay and tubulin in the calmodulin assay demonstrated no cross-reactivity between tubulin antibody and calmodulin, and between calmodulin antibody and tubulin, respectively, and produced essentially identical curves to those for no added inhibitor protein ( ●——● ).

laboratory to activate $Ca^{2+}$-stimulated phosphodiesterase activity and synaptic vesicle protein phosphorylation (Table III). The absolute degree of stimulation of endogenous phosphorylation produced by added calmodulin in tubulin A varied slightly from preparation to preparation, depending in part on the amount of endogenous calmodulin in this preparation.

Tubulin B did not contain detectable amounts of calmodulin as determined by protein staining, direct isolation procedures, and radioimmunoassay. Furthermore, calmodulin alone did not restore $Ca^{2+}$-stimulated endogenous phosphorylation to the tubulin B preparation, but did stimulate the effect of $Ca^{2+}$ on the phosphorylation of tubulin when tubulin A extract was added back to this preparation (Table III, Fig. 4). These results suggest that further purification

270

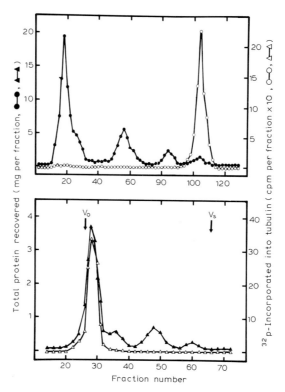

Fig. 9. Isolation of calcium-stimulated calmodulin-associated tubulin kinase activity by ion exchange chromatography on DEAE-cellulose and by molecular sieving chromatography on Sephadex G-200. A: Rat brains were homogenized (1 g brain/4 ml buffer) in 0.32 M sucrose, centrifuged at $100\,000 \times g$ for 1 h, and the resultant supernatant (cytoplasm, 120 mg) was applied to a 12 ml column of DEAE-cellulose (Whatman DE52) equilibrated with 160 mM KCl and 10 mM Tris–maleate buffer, pH 6.9. The column was eluted under pressure at 4 ml/min and 3 ml fractions were collected. After the sample was applied in a 35 ml volume the column was washed with 0.32 M sucrose in 10 mM Tris–maleate, pH 6.9 eluting fractions 10–39 (fraction Fa); at tube 40 the buffer was changed to 160 mM KCl plus 10 mM Tris–maleate and fractions 40–72 were eluted (fraction Fb); at fraction 73 the buffer was changed to 250 mM KCl plus 10 mM Tris–maleate and fractions 73–92 were eluted (fraction Fc); at fraction 92 the buffer was changed to 400 mM KCl plus 10 mM Tris–maleate pH 6.9 and fractions 92–112 were eluted (fraction Fd). Protein was determined for each fraction by the method of Lowry et al. (1951) (●——●). Endogenous [$^{32}$P]phosphate incorporation into tubulin for each fraction was determined by incubating equal aliquots under standard conditions in the presence of calcium and subjecting the stopped reaction mixture to SDS–PAGE, staining, and quantitation as described in Fig. 4 (○——○). The total recoveries of protein and calcium-stimulated phosphorylation of tubulin were 94% and 43%, respectively. Essentially all of the recovered calcium-dependent phosphorylation of tubulin was present in fractions 92–112. B: Gel filtration of fraction Fd containing the calcium-stimulated tubulin kinase activity from the DEAE column on Sephadex G-200. The peak fractions of calcium-stimulated tubulin kinase activity from the DEAE column (fractions 92–112) were pooled and 30 mg of this peak was applied to a 1.5 cm × 40 cm column of Sephadex G-200 equilibrated with 160 mM KCl plus 10 mM Tris–maleate, pH 6.9 and eluted with the same buffer, collecting 3 ml fractions. The void volume ($V_o$) and the salt volume ($V_s$) are indicated by arrows. Each fraction was assayed for protein and endogenous calcium-stimulated tubulin kinase activity as described above. Essentially 100% of the calcium-stimulated tubulin kinase activity (△——△) and 57% of the applied protein (▲——▲) eluted in fractions 22–32 near the void volume. SDS–PAGE of samples from peaks formed by pooling fractions 22–32, 33–40, 41–51, and 56–64 revealed that the main protein peak (fractions 22–32) contained 81% of the tubulin and 76% of the calmodulin staining from the starting Fd fraction applied to the column.

of tubulin not only removed calmodulin from the tubulin A preparation, but also other important components of the tubulin kinase system. Addition of calmodulin to brain cytoplasm caused only a negligible increase in the $Ca^{2+}$-dependent phosphorylation of tubulin in this preparation, since the cytoplasm has saturating levels of calmodulin, representing approximately 1% of the total soluble protein.

## ISOLATION OF THE $Ca^{2+}$ AND CALMODULIN TUBULIN KINASE SYSTEM

If some of the effects of $Ca^{2+}$ on tubulin-containing systems are mediated by calmodulin and $Ca^{2+}$-stimulated phosphorylation of tubulin, it might be expected that calmodulin and the $Ca^{2+}$ tubulin kinase would be associated with tubulin in brain cytoplasm in the form of a $Ca^{2+}$ calmodulin tubulin kinase complex. During the polymerization of microtubules from brain cytoplasm, it is possible that the presence of EGTA in the polymerization mixture may cause the dissociation of calmodulin and possibly some of the tubulin kinase from tubulin, resulting in the large proportion of calmodulin in the supernatant fraction following the first microtubule polymerization (Table III). To evaluate the possible existence in brain cytoplasm of a calmodulin-$Ca^{2+}$ tubulin kinase system, brain cytoplasm that was not treated with EGTA was subjected to ion exchange chromatography on DEAE-cellulose and by molecular sieving on Sephadex G-200 (Fig. 9A,B).

Fractionation of brain cytoplasm by DEAE-cellulose chromatography revealed that the endogenous $Ca^{2+}$-stimulated tubulin kinase system was retained on the column and finally eluted at 300–350 mM ionic strength in a single peak containing over 96% of the recovered $Ca^{2+}$-stimulated endogenous phosphorylation of tubulin and less than 7% of the starting cytoplasmic protein (fractions 96–112, Fd, Fig. 9A). The distribution of total protein, tubulin, calmodulin, and $Ca^{2+}$-stimulated phosphorylation of tubulin in each fraction from the DEAE column is presented in Table IV and the SDS–PAGE protein patterns and the autoradiographs

TABLE IV

DISTRIBUTION OF TOTAL PROTEIN, TUBULIN, CALMODULIN, AND CALCIUM-STIMULATED TUBU-LIN PHOSPHORYLATION IN EACH FRACTION OBTAINED FROM THE PREPARATION OF THE CAL-MODULIN TUBULIN KINASE SYSTEM BY DEAE-CELLULOSE COLUMN CHROMATOGRAPHY

| Fraction | Total protein (%) | Tubulin (%) | Calmodulin (%) | Calcium-stimulated tubulin phosphorylation | |
|---|---|---|---|---|---|
| | | | | % | RSA |
| Cytoplasm | 100 | 100 | 100 | 100 | 100 |
| Fa | $56.9 \pm 6.3$ | $6.2 \pm 1.3$ | $1.3 \pm 0.4$ | $0.9 \pm 0.2$ | 0.02 |
| Fb | $26.0 \pm 4.1$ | $3.4 \pm 1.8$ | $0.7 \pm 0.5$ | $0.6 \pm 0.1$ | 0.02 |
| Fc | $8.9 \pm 1.6$ | $2.0 \pm 0.9$ | $1.2 \pm 0.9$ | $0.3 \pm 0.1$ | 0.03 |
| Fd | $6.6 \pm 1.8$ | $82.1 \pm 9.6$ | $90.7 \pm 4.2$ | $43.5 \pm 8.1$ | 6.59 |

Rat brain cytoplasm was subjected to column chromatography on DEAE-cellulose and fractions Fa, Fb, Fc, and Fd were obtained as des described in Fig. 10. Cytoplasm total protein, tubulin, calmodulin, and calcium-stimulated tubulin phosphorylation were determined as described in Table III for four separate isolation procedures. Mean values of each determination in the starting cytoplasm are expressed as 100%, corresponding to mean absolute values of 125 mg, 6.3 mg, 0.83 mg, and $9.3 \times 10^5$ cpm, respectively. Total protein, tubulin, calmodulin, and calcium-stimulated tubulin phosphorylation for fractions Fa, Fb, Fc, and Fd are expressed as the means of four separate experiments $\pm$ S.E.M. and are expressed as percentage of the starting cytoplasmic values. RSA is expressed as described in Table III.

272

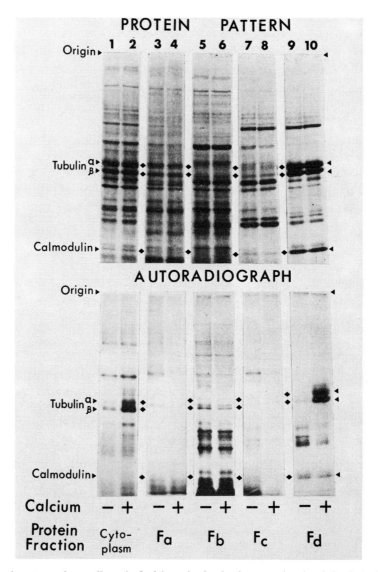

Fig. 10. Protein pattern and autoradiograph of calcium-stimulated endogenous phosphorylation for brain cytoplasm and each major protein peak from the DEAE column chromatograph of brain cytoplasm (Fig. 9A). Protein fractions Fa, Fb, Fc, and Fd correspond to the protein peaks composed of fractions 12–30, 48–68, 78–90, and 96–112, respectively, from the DEAE column chromatograph shown in Fig. 9A. Each protein fraction from the column and the starting cytoplasm was dialyzed against Iso-KCl plus EDTA, incubated under standard conditions for 30 sec in the presence or absence of 0.5 mM calcium, stopped with SDS stop solution, and subjected to SDS–PAGE, protein staining, and autoradiography as described in Fig. 4. The protein patterns illustrate the marked enrichment of the cytoplasmic protein staining of tubulin and calmodulin in fraction Fd (arrows). Tubulin and calmodulin accounted for over 73 % of the total protein staining in fraction Fd. The autoradiographs demonstrate that essentially all of the recovered calcium-stimulated phosphorylation of tubulin was also present in fraction Fd (arrows). Fractions Fa, Fb, and Fc showed essentially no calcium-stimulated phosphorylation of tubulin or protein staining for tubulin and calmodulin. The results shown are representative of six separate experiments.

of endogenous $Ca^{2+}$-stimulated protein phosphorylation in each major fraction from the DEAE column in comparison to the starting cytoplasm are shown in Fig. 10. Over 90% and 82% of the cytoplasmic protein staining of calmodulin and tubulin, respectively, were recovered in fraction Fd along with essentially all of the recovered endogenous $Ca^{2+}$-stimulated phosphorylation of tubulin (Table IV), indicating that tubulin, calmodulin and the tubulin kinase system co-purified. Calmodulin and tubulin comprised approximately 73% of the total protein in the Fd fraction. The presence of calmodulin and tubulin in the tubulin kinase fraction were confirmed by 2D gel electrophoresis (Fig. 5) and RIA for tubulin and calmodulin (Fig. 8). The mean RSA of $Ca^{2+}$-stimulated phosphorylation of tubulin in fraction Fd was increased by 6.59-fold in comparison to the starting cytoplasm (Table IV). The mean total recovery of cytoplasmic $Ca^{2+}$-stimulated phosphorylation of tubulin from the column was 45.3%, indicating that some of the total activity was lost during column chromatography. However, essentially all of the recovered activity was associated with the majority of calmodulin and tubulin in fraction Fd (Table IV). Addition of calmodulin to fraction Fd did not significantly stimulate $Ca^{2+}$ tubulin kinase activity since this preparation has a saturating level of calmodulin (Table IV).

To exclude the possibility that tubulin, calmodulin, and the tubulin kinase system in fraction Fd were merely eluting together from the DEAE column because they possessed similar net charges under the conditions of chromatography, fraction Fd was subjected to molecular sieving on Sephadex G-200 (Fig. 9B). Essentially all over the recovered endogenous $Ca^{2+}$-stimulated phosphorylation of tubulin eluted near the void volume of the Sephadex column (fractions 22–32, Fig. 9B) and contained a significant portion of the tubulin and calmodulin and several of the other protein components initially applied to the column (Fig. 10). These results indicate that tubulin, calmodulin, and the $Ca^{2+}$ tubulin kinase system co-purify. The total recovery of $Ca^{2+}$-stimulated phosphorylation of tubulin applied to the column was about 38% and essentially 100% of this recovered activity was associated with fractions 22–32 (Fig. 9B). Calmodulin caused a slight but significant stimulation of the tubulin kinase system related by Sephadex chromatography, confirming that some of the calmodulin originally associated with the tubulin kinase system had dissociated during the isolation procedure.

Incubation of the calmodulin tubulin kinase system (fraction Fd) with 5.0 mM EGTA prior to Sephadex chromatography caused the majority of the calmodulin to dissociate from the tubulin kinase system in the void volume peak and elute according to apparent column molecular weight of 25 000–30 000. The calmodulin-depleted tubulin kinase system eluted near the void volume of the column, but showed very low levels of $Ca^{2+}$-stimulated endogenous phosphorylation. Addition of calmodulin to the preparation restored the ability of $Ca^{2+}$ to stimulate the incorporation of [$^{32}$P]phosphate into tubulin by the tubulin system. The $Ca^{2+}$ tubulin kinase did not significantly separate from the void volume peak following EGTA treatment. Preliminary attempts to isolate the tubulin kinase from this fraction by various methods of chromatography have been unsuccessful, since enzyme activity is lost upon prolonged purification procedures. The results demonstrate that concentrations of EGTA employed in microtubule polymerization procedures (0.5–5 mM) can dissociate calmodulin from the tubulin kinase system, further indicating that EGTA releases the calmodulin from the tubulin kinase system.

Kinetic studies on the calmodulin tubulin kinase system isolated by column chromatography (Fig. 9) provide further evidence indicating that the proteins involved in this fraction, existed in the form of a complex. When different protein concentrations of the tubulin kinase system were incubated under standard reaction conditions (Fig. 4) in the presence or absence of $Ca^{2+}$, the time required to reach half-maximal levels of endogenous $Ca^{2+}$-stimulated phosphoryla-

274

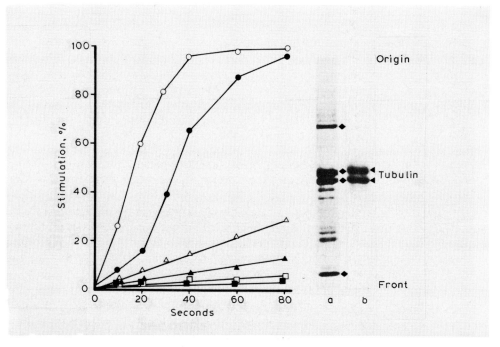

Fig. 11. Time course of endogenous tubulin phosphorylation and formation of microfilaments from the TK system. TK preparations from DEAE chromatography (Fig. 9A) were incubated at different time intervals under standard conditions except for the presence of 10 $\mu$M $Ca^{2+}$ plus 4 mM $Mg^{2+}$ ( O——O ), 4 M $Mg^{2+}$ ( △——△ ), and no divalent cations ( □——□ ) with 1.5 mg/ml TK protein in a reaction volume of 1 ml and the incorporation of [$^{32}$P]phosphate into tubulin was quantitated as described in Table III. To study the formation of microfilaments from the TK system, TK protein (1.5 mg/ml) was incubated exactly as described for the phosphorylation reaction, except that non-radioactive ATP was employed. The formation of microfilaments in the presence of 10 $\mu$M $Ca^{2+}$ plus 4 mM $Mg^{2+}$ ( ●——● ), 4 mM $Mg^{2+}$ ( ▲——▲ ), and no divalent cations ( ■——■ ) was followed by measuring absorbance at 350 nM for each reaction tube in a Gilford 2000 recording spectrophotometer. Samples at different time points were examined by electron microscopy (Fig. 12) and the changes in absorbance at 350 nM were shown to be proportional to the formation of microfilaments. The data for phosphorylation and changes in absorption are expressed as a percentage of maximal stimulation for comparison. The data give the mean values of four determinations and represent three separate experiments. The largest S.E.M. was 6 % and thus they were omitted for clarity. Centrifugation of the reaction tubes at 50 000 × g for 10 min produced a significant pellet and a clear supernatant for the $Ca^{2+}$ plus $Mg^{2+}$ condition, but little or no pellet was formed for the other conditions. Examination of this pellet by EM (Fig. 13) revealed that it was composed of microfilaments. The protein pattern (insert) for the whole reaction mixture (a) and the $Ca^{2+}$ plus $Mg^{2+}$ pellet (b) revealed that over 90 % of the total protein in the pellet was tubulin. Minor traces of calmodulin and the 100 000 dalton protein could also be found in the 10 nm filament pellet. Prolonged incubation of the TK system in the presence of 10 $\mu$M $Ca^{2+}$ caused the gradual breakdown of the tubulin doublet with formation of lower molecular weight proteins. This breakdown could be inhibited by iodoacetate, a known inhibitor of protease activity. The microfilament pellet was also found to contain over 86 % of the [$^{32}$P]phosphate incorporated into tubulin in the reaction mixture. Addition of EGTA (5 mM) and EDTA (10 mM) to the filament preparation after 2 min of incubation had no effect on the stability of the filaments, suggesting that $Ca^{2+}$ was not involved in maintaining the structures of the filaments. Treatment of these filaments with low and high (1 M) salt concentrations (either NaCl or KCl) also did not cause any significant breakdown of the 10 nm filament structure. Several attempts to form microtubules from the TK system employing standard polymerization procedures were not successful. Preliminary attempts to form microtubules from the TK system employing higher concentrations of EGTA (5–10 mM) in the polymerization media resulted in the formation of a few microtubules. These results suggest that the TK system can form microfilaments from phosphorylated tubulin, but does not appear to be able to form microtubules under standard conditions. The formation of microfilaments from the TK system xas shown not to be the result of minor pH changes in the reaction mixture due to the addition of divalent cations in the presence of EGTA and ADTA. The pH of each reaction tube was determined by pH electrode (Orion) before and after incubation under different conditions. Addition of $Ca^{2+}$ alone to the TK system (in the absence of $Mg^{2+}$) did not stimulate the phosphorylation of tubulin or the formation of microfilaments, suggesting further that the formation of the filaments required the phosphorylation of tubulin.

tion of tubulin were essentially independent of the concentration of the protein fraction added to the reaction mixture. These results indicate that the enzymes, substrates, and modulators involved in this $Ca^{2+}$-stimulated phosphorylating system are associated in the form of a complex ready to be activated by $Ca^{2+}$, and are not freely dispersed in the reaction media.

## $Ca^{2+}$-STIMULATED FORMATION OF MICROFILAMENTS FROM THE TUBULIN KINASE SYSTEM

Since we have shown that a considerable portion of tubulin and calmodulin in brain cytoplasm is associated with the $Ca^{2+}$-stimulated tubulin kinase system, it would be important to determine the possible function of this $Ca^{2+}$-activated complex. For example, does the activation of the tubulin kinase system cause the assembly or association of phosphorylated tubulin kinase reaction mixtures became turbid when incubated under standard conditions in the presence of $Ca^{2+}$ (DeLorenzo, 1981b,c; Burke and DeLorenzo, 1981a,b). By simultaneously quantitating the endogenous phosphorylation of tubulin and the turbidity changes in the reaction mixtures under various incubation conditions, it was found that conditions producing maximal levels of phosphorylation of tubulin also caused the greatest increase in turbidity (Fig. 11). The increase in turbidity was detected within seconds after the addition of $Ca^{2+}$, but lagged slightly behind the incorporation of [$^{32}$P]phosphate into tubulin (Fig. 11). Centrifugation of the turbid reaction mixtures after 2 min of incubation at $60\,000 \times g$ at $4°C$ for 20 min produced a pellet and a clear supernatant. The pellet contained only $14.3 \pm 6.1\%$ of the total protein in the reaction mixture, but accounted for $86.3 \pm 8.1\%$ of the $Ca^{2+}$-dependent phosphorylation of tubulin, representing the mean $\pm$ S.E.M. for 5 separate experiments. The molar ratios of [$^{32}$P]phosphate $\beta$-tubulin)/($\beta$-tublin) in the whole reaction mixture, supernatant and pellet were 0.21, 0.04, and 0.93, respectively. Increasing the ATP concentration in the standard reaction mixture from 10 to 100 $\mu$M produced a corresponding increase in the phosphorylation of tubulin. This increase in phosphorylated tubulin resulted in increased tubulin protein in the pellet fraction. SDS–PAGE (Fig. 11) and 2D gel electrophoresis of the pellet demonstrated that it was composed primarily of $\alpha$- and $\beta$-tubulin with minor amounts of a 98 000–104 000 dalton protein and minimal amounts of calmodulin (Fig. 11). The concentrations of free $Ca^{2+}$ required to produce half-maximal levels of phosphorylation and turbidity changes were essentially identical, 0.41 and 0.53 $\mu$M, respectively. These results indicate that activation of the $Ca^{2+}$ tubulin kinase system not only initiates the phosphorylation of tubulin, but also results in the aggregation of phosphorylated tubulin that could be separated by centrifugation from unphosphorylated tubulin.

Electron microscopy observation by negative staining of the turbid reaction mixture incubated for 1 min containing phosphorylated tubulin showed that it contained numerous microfilaments of approximately 10–12 nm diameter, distributed randomly across the grid (Fig. 12). No microtubules or ring structures were observed in the tubulin kinase filament preparation, but occasional globular particles of 4–8 nm diameter were also observed. Electron microscopy examination of reaction mixtures that did not become turbid or demonstrate endogenous phosphorylation of tubulin (Fig. 11) demonstrated that they were composed of numerous globular particles of 4–8 nm diameter. Few if any microfilaments were seen in these reaction mixtures. Moreover, incubation under standard conditions of the calmodulin-depleted tubulin kinase system in the presence of $Ca^{2+}$ and calmodulin also caused the solution to become cloudy forming microfilaments. However, the formation of these filaments did not occur with $Ca^{2+}$ alone, demonstrating that like phosphorylation, the $Ca^{2+}$-dependent formation of tubulin microfilaments was also dependent on the presence of calmodulin.

Phosphorylation of tubulin by the $Ca^{2+}$-calmodulin kinase system thus causes marked changes in the physicochemical properties of tubulin, resulting in the formation of non-random, insoluble structures clearly distinct from microtubules when viewed by electronmicroscopy (Fig. 13). This process is shown schematically in Fig. 14. These microfilaments were not solubilized by treatment with cold temperatures, high salt (2 M NaCl), $ZnCl_2$, or EGTA and EDTA (5 mM). The smallest filaments measured approximately 10–12 nM in diameter and were also seen at diameters of 21–23 and 41–42 nM. In cross section these structures were solid and easily distinguished from microtubules. The filaments were twisted in appearance and the 10–12 nM structures appeared to be twisted together in multiples of two or four to form the 21–23 and 41–42 nM filaments. The pH in the reaction tube was stable and the $Ca^{2+}$-calmodulin-dependent tubulin filaments were compared to and found to be distinct from the pH-dependent formation of tubulin ribbons (Burton and Himes, 1978) or the $ZnCl_2$ formation of tubulin structures (Gaskin and Kress, 1977). The exact structure of these microfilaments must still be determined. Whether these $Ca^{2+}$-calmodulin-modulated physicochemical changes in tubulin play an active role in synaptic function is currently under investigation. However, the ability of $Ca^{2+}$ and calmodulin to produce a physical change in the state of the tubulin molecule at the synapse could provide a biochemical motor force for mediating the $Ca^{2+}$ signal.

The tubulin component in the filament fraction accounted for the vast majority of protein in this preparation, as determined by SDS–PAGE (Fig. 11) and 2D gel electrophoresis and was shown to be immunologically identical to tubulin from microtubule preparations by our radioimmunoassay (RIA) for tubulin (Fig. 8A). Tubulin is a major structural component of these filaments (Fig. 11), but at this time it is not possible to rule out the presence of other associated proteins. The model shown in Fig. 14 demonstrates that as $Ca^{2+}$ binds to calmodu-

Fig. 12. Electron microscopy of negatively stained specimens of microfilaments isolated from phosphorylated tubulin A (A) and the TK system incubated under standard conditions in the absence (B) and presence (C) of 10 $\mu$M $Ca^{2+}$. Negative staining of each sample was performed as described in Fig. 3. All material was examined in a Phillips 300 electron microscope. The negatively stained preparation of phosphorylated tubulin A (A) revealed many flexible microfilaments distributed evenly across the grid surface. The TK system isolated by DEAE chromatography (Fig. 9A) was incubated under standard conditions for 1 min in the presence or absence of 10 $\mu$M $Ca^{2+}$ (Fig. 11) and then immediately applied to grids and prepared for negative staining. In the absence of $Ca^{2+}$ (B) the reaction mixture remained clear and no microtubules or filaments were observed. However, the $Ca^{2+}$-treated preparation became turbid in appearance and demonstrated many flexible microfilaments distributed evenly across the grid. Essentially identical results were obtained when reactions were terminated at 1 min with glutaraldehyde (1 % final concentration) and fixed for 1 h prior to negative staining. The filaments observed by negative staining were also pelleted by centrifugation, fixed in glutaraldehyde (1 %) for 1 h; then dehydrated and embedded in epon, sectioned, and stained with lead citrate and uranyl acetate. Examination of these thin-sectioned specimens revealed the presence of microfilament structures (Fig. 13). The bar in each electromicrograph is 0.1 $\mu$M.

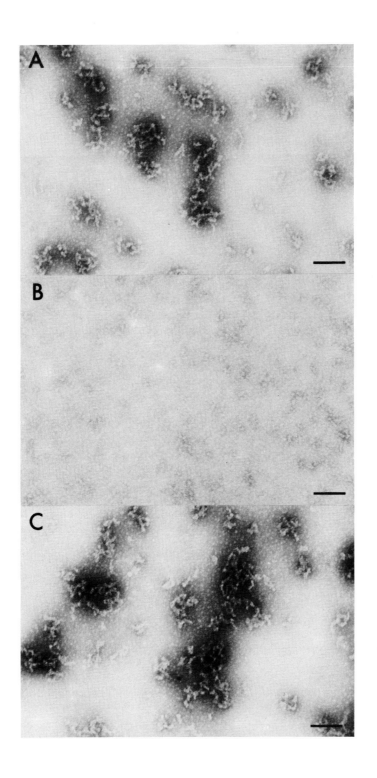

278

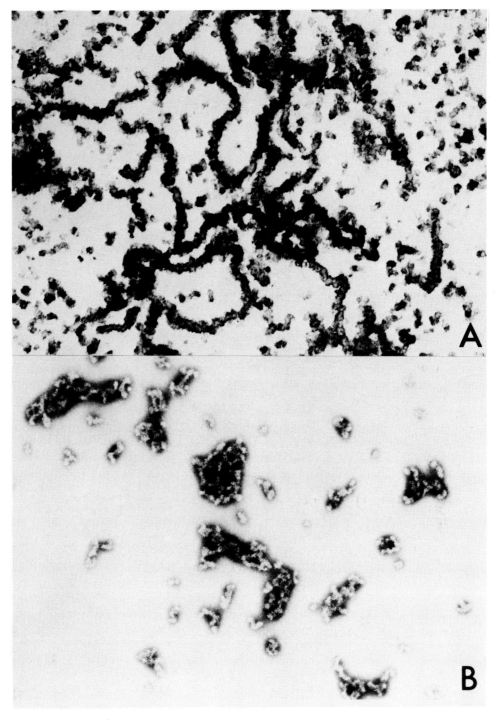

Fig. 13. Effects of $Ca^{2+}$- and calmodulin-stimulated phosphorylation on the morphology of tubulin. Following phosphorylation by the $Ca^{2+}$-calmodulin tubulin kinase, tubulin became insoluble as determined by turbidity measurements and centrifugation (Fig. 12). A: Glutaraldehyde–osium-fixed pellet of the phosphorylated tubulin following dehydration, epon embedding, and thin sectioning ($\times 148\,000$). The fibril-like structures were uniformly seen in the pellet. B: Negatively stained phosphorylated tubulin showing the same fibril-like structure seen in A ($\times 74\,000$) (from DeLorenzo, 1981c).

lin associated with the tubulin kinase system, it activates the complex, resulting in the phosphorylation of tubulin and the formation of microfilaments. Calmodulin and possibly the enzyme appear to be released from the complex based on the relative enrichment of tubulin in the filament fractions (Fig. 11). The microfilaments formed by the activation of the tubulin kinase system were essentially identical in appearance to some of the filaments described in the cold-stable microtubule fractions from brain (Berkowitz et al., 1977). The microfilaments formed from the tubulin kinase system are primarily composed of tubulin and do not contain detectable amounts of the 68 000, 160 000, and 210 000 dalton protein triad reported with other neurofilaments (Hoffman and Lasek, 1975). These results indicate that tubulin can form microfilaments, and that the large amount of tubulin seen in previously reported preparations of neurofilaments (Hoffman and Lasek, 1975; Schlaepfer, 1977) may also be part of the filament structure.

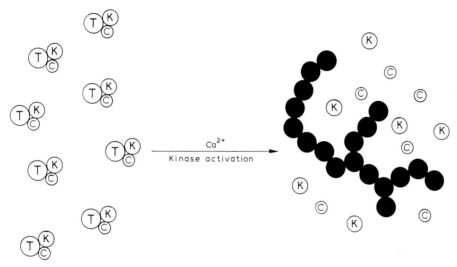

Fig. 14. Schematic model for the activation of the calmodulin tubulin kinase complex. In the presence of $\mu$M $Ca^{2+}$, calmodulin (C) bound to the tubulin kinase system binds $Ca^{2+}$ and activates the tubulin kinase (K), phosphorylating the tubulin (T) molecule. The tubulin kinase, calmodulin, tubulin, $Mg^{2+}$, and ATP are all present in brain cytoplasm, as a complex. The only requirement to activate the kinase system is an increase in $Ca^{2+}$ concentration. Thus, this enzyme complex is well suited to respond to the $Ca^{2+}$ signal. Initial studies suggest that both calmodulin and the calmodulin kinase are released from the enzyme complex during the phosphorylation of tubulin (black circles represent phosphorylated tubulin). This reaction is very rapid and occurs in less than 0.1 sec. The exact structure of the microfilaments formed by phosphorylated tubulin is currently being investigated (see Figs. 12 and 13).

It has been suggested that more than one kind of mammalian neurofilament is present in nervous tissue (Berkowitz et al., 1977; Johnson and Sinex, 1974; Schlaepfer, 1977). Our results indicate that one type of microfilament is formed follwing the activation by $Ca^{2+}$ of the tubulin kinase system and that these resultant filaments are composed primarily of phosphotubulin. Attempts to form microtubules from the tubulin kinase system in this laboratory were not successful, unless very high concentrations of EGTA were employed in the polymerization media. These results suggest that a significant portion of neurotubulin exists in the form of a $Ca^{2+}$ tubulin kinase system that can form microfilaments inthe presence of $Ca^{2+}$ and may only form microtubules when calmodulin is dissociated from this enzyme complex in the presence of EGTA or low $Ca^{2+}$ concentrations. In the presence of calmodulin, $Ca^{2+}$ in $\mu$M concentrations can prevent the polymerization of partially purified tubulin into microtubules (Marcum et al., 1978), suggesting that the presence of calmodulin with the tubulin kinase system in the form of a tightly bound complex may account for the difficulty in forming microtubules from this system unless high concentrations of EGTA are employed. Tubulin isolated by microtubule polymerization does not demonstrate tubulin kinase activity (Table IV). The effects observed by Marcum et al. (1978) may be accounted for by the association of calmodulin and tubulin in the absence of the tubulin kinase, but under these conditions $Ca^{2+}$ does not cause the aggregation of tubulin into specific structures. Our results demonstrate that the association of the tubulin kinase with calmodulin and tubulin in the form of an enzyme complex results in the formation of a $Ca^{2+}$-sensitive system that rapidly phosphorylates tubulin and forms microfilaments in the presence of $\mu$M concentrations of $Ca^{2+}$. Phosphorylation of tubulin in the presence of cAMP does not initiate the formation of microfilaments, indicating that the $Ca^{2+}$ tubulin kinase system phosphorylates a different site on the tubulin molecule which may initiate the polymerization of tubulin into neurofilaments.

## ROLE OF THE $Ca^{2+}$-CALMODULIN TUBULIN KINASE SYSTEM IN MEDIATING THE $Ca^{2+}$ SIGNAL

Our results elucidate a novel biochemical effect of $Ca^{2+}$ on tubulin. $Ca^{2+}$ significantly stimulates the endogenous phosphorylation of tubulin in brain cytoplasm and microtubule preparations. Although it has been suggested that $Ca^{2+}$-stimulated protein phosphorylation in brain may mediate some of the physiological effects of $Ca^{2+}$ on the nervous system (DeLorenzo, 1976; DeLorenzo, 1977), little was known about the identity or possible function of the phosphoprotein substrates of $Ca^{2+}$-activated protein kinases. The results reported here demonstrate that neurotubulin is a major substrate for $Ca^{2+}$- and calmodulin-stimulated protein kinase activity in brain, providing the first identification of a major cytoskeletal protein substrate for this calmodulin enzyme system. The important functions of tubulin and the role of $Ca^{2+}$ in modulating tubulin-containing systems in brain have been well documented. Results from this laboratory summarized in this presentation also demonstrate that the $Ca^{2+}$-calmodulin-stimulated phosphorylation of proteins DPH-L and DPH-M, as well as $\alpha$- and $\beta$-tubulin, correlated with neurotransmitter release and vesicle membrane interactions in isolated and intact synaptosome preparations (DeLorenzo et al., 1979; DeLorenzo, 1980a,b, 1981a–e). These results suggest the hypothesis that $Ca^{2+}$-stimulated endogenous phosphorylation of tubulin may be an underlying molecular mechanism regulating some of the actions of calcium on tubulin and may play a significant role in mediating some of the effects of calcium on cell function and neurotransmission.

The concentration or availability of calmodulin and/or the tubulin kinase in a cell may regulate the proportion of tubulin that exists in the form of the $Ca^{2+}$ tubulin kinase system. In brain cytosol, a significant fraction, but not all of the tubulin was associated with the tubulin kinase complex (Table IV). The amount of tubulin in the free form or associated with the tubulin kinase system may determine whether tubulin forms microtubules or manifests $Ca^{2+}$-stimulated phosphorylation and formation of microfilaments.

Tubulin is found in high concentrations in preparations of the nerve terminals (Blitz and Fine, 1974; Burke and DeLorenzo, 1981a) but microtubules are rarely seen in the presynaptic terminal, except under special circumstances. Tubulin or tubulin-like proteins have also been shown to be major protein components in synaptosome cytosol (Blitz and Fine, 1974; Feit et al., 1971), synaptic membrane (Kelly and Cotman, 1978), synaptic vesicles (Zisapel et al.,

1980), synaptic junctional complexes (Cotman, 1972), and the postsynaptic density (Kelly and Cotman, 1978). Since $Ca^{2+}$ plays a major role in synaptic function, it is possible that almost all of the tubulin in the nerve terminal is associated with the $Ca^{2+}$ tubulin kinase complex and thus not readily available to form microtubules. Results from this laboratory demonstrated that the majority of the tubulin found in the cytosol of synaptosome was associated with calmodulin in the form of a tubulin kinase complex (Burke and DeLorenzo, 1981b), suggesting that this endogenous calmodulin kinase system may play an important role in synaptic modulation. Synaptic vesicle proteins DPH-L and DPH-M were identified as $\alpha$- and $\beta$-tubulin (Burke and DeLorenzo, 1981c). Tubulin associated with synaptic membrane and synaptic junctional complexes (Cotman and Taylor, 1972; Kelly and Cotman, 1978) has also been recently shown to be phosphorylated by an endogenous membrane-bound tubulin kinase system (Burke and DeLorenzo, in preparation). The $Ca^{2+}$-calmodulin tubulin kinase system is present in synaptic membrane, synaptic vesicle, synaptic cytosol, and synaptic junction preparations. Thus, this enzyme system is well situated both pre- and postsynaptically to mediate the $Ca^{2+}$ signal at the synapse.

Unpublished results from this laboratory (Goldenring and DeLorenzo) have demonstrated that the calmodulin tubulin kinase phosphorylated the same peptide fragment of tubulin in tubulin prepared from brain cytosol, synaptoplasm, synaptic membrane, or synaptic vesicles. Thus, the marked allosteric changes produced in tubulin by phosphorylation forming microfilaments is likely to be occurring not only in soluble, but also in membrane-associated forms of the tubulin kinase complex. It has been demonstrated that $Ca^{2+}$ and calmodulin initiate vesicle and membrane interactions (DeLorenzo, 1980a,b, 1981b–e). These membrane interactions were also shown in these studies to correlate with membrane protein phosphorylation according to several parameters, including time course, substrate requirements, heat sensitivity, and inhibition by calmodulin and calmodulin kinase inhibitors. Thus, it was suggested from these results that $Ca^{2+}$-calmodulin-stimulated protein phosphorylation modulates vesicle–membrane interactions.

The membrane tubulin kinase system provides a unique biochemical mechanism for converting the $Ca^{2+}$ signal into a motor force by inducing an allosteric change in the tubulin molecule. The marked aggregation of phosphorylated tubulin into microfilaments (Figs. 12 and 13) represents a $Ca^{2+}$-dependent mechanism for regulating cytoskeletal elements in nervous tissue. Membrane-associated tublin may not form microfilaments upon phosphorylation; however, this form of tubulin may be able to interact with cytoplasmic tublin or vesicular tubulin upon phosphorylation. Fig. 15 presents a schematic model for the possible role of the membrane tubulin kinase system in mediating vesicle–membrane, or membrane–cytoskeletal interactions. In addition, it is also reasonable to suggest that upon phosphorylation, membrane-associated tubulin may alter its position or orientation in the membrane. Thus, the membrane-bound tubulin kinase system provides a $Ca^{2+}$-regulated biochemical mechanism for physicalle altering membrane structure or composition. This system could allow $Ca^{2+}$ to modulate membrane permeability changes, enzyme activation, or receptor availability (Fig. 16). The $Ca^{2+}$-regulated physical change in the tubulin molecule may provide a generalized mechanism for creating a motor force for mediating the $Ca^{2+}$ signal.

In conclusion, the fact that tubulin is a major "functional" and "structural" protein in nerve cells indicates that the $Ca^{2+}$-regulated phosphorylation of tubulin, especially at the synaptic level, may be of importance in the control of some aspects of neuronal function. The ability of tubulin to serve as a substrate for the $Ca^{2+}$-calmodulin kinase is a property of tubulin that may serve to regulate the state of aggregation and/or functional properties of the soluble and membrane-bound forms of tubulin. The suggested role of tubulin, calmodulin, and $Ca^{2+}$-de-

282

pendent protein phosphorylation in neurotransmitter release and synaptic modulation indicate that the $Ca^{2+}$-calmodulin-regulated phosphorylation of tubulin in the presynaptic nerve terminal may mediate some of the effects of calcium on synaptic function and delineate a dynamic role for tubulin in synaptic events and information processing in the mammalian brain.

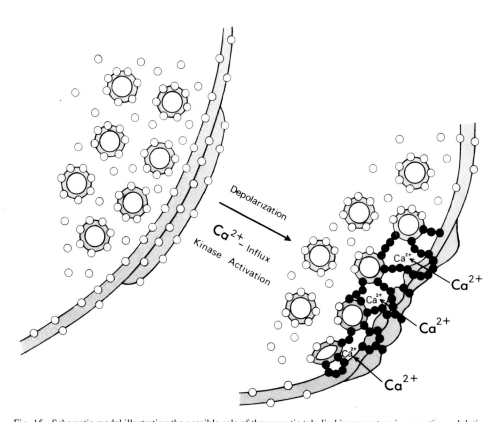

Fig. 15. Schematic model illustrating the possible role of the synaptic tubulin kinase system in synaptic modulation. In the resting nerve terminal (left) the tubulin kinase complex (white circles) is shown to be present in synaptoplasm, synaptic vesicle membrane, synaptic membrane, the synaptic junction, and the postsynaptic density. This kinase complex is primed to be activated by $Ca^{2+}$ as described in Fig. 14. The $Ca^{2+}$ receptor (calmodulin), tubulin, tubulin kinase, $Mg^{2+}$, and ATP are all present in the complex. Thus, during depolarization (right), the $Ca^{2+}$ influx into the nerve terminal immediately binds to calmodulin attached to this system and activates the phosphorylation of tubulin (black circles). The model illustrates that only the calmodulin tubulin kinase system near the synaptic membrane will be activated by the rapid and transient influx of $Ca^{2+}$. Following the phosphorylation of tubulin by the kinase (Fig. 14), the tubulin undergoes a rapid allosteric alteration and interacts with other adjacent phosphorylated tubulin molecules (black circles). This process results in the association of (1) vesicle–membrane tubulin, (2) vesicle–cytoplasm tubulin, (3) membrane–cytoplasm tubulin, (4) cytoplasm–cytoplasm tubulin, and (5) membrane–membrane tubulin. Thus, the phosphorylation of tubulin at the synapse provides a dynamic molecular process that may modulate the $Ca^{2+}$-calmodulin-dependent vesicle–membrane interactions at the synapse. The possible role of this system in holding the vesicles at the synapse, initiating exocytosis, altering membrane function, and allowing for cytoskeletal–membrane interactions is being actively investigated.

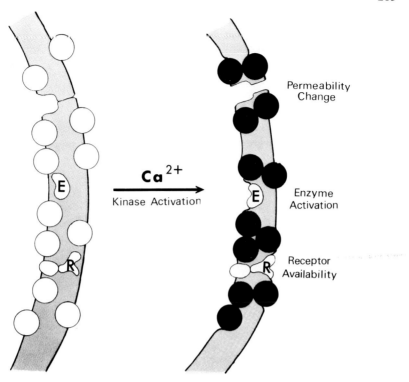

Fig. 16. Model illustrating the role of the tubulin kinase system in modulating membrane function. In the resting state (left) the tubulin kinase system is inactive (white circles) and several membrane parameters such as permeability, receptor availability, and enzyme activity are at the basal levels. In the presence of $Ca^{2+}$ (right), the tubulin kinase system is activated (black circles) and the phosphorylated tubulin associated with the membrane undergoes a rapid allosteric change. The altered form of phosphorylated tubulin causes a rearrangement of the fluid membrane system with the possible opening of membrane channels, exposure of enzyme systems (E), and the increased availability of receptor molecules (R). The tubulin kinase system provides a $Ca^{2+}$-regulated molecular system that may modulate membrane function.

## SUMMARY

$Ca^{2+}$ plays a major role in neurotransmission and synaptic modulation. Evidence is presented to support the calmodulin hypothesis of neurotransmission developed in this laboratory stating that calmodulin, a major $Ca^{2+}$-binding protein in brain, mediates the effects of $Ca^{2+}$ on neurotransmission. Calmodulin was isolated from highly enriched preparations of synaptic vesicles and nerve terminal cytoplasm. $Ca^{2+}$ and calmodulin were shown to regulate several synaptic processes in isolated and intact preparations, including endogenous synaptic $Ca^{2+}$-calmodulin protein kinase activity, neurotransmitter release, and synaptic vesicle and synaptic membrane interactions. Evidence for a role of $Ca^{2+}$-calmodulin protein kinase activity in synaptic activity is presented.

Depolarization-dependent $Ca^{2+}$ influx stimulated the phosphorylation of several synaptic proteins in whole synaptosomes, synaptic vesicles, and synaptic junctions in intact synaptosomes. Evidence is presented to demonstrate that $Ca^{2+}$-calmodulin-regulated synaptic protein phosphorylation plays a role in regulating neurotransmitter release in intact synaptosome and isolated vesicle preparations. Synaptic vesicle and synaptic membrane interactions in isolated systems were mediated by $Ca^{2+}$ and calmodulin and occurred under conditions that simultaneously stimulated neurotransmitter release and protein phosphorylation. $Ca^{2+}$ and calmodulin stimulated the activity of a synaptic tubulin kinase system that was shown to be a distinct enzyme system from the cAMP protein kinases.

The endogenous phosphorylation of tubulin from rat brain is stimulated by $Ca^{2+}$ and calmodulin. Calmodulin is associated with tubulin in brain cytoplasm in the form of a $Ca^{2+}$-activated tubulin kinase system. $Ca^{2+}$-stimulated endogenous phosphorylation of tubulin is lost when tubulin is highly purified by multiple cycles of microtubule assembly–disassembly and column chromatography. The ability of $Ca^{2+}$ to stimulate phosphorylation of tubulin is restored when calmodulin and other components that were removed from tubulin kinase complex during purification of tublin are added back to highly purified tubulin. Synaptosomal tubulin was also shown to be the major substrate for a $Ca^{2+}$-calmodulin-regulated protein kinase in synaptosome soluble fractions as determined by two-dimensional gel electrophoresis and peptide mapping. $Ca^{2+}$ activated this endogenous tubulin kinase system in presynaptic nerve terminal preparations. The $Ca^{2+}$-dependent activation of the tubulin kinase system was mediated by the $Ca^{2+}$-binding protein, calmodulin. The calmodulin-regulated phosphorylation of tubulin was found to cause marked alterations in the properties of tubulin, resulting in the formation of insoluble tubulin fibrils. The possible role of the tubulin kinase in converting the $Ca^{2+}$ signal into a motor force at the synapse is discussed. The activation of the tubulin kinase by $Ca^{2+}$ and calmodulin may play a role in the functional utilization of tubulin in the nerve terminal and may mediate some of the effects of $Ca^{2+}$ on synaptic function.

## ACKNOWLEDGEMENTS

This research was supported by U.S. Public Health Service Grant NS 136 32 and Research Career Development Award 5-KO4 NS00245 from the National Institute of Neurological and Communicative Disorders and Stroke to RJD.

The suggestions and discussions of Carl Cotman, Robert Yu, and George Palade were greatly appreciated. The technical assistance of Steven Maurer and Diana Hunt in preparing tubulin preparations is acknowledged.

## REFERENCES

Adelstein, R.S., Conti, M.A. and Pato, M.O. (1980) Regulation of myosin light chain kinase by reversible phosphorylation and calcium-calmodulin. *Ann. N.Y. Acad. Sci.*, 356: 142–150.

Berkowitz, S.A., Katagiri, J., Binder, H.K. and Williams, R.C. (1977) Separation and characterization of microtubule proteins from calf brain. *Biochemistry*, 16: 5610–5617.

Blitz, A.L. and Fine, R.E. (1974) Muscle-like contractable proteins and tubulin in synaptosomes. *Proc. nat. Acad. Sci. (Wash.)*, 71: 4472–4476.

Borisy, G.G. and Taylor, E.W. (1967) The mechanism of action of colchicine. *J. Cell Biol.*, 34: 525–533.

Burdette, S. and DeLorenzo, R.J. (1980) Benzodiazepine inhibition of calcium-dependent protein phosphorylation in synaptosome and synaptic vesicle preparations. *Neurology*, 30: 449.

Burke, B.E. and DeLorenzo, R.J. (1981a) Calcium and calmodulin dependent phosphorylation of neurotubulin. *Proc. nat. Acad. Sci. (Wash.)*, 78: 991–995.

Burke, B.E. and DeLorenzo, R.J. (1981b) $Ca^{2+}$ and calmodulin regulated endogenous tubulin kinase activity in presynaptic nerve terminal preparations. *Brain Res.*, in press.

Burke, B.E. and DeLorenzo, R.J. (1981c) $Ca^{2+}$ and calmodulin dependent phosphorylation of endogenous synaptic vesicle tubulin by a vesicle-bound calmoculin kinase system. *J. Neurochem.*, in press.

Burns, R. (1978) Rings, MAPs, and microtubules. *Nature (Lond.)*, 273: 709–710.

Burton, P.R. and Himes, R.H. (1978) Electron microscope studies of pH effects on assembly of tubulin free of associated proteins. *J. Cell Biol.*, 77: 120–133.

Cheung, W.Y. (1980) Calmodulin plays a pivotal role in cellular regulation. *Science*, 207: 19–27.

Cohen, P., Klee, C.B., Picton, C. and Shenolikar, S. (1980) Calcium control of muscle phosphorylase kinase through the combined action of calmodulin and troponin. *Ann. N.Y. Acad. Sci.*, 356: 151–161.

Connolly, J.A., Kalnins, V.I., Cleveland, D.W. and Kirschner, M.W. (1978) Intracellular localization of the high molecular weight microtubule accessory protein by indirect immunofluorescence. *J. Cell Biol.*, 76: 781–786.

Cotman, C.W. and Taylor, D. (1972) Isolation and structural studies on synaptic complexes from rat brain. *J. Cell Biol.*, 55: 696–711.

Del Castillo, J. and Stark, L. (1952) The effects of calcium ions on the motor endplate potentials. *J. Physiol.*, 124: 553–559.

DeLorenzo, R.J. (1976) Calcium-dependent phosphorylation of specific synaptosomal fraction proteins: possible role of phosphorylation in mediating neurotransmitter release. *Biochem. biophys. Res. Commun.*, 71: 590–597.

DeLorenzo, R.J. (1977) Antagonistic action of diphenylhydantoin and calcium on the level of phosphorylation of particular rat and human brain proteins. *Brain Res.*, 134: 125–138.

DeLorenzo, R.J. (1980a) Role of calmodulin in neurotransmitter release and synaptic function. *Ann. N.Y. Acad. Sci.*, 356: 92–109.

DeLorenzo, R.J. (1980b) Phenytoin: Calcium and calmodulin dependent protein phosphorylation and neurotransmitter release. In *Antiepileptic Drugs: Mechanisms of Action*, G.H. Glaser, J.K. Penry and D.M. Woodbury (Eds.), Raven Press, New York, pp. 399–414.

DeLorenzo, R.J. (1981a) Calcium, calmodulin, and synaptic function: modulation of neurotransmitter release, nerve terminal protein phosphorylation and synaptic vesicle morphology by calcium and calmodulin. In *Regulatory Mechanisms of Synaptic Transmission*, R. Tapia and C.W. Cotman (Eds.), Plenum Press, New York and London, pp. 205–240.

DeLorenzo, R.J. (1981b) The calmodulin hypothesis of neurotransmission. *Cell Calcium*, in press.

DeLorenzo, R.J. (1981c) Calmodulin in neurotransmitter release and synaptic function. *Fed. Proc.*, in press.

DeLorenzo, R.J. (1981d) Calcium-calmodulin protein phosphorylation in neuronal transmission. In *Status Epilepticus*, C. Waserlain and A.V. Delgado-Escueta (Eds.), Raven Press, New York, in press.

DeLorenzo, R.J. (1981e) Calmodulin modulation of the calcium signal in synaptic transmission. In *Compartmentation and Transmitter Interaction*, H.F. Bradford (Ed.), Plenum Press, New York and London, in press.

DeLorenzo, R.J. and Freedman, S.D. (1977a) Calcium-dependent phosphorylation of synaptic vesicle proteins and its possible role in mediating neurotransmitter release and vesicle function. *Biochem. biophys. Res. Commun.*, 77: 1036–1043.

DeLorenzo, R.J. and Freedman, S.D. (1977b) Possible role of calcium-dependent protein phosphorylation in mediating neurotransmitter release and anticonvulsant action. *Epilepsia*, 18: 357–365.

DeLorenzo, R.J. and Freedman, S.D. (1978) Calcium-dependent neurotransmitter release and protein phosphorylation in synaptic vesicles. *Biochem. biophys. Res. Commun.*, 80: 183–192.

DeLorenzo, R.J. and Glaser, G.H. (1976) Effects of diphenyldantoin on the endogenous phosphorylation of brain protein. *Brain Res.*, 105: 381–386.

DeLorenzo, R.J., Emple, G.P. and Glaser, G.H. (1977) Regulation of the level of endogenous phosphorylation of specific brain proteins by diphenylhydantoin. *J. Neurochem.*, 28: 21–30.

DeLorenzo, R.J., Freedman, S.D., Yohe, W.B. and Maurer, S.C. (1979) Stimulation of $Ca^{2+}$-dependent neurotransmitter release and presynaptic nerve terminal protein phosphorylation by calmodulin and a calmodulin-like protein isolated from synaptic vesicles. *Proc. nat. Acad. Sci. (Wash.)*, 76: 1838–1842.

DeLorenzo, R.J., Burdette, S. and Holderness, J. (1981) Benzodiazepine inhibition of the calcium-calmodulin protein kinase systems in brain membrane. *Science*, 212: 1157–1159.

Dentler, W.L., Granett, S. and Rosenbaum, J.L. (1975) Ultrastructural localization of the high molecular weight proteins associated with in vitro-assembled brain microtubules. *J. Cell Biol.*, 65: 237–241.

Douglas, W.W. (1968) Stimulus-secretion coupling: The concept and clues from chromaffin and other cells. *Brit. Pharmacol.*, 34: 451–474.

Ehrlich, Y.H. (1978) Phosphoproteins as specifiers for mediators and modulators in neuronal function. In *Modulators, Mediators and Specifiers in Brain Function*, Y.H. Ehrlich, J. Volarka, L.O. Davis and E.G. Brunngraber (Eds.), Plenum Press, New York and London, pp. 75–101.

Feit, H., Dutton, G.R., Barondes, S.H. and Shelanski, M.L. (1971) Microtubule protein: Identification in and transport to nerve endings. *J. Cell Biol.*, 51: 138–146.

Gaskin, F. and Kress, Y. (1977) Zinc ion-induced assembly of tubulin. *J. biol. Chem.*, 252: 6918–6924.

Grab, D.J., Carlin, R.K. and Siekevitz, P. (1980) The presence and functions of calmodulin in the postsynaptic density. *Ann. N.Y. Acad. Sci.*, 356: 55–72.

Himes, H.R., Burton, P.R. and Gaito, G.M. (1977) The dimethylsulfoxide-induced self-assembly of tubulin lacking associated proteins. *J. biol. Chem.*, 252: 6222–6228.

Hoffman, P.N. and Lasek, R.J. (1975) The slow component of axonal transport. Identification of major structural polypeptides of the axon and their generality among mammalian neurons. *J. Cell Biol.*, 66: 351–366.

Jameson, L., Frey, T., Zeeburg, B., Dalldouf, F. and Caplow, M. (1980) Inhibition of microtubule assembly by phosphorylation of microtubule associated proteins. *Biochemistry*, 19: 2472–2479.

Johnson, L.S. and Sinex, F.M. (1974) On the relationship of brain filaments to microtubules. *J. Neurochem.*, 22: 321–326.

Katz, B. and Miledi, R. (1969) Spontaneous and evoked activity of motor nerve endings in calcium Ringer. *J. Physiol.*, 203: 689–706.

Katz, B. and Miledi, R. (1970) Further study of the role of calcium in synaptic transmission. *J. Physiol.*, 207: 789–801.

Kelly, P.T. and Cotman, C.W. (1978) Synaptic Proteins: Characterization of tubulin and action and identification of a distinct postsynaptic density polypeptide. *J. Cell Biol.*, 79: 173–183.

Kim, H., Binder, L.I. and Rosenbaum, J.L. (1979) The periodic association of $MAP_2$ with brain microtubules in vitro. *J. Cell Biol.*, 80: 266–276.

Klee, C.B., Crouch, T.H. and Richman, P.G. (1980) Calmodulin. *Annu. Rev. Biochem.*, 49: 489–515.

Krueger, B., Forn, S. and Greengard, P. (1977) Depolarization-induced phosphorylation of specific proteins mediated by calcium influx in rat brain synaptosomes. *J. biol. Chem.*, 252: 2764–2773.

Lowry, O.H., Rosebrough, N.J., Farr, A.L. and Randall, R.J. (1951) Protein measurement with the Folin phenol reagent. *J. biol. Chem.*, 193: 265–275.

Marcum, J.M., Dedman, J.R., Brinkley, B.R. and Means, A.R. (1978) Control of microtubule assembly and disassembly by calcium-dependent regulator protein. *Proc. nat. Acad. Sci. (Wash.)*, 75: 3771–3775.

Matus, A., Ng, M.L. and Jones, D.H. (1979) Immunohistochemical localization of neurofilament antigen in rat cerebellum. *J. Neurocytol.*, 8: 513–525.

Miledi, R. (1973) Transmitter release induced by injection of calcium ions into nerve terminals. *Proc. roy. Soc. Lond.*, 183: 421–425.

Miledi, R. and Slater, C.R. (1966) The action of calcium on neuronal synapses in the squid. *J. Physiol.*: 184: 473–478.

O'Farrell, P.H. (1975) High resolution two-dimensional electrophoresis of proteins. *J. biol. Chem.*, 250: 4007–4021.

Rasmussen, H. and Goodman, D.B.P. (1977) Relationships between calcium and cyclic nucleotides in cell activation. *Physiol. Rev.*, 57: 421–509.

Rubin, R.P. (1972) The role of calcium in the release of neurotransmitter substances and hormones. *Pharm. Rev.*, 22: 389–428.

Schlaepfer, W.W. (1977) Immunological and ultrastructural studies of neurofilaments isolated from rat peripheral nerve. *J. Cell Biol.*, 74: 226–240.

Schulman, H. and Greengard, P. (1978) Stimulation of brain membrane protein phosphorylation by calcium and an endogenous heat-stable protein. *Nature (Lond.)*, 271: 478–479.

Shelanski, M.L., Gaskin, R. and Cantor, C.R. (1973) Microtubule assembly in the absence of added nucleotides. *Proc. nat. Acad. Sci. (Wash.)*, 70: 765–768.

Soifer, D. (1975) Enzymatic activity in tubulin preparations: cyclic AMP dependent protein kinase activity of brain microtubule protein. *J. Neurochem.*, 24: 21–23.

Yamauchi, T. and Fujisawa, H. (1980) Evidence for 3 distinct forms of calmodulin-dependent protein kinases from rat brain. *FEBS Lett.*, 116: 141–144.

Yamazaki, R.K., Mickey, D.L. and Story, M. (1979) The calibration and use of a calcium ion-specific electrode for kinetic studies of mitochondrial calcium transport. *Anal. Biochem.*, 93: 430–441.

Zisapel, N., Levi, M. and Gozes, D. (1980) Tubulin: An integral protein of mammalian synaptic vesicle membranes. *J. Neurochem.*, 34: 26–32.

# Membrane Phospholipid Turnover, Receptor Function and Protein Phosphorylation

YOSHIMI TAKAI, RYOJI MINAKUCHI, USHIO KIKKAWA, KIMIHIKO SANO, KOZO KAIBUCHI, BINZU YU*, TSUKASA MATSUBARA** and YASUTOMI NISHIZUKA

*Department of Biochemistry, Kobe University School of Medicine, Kobe 650, and Department of Cell Biology, National Institute for Basic Biology, Okazaki 444, Japan*

## 1. INTRODUCTION

A variety of cellular activities are often regulated by two opposing groups of extracellular messengers. In many tissues it seems plausible that cyclic AMP (cAMP) plays a role in the inhibitory cellular processes which may be induced by a group of hormones, neurotransmitters, prostaglandins and many other extracellular messengers. On the other hand, $Ca^{2+}$ has been proposed to play a role of crucial importance in the activiation of cellular functions, although the precise mechanism of this transmembrane signaling has not yet been clarified. We wish to describe in this article a new receptor function that is recently found in this laboratory. This receptor function appears to be directly related to phosphatidylinositol turnover which is induced by another group of extracellular messengers such as acetylcholine (muscarinic), catecholamines ($\alpha$), various peptide hormones and many other biologically active substances, whose actions are not mediated by cAMP but are implicated in $Ca^{2+}$ gating or movement. In a manner analogous to the cAMP-dependent signal pathway, a new species of protein kinase is involved as an essential ingredient in this receptor function as schematically shown in Fig. 1. This protein kinase, that is referred to as protein kinase C, is found widely in mammalian tissues, and has been purified from rat brain to near homogeneity. The enzyme absolutely requires $Ca^{2+}$ and membrane phospholipid for its activation. In addition, a small quantity of diacylglycerol derived from the receptor-linked cleavage of phosphatidylinositol dramatically increases the affinity of enzyme for $Ca^{2+}$ as well as for phospholipid, and thereby initiates the activation of enzyme at less than micromolar concentrations of $Ca^{2+}$. The enzyme activated in this way reveals catalytic properties distinctly different from those of cAMP-dependent protein kinase, and regulates several events probably related to cellular activation, although the precise relationship between this protein kinase and $Ca^{2+}$ gating is unknown at present. It will also be shown in this article that, in some tissues, both cAMP and cyclic GMP (cGMP) block the receptor-linked cleavage of phosphatidylinositol and thus counteract the activation of protein kinase C probably through actions of cyclic nucleotide-dependent protein kinases. Possible roles of several protein kinases in transmission of information across cell membranes will be discussed. Other aspects of protein kinase C have been reviewed elsewhere (Nishizuka et al., 1979; Nishizuka, 1980; Nishizuka and Takai, 1981; Takai et al., 1981b, 1982a,b). cAMP-dependent protein kinase and cGMP-dependent protein kinase will be referred to hereafter as protein kinase A and protein kinase G, respectively.

---

* On leave from Department of Biochemistry, Chinese Medical College, Shinyan, China.
** On leave from Department of Orthopedic Surgery, Kobe University School of Medicine, Kobe 650, Japan.

288

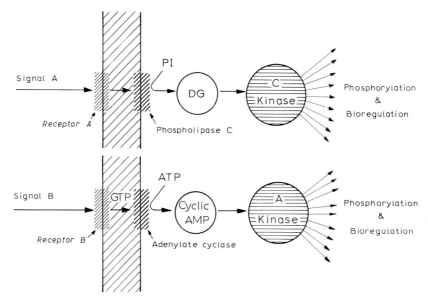

Fig. 1. Two receptor functions present in many mammalian tissues. PI, phosphatidylinositol; DG, diacylglycerol; C kinase, protein kinase C; A kinase, protein kinase A.


## 2. ENZYMOLOGY OF NEW PROTEIN KINASE

### 2.1. Physical and kinetic properties

Protein kinase C has been found in all tissues and organs examined, and in most tissues the activity exceeds that of protein kinase A when assayed with calf thymus H1 histone as phosphate acceptor as shown in Table I (Nishizuka, 1980; Kuo et al., 1980; Minakuchi et al.,

TABLE I

TISSUE DISTRIBUTION OF PROTEIN KINASES C AND A

Rat tissues were employed except for platelets, lymphocytes, and granulocytes which were obtained from human volunteers. The enzymes were assayed under comparable conditions with calf thymus H1 histone as phosphate acceptor. Detailed conditions are described elsewhere (Minakuchi et al., 1981). Values are units/mg of protein. One unit is defined as the amount of enzyme that transferred 1 pmole of phosphate from ATP to histone per min.

| Tissue | Protein kinase C | Protein kinase A |
|---|---|---|
| Platelets | 6 300 | 340 |
| Brain | 3 270 | 250 |
| Lymphocytes | 1 060 | 320 |
| Small intestinal smooth muscle | 770 | 560 |
| Granulocytes | 530 | 100 |
| Lung | 360 | 290 |
| Kidney | 280 | 150 |
| Liver | 180 | 130 |
| Adipocytes | 170 | 270 |
| Heart | 110 | 230 |
| Skeletal muscle | 80 | 110 |

1981). In brain tissues the activity of this enzyme is more than 10 times higher than that of protein kinase A, and it is found not only in soluble but also in particulate fractions. Subcellular fractionation analysis indicates that a large portion of enzyme in this particulate fraction is associated with synaptosomal membranes. This membrane-associated enzyme, that can be extracted by non-ionic detergent, is indistinguishable from soluble cytosolic enzyme, and enzymes from several mammalian tissues such as rat brain (Inoue et al., 1977), rat liver (Takai et al., 1977), human platelets (Kawahara et al., 1980a), and human peripheral lymphocytes (Ogawa et al., 1981; Ku et al., 1981) appear to show no tissue and species specificity at least in their kinetic and catalytic properties. The enzyme has been recently purified from rat brain soluble fraction to near homogeneity as judged by sodium dodecyl sulfate–polyacrylamide gel electrophoresis. The enzyme shows an approximate molecular weight of about 77 000, and is composed of a single polypeptide with at least two functionally different domains, namely hydrophobic membrane-binding and hydrophilic catalytic domains. Upon limited proteolysis with $Ca^{2+}$-dependent neutral protease, these two domains are separated, and a catalytically fully active fragment is obtained (Inoue et al., 1977; Takai et al., 1977; Kishimoto et al., 1981).

### 2.2. Mode of activation

Protein kinase C per se is catalytically inactive and requires the simultaneous presence of phospholipid, diacylglycerol and $Ca^{2+}$ for the enzymatic reaction. A series of experiments indicates that none of these factors is needed for the enzyme catalysis, since the fragment carrying catalytic domain obtained by limited proteolysis as described above is fully active without any one of these factors. Thus, phospholipid, diacylglycerol and $Ca^{2+}$ are all required for the activation process rather than the catalytic process of the enzyme. For this activation process $Ca^{2+}$ is indispensable and none of the other divalent cations is able to substitute for $Ca^{2+}$ except for $Sr^{2+}$ that is only less than 8 % as active as $Ca^{2+}$ under similar conditions. $Mg^{2+}$ is always necessary for the catalytic process.

Further analysis of the mode of activation of the enzyme reveals that, in the presence of large excess of phospholipid and at unusually higher concentrations ($10^{-4}$–$10^{-3}$ M) of $Ca^{2+}$, the enzyme is active without diacylglycerol. Kinetically, the addition of a small amount of diacylglycerol greatly increases the affinity of the enzyme for phospholipid, and concomitantly decreases the $K_a$ value for $Ca^{2+}$, the concentration necessary for the half-maximum activation, dramatically from $10^{-4}$ M to less than $10^{-6}$ M (Takai et al., 1979; Kishimoto et al., 1980). Diolein, dilinolein and diarachidonin are equally active, whereas diacylglycerols possessing saturated fatty acids such as dipalmitin and distearin are far less effective. A series of analyses has indicated that diacylglycerols containing at least one unsaturated fatty acid at either position 1 or 2 are active in this capacity irrespective of the chain length of the other fatty acyl moiety as shown in Table II. Mono- and triacylglycerols and free fatty acids are totally inactive, and the diacylglycerol structure is essential for enzyme activation (Mori et al., 1982).

Another set of experiments indicates that at physiologically low concentrations of $Ca^{2+}$ protein kinase C is activated selectively by phosphatidylserine. However, other species of phospholipids considerably modulate the enzyme activation. When phosphatidylethanolamine is supplemented to phosphatidylserine, further enhancement of the enzymatic activity is observed. Inversely, the addition of phosphatidylcholine or sphingomyelin markedly diminishes the phosphatidylserine-dependent activation of the enzyme. Neither phosphatidylinositol that serves as the source of unsaturated diacylclycerol, nor phosphatidic acid that is an intermediate of phosphatidylinositol turnover shows significant effects. Thus, each species of various membrane phospholipids plays a specific role with positive or negative cooperativity

TABLE II

EFFECTS OF VARIOUS SYNTHETIC DIACYLGLYCEROLS ON THE ACTIVATION OF PROTEIN KINASE C

The $K_a$ value for $Ca^{2+}$ and enzymatic activity at $4 \times 10^{-6}$ M $CaCl_2$ were obtained under conditions described elsewhere (Mori et al., 1982). Enzyme assay was made with 0.8 $\mu$g/ml of each diacylglycerol indicated.

| Diacylglycerol added | | $K_a$ for $Ca^{2+}$ ($\mu$M) | Enzyme activity ($^{32}P$ incorp./pmole/min) |
|---|---|---|---|
| R1–CO–* | R2–CO–* | | |
| none | | 90 | 4 |
| $C_{18:1}$ | $C_{18:1}$ | 8 | 26 |
| $C_{18:0}$ | $C_{18:0}$ | 90 | 5 |
| $C_{18:1}$ | $C_{18:0}$ | 2 | 53 |
| $C_{18:1}$ | $C_{10:0}$ | 1 | 48 |
| $C_{18:1}$ | $C_{6:0}$ | 1 | 50 |
| $C_{18:1}$ | $C_{2:0}$ | 1 | 42 |
| $C_{18:0}$ | $C_{18:1}$ | 8 | 28 |
| $C_{10:0}$ | $C_{18:1}$ | 3 | 40 |
| $C_{6:0}$ | $C_{18:1}$ | 1 | 58 |
| $C_{2:0}$ | $C_{18:1}$ | 1 | 44 |

* R1–CO– and R2–CO– indicate acyl moieties esterified to positions 1 and 2 of glycerol, respectively.

in the activation of protein kinase C, and presumably asymmetric distribution of various phospholipids in lipid bilayer of biological membranes seems to be favorable for making the enzyme more active (Kaibuchi et al., 1981).

## 3. POSSIBLE COUPLING TO RECEPTOR FUNCTION

### 3.1. Phosphatidylinositol turnover

Although phosphatidylinositol is usually a minor component that is located mainly in the inner monolayer of plasma membranes (for reviews, see Rothman and Lenard, 1977; Bergelson and Barsukov, 1977), this phospholipid turns over very rapidly upon stimulation by a variety of extracellular messengers (for reviews, see Michell, 1975, 1979; Hawthorne, 1960; Hawthorne and White, 1975; Berridge, 1980). This phospholipid turnover has been described first by Hokin and Hokin (1954) for acetylcholine-sensitive exocrine tissues. Upon stimulation of these tissues inorganic phosphate is rapidly incorporated into phosphatidylinositol and phosphatidic acid with little or no significant labeling of other major phospholipids. For exploring this labeling pattern it has been clarified later that the phospholipid is cleaved by phospolipase C to produce diacylglycerol and inositol phosphate. The diacylglycerol is rapidly phosphorylated to phosphatidic acid which then reacts with CTP to produce CDP-diacylglycerol. The latter compound finally reacts with inositol to reform phosphatidylinositol (for reviews, see Hawthorne and White, 1975; Michell, 1975). Since one of the primary products that is inositol phosphate is produced largely as inositol 1,2-cyclic phosphate (Dawson et al., 1971), a possible role of this material as a second messenger has been sometimes discussed in analogy to cAMP. However, virtually no evidence has been obtained implying such a biological role of this cyclic compound. Instead, based on the foregoing discussions, an alternative possibility may arise that diacylglycerol plays some role during the transmission of information across cell membranes. It has been established that phosphatidylinositol in mammalian tissues is not a single chemical entity but is a mixture of molecular species possessing different fatty acyl moieties. However, the fatty acid esterified at position 2 is most often arachidonic acid (Holub et al., 1970) and, therefore, the diacylglycerol produced from the receptor-linked cleavage of phosphatidylinositol must contain at least one unsaturated fatty acid that is active to support the activation of protein kinase C as described above. To obtain evidence for the coupling between phosphatidylinositol turnover and activation of protein kinase C, several sets of experiments have been conducted with various types of cells which respond to extracellular messengers, and so far the best results have been obtained with human platelets stimulated by thrombin (Kawahara et al., 1980a,b).

## 3.2. Role of protein kinase in cellular activation

Platelets respond to several extracellular messengers such as thrombin, ADP and collagen to aggregate and release serotonin, and this response is well known to be inhibited by cAMP-elevating agents including prostaglandin $E_1$, prostacyclin and adenosine (for review, see Haslam et al., 1978). Such activation and inhibition reactions of platelets may provide an ideal model for approaching to molecular basis of hormonal control of cellular activities. In addition, it has been described that thrombin induces rapid turnover of phosphatidylinositol in platelet membranes resulting in the transient accumulation of diacylglycerol (Rittenhouse-Simmons, 1979; Bell and Majerus, 1980). Another line of evidence indicates that when platelets are stimulated by thrombin at least two endogenous proteins having approximate molecular weights of 40 000 (or 47 000, Haslam et al., 1980) and 20 000 are heavily phosphorylated. The latter protein (20 K protein) has been identified as myosin light chain, and a calmodulin-dependent myosin light chain kinase has been proposed to be responsible for this reaction (Daniel et al., 1977). On the other hand, the enzyme responsible for 40 K protein phosphorylation has not yet been

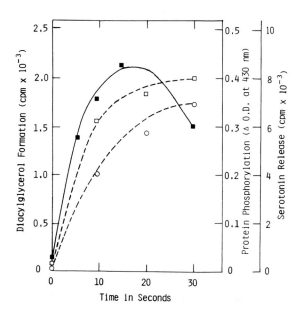

Fig. 2. Rapid formation of diacylglycerol, phosphorylation of 40 K protein, and release of serotonin in human platelets stimulated by thrombin. Detailed experimental conditions are described elsewhere (Kawahara et al., 1980a; Takai et al., 1981b). ■——■, diacylglycerol formation; □---□, 40 K protein phosphorylation; ○---○, serotonin release.

identified, although the phosphorylation of this protein is intimately related to the release reaction (Lyons et al., 1975; Haslam and Lynham, 1977; Wallace and Bensusan, 1980).

In confirmation of these observations, Fig. 2 shows that diacylglycerol is rapidly produced when platelets are stimulated by thrombin. This reaction is immediately followed by phosphorylation of 40 K protein and also by release of serotonin. This diacylglycerol appears to be derived from phosphatidylinositol, but a more quantitative analysis shows that the disappearance of this phospholipid exceeds by far the accumulation of diacylglycerol. This poor stoichiometry is presumably due to the rapid conversion of this neutral lipid back to phosphatidylinositol by way of phosphatidic acid as mentioned above, and also to further degradation to free arachidonic acid and its derivatives as discussed below. In fact, as shown in this figure, diacylglycerol once produced rapidly disappears. In any case the formation of diacylglycerol is always accompanied with 40 K protein phosphorylation as well as serotonin release. In another set of experiments, it is shown that 40 K protein purified from platelets serves as a preferable phosphate acceptor for homogeneous preparation of protein kinase C (manuscript in preparation). These results together with those described elsewhere (Kawahara et al., 1980a,b; Takai et al., 1981b, 1982a,b; Nishizuka and Takai, 1981) strongly suggest that in platelet system phosphatidylinositol turnover induced by thrombin is directly coupled to activation of protein kinase C, and that the enzyme thus activated phosphorylates 40 K protein to lead eventually to release of serotonin.

## 4. RELATION TO CYCLIC NUCLEOTIDES

### 4.1. Relationships between receptor functions

Although evidence that phosphatidylinositol turnover is directly coupled to the activation of protein kinase C is just beginning to accumulate, it is suggestive that the enzyme may play a role of crucial importance in the transmission of information of a large number of extracellular messengers. Presumably, these messengers include $\alpha$-adrenergic and muscarinic cholinergic stimulators, peptide hormones such as vasopressin and angiotensin II, mitogenic substances such as growth factors and plant lectins, and many active substances which are known to induce phosphatidylinositol turnover in their respective target cell membranes. This class of receptor functions generally seem to be implicated in $Ca^{2+}$ actions which control contractions, exocytosis, endocytosis, membrane permeability, metabolism, cell division and proliferation, and other biological processes. In addition, various extracellular messengers in this group usually increase cGMP but not cAMP in their target tissues, although such generalization may not always be possible, as shown in Table III. Thus, phosphatidylinositol turnover, $Ca^{2+}$ and cGMP appear to be integrated together in a single receptor cascade system. Michell (1975, 1979) has proposed a possible role of this phospholipid turnover in the regulation of $Ca^{2+}$ gating, but the biochemical basis for this hypothesis has not yet been clarified. Similarly, no evidence is available at present indicating a possible involvement of protein kinase C in $Ca^{2+}$ gating. Nevertheless, a large body of circumstantial evidence in the literature is consistent with the supposition that phosphatidylinositol turnover may be an important transduction step in the signal pathway leading to the opening of $Ca^{2+}$ gates (for reviews, see Michell, 1975, 1979; Berridge, 1980). Another point to be made here is that, although this phospholipid turnover is often associated with the formation of cGMP as mentioned above, the signal pathway for generating this cyclic nucleotide has again not yet been clarified. One possibility is that sometimes $Ca^{2+}$ causes the direct activation of guanylate cyclase (for review, see Murad et al., 1979). Another possibility is that arachidonic acid peroxide and prostaglandin endoperoxide

TABLE III

EFFECTS OF VARIOUS EXTRACELLULAR MESSENGERS ON PHOSPHATIDYLINOSITOL TURNOVER, $Ca^{2+}$, cGMP AND cAMP

| Stimulant | Target tissue | PI* turnover | $Ca^{2+}$ | cGMP | cAMP |
|---|---|---|---|---|---|
| Adrenalin ($\alpha$) | Various | ↑ | ↑ | ↑ | → or ↓ |
| Acetylcholine (m) | Various | ↑ | ↑ | ↑ | → or ↓ |
| Histamine (Hl) | Smooth muscle, brain | ↑ | ↑ | ↑ | → |
| Angiotensin | Liver | ↑ | ↑ | ? | → |
| Vasopressin | Liver | ↑ | ↑ | ? | → |
| Thrombin | Platelets | ↑ | ↑ | ↑ | → |
| fMet-Leu-Phe | Leukocytes | ↑ | ↑ | ↑ | → |
| Plant lectin | Lymphocytes | ↑ | ↑ | ↑ | → or ↓ |
| Glucagon | Liver, fat cells | → | → | → | ↑ |
| Adrenalin ($\beta$) | Various | → | → or ↓ | → | ↑ |
| Histamine (H2) | Smooth muscle, brain | → | → | → | ↑ |

* PI, phosphatidylinositol.

activate guanylate cyclase (Hidaka and Asano, 1977; Graff et al., 1978). Arachidonic acid may be derived from phosphatidylinositol through reactions catalyzed by phospholipase C followed by diacylglycerol lipase (Bell et al., 1979; Rittenhouse-Simmons, 1979, 1980; Bell and Majerus, 1980; Billah et al., 1980), although it may also be produced from phosphatidylcholine by reaction of phospholipase $A_2$ (Bills et al., 1976; Blackwell et al., 1977).

In marked contrast, another class of receptor functions that increase cAMP do not induce phosphatidylinositol turnover nor elevate cGMP. Axelrod and his coworkers (for review, see Hirata and Axelrod, 1980) have proposed that enzymatic methylation of phosphatidylethanolamine to produce phosphatidylcholine may occur in the plasma membrane that is activated by $\beta$-adrenergic stimulators, and that this phospholipid methylation is coupled to the activation of adenylate cyclase. The precise nature as well as the mechanism of this coupling remain largely unexplored.

Based on the foregoing discussions it seems likely that there are at least two major receptor functions in most tissues; one is related to phospholipid turnover, $Ca^{2+}$ and cGMP, and the other is mediated by cAMP. Thus, the next discussion will be devoted to the relationship between these two major receptor functions.

## 4.2. Inhibitory action of cAMP

In mammalian tissues the mode of cellular response may be roughly divided into two groups; in most systems such as platelets, lymphocytes, polymorphonuclear leukocytes, smooth muscles, nervous tissues and many others, the receptors that induce phosphatidylinositol turnover generally promote activation of cellular functions, whereas the receptors that produce cAMP usually antagonize such activation. In contrast, in another group of systems the two classes of receptors do not appear to interact with each other but function independently. For instance, in hepatic tissue $\alpha$- and $\beta$-adrenergic stimulators, that induce the phospholipid turnover and cAMP formation, respectively, equally enhance glycogenolysis. For the approach to such receptor interactions, human platelets again share with other systems extensive studies on the mode of response to various extracellular messengers.

294

It seems established that inhibitory action of prostaglandin $E_1$ on thrombin-induced activation of platelets is mediated by cAMP, presumably through action of protein kinase A (for review, see Haslam et al., 1978). Two possible mechanisms for this inhibition have thus far been postulated. First, protein kinase A phosphorylates microsomal proteins having molecular weights of about 24 000 (24 K protein) and 22 000 (22 K protein) resulting in the activation of $Ca^{2+}$-activated ATPase followed, in due course, by the decrease in cytosolic $Ca^{2+}$ that is available for platelet activation (Berridge, 1975; Katz et al., 1975; Haslam et al., 1980). Second, protein kinase A phosphorylates $Ca^{2+}$-activated myosin light chain kinase resulting in the inactivation of its catalytic activity (Adelstein et al., 1978). Myosin light chain kinase specifically phosphorylates this particular protein, and this reaction leads to the activation of myosin ATPase (Adelstein and Conti, 1975). In another line of experiments, it has been shown that dibutyryl cAMP inhibits thrombin-induced diacylglycerol formation (Rittenhouse-Simmons, 1979; Kawahara et al., 1980a). It has also been described that, when intact platelets are treated with dibutyryl cAMP, phospholipase C activity is decreased as measured by the conversion of endogenous phosphatidylinositol to diacylglycerol using deoxycholate-solubilized preparations (Billah et al., 1979). Extending these observations Fig. 3 shows that thrombin-induced diacylglycerol formation, 40 K protein phosphorylation and serotonin release described in section 3 are all progressively inhibited in parallel manners by increasing amounts of prostaglandin $E_1$, and this inhibition appears to be proportional to the amount of cAMP produced. In fact, dibutyryl cAMP reproduces the inhibitory effects on the three reactions mentioned above. In contrast to such inhibition of 40 K protein phosphorylation, at least four distinct proteins having molecular weights of 240 000 (240 K protein), 50 000 (50 K protein), 24 000 (24 K protein) and 22 000 (22 K protein) are increasingly phosphorylated by incubation with prostaglandin $E_1$ or dibutyryl cAMP. Densitometric analysis of a series of autoradiographs prepared under different conditions indicates that the phosphorylation of various platelet proteins described above are opposingly regulated by the two distinctly

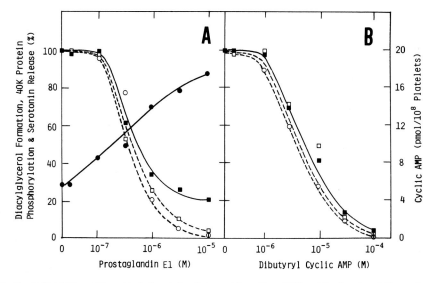

Fig. 3. Parallel inhibition of thrombin-induced diacylglycerol formation, 40 K protein phosphorylation and serotonin release by prostaglandin $E_1$ (A) and dibutyryl cAMP (B) in human platelets. Detailed experimental conditions are described elsewhere (Kawahara et al., 1980a; Takai et al., 1982b). ■——■, diacylglycerol formation; □ - - □, 40 K protein phosphorylation; ○ - - ○, serotonin release; ●——●, cAMP.

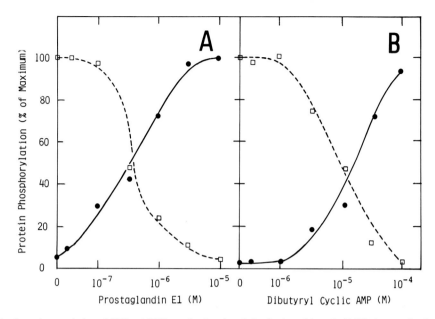

Fig. 4. Opposing regulation of 40 K and 50 K protein phosphorylation by thrombin and cAMP in human platelets (A), by prostaglandin E₁, and (B), by dibutyryl cAMP. Detailed experimental conditions are described elsewhere (Kawahara et al., 1980a; Takai et al., 1982b). ●——●, 50 K protein phosphorylation; □‑‑‑□, 40 K protein phosphorylation.

different receptor functions elicited by thrombin and prostaglandin $E_1$. 240 K protein is suggested to be an actin-binding protein, probably filamin (Wallach et al., 1978), and 24 K and 22 K proteins are proposed to be regulator proteins for microsomal $Ca^{2+}$-activated ATPase (Haslam et al., 1979, 1980) as already mentioned. Although the role of 50 K protein has not yet been identified, the phosphorylation of this protein is inversely proportional to 40 K protein phosphorylation as shown in Fig. 4. These results strongly suggest that cAMP blocks the phospholipid turnover probably through the action of protein kinase A, and thereby counteracts the activation of protein kinase C.

The interaction of the two receptor functions described above is also observed in other cell types which may be activated by various extracellular messengers but inhibited by another group of extracellular messengers that increase cAMP. For instance, Table IV shows that in human peripheral lymphocytes and rat polymorphonuclear leukocytes that are activated by phytohemagglutinin and fMet-Leu-Phe, a chemoattractant, respectively, phosphatidylinositol turnover is blocked by dibutyryl cAMP as well as by prostaglandin $E_1$ that markedly elevates cAMP (Takai et al., 1982b). It has been shown recently that in mast cells prostaglandin $E_1$ inhibits phosphatidylinositol turnover as well as histamine release which are induced by concanavalin A plus phosphatidylserine (Kennerly et al., 1979).

The observations briefly mentioned above raise a question as to whether cAMP inhibits the phospholipid turnover in another group of systems such as hepatocytes. In this tissue it seems established that glycogenolysis is enhanced by glucagon and $\beta$-adrenergic stimulators through a cAMP-dependent pathway. It is also well known that $\alpha$-adrenergic stimulators, vasopressin and angiotensin II induce glycogenolysis as well as phosphatidylinositol turnover without any detectable increase in cAMP levels and without protein kinase A activation (for review, see Michell, 1979). In isolated hepatocytes this enhanced phospholipid turnover appears to be

TABLE IV

INHIBITION OF PHOSPHATIDYLINOSITOL TURNOVER BY cAMP

Human peripheral lymphocytes and rat peritoneal polymorphonuclear leukocytes were employed. The activation of lymphocytes was assayed by measuring the rate of incorporation of [$^3$H]thymidine into DNA at 72 h after phytohemagglutinin challenge. The activation of leukocytes was assayed by measuring the release of $N$-acetylglucosaminidase into medium upon stimulation by fMet-Leu-Phe. Phosphatidylinositol turnover was assayed by measuring the incorporation of $^{32}$Pi into this phospholipid immediately after the addition of each stimulator. cAMP was determined by radioimmunoassay. Detailed experimental conditions are described elsewhere (Takai et al., 1982b).

| Cell type | Addition | Cellular activation (cpm) | PI turnover (cpm) | cAMP (pmoles/1 × 10$^7$ cells) |
|---|---|---|---|---|
| Lymphocytes | None | 420 | 1 090 | 2.2 |
| | PHA | 1 710 | 2 730 | 2.0 |
| | PHA + PGE$_1$ | 560 | 1 250 | – |
| | PHA + DbcAMP | 670 | 1 450 | – |
| | PGE$_1$ | 510 | 790 | 22.0 |
| | DbcAMP | 430 | 820 | – |
| | | (%*) | (cpm) | (pmoles/1 × 10$^7$ cells) |
| Polymorphonuclear leukocytes | None | 16.5 | 160 | 1.7 |
| | fMLP | 47.2 | 420 | 1.9 |
| | fMLP + PGE$_1$ | 22.4 | 200 | – |
| | fMLP + DbcAMP | 19.4 | 180 | – |
| | PGE$_1$ | 22.1 | 180 | 3.5 |
| | DbcAMP | 22.7 | 190 | – |

* The numbers indicate percentages of the enzymatic activity released into the medium with the total activity as 100. PI, phosphatidylinositol; PHA, phytohemagglutinin; fMLP, fMet-Leu-Phe; PGE$_1$, prostaglandin E$_1$; DbcAMP, dibutyryl cAMP.

insusceptible to cAMP (unpublished observation). Although our current knowledge has been obtained from studies with a limited number of limited tissues, it seems attractive to suggest that in a group of systems such as platelets the receptor-linked activation of protein kinase C is blocked by cAMP presumably through the action of protein kinase A, whereas in another group of systems such as hepatocytes protein kinases C and A function independently to promote their specific roles in controlling cellular activities. The inhibition of phosphatidylinositol turnover by protein kinase A does not appear to be simply due to the phosphorylation of phospholipase C, and the molecular basis of this tissue difference remains unknown.

### 4.3. A possible role of cGMP

It has been thought for many years that cGMP is a possible messenger for various hormones, neurotransmitters and other biologically active substances as briefly described above (for review, see also Goldberg and Haddox, 1977), but its definitive role in biological regulation has not yet been fully understood. It remains also puzzling that protein kinase G shows very similar, if not identical, catalytic properties to those of protein kinase A as far as tested in in vitro systems as first reported from this laboratory (Hashimoto et al., 1976). Schultz et al. (1977) have proposed that cGMP may be a feedback inhibitor rather than a positive messenger of muscarinic cholinergic transmitter for smooth muscle contraction. This assumption has been based on the observation that cGMP-elevating agents such as sodium nitroprusside cause

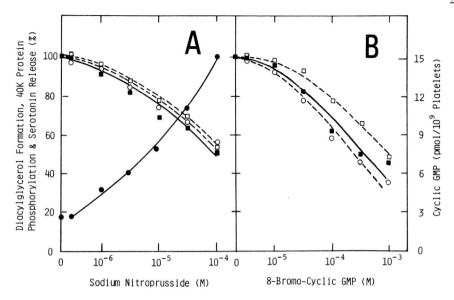

Fig. 5. Parallel inhibition of thrombin-induced diacylglycerol formation, 40 K protein phosphorylation and serotonin release by sodium nitroprusside (A) and 8-bromo-cGMP (B). Detailed experimental conditions are described elsewhere (Takai et al., 1981a). ■——■, diacylglycerol formation; □---□, 40 K protein phosphorylation; ○---○, serotonin release; ●——●, cGMP.

muscle relaxation, although muscarinic cholinergic stimulators enhance cGMP as well as phosphatidylinositol turnover upon muscle contraction. Analogously, Haslam et al., (1980) have proposed more recently that, although cGMP is increased in human platelets stimulated by thrombin and collagen, this cyclic nucleotide probably serves as an inhibitor for platelet activation, since sodium nitroprusside markedly increases cGMP and strongly inhibits platelet activation.

Extending these observations, the experiments given in Fig. 5 indicate that, in platelets stimulated by thrombin, diacylglycerol formation, 40 K protein phosphorylation and serotonin release are again progressively and concurrently inhibited by the addition of increasing amounts of sodium nitroprusside (Takai et al., 1981a). Under these conditions cGMP is markedly increased, and 8-bromo-cGMP shows similar effects. Neither sodium nitroprusside nor 8-bromo-cGMP alone affects resting platelets. In another set of experiments both compounds stimulate the phosphorylation of a selectively distinct protein having a molecular weight of about 50 000, that is apparently indistinguishable from 50 K protein already mentioned above. Other proteins such as 240 K, 24 K and 22 K protein are not significantly phosphorylated by these compounds. However, sodium nitroprusside is known to enhance also cAMP levels slightly, at most 2-fold. Nevertheless, a series of analyses suggests that the observed inhibitory effect of this compound is most likely mediated by cGMP, since under the condition where cAMP is not significantly increased sodium nitroprusside causes a marked increase in cGMP levels and concomitant inhibition of platelet activation. Presumably, a slight increase in cAMP caused by sodium nitroprusside may not account for more than a fraction of this inhibitory activity (Haslam et al., 1980). The phosphorylation of 50 K protein under these conditions is again inversely proportional to the phosphorylation of 40 K protein that is stimulated by thrombin.

298

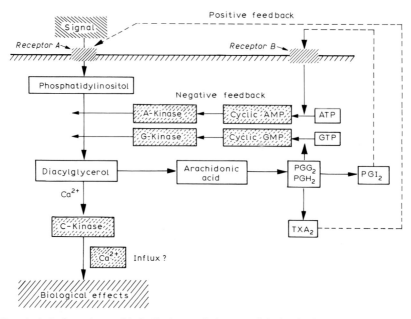

Fig. 6. Hypothetical scheme for possible feedback control of receptor-linked activation of protein kinase C by cyclic nucleotides in platelets. PGG2, prostaglandin $G_2$; PGH2, prostaglandin $H_2$; PGI2, prostacyclin; TXA2, thromboxane $A_2$; A Kinase, protein kinase A; G Kinase, protein kinase G; C Kinase, protein kinase C.


The experimental evidence presented above is not sufficient, but is suggestive that in a receptor cascade system occurring in the activated platelets cGMP may be involved in an intracellular circuit leading to the feedback inhibition of cellular activation. Fig. 6 illustrates such a hypothetical scheme that is outlined for the platelet system, and here both cAMP and cGMP may block the receptor-linked cleavage of phosphatidylinositol, and thereby counteract the activation of protein kinase C. Although this inhibition of phospholipid turnover is probably mediated through the actions of protein kinases A and G, the molecular basis of such inhibitory actions is not clear at present.


## 5. CONCLUDING REMARKS

In receptor functions there should be dramatic variations and heterogeneity from tissue to tissue. Nevertheless, using human platelets as a model system, the present article briefly outlines the properties and possible roles of protein kinase C that is found recently in this laboratory. The supporting evidence currently available is obviously limited, but it is suggestive that this protein kinase is potentially important in cellular activation, particularly in the transmission of information across the cell membrane. It seems plausible that $Ca^{2+}$ and diacylglycerol, that is derived from the receptor-linked cleavage of phosphatidylinositol, play key roles in the activation of this enzyme. In addition, various other membrane phospholipids appear to show positive and negative cooperative roles in this process, and arachidonic acid cascade may also be related directly or indirectly to the regulation of protein kinase C probably through actions of various prostaglandins. It is also suggestive that in some tissues cAMP and cGMP appear to be integrated in the extracellular and intracellular circuits, respectively, leading to the feedback inhibition of this unique protein kinase system. At present, there is virtually no evidence for discussing the mechanism of action of phospholipase C in stimulated plasma membranes. Also, we are ignorant concerning the physiological functions of this protein kinase in a variety of mammalian tissues. It is hoped that the new receptor function outlined in this article may open ways to elucidate the mode of action of a large number of hormones, neurotransmitters as well as of many other biologically active substances. The principles and mechanisms proposed in this article may undoubtedly be modified in the next few years by the sum of individual pieces of knowledge, which will be expanded rapidly by analysis of the receptor functions in a wide variety of tissues and organs including nervous tissues.

## ACKNOWLEDGEMENTS

This article has been presented at the Symposium on Brain Phosphoproteins at Utrecht, September 2–5, 1981 by one of the authors (Y.N.) who expresses his deep gratitude to Prof. W.H. Gispen as well as to other committee members for the invitation which made this talk possible. The authors are also grateful to Mrs. S. Nishiyama and Miss K. Yamasaki for their skillful secretarial assistance.

This investigation has been supported in part by research grants from the Scientific Research Fund of the Ministry of Education, Science and Culture, the Intractable Diseases Division, Public Health Bureau, the Ministry of Health and Welfare, a Grant-in-Aid of New Drug Development from the Ministry of Health and Welfare, the Yamanouchi Foundation for Research on Metabolic Disorders, and the Research Fund of Takeda Chemical Industries, Ltd., Japan.

## REFERENCES

Adelstein, R.S. and Conti, M.A. (1975) Phosphorylation of platelet myosin increases actin-activated myosin ATPase activity. *Nature (Lond.)*, 256: 597–598.

Adelstein, R.S., Conti, M.A., Hathaway, D.R. and Klee, C.B. (1978) Phosphorylation of smooth muscle myosin light chain kinase by the catalytic subunit of adenosine $3':5'$-monophosphate-dependent protein kinase. *J. biol. Chem.*, 253: 8347–8350.

Bell, R.L. and Majerus, P.W. (1980) Thrombin-induced hydrolysis of phosphatidylinositol in human platelets. *J. biol. Chem.*, 255: 1790–1792.

Bell, R.L., Kennerly, D.A., Stanford, N. and Majerus, P.W. (1979) Diglyceride lipase: a pathway for arachidonate release from human platelets. *Proc. nat. Acad. Sci. (Wash.)*, 76: 3238–3241.

Bergelson, L.D. and Barsukov, L.I. (1977) Topological asymmetry of phospholipids in membranes. *Science*, 197: 224–230.

Berridge, M.J. (1975) The interaction of cyclic nucleotides and calcium in the control of cellular activity. *Adv. cycl. Nucleot. Res.*, 6: 1–98.

Berridge, M.J. (1980) Receptors and calcium signalling. *Trends pharmacol. Sci.*, 1: 419–424.

Billah, M.M., Lapetina, E.G. and Cuatrecasas, P. (1979) Phosphatidylinositol-specific phospholipase-C of platelets: association with 1,2-diacylglycerol-kinase and inhibition by cyclic-AMP. *Biochem. biophys. Res. Commun.*, 90: 92–98.

Billah, M.M., Lapetina, E.G. and Cuatrecasas, P. (1980) Phospholipase $A_2$ and phospholipase C activities of platelets. Differential substrate specificity, $Ca^{2+}$ requirement, pH dependence, and cellular localization. *J. biol. Chem.*, 255: 10227–10231.

Bills, T.K., Smith, J.B. and Silver, M.J. (1976) Metabolism of [$^{14}$C]arachidonic acid by human platelets. *Biochim. biophys. Acta*, 424: 303–314.

Blackwell, G.J., Duncombe, W.G., Flower, R.J., Parsons, M.F. and Vane, J.R. (1977) The distribution and metabolism of arachidonic acid in rabbit platelets during aggregation and its modification by drugs. *Brit. J. Pharmacol.*, 59: 353–366.

Daniel, J.L., Holmsen, H. and Adelstein, R.S. (1977) Thrombin-stimulated myosin phosphorylation in intact platelets and its possible involvement in secretion. *Thrombos. Haemostas.,* 38: 984–989.

Dawson, R.M.C., Freinkel, N., Jungalwala, F.B. and Clarke, N. (1971) The enzymic formation of *myo* inositol 1:2-cyclic phosphate from phosphatidylinositol. *Biochem. J.,* 122: 605–607.

Goldberg, N.D. and Haddox, M.K. (1977) Cyclic GMP metabolism and involvement in biological regulation. *Annu. Rev. Biochem.,* 46: 823–896.

Graff, G., Stephenson, J.H., Glass, D.B., Haddox, M.K. and Goldberg, N.D. (1978) Activation of soluble splenic cell guanylate cyclase by prostaglandin endoperoxides and fatty acid hydroperoxides. *J. biol. Chem.,* 253: 7662–7676.

Hashimoto, E., Takeda, M., Nishizuka, Y., Hamana, K. and Iwai, K. (1976) Studies on the sites in histones phosphorylated by adenosine 3',5'-monophosphate-dependent and guanosine 3',5'-monophosphate-dependent protein kinases. *J. biol. Chem.,* 251: 6287–6293.

Haslam, R.J. and Lynham, J.A. (1977) Relationship between phosphorylation of blood platelet proteins and secretion of platelet granule constituents. I. Effects of different aggregating agents. *Biochem. biophys. Res. Commun.,* 77: 714–722.

Haslam, R.J., Davidson, M.M.L., Davies, T., Lynham, J.A. and McClenaghan, M.D. (1978) Regulation of blood platelet function by cyclic nucleotides. *Adv. cycl. Nucleot. Res.,* 9: 533–552.

Haslam, R.J., Lynham, J.A. and Fox, J.E.B. (1979) Effects of collagen, ionophore A23187 and prostaglandin E$_1$ on the phosphorylation of specific proteins in blood platelets. *Biochem. J.,* 178: 397–406.

Haslam, R.J., Salama, S.E., Fox, J.E.B., Lynham, J.A. and Davidson, M.M.L. (1980) Roles of cyclic nucleotides and of protein phosphorylation in the regulation of platelet function. In *Platelets: Cellular Response Mechanisms and their Biological Significance,* A. Rotman, F.A. Meyer, C. Gitler and A. Silberberg (Eds.), John Wiley, New York, pp. 213–231.

Hawthorne, J.N. (1960) The inositol phospholipids. *J. Lipid Res.,* 1: 255–280.

Hawthorne, J.N. and White, D.A. (1975) Myo-inositol lipids. *Vitam. Horm.,* 33: 529–573.

Hidaka, H. and Asano, T. (1977) Stimulation of human platelet guanylate cyclase by unsaturated fatty acid peroxides. *Proc. nat. Acad. Sci. (Wash.),* 74: 3657–3661.

Hirata, F. and Axelrod, J. (1980) Phospholipid methylation and biological signal transmission. *Science,* 209: 1082–1090.

Hokin, M.R. and Hokin, L.E. (1954) Effects of acetylcholine on phospholipids in the pancreas. *J. biol. Chem.,* 209: 549–558.

Holub, B.J., Kuksis, A. and Thompsom, W. (1970) Molecular species of mono-, di-, and triphosphoinositides of bovine brain. *J. Lipid Res.,* 11: 558–564.

Inoue, M., Kishimoto, A., Takai, Y. and Nishizuka, Y. (1977) Studies on a cyclic nucleotide-independent protein kinase and its proenzyme in mammalian tissues. II. Proenzyme and its activation by calcium-dependent protease from rat brain. *J. biol. Chem.,* 252: 7610–7616.

Kaibuchi, K., Takai, Y. and Nishizuka, Y. (1981) Cooperative roles of various membrane phospholipids in the activation of calcium-activated, phospholipid-dependent protein kinase. *J. biol. Chem.,* 256: 7146–7149.

Katz, A.M., Tada, M. and Kirchberger, M.A. (1975) Control of calcium transport in the myocardium by the cyclic AMP-protein kinase system. *Adv. cycl. Nucleot. Res.,* 5: 453–472.

Kawahara, Y., Takai, Y., Minakuchi, R., Sano, K. and Nishizuka, Y. (1980a) Phospholipid turnover as a possible transmembrane signal for protein phosphorylation during human platelet activation by thrombin. *Biochem. biophys. Res. Commun.,* 97: 309–317.

Kawahara, Y., Takai, Y., Minakuchi, R., Sano, K. and Nishizuka, Y. (1980b) Possible involvement of Ca$^{2+}$-activated, phospholipid-dependent protein kinase in platelet activation. *J. Biochem.,* 88: 913–916.

Kennerly, D.A., Secosan, C.J., Parker, C.W. and Sullivan, T.J. (1979) Modulation of stimulated phospholipid metabolism in mast cells by pharmacologic agents that increase cyclic 3',5'-adenosine monophosphate levels. *J. Immunol.,* 123: 1519–1524.

Kishimoto, A., Takai, Y., Mori, T., Kikkawa, U. and Nishizuka, Y. (1980) Activation of calcium and phospholipid-dependent protein kinase by diacylglycerol, its possible relation to phosphatidylinositol turnover. *J. biol. Chem.,* 255: 2273–2276.

Kishimoto, A., Kajikawa, N., Tabuchi, H., Shiota, M. and Nishizuka, Y. (1981) Calcium-dependent neutral protease, widespread occurrence of a species of protease active at lower concentrations of calcium. *J. Biochem.,* 90: 889–892.

Ku, Y., Kishimoto, A., Takai, Y., Ogawa, Y., Kimura, S. and Nishizuka, Y. (1981) A new possible regulatory system for protein phosphorylation in human peripheral lymphocytes. II. Possible relation to phosphatidylinositol turnover induced by mitogens. *J. Immunol.,* 127: 1375–1379.

Kuo, J.F., Andersson, R.G.G., Wise, B.C., Mackerlova, L., Salomonsson, I., Brackett, N.L., Katoh, N., Shoji, M.

and Wrenn, R.W. (1980) Calcium-dependent protein kinase: widespread occurrence in various tissues and phyla of the animal kingdom and comparison of effects of phospholipid, calmodulin, and trifluoperazine. *Proc. nat. Acad. Sci. (Wash.)*, 77: 7039–7043.

Lyons, R.M., Stanford, N. and Majerus, P.W. (1975) Thrombin-induced protein phosphorylation in human platelets. *J. clin. Invest.*, 56: 924–936.

Michell, R.H. (1975) Inositol phospholipids and cell surface receptor function. *Biochim. biophys. Acta*, 415: 81–147.

Michell, R.H. (1979) Inositol phospholipids in membrane function. *Trends biochem. Sci.*, 4: 128–131.

Minakuchi, R., Takai, Y., Yu, B. and Nishizuka, Y. (1981) Widespread occurrence of calcium-activated, phospholipid-dependent protein kinase in mammalian tissues. *J. Biochem.*, 89: 1651–1654.

Mori, T., Takai, Y., Yu, B., Takahashi, J., Nishizuka, Y. and Fujikura, T. (1982) Specificity of the fatty acyl moieties of diacylglycerol for the activation of calcium-activated, phospholipid-depedent protein kinase. *J. Biochem.*, 91: 427–431.

Murad, F., Arnold, W.P., Mittal, C.K. and Braughler, J.M. (1979) Properties and regulation of guanylate cyclase and some proposed functions for cyclic GMP. *Adv. cycl. Nucleot. Res.*, 11: 175–204.

Nishizuka, Y. (1980) Three multifunctional protein kinase systems in transmembrane control. *Mol. Biol. Biochem. Biophys.*, 32: 113–135.

Nishizuka, Y. and Takai, Y. (1981) Calcium and phospholipid turnover in a new receptor function for protein phosphorylation. In *Cold Spring Harbor Conf. Cell Prolif.*, 8: 237–249.

Nishizuka, Y., Takai, Y., Hashimoto, E., Kishimoto, A., Kuroda, Y., Sakai, K. and Yamamura, H. (1979) Regulatory and functional compartment of three multifunctional protein kinase systems. *Mol. cell. Biochem.*, 23: 153–165.

Ogawa, Y., Takai, Y., Kawahara, Y., Kimura, S. and Nishizuka, Y. (1981) A new possible regulatory system for protein phosphorylation in human peripheral lymphocytes. I. Characterization of a calcium-activated, phospholipid-dependent protein kinase. *J. Immunol.*, 127: 1369–1374.

Rittenhouse-Simmons, S. (1979) Production of diglyceride from phosphatidylinositol in activated human platelets. *J. clin. Invest.*, 63: 580–587.

Rittenhouse-Simmons, S. (1980) Indomethacin-induced accumulation of diglyceride in activated human platelets. The role of diglyceride lipase. *J. biol. Chem.*, 255: 2259–2262.

Rothman, J.E. and Lenard, J. (1977) Membrane asymmetry. *Science*, 195: 743–753.

Schultz, K.-D., Schultz, K. and Schultz, G. (1977) Sodium nitroprusside and other smooth muscle-relaxants increase cyclic GMP levels in rat ductus deferens. *Nature (Lond.)*, 265: 750–751.

Takai, Y., Yamamoto, M., Inoue, M., Kishimoto, A. and Nishizuka, Y., (1977) A proenzyme of cyclic nucleotide-independent protein kinase and its activation by calcium-dependent neutral protease from rat liver. *Biochem. biophys. Res. Commun.*, 77: 542–550.

Takai, Y., Kishimoto, A., Kikkawa, U., Mori, T. and Nishizuka, Y. (1979) Unsaturated diacylglycerol as a possible messenger for the activation of calcium-activated, phospholipid-dependent protein kinase system. *Biochem. Biophys. Res. Commun.*, 91: 1218–1224.

Takai, Y., Kaibuchi, K., Matsubara, T. and Nishizuka, Y. (1981a) Inhibitory action of guanosine 3′,5′-monophosphate on thrombin-induced phosphatidylinositol turnover and protein phosphorylation in human platelets. *Biochem. biophys. Res. Commun.*, 101: 61–67.

Takai, Y., Kishimoto, A., Kawahara, Y., Minakuchi, R., Sano, K., Kikkawa, U., Mori, T., Yu, B., Kaibuchi, K. and Nishizuka, Y. (1981b) Calcium and phosphatidylinositol turnover as signalling for transmembrane control of protein phosphorylation. *Adv. cycl. Nucleot. Res.*, 14: 301–313.

Takai, Y., Kishimoto, A. and Nishizuka, Y. (1982a) Calcium and phospholipid turnover as transmembrane signalling for protein phosphorylation. In *Calcium and Cell Function*, Vol. 2, W.Y. Cheung (Ed.), Academic Press, New York, pp. 385–412.

Takai, Y., Kaibuchi, K., Matsubara, T., Sano, K., Yu, B. and Nishizuka, Y. (1982b) Two transmembrane control mechanisms for protein phosphorylation in bidirectional regulation of cell function. In *Recent Advances in Calcium and Cell Functions*. S. Kakiuchi, H. Hidaka and A.R. Means (Eds.), Plenum Press, New York, pp. 333–347.

Wallace, W.C. and Bensusan, H.B. (1980) Protein phosphorylation in platelets stimulated by immobilized thrombin at 37 and 4°C. *J. biol. Chem.*, 255: 1932–1937.

Wallach, D., Davies, P.J.A. and Pastan, I. (1978) Purification of mamalian filamin. Similarity to high molecular weight actin-binding protein in macrophages, platelets, fibroblasts, and other tissues. *J. biol. Chem.*, 253: 3328–3335.

# B-50 Protein Kinase and Kinase C in Rat Brain

V.J. ALOYO, H. ZWIERS and W.H. GISPEN

*Division of Molecular Neurobiology, and Institute of Molecular Biology,*
*Rudolf Magnus Institute for Pharmacology, State University of Utrecht,*
*Padualaan 8, 3508 TB Utrecht, The Netherlands*

## INTRODUCTION

ACTH and some of its fragments are known to affect both brain metabolism and behavior (Schotman et al., 1976; De Wied and Gispen, 1977; Gispen 1981). Neurochemical studies revealed that such peptides can modify RNA and protein metabolism, polyamine metabolism, cyclic nucleotide levels, catecholamine turnover and phosphorylation of both membrane proteins and lipids (Schotman et al., 1976; Dunn and Gispen, 1977; Jolles et al., 1981).

With regard to the in vitro phosphorylation of synaptic plasma membranes (SPM) it was found that synthetic $ACTH_{1-24}$ selectively inhibited the endogenous phosphorylation of certain protein bands as separated by SDS–PAGE (Zwiers et al., 1976). Further experiments revealed that the structure–activity relationship between ACTH-induced inhibition of SPM phosphorylation and ACTH-induced excessive grooming in the rat are very similar (Gispen et al., 1979; Zwiers et al., 1977, 1978, 1981). For at least one SPM protein (B-50) the inhibition of the phosphorylation by ACTH is the result of a direct action of the peptide on the protein kinase activity in the membrane (Zwiers et al., 1978).

Further characterization of the endogenous phosphorylation of the B-50 protein in SPM revealed that it is insensitive to cyclic AMP (cAMP) or cyclic GMP (cGMP) (Zwiers et al., 1976). Furthermore the endogenous phosphorylation of B-50 requires both $Ca^{2+}$ and $Mg^{2+}$ (Gispen et al., 1979).

Another cyclic nucleotide–insensitive, calcium–requiring protein kinase, kinase C, has been isolated from rat brain (Inoue et al., 1977). Although this kinase was originally isolated from the soluble fraction of rat brain homogenate (Inoue et al., 1977) it has recently been found in the particulate fraction as well (Kuo et al., 1980). The activity of kinase C is stimulated by either partial proteolysis by trypsin or a calcium-dependent protease isolated from rat brain (Inoue et al., 1977) or by any of several phospholipids, such as phosphatidylserine (PS) (Takai et al., 1979a). It would appear that in the presence of calcium the soluble kinase binds to membranes resulting in its activation (Takai et al., 1979b).

During our studies on the B-50 protein kinase, we noted several apparent similarities between this kinase and kinase C. Our present paper details the experiments which lead us to conclude that B-50 kinase is indeed very similar if not identical to kinase C. The implication of this finding with regard to the role of ACTH and of lipid metabolism in brain cell function is discussed.

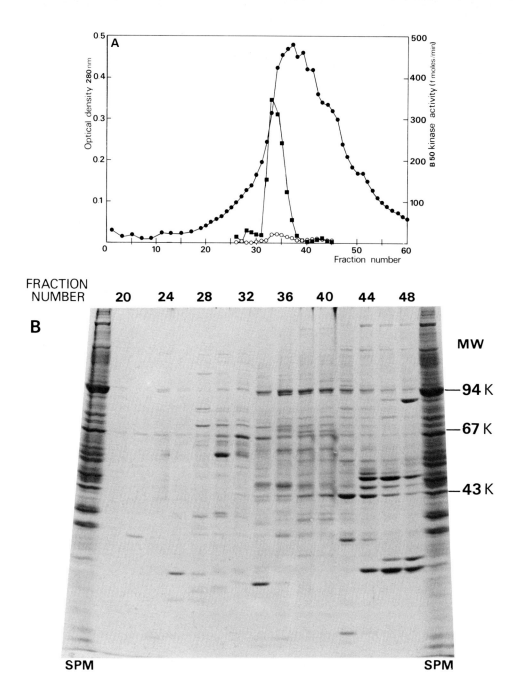

Fig. 1. Purification of B-50 protein and B-50 kinase by DEAE-cellulose chromatography. The Triton X-100/KCl-solubilized material was mixed with DEAE-cellulose and stirred for 15 min to allow the proteins to bind. The unbound proteins were removed by filtration through a sintered glass funnel followed by 5 washes of buffer A (10 mM Tris–HCl, 0.1 mM dithiothreitol, pH 7.4) without detergent (200 ml per wash). The washed DEAE-cellulose was poured into a column and eluted with a linear NaCl gradient (0–0.4 M NaCl in buffer A). A: Optical density and activity profile. The optical density at 280 nm was determined for each fraction (●). The fractions were assayed for endogenous phosphorylation of B-50 protein under the following conditions: 10 $\mu$l of each fraction, 10 mM Na$^+$-acetate, 10 mM Mg$^{2+}$-acetate, 0.1 mM Ca$^{2+}$-acetate, 6 mM Tris–HCl, 10 $\mu$M ATP, 2$\mu$Ci [$\gamma$-$^{32}$P]ATP, with (■) or without (○) 0.5 $\mu$g PS, pH 7.4, final volume 25 $\mu$l. The mixture was prewarmed at 30°C for 5 min and then the reaction was initiated by the addition of ATP. After incubating at 30°C for 10 min the reaction was terminated by the addition of a denaturing solution giving a final concentration of 2% SDS. The proteins were separated by SDS–PAGE and the incorporation of $^{32}$P into B-50 protein was determined. B: Protein-staining pattern of fractions. An aliquot of each fraction was applied to an SDS–PAGE slab gel. After electrophoresis the gel was fixed and stained with Fast Green.

# PURIFICATION OF B-50 AND B-50 PROTEIN KINASE

An attempt was made to solubilize the protein kinase from rat brain synaptosomal plasma membranes which is responsible for the phosphorylation of a membrane-bound protein substrate (MW 48 K; B-50) and is modulated by the behaviorally active peptide ACTH$_{1-24}$.

In pilot experiments it was found that the extraction procedure (0.1% Triton) described by Uno et al. (1976, 1977) did yield some solubilized B-50 protein kinase activity but its sensitivity to ACTH$_{1-24}$ was not preserved. Therefore alternative extraction procedures were studied. The detergent procedures used (Table I) all solubilized between 75 and 88% of the membrane protein, yielding extracts of a rather similar protein composition. However, only the Triton X-100/KCl treatment yielded soluble ACTH-sensitive, B-50 protein kinase activity. Due to our interest in ACTH-sensitive protein kinase, the recovery of enzyme activity was determined only in the Triton/KCl extract and residue. It was found that only 15% of the membrane-bound B-50 protein kinase activity was solubilized by the Triton X-100/KCl treatment while 85% of the activity remained in the residue (Table I). Why the addition of KCl preserved the sensitivity of the kinases to ACTH is not clear.

The Triton/KCl-solubilized ACTH-sensitive, B-50 protein kinase was further purified by DEAE-cellulose chromatography (Fig. 1). The endogenous phosphorylation of B-50 in the eluate fractions was assayed with or without PS. This activity was markedly stimulated by PS and the peak of activity eluted at about 0.2 M NaCl (Fig. 1). The fractions containing both the B-50 kinase and the B-50 protein were combined and subjected to ammonium sulfate fractionation. As discussed in detail previously (Zwiers et al., 1980) the B-50 kinase and B-50 protein were obtained in the material precipitating between 57 and 82% saturation.

Table II shows the quantitative aspects of the isolation of the B-50 protein kinase while Fig. 2 summarizes the qualitative aspects as visualized by protein patterns and autoradiographs after separation by SDS–PAGE. Throughout the purification procedure, the B-50 phosphorylating activity could be inhibited by ACTH$_{1-24}$.

In order to identify the B-50 protein kinase as well as to obtain purified B-50 protein,

TABLE I

THE EFFECT OF DIFFERENT SOLUBILIZATION PROCEDURES AND ACTH$_{1-24}$ ON RAT BRAIN SPM B-50 PROTEIN KINASE

| Fraction* | Total protein † (mg) | B-50 protein kinase (units)** | Inhibition by ACTH$_{1-24}$ (%) *** |
|---|---|---|---|
| SPM | 8.0±0.1 | 102.0±5.2 | −52 |
| Triton X-100/KCl extract | 6.0±0.1 | 16.0±0.4 | −52 |
| Triton X-100/KCl residue | 2.2±0.1 | 86.4±3.2 | −51 |
| Triton X-100 extract | 6.4±0.2 | n.d. | −5 |
| Deoxycholate (DOC) extract | 7.0±0.1 | n.d. | +5 |
| Triton X-100/DOC extract | 7.0±0.1 | n.d. | −2 |

\* SPM was extracted with the following reagents: 0.5% Triton X-100 plus 75 mM KCl; 0.5% Triton X-100; 0.5% DOC; 0.5% Triton X-100 plus 0.5% DOC.
\*\* The total B-50 protein kinase activity was determined using linear incorporation conditions (10 μg protein, 200 μM ATP, 4–5 μCi [γ-$^{32}$P]ATP, 10 mM Mg$^{2+}$-acetate, 50 mM Na$^+$-acetate, pH 6.5, total volume 25 μl) with a phosphorylation time of 15 sec.
\*\*\* The inhibition by ACTH$_{1-24}$ (10$^{-4}$ M, final concentration) is expressed as the percentage difference from control.
† Protein was determined by the method of Lowry et al. (1951). Each value is the mean (± S.E.M.) for three determinations.

TABLE II

SUMMARY OF ISOLATION OF ACTH-SENSITIVE PROTEIN KINASE FROM
RAT BRAIN MEMBRANES

| Step* | Volume (ml) | Protein (mg) | Specific activity (pmoles/mg/min) | Total activity (units**) |
|---|---|---|---|---|
| Triton/KCl extract | 220 | 225 | 1.8 | 405 |
| DEAE-pool | 24 | 12 | 5.5 | 65 |
| Ammonium sulfate (0–57) | 4 | 11 | 0.9 | 11 |
| Ammonium sulfate (57–82) | 0.8 | 0.4 | 148 | 53 |

\* Samples (1 ml) of all purification steps were dialyzed overnight against 1 l of buffer A. 15 $\mu$g total protein from each step (in triplicate) was used in the phosphorylation assay (as in Fig. 1).
\*\* One unit is defined as the amount of endogenous B-50 kinase activity transfering 1 pmole phosphate to B-50 in 1 min at 30°C.

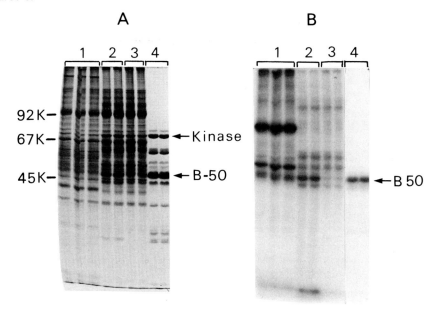

Fig. 2. A: Protein-staining pattern of different steps of the purification of protein kinase and B-50 protein. The numbers on top refer to the following steps: (1) Triton X-100/KCl extract; (2) DEAE-pooled fractions; (3) 0–57% ammonium sulfate precipitate; (4) 57–82% ammonium sulfate precipitate. Tracks 1–3 contain 12 $\mu$g of total protein. Track 4 contains 6 $\mu$g of total protein. At the left the position of three molecular weight marker proteins; at the right the position of B-50 and kinase is indicated. B: Autoradiogram showing the corresponding endogenous phosphorylation profile. Phosphorylation was carried out for 1 min with 7.5 $\mu$M ATP, using 1 $\mu$Ci [$\gamma$-$^{32}$P]ATP. Autoradiography took 16 h; because of high incorporation into B-50 (step 4) these tracks are from an autoradiogram which was exposed for 2 h.

samples of ASP$_{57-82}$ were subjected to IEF on a 5% acrylamide slab gel as described by Zwiers et al. (1980). After focusing the gel was cut into several lanes. One lane was used for pH determination, another was used for two-dimension SDS–PAGE (Fig. 3A). The remaining lanes were cut into 5 mm slices, eluted and dialyzed against buffer A. Each fraction was studied for endogenous phosphorylating activity as well as for its capacity to phosphorylate

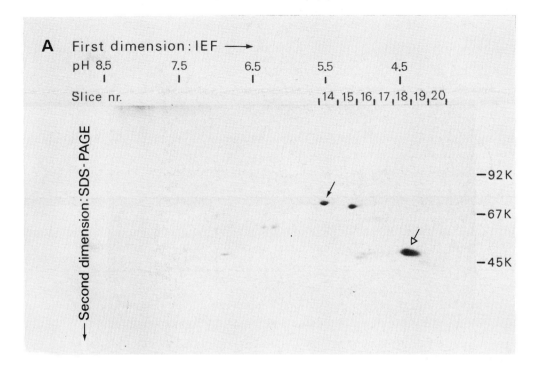

**A**   First dimension: IEF ⟶

pH 8.5          7.5          6.5          5.5          4.5

Slice nr.                              |14|15|16|17|18|19|20|

Second dimension: SDS-PAGE ⟶

—92 K

—67 K

—45 K

**B**

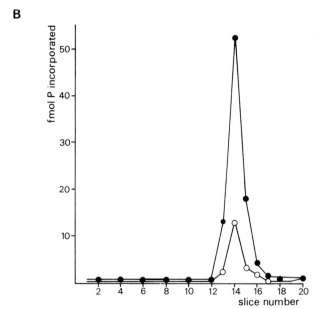

Fig. 3.  A: Protein-staining pattern of $ASP_{57-82}$ after two-dimensional separation of proteins. Samples were applicated on an IEF slab gel for separation in the first dimension. After running a whole track was cut out and mounted on top of an SDS slab gel for separation in the second dimension. After running, the gel was stained for proteins. At the top, the pH in the IEF gel is indicated as measured in a corresponding track of the same gel. Furthermore, the slice numbers are indicated, corresponding to fractions of the remaining part of the IEF gel which were used to identify the location of the protein kinase (see below). At the right the position of three molecular weight marker proteins are indicated. Arrows indicate the location of B-50 (48 K; open arrow) and kinase (70 K; closed arrow). B: Detection of B-50 kinase by IEF–PAGE. Proteins of $ASP_{57-82}$ were separated on an IEF slab gel. The gel was cut into slices and the proteins were eluted. All fractions were phosphorylated with added B-50 or histone. After phosphorylation, the proteins were separated on an SDS–PAGE slab gel and stained for protein. Incorporation of $^{32}P$ into B-50 (o——o) and into histone (●——●) was quantified by liquid scintillation counting of the excised gel band. No endogenous phosphorylation was observed in any slice.

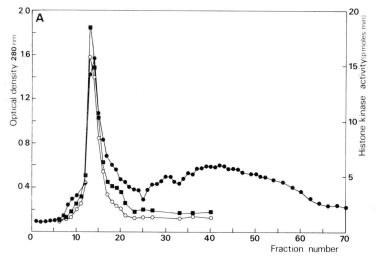

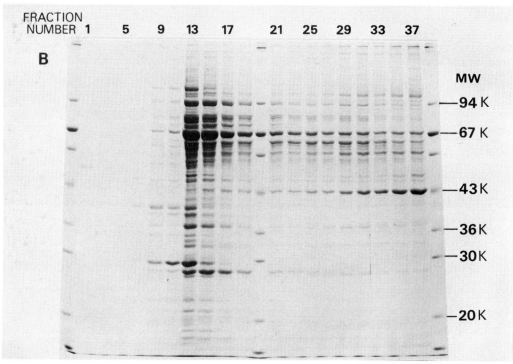

Fig. 4. Purification of kinase C by DEAE-cellulose chromatography. The 80 000 × g supernatant was mixed with 80 ml of DEAE-cellulose, pre-equilibrated with buffer B (20 mM Tris–HCl, pH 7.5, 50 mM 2-mercaptoethanol, 2 mM EDTA and 5 mM EGTA) and allowed to stir for 15 min. The unbound proteins were removed by filtration through a sintered glass funnel followed by 5 washes of buffer B (200 ml per wash). The DEAE-cellulose was poured into a column and the bound proteins were eluted with a linear NaCl gradient (0–400 mM NaCl in buffer B, 1 l total volume). A: Optical density and activity profile of eluate fractions. The optical density at 280 nm was determined for each fraction (●). The fractions were assayed for phospholipid-stimulated histone kinase activity under the following conditions: 10 $\mu$l of each fraction was added to 50 $\mu$l of a mixture containing 30 $\mu$g of whole histone (Sigma H-9250) and giving a final concentration of 40 mM Tris–HCl pH 7.5, 10 mM $Mg^{2+}$-acetate, 1 mM $Ca^{2+}$-acetate, 10 $\mu$M ATP, 0.5 $\mu$Ci [$^{32}$P]ATP with (■) or without (○) 0.6 $\mu$g of phosphatidylserine. The mixture was prewarmed at 30°C for 5 min before the reaction was initiated by the addition of $^{32}$P and was assayed by the filter paper method (Corbin and Reimann, 1974). B: Protein-staining pattern of fractions. An aliquot of each fraction was applied to an SDS–PAGE slag gel. After electrophoresis the gel was fixed and stained with Fast Green.

both B-50 protein (isolated from a similar IEF gel) and whole histone (Sigma H-9250). As can be seen in Fig. 3B, the protein kinase activity phosphorylating exogenous B-50 and histone was for a major part recovered in slice 14. No endogenous phosphorylation could be detected in the slice containing the B-50 protein (slice 18). As is shown in Fig. 3A, slice 14 contained only one protein after two-dimensional gel electrophoresis. The purified B-50 protein kinase has an estimated molecular weight in SDS of 70 K and an IEP of 5.5.

In order to compare the properties of partially purified B-50 protein kinase with those of kinase C, kinase C was prepared by the method of Inoue et al. (1977). Whole rat brain (minus cerebellum) was homogenized in ice-cold buffer containing 20 mM Tris–HCl, 0.25 M sucrose, 2 mM EDTA and 10 mM EGTA, pH 7.5. After centrifugation at $80\,000 \times g$ for 90 min, the supernatant proteins were separated by DEAE-cellulose chromatography (Fig. 4). The fractions containing kinase C activity were pooled, concentrated and further purified by Sephadex G-100 column chromatography (Fig. 5). Fraction 27, which contained the peak of kinase C activity (Fig. 5) was used for all further experiments. When compared to the initial homogenate the above procedure led to an enhancement of specific activity of about 200-fold. During the two–step purification procedure, kinase C activity was assayed after activation with both PS (see Figs. 4 and 5) and $Ca^{2+}$-dependent protease (partially purified by the method of Inoue et al. (1977) (data not shown). The peak of the kinase C activity after both activation procedures coincided with that of the non-activated kinase activity for both the eluates of the DEAE column and the Sephadex G-100 column. Furthermore, we have confirmed that neither cAMP nor cGMP affect the activity of this kinase while chlorpromazine is an inhibitor. Based on these criteria we conclude that we have indeed partially purified the kinase specified by Inoue et al. (1977).

## COMPARISON OF B-50 KINASE AND KINASE C

Previously, Inoue et al. (1977) have reported that kinase C has a molecular weight of 77 K as determined by sucrose density gradient centrifugation analysis and an isoelectric point of 5.6 obtained by isoelectric focusing electrophoresis. An analysis of the elution profile of the kinase C activity from the Sephadex G-100 column (Fig. 5) shows that the peak of activity corresponds to a molecular weight of about 80 K. However, molecular weight determination of the kinase C preparation by SDS–PAGE results in a value of 70 K (Fig. 6). B-50 kinase (from $ASP_{57-82}$) and kinase C have identical molecular weights by SDS–PAGE. Fig. 6 also shows that the $ASP_{57-82}$ contains several proteins, including the endogenous substrate protein B-50 and the B-50 breakdown product B-60. The corresponding autoradiogram shows that both kinases are able to phosphorylate B-50 (Fig. 6B). In addition, $ACTH_{1-24}$ inhibits the phosphorylation of B-50 by both kinases (Fig. 6B).

A comparison of these two kinases by two-dimensional PAGE, using IEF–PAGE for the first dimension and SDS–PAGE in the second dimension, showed that they have identical mobilities (see Fig. 7). These kinases were further characterized by peptide mapping analysis. The proteins of the two preparations were first separated by IEF–PAGE before being subjected to limited proteolysis. The resulting peptides were separated by SDS–PAGE, thus allowing a comparison of the molecular weights of the peptides. Fig. 7 shows that the protein staining pattern of the digestion fragments of B-50 kinase and kinase C are identical.

B-50 protein kinase as first described by Zwiers et al. (1980) is characterized by its ability to phosphorylate B-50 protein. Therefore, kinase C and three preparations of cAMP-dependent protein kinase (type I, rabbit muscle, Sigma P4890; type II, beef heart, Sigma P5511; catalytic

310

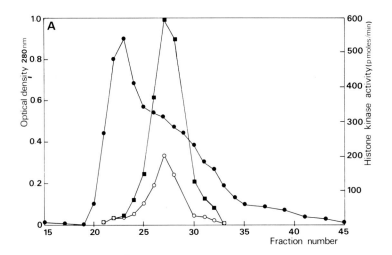

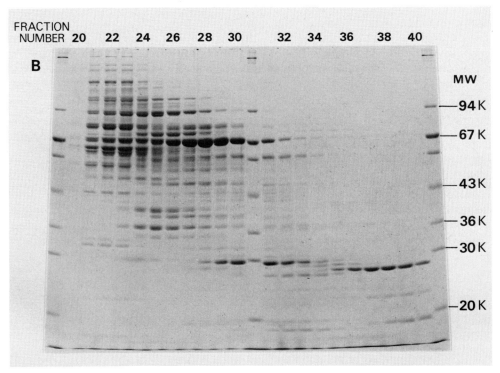

Fig. 5. Purification of kinase C by Sephadex G-100 chromatography. The DEAE-cellulose fractions containing kinase C activity (see Fig. 4) were pooled and concentrated by ultrafiltration (Amicon PM10). The concentrate was applied to a Sephadex G-100 column (100 cm × 2 cm) pre-equilibrated with buffer C (20 mM Tris–HCl, pH 7.5, 50 mM 2-mercaptoethanol and 0.5 mM EGTA). The column was eluted at 20 ml/h with buffer C and 5.4 ml fractions were collected. A: Optical density and activity profile. The optical density at 280 nm was determined for each fraction (●). The fractions were assayed for phospholipid-stimulated histone kinase activity under the following conditions: 1 $\mu$l of each fraction was added to 59 $\mu$l of a mixture containing 30 $\mu$g whole histone and giving a final concentration of 5 mM Tris–HCl pH 7.5, 10 mM Na$^+$-acetate, 10 mM Mg$^{2+}$-acetate, 1 mM Ca$^{2+}$-acetate, 10 $\mu$M ATP, 0.5 $\mu$Ci [$^{32}$P]ATP with (■) or without (○) 0.6 $\mu$g of phosphatidylserine. The mixture was prewarmed at 30°C for 5 min and then the reaction was initiated by the addition of ATP. After incubation for 10 min at 30°C the reaction was terminated and the incorporated $^{32}$P was assayed by the filter paper method. B: Protein-staining pattern of fractions. An aliquot of each fraction was applied to an SDS–PAGE slab gel. After electrophoresis the gel was fixed and stained with Fast Green.

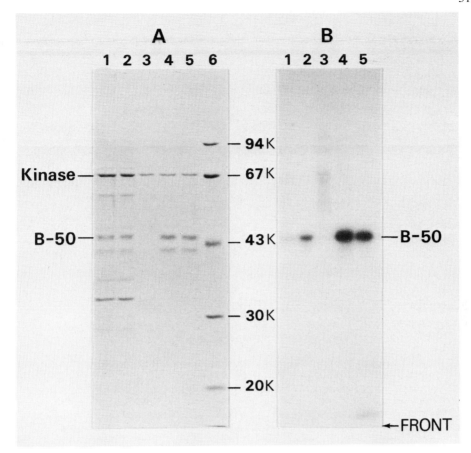

Fig. 6. Phosphorylation of B-50 by B-50 kinase and kinase C. $ASP_{57-82}$ proteins (2.5 μg total protein) plus $10^{-5}$ M $ACTH_{1-24}$ (track 1); $ASP_{57-82}$ proteins (as in track 1) (track 2); kinase C (track 3, 0.13 μg total protein); kinase C (as in track 2) plus B-50 (0.5 μg protein, including the breakdown product B-60; track 4); kinase C plus B-50 (as in track 4) plus $10^{-5}$ M $ACTH_{1-24}$ (track 5) were incubated with $[^{32}P]$ATP for 10 min. Phosphatidylserine (20 μg/ml) was present in the incubation mixtures (for details see legend Fig. 1). Part A shows the protein-staining pattern after SDS–PAGE. The position of the kinases (70 K) and of B-50 (48 K) are indicated. Track 6 shows the molecular weight of several standard proteins. The corresponding autoradiography (part B) shows the phosphorylation of B-50 and its inhibition by $ACTH_{1-24}$.

subunit from beef heart, Sigma P2645) were compared for their ability to use purified B-50 protein as a substrate. Table III shows that the B-50 protein is poorly phosphorylated by the cAMP-dependent kinases, whereas kinase C phosphorylates B-50. A further characteristic of B-50 protein kinase is the inhibition of its activity by ACTH and other behaviorally active neuropeptides (Zwiers et al., 1980, 1981). Similar to B-50 protein kinase, kinase C (using B-50 protein as a substrate) was inhibited 79% by $ACTH_{1-24}$ and 63% by $ACTH_{5-18}$ but not by $ACTH_{1-10}$. The same structure–activity relationship was found when endogenous B-50 phosphorylation was assayed in SPM (Zwiers et al., 1978). The phosphorylation of B-50 by kinase C is not affected by $10^{-5}$ M cAMP or cGMP. Chlorpromazine ($10^{-4}$ M) inhibited the phosphorylation of B-50 by about 85%.

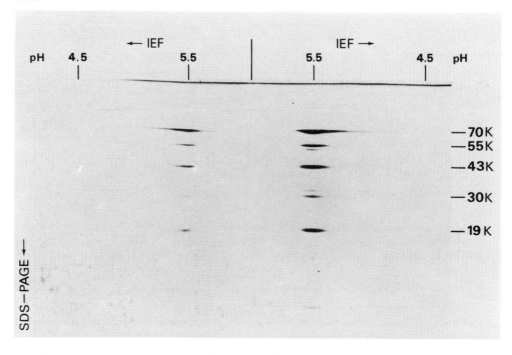

Fig. 7. Peptide mapping of B-50 protein kinase (left) and of kinase C (right). Peptide mapping with *Staphylococcus aureus* V8 protease was performed with a two-domensional method essentially as described by Bordier and Crettol-Järvinen (1979). Separation in the first dimension of B-50 kinase and kinase C was performed on a polyacrylamide slab gel (5 % acrylamide) containing 2.5 % (w/v) ampholine 3.5–10.0. The two gel tracks containing the samples were cut out and mounted on a single SDS slab gel (15 % acrylamide). Digestion was performed with 3 $\mu$g of *Staphylococcus aureus* V8 protease. Polypeptides were detected with a silver stain method (Merril et al., 1981). The pH of the IEF gel lanes is indicated at the top of the photograph and the molecular weights of the undigested protein kinases (70 K) and of four major digestion products are indicated on the right.

TABLE III

ABILITY OF SEVERAL KINASES TO PHOSPHORYLATE B-50 PROTEIN

| Kinase | Activity (fmoles/min) |
| --- | --- |
| cAMP-Dependent (beef heart) (0.607 $\mu$g) | $0.36 \pm 0.13$ |
| cAMP-Dependent (rabbit muscle) (2.33 $\mu$g) | $0.10 \pm 0.20$ |
| Catalytic subunit of cAMP-dependent kinase (beef heart) (0.056 $\mu$g) | $0.06 \pm 0.21$ |
| Kinase C (1.56 $\mu$g) | $37.90 \pm 0.81$ |

The kinases were assayed using 0.1 $\mu$g B-50 as the substrate under the conditions used in Fig. 1, except 5 $\mu$M cAMP (final concentration) was added to the cAMP-dependent protein kinases and 20 $\mu$g PS/ml (final concentration) was added to kinase C. Under identical conditions the amounts of kinase used incorporated 5–6 pmoles of phosphate/min into 30 $\mu$g histone.

The distinguishing characteristics of kinase C are its activation by PS and the $Ca^{2+}$-dependent protease and its inhibition by chlorpromazine (Inoue et al., 1977; Takai et al., 1979a; Mori et al., 1980). Therefore we tested the effects of these compounds on $ASP_{57-82}$. The endogenous phosphorylation of B-50 in $ASP_{57-82}$ is stimulated 4-fold by treatment with the $Ca_{2+}$-dependent protease. A similar 4-fold stimulation of B-50 phosphorylation was observed after the addition of PS (20 $\mu$g/ml, final concentration) to $ASP_{57-82}$. The addition of PS, while stimulating the endogenous B-50 phosphorylation did not affect the percentage inhibition observed after the addition of $ACTH_{1-24}$. Chlorpromazine ($10^{-4}$ M) is an inhibitor of B-50 phosphorylation in $ASP_{57-82}$ resulting in 80% inhibition.


## CONCLUSIONS AND DISCUSSION

By the physical and enzymatic criteria used, B-50 protein kinase and kinase C appear to be identical. This identity leads to questions about the role of this kinase in the regulation of brain function. Kinase C has been reported to occur in a wide variety of tissues (including brain) in both soluble and membrane-bound form (Kuo et al., 1980). In addition, kinase C has been shown to phosphorylate a variety of substrate proteins of nuclear, cytoplasmic and membrane origins (Wrenn et al., 1980; Nishizuka, 1980). In view of this enzyme's multifunctional properties, what then may be the physiological significance of the inhibition of this enzyme by behaviorally active peptides such as $ACTH_{1-24}$? It is important to note that $ACTH_{1-24}$ has been reported to inhibit the phosphorylation of several proteins in addition to B-50 (Jolles et al., 1979; Zwiers et al., 1979). In brain, B-50 may be a natural substrate for the kinase since the kinase and the B-50 protein copurify (Zwiers et al., 1979, 1980). Thus, in brain it may be that at least part of the B-50 protein kinase or kinase C is associated with the membrane-bound B-50 protein. Evidence for such a complex is obtained from the DEAE-cellulose column elution profiles (Figs. 1 and 4). Kinase C elutes at about 70 mM NaCl (Fig. 4), while both the B-50 protein and the B-50 protein kinase elute at about 200 mM NaCl (Fig. 1). This retarded elution may be due to the interaction of the kinase with the B-50 protein. Furthermore, the B-50 protein appears to be a brain–specific protein (Kristjansson et al., 1982), which is presynaptically located (Sorensen et al., 1981). Therefore, the interaction of $ACTH_{1-24}$ and kinase C (B-50 protein kinase) may only be of importance in those brain subcellular areas where the B-50 protein is located.

Another question which arises from the proposed identity of B-50 protein kinase and kinase C is the role of lipids in the regulation of protein phosphorylation. Nishizuka (1980) has suggested that kinase C is activated by the breakdown of phosphoinositides (PI) to diglyceride. The proposed scheme is that hormones interact with a receptor to stimulate a phospholipase C. This phospholipase C then cleaves PI to give a diglyceride which activates membrane-bound kinase C, which then inturn phosphorylates its substrate protein(s). On the other hand, Jolles et al. (1979, 1980) have reported that the phosphorylation of DPI to TPI by DPI kinase is dependent upon the state of B-50 phosphorylation due to the activity of B-50 kinase. Thus, it was concluded that the phosphorylation state of B-50 protein may effect the metabolism of polyphosphoinositides in brain cell membranes (Zwiers et al., this volume). An important avenue of future research will involve what the actual sequence of events is: is the breakdown of PI followed by the activation of kinase C/B-50 kinase (Nishizuka, 1980), or is the change in the phosphorylation state of B-50 a regulating event in polyphosphoinositide metabolism (Jolles et al., 1979, 1980).

314

## ACKNOWLEDGEMENTS

Dr. Henry R. Mahler (Department of Biochemistry, Indiana University, Bloomington) is gratefully acknowledged for his helpful discussions. We thank Dr. B. Poorthuis (Department of Biochemistry, University of Utrecht) for the generous gift of purified pig brain phosphatidylserine. We also thank M.A. Hoogkamer for excellent technical assistance. The authors wish to express their gratitude to Ed Kluis and Lia Claessens for their help in preparing this manuscript. V.J. Aloyo was supported by a NATO postdoctoral fellowship.

## REFERENCES

Bordier, C. and Crettol-Järvinen, A. (1979) Peptide mapping of heterogenous protein samples. *J. biol. Chem.*, 254: 2565–2567.

Corbin, J.D. and Reimann, E.M. (1974) Assay of cyclic AMP-dependent protein kinases. In *Methods of Enzymology*, Vol. 38C, S.P. Colowick and N.O. Kaplan (Eds.), Academic Press, New York, pp. 287–291.

De Wied, D. and Gispen, W.H. (1977) Behavioral effects of peptides. In *Peptides in Neurobiology*, H. Gainer (Ed.), Plenum Press, New York, pp. 397–448.

Dunn, A.J. and Gispen, W.H. (1977) How ACTH acts on the brain. *Biobehav. Rev.*, 1: 15–23.

Gispen, W.H. (1981) On the neurochemical mechanism of action of ACTH. *Progr. Brain Res.*, 53: 194–206.

Gispen, W.H., Zwiers, H., Wiegant, V.M., Schotman, P. and Wilson, J.E. (1979) The behaviorally active neuropeptide ACTH as neurohormone and neuromodulator: The role of cyclic nucleotides and membrane phosphoproteins. *Adv. exp. Med. Biol.*, 116: 199–224.

Inoue, M., Kishimoto, A., Takai, Y. and Nishizuka, Y. (1977) Studies on a cyclic nucleotide-independent protein kinase and its proenzyne in mammalian tissues. *J. biol. Chem.*, 252: 7610–7616.

Jolles, J., Wirtz, K.W.A., Schotman, P. and Gispen, W.H. (1979) Pituitary hormones influence polyphosphoinositide metabolism in rat brain. *FEBS Lett.*, 105: 110–114.

Jolles, J., Zwiers, H., van Dongen, C., Schotman, P., Wirtz, K.W.A. and Gispen, W.H. (1980) Modulation of brain polyphosphoinositide metabolism by ACTH-sensitive protein phosphorylation. *Nature (Lond.)*, 286: 623–625.

Jolles, J., Aloyo, V.J. and Gispen, W.H. (1982) Molecular correlates between pituitary hormones and behavior. In *Molecular Approaches to Neurobiology*, I.R. Brown (Ed.), Academic Press, New York, pp. 285–316.

Kristjansson, G.I., Zwiers, H., Oestreicher, A.B. and Gispen, W.H. (1982) Is the synaptic phosphoprotein B-50 specific for nervous tissue? In press.

Kuo, J.F., Anserssson, R.G.G., Wise, B.C., Mackerlova, L., Salomonsson, I., Brackett, M.L., Katoh, N., Shoji, M. and Wrenn, R.W. (1980) Calcium-dependent protein kinase: Widespread occurrence in various tissues and phyla of the animal kingdom and comparison of effects of phospholipid, calmodulin and trifluoperazine. *Proc. nat. Acad. Sci. (Wash.)*, 77: 7039–7043.

Lowry, O.H., Rosebrough, N.J., Farr, A.L. and Randall, R.J. (1951) Protein measurement with the Folin phenol reagent. *J. biol. Chem.*, 193: 265–275.

Merril, C.R., Goldman, D., Sedman, S.A. and Ebert, M.H. (1980) Ultrasensitive stain for proteins in polyacrylamide gels shows regional variation in cerebrospinal fluid proteins. *Science*, 211: 1437–1438.

Mori, T., Takai, Y., Minakuchi, R., Yu, B. and Nishizuka, Y. (1980) Inhibiting action of chlorpromazine dibucaine, and other phospholipid-interacting drugs on calcium-activated, phospholipid-dependent protein kinase. *J. biol. Chem.*, 255: 8378–8380.

Nishizuka, Y. (1980) Three multifunctional protein kinase systems in transmembrane control. *Mol. Biol. Biochem. Biophys.*, 32: 113–135.

Schotman, P., Reith, M.E.A., van Wimersma Greidanus, Tj.B., Gispen, W.H. and de Wied, D. (1976) Hypothalamic and pituitary peptide hormones and the central nervous system: with special reference to the neurochemical effects of ACTH. In *Molecular and Functional Neurobiology*, W.H. Gispen (Ed.), Elsevier, Amsterdam, pp. 309–344.

Sörensen, R.G., Kleine, L.P. and Mahler, H.R. (1981) Presynaptic localization of phosphoprotein B-50. *Brain Res. Bull.*, 7: 57–61.

Takai, Y., Kishimoto, A., Iwasa, Y., Kawahara, Y., Mori, T., Nishizuka, Y., Tamura, A. and Fukii, T. (1979a) A role of membranes in the activation of a new multifunctional protein kinase system. *J. Biochem.*, 86: 575–578.

Takai, Y., Kishimoto, A., Iwasa, Y., Kawahara, Y., Mori, T. and Nishizuka, Y. (1979b) Calcium-dependent activation of a multifunctional protein kinase by membrane phospholipids. *J. biol. Chem.*, 254: 3692–3695.

Uno, I., Ueda, T. and Greengard, P. (1976) Differences in properties of cytosol and membrane-derived protein kinases. *J. biol. Chem.*, 251: 2192–2195.

Uno, I., Ueda, T. and Greengard, P. (1977) Adenosine 3′,5′-monophosphate-regulated phosphoprotein system of neuronal membranes. II. Solubilization, purification and some properties of an endogenous adenosine 3′,5′-monophosphate-dependent protein kinase. *J. biol. Chem.*, 252: 5164–5174.

Wrenn, R.W., Katoh, N., Wise, B.C. and Kuo, J.F. (1980) Stimulation by phosphatidylserine and calmodulin of calcium-dependent phosphorylation of endogenous proteins from cerebral cortex. *J. biol. Chem.*, 255: 12042–12046.

Zwiers, H., Veldhuis, D., Schotman, P. and Gispen, W.H. (1976) ACTH, cyclic nucleotides and brain protein phosphorylation in vitro. *Neurochem. Res.*, 1: 669–677.

Zwiers, H., Wiegant, V.M., Schotman, P. and Gispen, W.H. (1977) Intraventricular administered ACTH and changes in rat brain protein phosphorylation: A preliminary report. In *Mechanism, Regulation and Special Functions of Protein Synthesis in the Brain*, S. Roberts, A. Lajtha and W.H. Gispen (Eds.), Elsevier/North-Holland Biomedical Press, Amsterdam, pp. 267–272.

Zwiers, H., Wiegant, V.M., Schotman, P. and Gispen, W.H. (1978) ACTH-induced inhibition of endogenous rat brain protein phosphorylation in vitro; Structure-activity. *Neurochem. Res.*, 3: 455–463.

Zwiers, H., Tonnaer, J., Wiegant, V.M., Schotman, P. and Gispen, W.H. (1979) ACTH-sensitive protein kinase from rat brain membranes. *J. Neurochem.*, 33: 247–256.

Zwiers, H., Schotman, P. and Gispen, W.H. (1980) Purification and some characteristics of an ACTH-sensitive protein kinase and its substrate protein in rat brain membranes. *J. Neurochem.*, 34: 1689–1700.

Zwiers, H., Aloyo, V.J. and Gispen, W.H. (1981) Behavioral and neurochemical effects of the new opioid peptide dynorphini (1-13): Comparison with other neuropeptides. *Life Sci.*, 28: 2545–2551.

# Evidence that High Frequency Stimulation Influences the Phosphorylation of Pyruvate Dehydrogenase and that the Activity of this Enzyme is Linked to Mitochondrial Calcium Sequestration

M. BROWNING[1], M. BAUDRY and G. LYNCH

[1] *Department of Pharmacology, Yale University School of Medicine, 333 Cedar Street, New Haven, CT 06510, and Psychobiology Department, University of California, Irvine, CA 92717, U.S.A.*

## INTRODUCTION

Memory is a phenomenon that has fascinated philosophers and scientists for centuries. It is difficult to imagine how transient events, which apparently leave only subtle biological traces, can produce permanent modifications in the behavior of an animal. Nevertheless, animals do learn and remember, and we must assume that this is isomorphic with alterations in the operating properties of the brain. In 1949, D.O. Hebb suggested, in his still influential model for the cellular basis of memory, that the most likely locus of the physiological substrate of memory would be a synaptic system which shows long-lasting changes in efficiency following brief periods of use. Consequently considerable interest attended the demonstration by Bliss and Lomo (1973) that a brief burst of high frequency stimulation produced a long-lasting increase in the efficiency of the stimulated synapses. Subsequent work revealed that such long-term potentiation (LTP) may persist for weeks or even longer (Douglas and Goddard, 1975) and that it can be elicited by as few as 10–20 stimuli delivered at 100–300 sec$^{-1}$ (Goddard, personal communication; also unpublished observations). Thus in brain, at least in the hippocampus, it is possible to produce extremely long-lasting increases in synaptic efficacy following a brief period of use. When it was subsequently demonstrated that LTP could be elicited in the in vitro hippocampal slice (Alger and Tyler, 1976; Andersen et al., 1977; Schwartzkroin and Wester, 1975; Deadwyler et al., 1976), it became possible to use the analytical power offered by in vitro methodologies to dissect a physiological process which possessed properties thought to be characteristic of the cellular substrates of memory.

## LONG-TERM POTENTIATION IN THE HIPPOCAMPAL SLICE

The hippocampal slice contains the major afferent input and the trisynaptic circuitry characteristic of the hippocampus (Fig. 1). Approximately 1 h after preparation of the slice, a bipolar stimulating electrode is placed where it will activate the massive Schaffer-commissural input to the CA-1 pyramidal cells. A recording electrode is placed in the terminal field of these axons where it can record the extracellular representation of the EPSP produced when the Schaffer-commissural axons are stimulated. Single pulses are then delivered until a stable

318

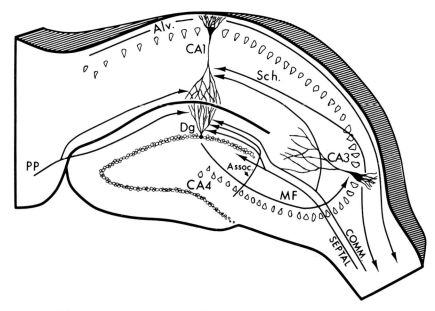

Fig. 1. Diagram of the cellular arrangement of the hippocampal formation. This schematic represents a typical in vitro tissue section cut perpendicular to the septo-temporal axis of the hippocampal formation. Alv, alveus, containing axons of CA1 cells exiting the hippocampus; Assoc., ipsilateral associational axons arising from CA3 cells and terminating in middle molecular layer of the dentate gyrus and CA1; CA1, CA3, and CA4, subfields of pyramidal cells; COMM., hippocampal commissural axons from contralateral CA3 cells, terminating in same dendritic fields as Assoc.; Dg, dentate gyrus (granule cell layer); MF, mossy fiber axons of the granule cells innervating the inner molecular layer of CA3 cells; PP, perforant path, containing axons originating in cells of the entorhinal cortex and terminating in dentate gyrus and CA1 outer molecular layers; Sch., Schaffer correlates of CA3 axons, terminating in middle dendritic zone of CA1 cells; SEPTAL, spetal axons terminating in the inner molecular layer of the dentate gyrus. (From Lynch et al., 1975.)

baseline response is obtained and held for 30 min. Then a 1 sec burst of high frequency (100 pulses sec$^{-1}$) stimulation is delivered for 1 sec and then testing is resumed with stimulation at 1 pulse sec$^{-1}$. A short-term form of potentiation (STP) can be detected within seconds of the cessation of the high frequency stimulation (Fig. 2); and, like the post-tetanic potentiation seen at the neuromuscular junction, this STP decays rapidly. However, the potentiated response does not return to baseline. Rather, within 2–3 min of the cessation of stimulation, the potentiated response is stabilized and this potentiated response typically persists for the life of the slice (4–6 h).

## MOLECULAR MECHANISMS OF LTP

Considerable evidence exists which localizes LTP to the synaptic mileau (Andersen et al., 1977; Schwartzkroin and Wester, 1975; Lynch et al., 1977); however, little if any information has appeared concerning the biochemical correlates of this process. A biochemical analysis of synaptic potentiation, while fascinating in its own right, could well have the added benefit of expanding our understanding of the sequence of events required to produce LTP (i.e., certain

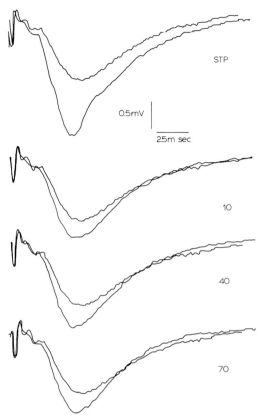

Fig. 2. Post-synaptic responses recorded in the regio superior of the CA1 pyramidal cells following stimulation of the Schaffer collateral-commissural projection to the region. Two responses are superimposed for each of the four conditions described (STP, 10, 40, 70). One trace is the control response that was obtained during a stable baseline period prior to the delivery of repetitive stimulation (100 pulses · sec⁻¹, for 1 sec). The second trace is the potentiated response obtained at various times following repetitive stimulation. Note the increase in both the slope and the amplitude of the potentiated response. The numbers adjacent to each pair of traces represent the time (min) between the repetitive stimulation and the collection of the second response (STP; post-tetanic potentiation, second response taken within seconds of cessation of the repetitive stimulation). Note that the marked potentiation present immediately after the repetitive stimulation (STP) shows a marked decay with time; however, the long-term potentiation (LTP) that is present at 10 min persists essentially without decrement for at least 70 min. (Lynch et al., 1979.)

biochemical correlates could predict other structural substrates of LTP). Beyond this it might be possible to test for chemical mechanisms in identified brain pathways during learning.

It is appropriate in beginning a study of the molecular mechanisms of LTP to consider what properties these mechanisms must have. The time course of the synaptic potentiation seen in the hippocampus requires a mechanism that can be triggered almost instantaneously and once initiated it must persist, or trigger changes that persist, indefinitely. Second, the mechanism should depend in some way on calcium since appropriate levels of this cation must be present to initiate LTP (Dunwiddie and Lynch, 1979). Finally the process must be shown to operate in synaptic regions. Protein phosphorylation is one process that fulfills these requirements. The process is a post-translational modification of protein which involves the enzyme (protein kinase) catalyzed transfer of the terminal phosphate from ATP to a serine or a theronine in the

320

protein. Protein phosphatases reverse the process by removing the covalently bound phosphate. This enzymatic process is widely considered to be the primary means of metabolic control in eukaryotes, and has received considerable attention in studies of synaptic events (Greengard, 1978). A series of papers from the laboratory of Paul Greengard have shown that protein kinases (Maeno et al., 1971), protein phosphatases (Maeno and Greengard, 1972), and the phosphoprotein substrates (Johnson et al., 1971) for these enzymes are all present in synaptic regions. Moreover, there have been numerous reports concerning possible roles for protein phosphorylation in regulation of neuronal function (Williams and Rodnight, 1974, 1975; Conway and Routtenberg, 1978; DeBlas et al., 1979; Ehrlich et al., 1978). A study by Williams and Rodnight (1975; see also Heald, 1957) was particularly interesting to us. These authors reported that field stimulation of cortical brain slices produced an increase in incorporation of $^{32}$P into total protein from neuronal membranes. The effect of such stimulation appeared to be a reversible phenomenon with a time course of approximately 10 min.

We proceeded, therefore, to test the possibility that protein phosphorylation might be involved in LTP by incubating hippocampal slices in $^{32}$P and then examining the effect of high frequency stimulation on protein phosphorylation (Browning et al., 1979). Our work differed from that of Williams and Rodnight (1975) in that we used potentiating stimulation of an identified pathway and verified the synaptic activation produced by this stimulation. In addition, we chose to look for stimulation-dependent changes in the phosphorylation of specific proteins rather than total membrane protein. However, as we soon realized, we were unable to obtain detectable levels of $^{32}$P in specific proteins without using an unacceptably high level of radioactivity during the preincubation and stimulation periods. We then turned to a "back-phosphorylation" assay (Ehrlich et al., 1976; Zwiers et al., 1976). Briefly, we used $[\gamma\text{-}^{32}P]$ATP in an in vitro assay conducted after subcellular fractionation of the stimulated and control slices. We hypothesized that if, as schematized in Fig. 3, stimulation produces an

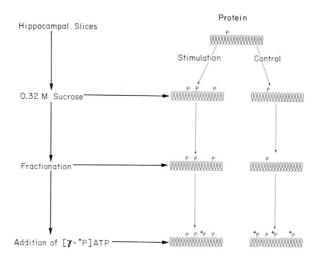

Fig. 3. Schematic of the hypothesis for the "back-phosphorylation" assay. A protein is depicted as containing a single phosphate (P) at rest in the slice. Stimulation increases the number of phosphates (P) on the protein. The protein from the control retains its single phosphate. The number of phosphates on the protein from the two samples is depicted as remaining constant through homogenization in 0.32 M sucrose and during subcellular fractionation. Finally when $[\gamma\text{-}^{32}P]$ATP is made available in the assay, only one radiolabeled phosphate (*P) can be incorporated into the protein from the stimulated sample. Three radiolabeled phosphates (*P) can be incorporated into the protein from the control sample.

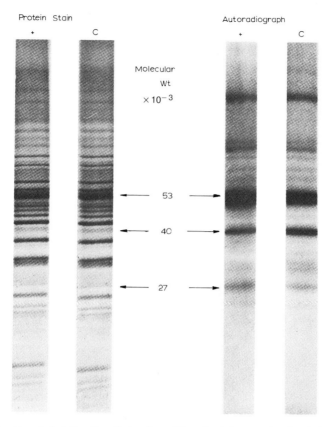

Protein Stain    Autoradiograph

+    C    +    C

Molecular
Wt
× 10⁻³

53

40

27

Fig. 4. Polyacrylamide gel depicting the effects of repetitive stimulation on phosphorylation of specific SPM components. +, stimulated sample; C, control sample. The molecular weight estimations were based on comparisons with the mobilities of standards of known molecular weight. Molecular weight values shown indicate bands in which significant stimulation-dependent changes in phosphorylation were observed (see Table I). (Browning et al., 1979.)

increase in the endogenous phosphorylation of a specific protein, and if this phosphate remains on the protein during the subsequent homogenization and fractionation, then when radiolabeled $[\gamma\text{-}^{32}P]ATP$ is made available in the in vitro assay, there should be fewer sites for the incorporation of label into the protein in the fraction prepared from the stimulated slices. The results of a typical experiment are presented in Fig. 4. As is apparent from visual inspection of the autoradiograph, a protein band with an apparent molecular weight of 40 000 dalton (40 K) incorporates less label in stimulated slices than in paired controls. Detailed analysis from 20 separate experiments revealed that the 40 K protein band incorported less label in the stimulated samples in 19 of the 20 experiments (Table I). Smaller and less consistent stimulation-dependent differences (increases) were also detected in bands with minimum molecular weights of 53 K and 27 K. We determined that the stimulation-dependent change in the phosphorylation of the 40 K protein was highly significant ($P < 0.001$) while the effects on the 53 K and 27 K bands were somewhat less significant ($P < 0.012$ and 0.01 respectively).

We next determined whether synaptic activation was required for these effects. Accordingly we repeated the experiments using slices that were incubated in medium from which the calcium had been omitted. In 8 separate experiments (Table II) we found no significant effect

TABLE I

STIMULATION-DEPENDENT ALTERATIONS IN PHOSPHORYLATION OF SPECIFIC SPM COMPONENTS

These data summarize the effects of stimulation at a rate of 100 pulses/sec for 1 sec in 20 experiments. The bands listed include only those which demonstrated detectable incorporation of label in 10 or more of the 20 experiments. Quantification of the incorporation of label into specific bands was based on densitometric scans of autoradiographs. (These values were in good agreement with radioactivity profiles obtained from scintillation counts made of 1 mm slices of the gels). Ratios between experimental and control values were determined for all detectable bands after normalization to control on the basis of total incorporation (as reflected by the densitometric values.) Percentage change is the average ratio for the 20 experiments. $N$, number of instances in which the stimulated value was greater (+) or less (−) than control.

| Molecular weight | Percentage change (mean) | $N$ | |
| --- | --- | --- | --- |
| | | + | − |
| 112 000 | + 3.6 | 10 | 4 |
| 85 000 | − 1.8 | 6 | 6 |
| 80 000 | + 7.9 | 12 | 5 |
| 68 000 | + 3.4 | 11 | 9 |
| 62 000 | − 0.9 | 5 | 8 |
| 53 000 | + 8.6 | 16 | 4* |
| 50 000 | − 0.7 | 10 | 10 |
| 45 000 | − 3.2 | 4 | 7 |
| 40 000 | − 25.9 | 1 | 19** |
| 33 000 | + 3.7 | 6 | 6 |
| 27 000 | + 16.0 | 15 | 2*** |

* $P < 0.012$.
** $P < 0.001$.
*** $P < 0.002$; two-tailed binomial test.

TABLE II

EFFECTS OF HIGH FREQUENCY STIMULATION, IN THE ABSENCE OF CALCIUM, ON ENDOGENOUS PHOSPHORYLATION OF SPECIFIC SPM COMPONENTS

These data summarize the effects of stimulation at 100 pulses/sec for 1 sec in 8 experiments. The bands listed include only those which demonstrated detectable incorporation in 4 or more of the 8 experiments. $n$, number of instances in which the stimulated value was greater (+) or less (−) than control. Quantification, as described in Methods, revealed no significant stimulation-dependent effects on any of the bands analyzed.

| Molecular weight (dalton) | % Change $\bar{X}$ | $n$ | |
| --- | --- | --- | --- |
| | | + | − |
| 112 000 | − 4.2 | 3 | 4 |
| 85 000 | − 2.1 | 4 | 4 |
| 80 000 | − 2.4 | 5 | 3 |
| 62 000 | + 5.3 | 5 | 1 |
| 53 000 | + 3.1 | 4 | 4 |
| 50 000 | − 6.2 | 3 | 5 |
| 40 000 | + 3.7 | 5 | 3 |
| 33 000 | + 5.3 | 3 | 2 |

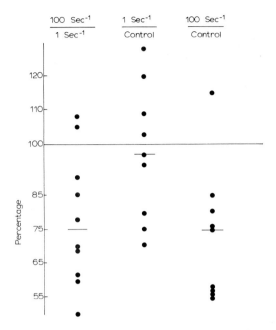

Fig. 5. A comparison of the effects of high frequency stimulation (100 pulses/sec for 1 sec), low frequency stimulation (1 pulse/sec for 100 sec), and no stimulation on the endogenous phosphorylation of the 40 K protein. We compared the effects of high and low frequency stimulation by calculating the ratio of incorporation into the 40 K protein in the two samples as follows: the incorporation following high frequency stimulation was divided by the incorporation following low frequency stimulation. This ratio was multiplied by 100 to give the percentage of incorporation for each experiment. A value less than 100 % indicates that there was less phosphorylation of the 40 K protein in the sample that received high frequency stimulation; a value greater than 100 % indicates less incorporation in the sample that received low frequency stimulation. Similarly in the comparison of high and low frequency stimulation with unstimulated controls, a percentage less than 100 indicates more phosphorylation of the 40 K band in the unstimulated sample. Each dot represents the percentage for a separate experiment.

of stimulation on the endogenous phosphorylation of the 40 K protein, nor were significant changes detected in any of the other bands we were able to analyze.

To assess whether the stimulation-dependent changes in phosphorylation of the 40 K protein were due to high frequency stimulation or merely to repetitive synaptic activation we compared the effects of high frequency stimulation (100 pulses sec$^{-1}$ for 1 sec) and low frequency non-potentiating stimulation (1 pulse sec$^{-1}$ for 100 sec). As shown in Fig. 5, high frequency stimulation produced a significant decrease in the phosphorylation of the 40 K protein when compared to matched samples stimulated at 1 pulse sec$^{-1}$ or unstimulated controls. However, low frequency, non-potentiating, stimulation had no effect on the 40 K protein when compared to unstimulated controls.

We were next interested in determining how long the stimulation-dependent effect on the 40 K protein would last. We therefore stimulated the slices at 100 pulses sec$^{-1}$ for 1 sec and then waited various periods of time before transferring the slices to cold sucrose. When 2 min were permitted to elapse before transfer of the slice to sucrose, a significant decrease in the phosphorylation of the 40 K protein was reliably detected (Fig. 6, $P < 0.001$, median decrease 25.9 %). Similarly, at the 5 min time point, a significant decrease was also detected although the magnitude of this effect was somewhat less than for the 2 min time point. No significant differences between stimulated and control samples were detected at the 15 and 30 min time

324

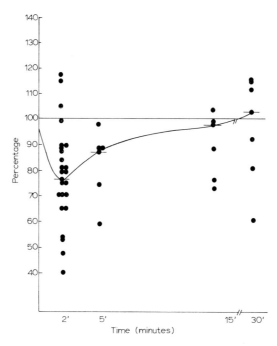

Fig. 6. A time course of the effects of high frequency stimulation on the endogenous phosphorylation of the 40 K protein. Tissue was transferred to ice cold sucrose at 2, 5, 14, and 30 min after the cessation of high frequency stimulation. The incorporation of label into the 40 K polypeptide in samples prepared from stimulated slices was compared with the incorporation into the unstimulated samples. The incorporation in the stimulated sample was divided by the corresponding value for the control sample to give a ratio which was multiplied by 100 to give the percentage of incorporation for each comparison. A value greather than 100 % indicated more incorporation into the 40 K protein from the stimulated fraction; a value less than 100 indicated greater incorporation into this band in the control sample. Each dot represents a separate experiment.

points. A 5 min time course has a number of implications concerning the possible role(s) played by the protein in potentiation. First, it appears unlikely that this phosphorylation change could be directly involved in producing LTP since this form of potentiation lasts considerably longer than the stimulation-dependent effects on the protein. Therefore, if the 40 K protein is involved in mediating LTP it would have to initiate events that persist long after the phosphorylation trigger has decayed. However, in the case of STP, the roles of trigger and effector would both be consistent with a 5 min time course since STP characteristically lasts only on the order of a few hundred seconds.

## CALMODULIN DEPENDENCE OF LTP AND THE 40 K PHOSPHOPROTEIN

As mentioned above, extracellular calcium is required for the induction of LTP and the production of the stimulation-dependent effects on the 40 K protein. We have, therefore, been particularly interested in the numerous reports indicating that many of the intracellular roles of calcium may be mediated by a calcium-binding protein called calmodulin (Cheung et al., 1978). To explore the possibility that calmodulin might be involved in the production of LTP, we examined the effect of trifluoperazine (TFP), a potent calmodulin inhibitor (Levin and

Weiss, 1976) on the induction of LTP in hippocampal slices (Finn et al., 1979). The results of a typical experiment are shown in Fig. 7. As is readily apparent, perfusion of the slice with 40 μM TFP produced a marked decrease in the magnitude of the potentiation seen following high frequency stimulation. In 15 experiments the mean increase in the slope of the evoked potential in the controls was 56% compared to only 8% for slices stimulated in the presence of TFP. It should be noted that TFP had no detectable effect on the evoked response obtained in the stabilization period, even at concentrations as high as 120 μM.

We next examined the effect of calmodulin and TFP on the phosphorylation of the 40 K protein. The data in Fig. 8 clearly show that TFP inhibits, and calmodulin stimulates, the phosphorylation of the 40 K protein. It is of interest to note that the concentration of TFP (40 μM) which half-maximally inhibits the phosphorylation of the 40 K protein and blocks the induction of LTP is close to the $K_i$ of TFP for calmodulin (Levin and Weiss, 1976). These data provide support for the hypothesis that calcium is the trigger for LTP and that the phosphorylation of the 40 K protein may be involved in this process.

## CHARACTERIZATION AND IDENTIFICATION OF THE 40 K PROTEIN

Given the potential importance of the 40 K protein to LTP, we have been particularly interested in establishing its identity. As a first step in characterizing this protein, we examined its subcellular distribution (Browning et al., 1981a). These studies (Fig. 9) demonstrated that

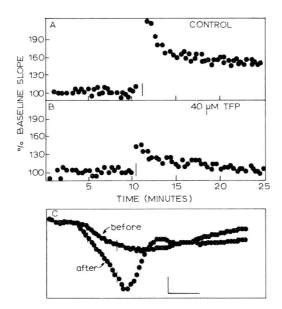

Fig. 7. A and B: typical experiments in the absence of (A) and in the presence of (B) 40 μM TFP. The high frequency trains were given at the arrows. The mean of all prestimulus-train slopes was set to 100%. C: evoked potentials obtained in normal medium before and after the high frequency trains. A MINC-11 analyzes the potentials in 85 μsec bins and performs a least squares linear regression on all points within the preset window. In this case the before-potentiation slope was −0.724 MV/msec ($r = −0.9956$) and 11 min after the high frequency trains was −1.299 MV/msec ($r = −0.9992$) for a slice tested in the absence of TFP. Calibration lines are 0.5 mV and 1 msec. (Finn et al., 1980.)

326

although the protein was present in synaptic plasma membrane fractions, it was highly enriched in the mitochondrial fraction. It is known that the $\alpha$ subunit of pyruvate dehydrogenase (PDH) is the predominant mitochondrial phosphopeptide at that $M_r$ range (Hughes and Denton, 1976). In addition, Seals et al. (1979) have reported that the $\alpha$ subunit of PDH, like the 40 K brain protein, is commonly found in purified plasma membrane fractions. To explore the possibility that the 40 K protein might be the $\alpha$ subunit of PDH, we compared the mobility of the 40 K brain protein with PDH which had been purified from kidney (Linn et al., 1972) and which was a gift from Dr. Tracy Linn. The data in Fig. 10 show that the 40 K brain protein and $\alpha$-PDH comigrate.

We next compared the two proteins in one-dimensional and two-dimensional peptide mapping experiments. A typical comparison of the chymotryptic phosphopeptides of $\alpha$-PDH and the 40 K protein is shown in Fig. 11. The two-dimensional maps reveal identical migration patterns for two major and three minor phosphopeptide fragments of the 40 K protein and $\alpha$-PDH. One-dimensional maps of the phosphopeptide fragments produced by Staphylococcus

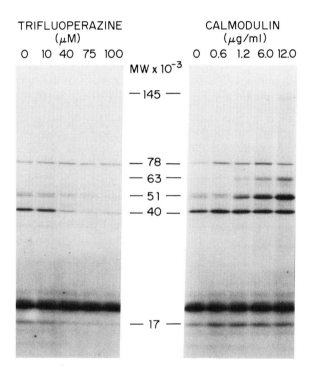

Fig. 8. Autoradiograph depicting the pattern of incorporation of $^{32}$P into specific polypeptides in the presence and absence of either TFP or calmodulin. Standard assay conditions included P2 protein at 0.33 mg/ml, 20 mM HEPES pH 7.4, 1 mM MgCl$_2$, 125 $\mu$M EGTA, 225 $\mu$M CaCl$_2$ (final volume 40 $\mu$l). Following a 1 min preincubation at 30° C, the reaction was initiated by the addition of 10 $\mu$l of [$\gamma$-$^{32}$P]ATP (10 $\mu$Ci/50 $\mu$moles final concentration). The reaction was terminated after 10 sec by the addition of a stop solution that yielded final concentrations of 2.3 % sodium dodecyl sulfate (w/v), 5 % $\beta$-mercaptoethanol (v/v), 62.5 mM Tris–HCl, 10 % glycerol (v/v), pH 6.8. TFP markedly inhibited the endogenous phosphorylation of proteins with molecular weights of 53 000, 51 000, 40 000 and 17 000. Calmodulin increased the phosphorylation of proteins with molecular weights of 78 000, 40 000 and 17 000 at the lowest dose tested (0.6 $\mu$g/ml). At higher doses, exogenous calmodulin enhanced the phosphorylation of proteins with molecular weights of 145 000, 62 000 and 51 000. Molecular weight estimations are based on comparisons with the mobilities of standards of known molecular weight. (Finn et al., 1980.)

$V_8$ protease (Cleveland et al., 1977) also indicate total homology between the 40 K protein and $\alpha$-PDH (data not shown).

We next compared the pharmacological properties of the phosphorylation of the 40 K brain protein and the $\alpha$ subunit of PDH. These data reveal (Fig. 12A) that dichloroacetate, which has been shown to selectively inhibit PDH kinase (Whitehouse et al., 1974), also inhibits the phosphorylation of the 40 K protein. Furthermore, phosphorylation of the 40 K protein can be effected in the presence of very low concentrations of $Mg^{2+}$ (Fig. 12B) as has been reported for $\alpha$-PDH in adipocytes (Seals et al., 1979; see also Hershkowitz, 1978).

## PDH ACTIVITY AND NEURONAL FUNCTION

Pyruvate dehydrogenase is part of a multi-enzyme complex which converts pyruvate and coenzyme A to acetyl-CoA in the mitochondrial matrix. Linn et al. (1969a,b) demonstrated that the activity of the kidney pyruvate dehydrogenase complex is inhibited by the phosphorylation of the $\alpha$ subunit of PDH, and a similar effect on brain PDH has also been observed (Seiss et al., 1971; Booth and Clark, 1978). The level of PDH in brain has been reported to be only minimally sufficient to maintain the normal flux of pyruvate through the oxidative pathway (Cremer and Teal, 1974; Blass and Gibson, 1978); this observation, combined with the fact that energy metabolism is almost totally dependent on glucose (McIlwain and Bachelard, 1971), suggests that changes in the phosphorylation of $\alpha$-PDH could have a major impact on mitochondrial functions such as ATP production and calcium sequestration. The demonstration of a link between potentiating stimulation and the phosphorylation of PDH raises the

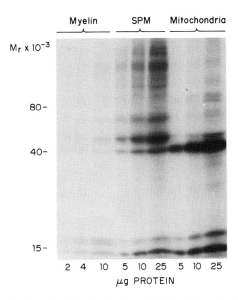

Fig. 9. Autoradiograph depicting the subcellular distribution of $^{32}$P-labeled proteins from brain. A $P_2$ fraction was prepared, phosphorylated with endogenous kniases and fractionated. Purified myelin, SPM and mitochondrial fractions were solubilized in SDS and subjected to electrophoresis in a one-dimensional polyacrylamide gel. Molecular weight estimations were based on comparisons with the mobility of standards of known $M_r$. (Browning et al., 1981a.)

328

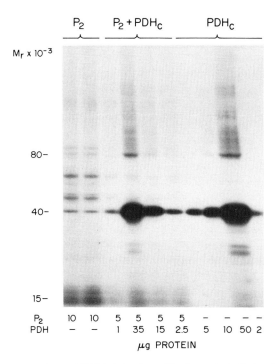

Fig. 10. Autoradiographic comparison of $^{32}$P-labeled polypeptides from a brain $P_2$ fraction and the bovine kidney pyruvate dehydrogenase complex (PDHc). The $P_2$ fraction and the complex were phosphorylated with endogenous kinases and [$\gamma$-$^{32}$P]ATP, solubilized in SDS, and electrophoresed in an SDS–polyacrylamide gel. The two wells at the left contain the $P_2$ fraction alone, while the next four wells contain various amounts of the PDHc mixed with the $P_2$ fraction. Various amounts of the pyruvate dehydrogenase complex were electrophoresed alone in the four wells at the right of the figure. (Browning et al., 1981a.)

question of how changes in the activity of this enzyme might influence the efficacy of synaptic transmission. In this light, it is particularly exciting to consider the possibility that changes in the phosphorylation of PDH might influence the ability of mitochondria to buffer the intracellular calcium load that is thought to result from high frequency stimulation. To explore this possibility, we have utilized dichloroacetate (which inhibits PDH phosphorylation) to examine the relationship between PDH phosphorylation and the ability of mitochondria to sequester calcium (Browning et al., 1981b). We first prepared purified mitochondria after Clark and Nicklas (1970) and examined the characteristics of pyruvate-supported calcium uptake in this preparation. Our purified preparation exhibited an apparent affinity for calcium of 1.0 $\mu$M, and significant cooperativity (Hill coefficient = 1.8) (Table III). Further, the pyruvate-supported uptake was stimulated by oxalate and almost totally inhibited by mitochondrial inhibitors, A23187, and EGTA. We next determined whether dichloroacetate (DCA) would in fact increase PDH activity via its effects on PDH phosphorylation as had been reported for liver and kidney PDH (Whitehouse et al., 1974; Cooper et al., 1974; Pratt and Roche, 1979; Hiraoka et al., 1980). DCA produced a dose-dependent activation of PDH and was half-maximally effective at a concentration of 0.3 mM (Fig. 13). Similarly, DCA half-maximally inhibited PDH phosphorylation at 0.2 mM.

Having confirmed that DCA could effectively activate PDH by inhibiting the phosphorylation of the 40 K brain protein ($\alpha$-PDH), we proceeded to study the effects of DCA on calcium

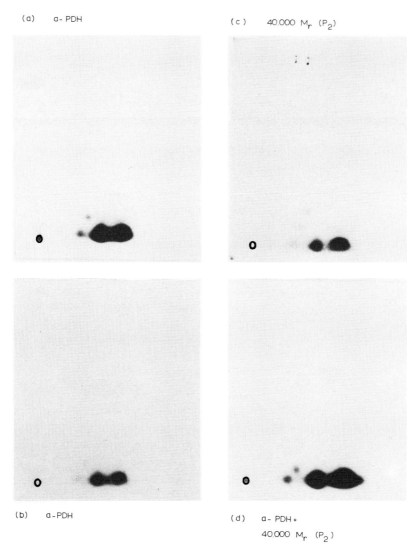

Fig. 11. Two-dimensional tryptic peptide map autodiagrams of the [32]P-mabeled $\alpha$ subunit of PDH and the $40\,000\,M_r$ brain protein. The pyruvate dehydrogenase complex and a $P_2$ fraction from brain were phosphorylated with endogenous kinases and electrophoresed in a one-dimensional polyacrylamide slab gel. The $40\,000\ M_r$ brain phosphoprotein and the $\alpha$ subunit of PDH ($\alpha$-PDH) were located by autoradiography, cut from the gel, and subjected to tryptic digestion followed by electrophoresis and chromatography. (a) [32]P-labeled tryptic peptides of the $\alpha$ subunit of PDH; total radioactivity 1000 dpm. (b) Same as in (a); total radioactivity 400 dpm. (c) Tryptic peptides of [32]P-labeled $40\,000\,M_r$ protein from a $P_2$ fraction; total radioactivity 400 dpm. (d) Equivalent amounts (400 dpm/sample) of (b) and (c) were mixed prior to application to the TLC plate. The open circle at the bottom left corner of each autoradiograph indicates the origin. Electrophoresis was carried out in the horizontal dimension from left (anode) to right (cathode). Chromatography was in the vertical dimension and the front traveled to within 2 mm of the upper edge of each autoradiogram. (Browning et al., 1981a.)

330

uptake by mitochondria. As the data in Fig. 14 clearly show, DCA markedly stimulated mitochondrial calcium uptake. The concentration of DCA that was half-maximally effective was 0.4 mM, a value comparable to that obtained for its inhibition of PDH phosphorylation (0.2 mM). These data suggest that alterations in the phosphorylation of the 40 K protein ($\alpha$-PDH) do in fact influence the ability of mitochondria to sequester calcium. However, it is possible that DCA or its metabolites might be enhancing calcium accumulation by a secondary action on some other aspect of the uptake mechanism. To control for such a possibility, we examined the effect of DCA on calcium uptake supported by either ATP or succinate, two substrates which do not require PDH activity to fuel calcium transport. DCA had no detectable effect on calcium uptake supported by these substrates. It appears therefore that pyruvate-supported calcium accumulation by brain mitochondria is tightly linked to PDH activity which is, in turn, significantly dependent on the phosphorylation state of its $\alpha$ subunit.

## A TRIGGERING MECHANISM FOR LTP

The data presented above indicate that potentiating synaptic stimulation of the Schaffer-commissural input to the CA-1 region in the hippocampal slice produces significant alterations in the subsequent endogenous phosphorylation of phosphoproteins with $M_r$ of 53 000, 40 000 and 27 000. The most reliable effect observed was a stimulation-dependent decrease in the phosphorylation of the 40 000 $M_r$ protein which we have shown to be the $\alpha$ subunit of pyruvate dehydrogenase (PDH). There are a number of possible explanations for this effect. There could be less of the 40 K protein in the stimulated fraction; however, such selective proteolysis in unlikely since the effect of stimulation is readily reversible. The decrease in phosphorylation

TABLE III

PROPERTIES OF PYRUVATE-SUPPORTED CALCIUM ACCUMULATION

Purified mitochondria were prepared and assayed for calcium accumulation under steady-state conditions supported by pyruvate (0.1 mM). Results are expressed as percentage of $^{45}$Ca accumulated in the absence of added agents.

| Treatment | $^{45}Ca$ accumulation (%) | Kinetic characteristics |
|---|---|---|
| Control | 100 | Maximal accumulation = 18 nmoles/mg protein/10 min |
| Oxalate (5 mM) | 250 | Apparent affinity = $1.0 \pm 0.2$ $\mu$M |
| EGTA (1 mM) | 0 | Hill coefficient = $1.8 \pm 0.1$ |
| A23187 (10 $\mu$M) | 0 | |
| Mitochondrial inhibitors* | 5 | |

* A combination of sodium azide, 0.1 mM; DNP, 0.1 mM; and oligomycin, 0.7 $\mu$g/ml (Browning et al., 1981b).

Fig. 12. Effects of dichloroacetate and magnesium on the endogenous phosphorylation of the 40 000 $M_r$ brain protein. A: The 40 000 $M_r$ brain protein from a crude mitochondrial fraction (P$_2$) was phosphorylated in the presence of various doses of dichloroacetate. Results are expressed as percentage of the phosphorylation of the 40 000 $M_r$ protein measured in the absence of dichloroacetate. B: The 40 000 $M_r$ protein from a P$_2$ fraction was phosphorylated in the presence of various concentrations of MgSO$_4$ in the absence or presence of 1.0 mM EDTA. (Browning et al., 1981a.)

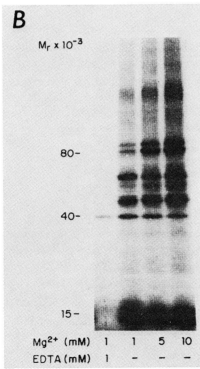

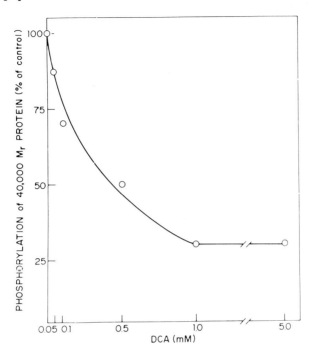

332

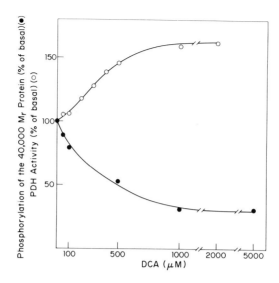

Fig. 13. Effects of dichloroacetate on the phosphorylation and activity of pyruvate dehydrogenase (PDH). Phosphorylation of the $40\,000\,M_r$ protein ($\alpha$-PDH) from purified mitochondria was measured in the presence of increasing doses of DCA. Similarly PDH activity from the same preparation was determined in the presence of DCA. Results are expressed as percentage of the phosphorylation or activity measured in the absence of DCA. Values expressed are the means of three separate experiments. (Browning et al., 1981b.)

could be due to increased PDH phosphatase activity; however, we can detect little if any of this enzyme under our assay conditions in the SPM fraction. This leaves only changes in PDH kinase activity or changes in the number of sites available on the 40 K protein ($\alpha$-PDH) as the likely causes of the stimulation-dependent decrease in the phosphorylation of PDH. We consider the latter hypothesis more attractive since, as mentioned before, the stimulation-dependent change must persist through homogenization and fractionation to be detectable in our assay. Thus we consider the phosphorylation of PDH, which is a covalent modification, as a better candidate for a persistent effect than PDH kinase activation which is thought to result from the allosteric effects of soluble factors (Cooper et al., 1974; Roche and Reed, 1974; Pratt and Roche, 1979; Cate and Roche, 1979). Thus, as our working model, we suggest that high frequency synaptic stimulation leads to the phosphorylation of PDH and that this increased phosphorylation persists until the subsequent assay, thus resulting in fewer sites being available for incorporation of label.

If, in fact, high frequency synaptic stimulation does lead to an increase in the phosphorylation of PDH, one question that immediately comes to mind concerns the mechanism of this effect. It is widely recognized that there are a variety of factors, including NADH/NAD, ATP/ADP, and acetyl CoA/CoA ratios, that influence the phosphorylation state of PDH (Kerbey et al., 1976; Cate and Roche, 1979). Recent work by Seals et al. (1979) provides evidence for an extra-mitochondrial regulation of the state of PDH phosphorylation. These authors report that insulin dephosphorylates PDH, presumably by interactions with a cell membrane receptor to produce an intracellular messenger that activates PDH phosphatase. Considerable precedent does therefore exist for modulation of PDH phosphorylation in response to changes in hormonal and metabolic state. Perhaps high frequency stimulation influences PDH phosphorylation via effects on systems such as those outlined above. An additional possibility that should be mentioned concerns our demonstration that calmodulin

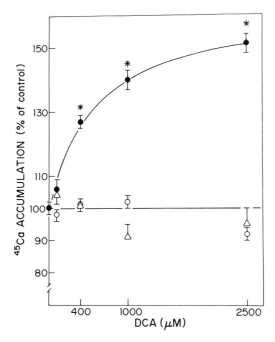

Fig. 14. Effect of various concentrations of dichloroacetate on calcium accumulation supported by pyruvate, succinate, or ATP. Calcium accumulation in rat brain mitochondria was measured after 10 min incubations in the presence of various DCA concentrations and either 0.1 mM pyruvate (closed circles), 5.0 mM succinate (open circles), or 1.0 mM ATP (open triangles). Results are mean ± S.E.M. of four to six different experiments and are expressed as percentage of the accumulation in the absence of added DCA (control values were pyruvate, 828 ± 25; succinate, 1890 ± 150; and ATP, 1420 ± 70 ng calcium/mg protein). *$P < 0.01$. (Browning et al., 1981b.)

stimulates PDH phosphorylation in vitro. Given the calcium dependence of LTP, it is tempting to hypothesize that high frequency stimulation leads to the phosphorylation of PDH via effects of calcium/calmodulin on PDH kinase. This hypothesis is made even more attractive by the fact that Trifluoperazine, a potent inhibitor of calmodulin, effectively blocks the LTP seen following high frequency stimulation. Finally, in a recent report, Sieghart (1981) demonstrated that micromolar concentrations of glutamate produced a 300% increase in the endogenous phosphorylation of PDH. Since glutamic acid is known to be released during high frequency stimulation (Baudry and Lynch, 1979), the possibility exists (as suggested by Sieghart, 1981) that the effects of potentiating stimulation on PDH phosphorylation could be mediated by glutamate. This would of course be consistent with the fact that neither LTP nor phosphorylation changes in PDH are produced by stimulation of brain slices incubated in the absence of calcium, a condition that blocks transmitter release.

The final point to be considered concerns the relationship between changes in PDH phosphorylation and the synaptic potentiation seen following high frequency stimulation. Our data linking the phosphorylation state of PDH to calcium sequestration by mitochondria may provide an explanation for some of the changes in synaptic physiology which follow repetitive stimulation. Such stimulation may, by altering PDH activity, lead to a decrease in the ability of mitochondria to sequester the elevated level of intracellular calcium that is thought to result from such stimulation. It must be emphasized that the data supporting this hypothesis are indirect; no data are yet available which show that high frequency stimulation influences pyruvate-supported mitochondrial calcium uptake. It is interesting in this regard that Alnaes and Rahamimoff (1975) have presented evidence that suggests that mitochondria can influence transmitter release by regulating calcium in the synaptic terminal. Furthermore, Rahamimoff et al. (1978) have suggested that post-tetanic potentiation, a short-term form of potentiation seen at the neuromuscular junction, may be caused by disturbances in mito-chondrial sequestration. Finally, it must be remembered with regard to the hypothesis outlined above, that the stimulation-dependent changes in PDH last only a few minutes. Thus changes in intraterminal calcium that result form a brief interruption in mitochondrial sequestration would be expected to be transitory. This short-term elevation in calcium could directly mediate the short-term potentiation seen after high frequency stimulation. However, these changes in calcium level could participate in the production of long-term potentiation only if they were to trigger cellular alterations of a more permanent nature.

## LONG-LASTING CORRELATES OF LTP

The data presented so far lead to the hypothesis that a short-lasting disturbance in free cytoplasmic calcium is the triggering mechanism for LTP. Where, among the multitude of cellular processes regulated by calcium, is (are) to be found the mechanims(s) ultimately resulting in the long-lasting alteration of synaptic transmission underlying LTP? Intuitively, it seems clear that changes in neurotransmitter release and/or neurotransmitter receptor function are the two immediate candidates. Therefore if we can reveal mechanisms linking calcium perturbation and long-lasting changes in neurotransmitter release or receptors, such me-chanisms could offer a valuable starting point to investigate potential cellular bases of LTP. In this context, it is worth mentioning that glutamate or a closely substance is very likely the neurotransmitter of the pathways exhibiting LTP (Storm-Mathisen, 1977). Hippocampal membranes have been shown to possess high-affinity, sodium-independent [$^3$H]glutamate-binding sites which exhibit properties expected of a postsynaptic glutamate receptor (Baudry and Lynch, 1981a,b). Interestingly enough, low concentrations of calcium (10–100 $\mu$M) are able to increase, in an irreversible manner, the number of these sites without changing their affinity for glutamate (Baudry and Lynch, 1979). Moreover, high frequency electrical stimu-lation of the Schaffer-commissural system also results in an increase in the number of these sites (Baudry et al., 1980), an effect which is not observed following low frequency stimula-tion or when the high frequency stimulation is given in a low calcium–high magnesium medium (Lynch et al., submitted). Although the time-course of this effect has not been extensively studied, the increase in binding occurs rapidly (5–10 min) and is still present at least 1 h following the "potentiating" trains. This led us to postulate that some patterns of synaptic activity are able to increase the number of glutamate receptors and consequently to increase the efficacy of synaptic transmission.

Another approach demonstrated that the same type of electrical stimulation resulted in two categories of ultrastructural changes in the synaptic field, target of the stimulated fibers: (i) an increase in the number of shaft synapses and (ii) a change in the shape of spine synapses, possibly due to a transition from a ellipsoidal to a spherical shape (Lee et al., 1980, 1981). Again it is possible, but not proven, that such a structural modification results in an increased strength of synaptic transmission. The question which naturally follows is whether or not these two types of modification, biochemical and ultrastructural, are simply by-products of some processes more directly related to the induction of LTP, or are indeed part of the alterations involved in the establishment of LTP. If the later hypothesis is correct, can the same mechanism be responsible for both types of modification? This is not unlikely because is would seem certainly possible that a change in the spine shape is accompanied by some reorganization of the synaptic membranes and consequently of its protein components, or conversely that a modification in the membrane chemistry can result in an alteration in the shape of the spine. For instance, it has been shown, in blood platelets, that a shape change is accompanied by a modification in the number of some cell surface receptors (Kao et al., 1981).

The study of the calcium regulation of [$^3$H]glutamate receptor binding in hippocampal membranes has revealed the existence of a mechanism which might well provide an answer to the above questions. Thus we found that several inhibitors of calcium-activated neutral thiol proteinases (CAPs) inhibit the stimulatory effect of calcium on glutamate binding (Baudry and Lynch, 1980). More recently we provided evidence that hippocampal as well as cortical membranes posses a calcium-sensitive proteolytic enzyme. Thus low concentrations of calcium (10–100 $\mu$M) induce the degradation of a high molecular weight doublet protein. The similarities between the calcium stimulation of glutamate binding and calcium stimulation of this proteolytic process led us to propose that the latter is responsible for the former (Baudry et al., 1981). In addition, although the nature of the doublet protein is not yet known, its characteristics suggest that it may be a neurofilament-related protein. In view of the involvement of the proteins in this family in the regulation of shape maintenance and cell surface receptor mobility (Edelman, 1976; Nicolson, 1979), we proposed that the calcium-induced stimulation of the proteolysis of this membrane component could be responsible for both the change in the number of glutamate receptors and the change in the spine shape (Lynch and Baudry, 1981).

In conclusion, it appears that we might be very close to a precise understanding of the various steps initiated by high frequency electrical stimulation and leading to a long-lasting increase in synaptic transmission. They should provide us various possible ways of interfering with the induction of LTP, and therefore to start extending the studies from test tubes and slices to the world of behaving animals.

## REFERENCES

Alger, B. and Tyler, T. (1976) Long-term and short-term plasticity in the CA$_1$, CA$_2$ and dentate regions of the hippocampal slice. *Brain Res.*, 110: 463–480.

Alnaes, E. and Rahamimoff, R. (1975) Role of mitochondria in transmitter release from motor terminals. *J. Physiol. (Lond.)*, 248: 285–306.

Andersen, P., Sandberg, S., Sveen O. and Wigström, H. (1977) Specific long-lasting potentiation of synaptic transmission in hippocampal slice. *Nature (Lond.)*, 226: 736–737.

Baudry, M. and Lynch, G. (1979) Regulation of glutamate receptors by cations. *Nature (Lond.)*, 282: 748–750.

Baudry, M. and Lynch, G. (1980) Regulation of hippocampal glutamate receptors: evidence for the involvement of a calcium-activated protease. *Proc. nat. Acad. Sci. (Wash.)*, 77: 2298–2302.

Baudry, M. and Lynch, G. (1981a) Characterization of two $^3$H-glutamate binding sites in rat hippocampal membranes. *J. Neurochem.*, 36(3): 811–820.

Baudry, M. and Lynch, G. (1981b) High affinity binding sites for $^3$H-glutamate in hippocampal membranes: The search for a glutamate receptor. In *Advances in Biochemical Psychopharmacology*, Vol. 29, F. De Feudis and P. Mandel (Eds.), Raven Press, New York, pp. 397–403.

Baudry, M., Oliver, M., Creager, R., Wieraszko, A. and Lynch, G. (1980) Increase in glutamate receptors following repetitive electrical stimulation in hippocampal slices. *Life Sci.*, 27: 325–330

Baudry, M., Bundman, M., Smith, E. and Lynch, G. (1981) Micromolar levels of calcium stimulate proteolytic activity and glutamate receptor binding in rat brain synaptic membranes. *Science*, 212: 937–938.

Blass, J. and Gibson, G. (1978) Studies of the pathophysiology of pyruvate dehydrogenase dfiency. *Adv. Neurol.*, 21: 181–194.

Bliss, T.V.P. and Lomo, T. (1973) Long-lasting potentiation of synaptic transmission in the dentate area of aneathesized rabbit following stimulation of the perforant path. *J. Physiol. (Lond.)*, 232: 331–356.

336

Booth, R. and Clark, J. (1978) The control of pyruvate dehydrogenase in isolated brain mitochondria. *J. Neurochem.,* 30: 1003–1008.

Browning, M., Dunwiddie, T., Bennett, W., Gispen, W. and Lynch, G. (1979) Synaptic phosphoproteins: Specific changes after repetitive stimulation of the hippocampal slice. *Science,* 203: 60–62.

Browning, M., Bennett, W., Kelly, P. and Lynch, G. (1981a) The 40,000 Mr phosphoprotein influenced by high frequency synaptic stimulation is the alpha subunit of pyruvate dehydrogenase. *Brain Res.,* 218: 255–266.

Browning, M., Baudry, M., Bennett, W. and Lynch, G. (1981b) Phosphorylation-mediated changes in pyruvate dehydrogenase activitry influence pyruvate-supported calcium accumulation by brain mitochondria. *J. Neurochem.,* 36: 1932–1940.

Cate, R. and Roche, T. (1978) A unifying mechanism for stimulation of mammalian pyruvate dehydrogenase kinase by reduced nicotinamide adenine dinucleotide, dehydrolipoamide, acetyl coenzyme A, or pyruvate. *J. biol. Chem.,* 253: 496–503.

Cheung, W., Lynch, T. and Wallace, R. (1978) An endogenous $Ca^{2+}$-dependent activator protein of brain adenylate cyclase and cyclic nucleotide phosphadiesterase. *Adv. cyclic Nucleot. Res.,* 9: 233–251.

Clark, J. and Nicklas, W. (1970) The metabolism of rat brain mitochondria. Preparation and characterization. *J. biol. Chem.,* 245: 4724–4731.

Cleveland, D., Fischer, S., Kirschner, J. and Laemmli, U. (1977) Peptide mapping by limited proteolysisin sodium sulphate and analysis by gel electrophoresis. *J. biol. Chem.,* 252: 1102–1106.

Conway, R. and Routtenberg, A. (1978) Endogenous phosphorylation in vitro: Selective effects of sacrifice methods on specific brain proteins. *Brain Res.,* 139: 366–373.

Cooper, R., Randle, P. and Denton, R. (1974) Regulation of heart muscle pyruvate dehydrogenase kinase. *Biochem. J.,* 143: 625–641.

Cremer, J. and Teal, H. (1974) The activity of pyruvate dehydrogenase in rat brain during postnatal development. *FEBS Lett.,* 39: 17–20.

Deadwyler, S., Gribkoff, V., Cotman, C. and Lynch, G. (1976) Long lasting changes in the spontaneous activity of hippocampal neurons following stimulation of the entorhinal cortex. *Brain Res. Bull.,* 1: 1–7.

DeBlas, A., Wang, Y., Sörensen, R. and Mahler, H. (1979) Protein phosphorylation in synaptic membranes regulated by adenosine 3',5'-monophosphate: regional and subcellular distribution of the endogenous substrates. *J. Neurochem.,* 33: 647–659.

Denton, R., Randle, P. and Martin, B. (1972) Stimulation by calcium ions of pyruvate dehydrogenase phosphate phosphatase. *Biochem. J.,* 128: 161–163.

Douglas, R.M. and Goddard, G.V. (1975) Long-term potentiation of the perforant path granule cell synapse in the rat hippocampus. *Brain Res.,* 86: 205–215.

Dunwiddie, T., Madison, D. and Lynch, G. (1978) Synaptic transmission is required for initiation of long-term potentiation. *Brain Res.,* 150: 413–417.

Edelman, G.M. (1976) Surface modulation in cell recognition and cell growth. *Science,* 192: 218–226.

Ehrlich, Y., Gilfoil, T. and Brunngraber, E. (1976) *Neurosci. Abstr.,* 2: 600.

Ehrlich, Y., Prasad, K., Sinha, R., Davis, L. and Brunngraber, E. (1978) Endogenous phosphorylation of specific proteins in subcellular fractions from malignang and cAMP-induced differentiated neuroblastoma cell in culture. *Neurochem. Res.,* 3: 803–814.

Finn, R., Browning, M. and Lynch, G. (1980) Trifluoperazine inhibits hippocampal long-term potentiations and the phosphorylation of a 40,000 dalton protein. *Neurosci. Lett.,* 19: 103–108.

Greengard, P. (1978) Phosphorylated proteins as physiological effectors. *Science,* 199: 146–152.

Heald, J. (1957) The incorporation of phosphate into cerebral phosphoprotein promoted by electrical impulses. *Biochem. J.,* 66: 659–663.

Hebb, D.O. (1949) *The Organization of Behavior.* Wiley, New York.

Hershkowitz, M. (1978) Influence of calcium on phosphorylation of a synaptosomal protein. *Biochim. biophys. Acta,* 542: 274–283.

Hiraoka, T., DeBuysere, M. and Olson, M. (1980) Studies of the effects of $\beta$-adrenergic agonists on the regulation of pyruvate dehydrogenase in the perforant path. *J. biol. Chem.,* 255: 7604–7609.

Hughes, W. and Denton, R. (1976) Incorporation of $^{32}P_i$ into pyruvate dehydrogenase phosphate in mitochondria from control and insulin-treated adipose tissue. *Nature (Lond.),* 264: 471–473.

Johnson, E., Maeno, H. and Greengard, P. (1971) Phosphorylation of endogenous protein of rat brain by cyclic adenosine 3',5'-monophosphate-dependent protein kinase. *J. biol. Chem.,* 246: 7731–7735.

Kao, K.-J., Sommer, J.R. and Pizzo, S.V. (1981) Modulation of platelets shape and membrane receptor binding by $Ca^{2+}$-calmodulin complex. *Nature (Lond.),* 292: 82–84.

Kerbey, A., Randle, P., Cooper, R., Whitehouse, S., Pask, H. and Denton, R. (1976) Regulation of pyruvate dehydrogenase in rat heart. *Biochem. J.,* 154: 327–348.

Lee, K., Schottler, F., Oliver, M. and Lynch, G. (1980) Brief bursts of high-frequency stimulation produce two types of structural change in rat hippocampus. *J. Neurophysiol.*, 44: 247–258.

Lee, K., Oliver, M., Schottler, F. and Lynch, G. (1981) Electron microscopic studies of brain slices: The effects of high frequency stimulation on dendritic ultrastructure. In *Electrical Activity in Isolated Mammalian CNS Preparations*, G. Kerkut (Ed.), in press.

Levin, R. and Weiss, B. (1976) Mechanism by which psychotropic drugs inhibit adenosine cyclic 3′,5′-monophosphate phosphodiesterase of brain. *Mol. Pharmacol.*, 12: 581–589.

Linn, T., Pettit, F. and Reed, L. (1969a) α-Keto acid dehydrogenase complexes. X. Regulation of the activity of the pyruvate dehydrogenase complex from beef kidney mitochondria by phosphorylation and dephosphorylation. *Proc. nat. Acad. Sci. (Wash.)*, 62: 234–241.

Linn, T., Pettit, F., Hucho, F. and Reed, L. (1969b) α-Keto acid dehydrogenase complexes. XI. Comparative studies of regulatory properties of the pyruvate dehydrogenase complexes from kidney, heart and liver mitochondria. *Proc. nat. Acad. Sci. (Wash.)*, 64: 227–234.

Linn, T., Pelley, J., Pettit, F., Hucho, F., Randall, D. and Reed, L. (1972) α-Keto acid dehydrogenase complexes. XV. Purification and properties of the component enzymes of the pyruvate dehydrogenase complexes from bovine kidney and heart. *Arch. Biochem. Biophys.*, 148: 327–342.

Lynch, G. and Baudry, M. (1981) Origins and manifestations of neuronal plasticity in the hippocampus. In *Clinical Neurosciences*, W. WIllis (Ed.), Churchill-Livingstone, Edinburgh, in press.

Lynch, G., Smith, R., Browning, M. and Deadwyler, S. (1975) Evidence for bidirectional dentritic transport of horseradish peroxidase. *Adv. Neurol.*, 12: 297–314.

Lynch, G., Dunwiddie, T. and Gribkoff, V. (1977) Heterosynaptic depression: A postsynaptic correlate of long-term potentiation. *Nature (Lond.)*, 266: 737–739.

Lynch, G.S., Browning, M. and Bennett, W. (1979) Biochemical and physiological studies of synaptic plasticity. *Fed. Proc.*, 38: 69–72.

McIlwain, H. and Bachelard, H. (1971) *Biochemistry and the Central Nervous System*, 4th edn., Churchill-Livingstone, Edinburgh.

Maeno, H. and Greengard, P. (1972) Phosphoprotein phosphatases from rat cerebral cortex: Subcellular distribution and characterization. *J. biol. Chem.*, 247: 3269–3273.

Maeno, H., Johnson, E. and Greengard, P. (1971) Subcellular distribution of adenosine 3′, 5′-monophosphate-dependent protein kinase in rat brain. *J. biol. Chem.*, 246: 134–140.

Nicolson, G.L. (1979) Topographic display of cell surface components and their role in transmembrane signaling. *Curr. Top. Dev. Biol.*, 13: 305–338.

Pratt, M. and Roche, T. (1979) Mechanisms of pyruvate inhibition of kidney pyruvate dehydrogenase kinase and synergistic inhibition by pyruvate and ADP. *J. biol. Chem.*, 254: 7191–17196.

Rahamimoff, R., Erulkar, S., Lev-Tov, A. and Meiri, H. (1978) Intracellular and extracellular calcium ions in transmitter release at the neuromuscular synapse. *Ann. N.Y. Acad. Sci.*, 307: 583–597.

Roche, T. and Reed, L. (1975) Monovalent cation requirement for ADP inhibition of pyruvate dehydrogenase kinase. *Biochem. Biophys. Res. Commun.*, 59: 1341–1348.

Schwartzkroin, P. and Wester, K. (1975) Long-lasting facilitation of a synaptic potential following tetanization in the in vitro hippocampal slice. *Brain Res.*, 89: 107–119.

Seals, J., McDonald, J. and Jarrett, L. (1979) Insulin effect on protein phosphorylation of plasma membranes and mitochondria in a subcellular system from rat adipocytes. *J. biol. Chem.*, 254: 6991–1996.

Seiss, E., Whittman, J. and Wieland, D. (1971) Interconversion and kinetic properties of pyruvate dehydrogenase from brain. *Hoppe-Seyler's Z. Physiol. Chem.*, 352: 447–452.

Sieghart, W. (1981) *J. Neurochem.*, 37: 1116–1124.

Storm-Mathisen, J. (1977) Localization of transmitter candidates in the brain: The hippocampal formation as a model. *Progr. Neurobiol.*, 8: 119–181.

Whitehouse, S., Cooper, R. and Randle, P. (1974) Mechanisms of activation of pyruvate dehydrogenase by dichloroacetate and other halogenated carboxylic acids. *Biochem. J.*, 141: 761–774.

Williams, M. and Rodnight, R. (1974) Evidence for a role for protein phosphorylation in synaptic function in the cerebral cortex mediated through a β noradrenergic receptor. *Brain Res.*, 77: 502–506.

Williams, M. and Rodnight, R. (1975) Stimulation of protein phosphorylation in brain slices by electrical pulses: Speed of response and evidence for net phosphorylation. *J. Neurochem.*, 24: 601–603.

Zwiers, H., Veldhuis, H., Schotman, P. and Gispen, W.H. (1976) ACTH, cyclic nucleotides and brain protein phosphorylation in vitro. *Neurochem. Res.*, 1: 669–681.

# Changes in Membrane Phosphorylation Correlated with Long-Lasting Potentiation in Rat Hippocampal Slices

F.H. LOPES DA SILVA[1], P.R. BÄR[2], A.M. TIELEN[3] and W.H. GISPEN[2]

[1] *Department of Animal Physiology, University of Amsterdam, Kruislaan 320, 1098 SM Amsterdam;* [2] *Institute of Molecular Biology and Rudolf Magnus Institute for Pharmacology, State University of Utrecht, Padualaan 8, 3508 TB Utrecht; and* [3] *Institute for Medical Physics, MFI-TNO, Da Costakade 45, 2861 PN Utrecht, The Netherlands*

## INTRODUCTION

Long-term potentiation is a well known phenomenon which has been used as an experimental model for plasticity at the synaptic level. Long-term potentiation (LTP) is characterized by the fact that a synaptic response to stimulation of the corresponding afferents with a pulse, becomes enhanced after the application of a train of pulses to the same afferents; this potentiation can last for many minutes, even hours as shown in many preparations (for review see Spencer and April, 1970). LTP is considered to be an analogue of a class of plastic phenomena in the nervous system which underlie learning processes. The latter imply of course behavioural modification which certainly involves more complex stimulus patterns than LTP. Nevertheless, it can be assumed that a study of the cellular processes underlying LTP may give some clues regarding the basic changes in neuronal activity accompanying learning processes.

## HYPOTHESES CONCERNING LTP

Several hypotheses have been advanced to explain LTP. Both presynaptic and postsynaptic processes have been implied. At the *presynaptic level* LTP may be caused by an increase in the amount of transmitter released, for example, induced by an enhancement of $[Ca^{2+}]_i$ or a modification of the local turnover of transmitter. At the *postsynaptic level* LTP may be related to a modification of receptor properties, to a change in the spike-generating capacity of postsynaptic neurons, and/or a change in input resistance of the dendrites of the postsynaptic neurons. These different possibilities are, of course, not mutually exclusive. Elsewhere, we have discussed that several of the factors indicated above, probably work in a complementary way in producing LTP (Lopes da Silva et al., 1982).

## INFLUENCE OF NEURONAL STIMULATION ON NEUROCHEMICAL PROCESSES

All the possibilities listed above imply changes in neuronal membrane processes. Therefore, we have been trying to elucidate whether it is possible to understand the changes occurring at the membrane level after the electrical stimulation and which may help clarify the basic

340

processes in the development of LTP. The influence of electrical stimulation upon biochemical processes within neurons has been investigated in relation to different subsystems: macromolecular synthesis, enzyme and receptor induction, etc. Although macromolecular synthesis has been implied in mediating the function of memory traces (Dunn, 1976) it is not likely that it is responsible for the rapid changes occurring in LTP. Indeed, it has been shown by Schwartz et al. (1971) that blocking protein synthesis does not alter the post-tetanic facilitation of the monosynaptic response in neurons in the abdominal ganglion of Aplysia. Thus, although plastic changes taking place in the course of days may depend on protein synthesis, phenomena such as LTP which is established in a few seconds are not dependent on such biochemical changes. Enzyme induction has received some attention as a possible biochemical mechanism for explaining long-term effects of neural activity. Indeed, electrical stimulation of the pre-ganglionic input to the rat superior cervical ganglion lasting 10–90 min increases tyrosine hydroxylase (TH) activity in the ganglion (Zigmond and Bowers, 1981). TH is responsible for the synthesis of DOPA from tyrosine. Whether such a mechanism plays a role in LTP induced by stimuli within the physiological range is not yet clear.

Recently, Baudry and Lynch (1980) suggested that LTP elicited in hippocampal slices may depend on the exposure of additional glutamate receptors in the dendrites of hippocampal neurons; they proposed a multiple-stage hypothesis for LTP: (a) the tetanus would cause an increase in intracellular $Ca^{2+}$; (b) this would lead to the activation of a membrane-bound protease which (c) would expose glutamate receptors. This hypothesis is attractive since it does not imply new protein synthesis and it could account for the speed with which LTP is established. Additional experimental evidence, however, is needed in order to establish this hypothesis on a firm basis.

Another interesting biochemical phenomenon which may constitue a basis for explaining LTP is the formation of the covalent bond between a phosphate group and a protein amino acid residue (serine, threonine), since this is a very fast reaction which takes place in seconds and can have an important influence on protein structure and enzyme activity (Weller, 1979). This comprises the phenomenon of protein phosphorylation. It is known (Heald, 1957, 1962) that electrical stimulation of brain cortex slices leads to changes in protein phosphorylation. Moreover, Forn and Greengard (1978) have shown that depolarization of cortical slices using high concentrations of $K^+$ or veratridine is correlated with the degree of phosphorylation of a specific neuronal membrane protein. These new facts led us (Bär et al., 1980a) and others (Browning et al., 1979a) to investigate whether the degree of synaptic protein phosphorylation was related to LTP.

## EXPERIMENTAL EVIDENCE ON THE RELATION BETWEEN LTP AND MEMBRANE PROTEIN PHOSPHORYLATION

The two initial studies on this topic were those of Browning et al. (1979a) and ours (Bär et al., 1980a). It is useful to discuss here the common aspects of those investigations and also the main differences. In both studies slices of hippocampus were used since in this preparation it is relatively easy to combine physiological and biochemical measurements. In the transversal slice of the hippocampus (Fig. 1) several sub-systems may be distinguished (Lopes da Silva and Arnolds, 1978); the main ones are the following: the perforant path → granule cell synapses, the mossy fibres (axons of granule cells) → CA3 pyramidal neurons, the Schaffer collaterals (collaterals of CA3 axons) → CA1 pyramidal neurons. Browning et al. (1979a) and Bär et al. (1980a) used two different sub-systems for their investigations: the former studied

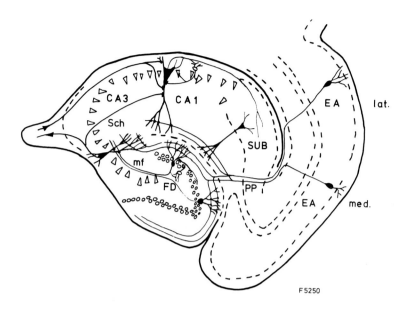

Fig. 1. Diagram of a section of the hippocampal region of a rat. Different fields and sub-fields are indicated. Two sub-systems, which we discussed in the text should be singled out; the Schaffer collaterals (Sch) projecting to the apical dendrites of sub-field Ca1 and the perforant path fibres (PP) projecting to the granular cells of the fascia dentata (FD).

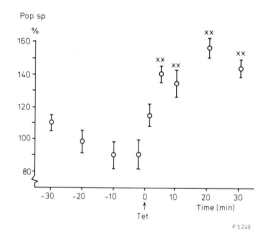

Fig. 2. Plot of the mean amplitude and the corresponding S.E.M. of the population spike (open circles) and the extracellularly recorded EPSP (closed circles) recorded from the fascia dentata and elicited by a short stimulus applied to the perforant path (5 slices). Note the time scale is logarithmic in order to emphasize the initial brief depression phase. The potentiation of both responses can be seen. "Controls" are values obtained before the tetanus. (Adapted from Tielen et al., 1982).

LTP of the synapses of the Schaffer collaterals → CA1 pyramidal neurons, whereas the latter used the perforant path → granule cell synapses in the dentate area (Fig. 2). In both systems LTP was found, although there were differences in some aspects which confirm results obtained previously (Alger and Teyler, 1976; Dudek et al., 1976; Schwartzkroin, 1975). The main difference appears to be that LTP in CA1 is established almost immediately after the cessation of the tetanus whereas in the dentate area LTP appears clearly after a brief phase of depression, i.e. about 8 or 10 min after the tetanus (Tielen et al., 1982). In both cases, however, it may persist for hours. The way the slices were stimulated was also not exactly the same; Browning et al. (1979a) used a tetanus consisting of 100 pulses/sec for 1 sec, whereas Bär et al. (1980) used 15 pulses/sec for 15 sec. It is appropriate to note that in both hippocampal sub-systems the same synaptic transmitters are present: glutamate and aspartate (DiLauro et al., 1981; Storm-Mathisen, 1977). An important difference between the two studies, however, is the fact that Browning et al. (1979a) took the slices 2 min after the application of the tetanus for biochemical analysis, whereas Bär et al. (1980a) left them in the incubation bath for 15 min after the tetanus and only then proceeded with the biochemical analysis. The reason for this delay was the fact that LTP in the dentate was established in most slices only 8 or 10 min after the tetanus. The biochemical assay was essentially the same but the following differences should be pointed out: in the study of Browning et al. $Mg^{2+}$ concentration was 1 mM, ATP was 50 $\mu$M and EGTA (125 $\mu$M) was included, whereas in that of Bär et al. 10 mM for $Mg^{2+}$ and 7.5 $\mu$M for ATP were used and no EGTA was added. Undoubtedly, this may have some influence on the endogenous phosphorylation of the hippocampal acceptor proteins. In both studies, however, the so-called post-hoc phosphorylation assay (Routtenberg et al., 1975) was used. In this way one determines post hoc the capacity of the protein to accept phosphate; this capacity will be larger if the protein, when entering the assay, has more sites available than if the sites are already occupied. This means that a protein that in the post-hoc assay shows strong phosphorylation was rather depleted from phosphate in vivo, and vice versa.

The main results of the two studies differed in that Browning et al. put all the emphasis on the decrease of phosphate incorporation of a protein with a molecular weight around 40 000 (40 K) present in a crude mitochondrial fraction and only mention an increase of phosphorylation of two other major phosphoprotein bands: one at 53 K and the other at 27 K. In the study of Bär et al., also using a mitochondrial fraction, the main finding was an increase in phosphorylation of a 50 K band whereas the 40 K band only showed a slight decrease of phosphorylation which did not reach a significant level. The most likely reason which may account for these differences is the fact that Browning et al. (this volume) have shown that the increase in phosphorylation of the 40 K band is of short duration; it reaches again control values around 10 min after the tetanus. This is probably the reason why Bär et al. did not find significant changes in this band since they analysed the slices only after 15 min. Nevertheless it should be stressed that in both studies a decrease in post-hoc phosphorylation of a 50–53 K band was observed, although it was clearer in the study of Bär et al. It is possible that here also the factor time may account for the difference in degree of phosphorylation of the 50–53 K band, but at the moment there is no further evidence to support such an explanation.

Since these original observations, progress has been achieved in identifying these protein bands more precisely. Browning et al. (1979b) found that the 40 K band was phosphorylated in vitro by phosphorylase kinase and on the basis of molecular weight and proteolytic fingerprinting they recently reported (Browning et al., 1981) that this band is the $\alpha$ subunit of the enzyme pyruvate dehydrogenase (PDH). It is also most interesting to note in this connection that phosphorylation of the same protein band was shown by Routtenberg et al. (1975) in vivo to be responsive to behavioural training; later they determined that the protein band in question (40–43 K or band F2) was also the $\alpha$ subunit of PDH (Morgan and Routtenberg, 1980). Furthermore, Morgan and Routtenberg (1981) have shown that an increase in post-hoc assayed phosphorylation of the protein band 40 K was correlated with a decrease of PDH enzyme activity.

Our own recent work revealed that the 50 K protein band in fact consists of two proteins with different biochemical properties and subcellular localization (Bär et al., 1981, 1982). Only one of the proteins is sensitive to electrical treatment and present in synaptosomal plasma membranes. By direct comparison of the 50 K phosphoprotein band of a crude mitochondrial/synaptosomal (P2) fraction and of a fraction enriched in synaptic membranes on the same gel, and by analysis of the autoradiograms using a slit width of 10 $\mu$m instead of 100 $\mu$m it became apparent that the 50 K band could be separated into two components with $M_r$ 50 K and 52 K. They run very close together and the 52 K band does not always appear as a distinct band, owing to the high incorporation of label into the nearby 50 K band; often the 50 K band which in

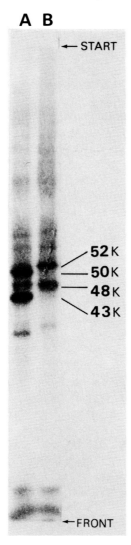

Fig. 3. Autoradiogram of separated proteins, phosphorylated in a crude mitochondrial/synaptosomal fraction (A) or in a purified synaptic membrane fraction (B) of rat hippocampal tissue. The numbers denote the position and apparent molecular weight of the phosphoproteins discussed in the text.

a P2 fraction is phosphorylated predominantly with respect to the 52 K band, overlaps the 52 K on the autoradiogram. In order to study the localization of these two phosphoproteins in more detail we prepared the following fractions of a rat hippocampal homogenate: a crude synaptosomal/mitochondrial fraction (P2), and a synaptosomal membrane–enriched fraction (SPM). These fractions were assayed for endogenous phosphorylation and attention was focussed on bands in the 40–55 K region.

In the P2 fraction (Fig. 3, lane A) all four major bands in this region are present: 43 K, 48 K, 50 K and 52 K. In this fraction, which still contains mitochondria, 43 K and 50 K are predominantly phosphorylated. The 48 K and 43 K phosphoprotein bands are also seen in other studies on brain phosphoproteins. The 48 K protein is phosphorylated by a calcium-sensitive protein kinase and is identical to the B-50 protein ($M_r$ 48 K, IEP 4.5). This protein was purified (Zwiers et al., 1979, 1980) and may correspond to $\gamma$-5 (Rodnight, 1979), F1 (Ehrlich and Routtenberg, 1974) and is identical to p54p (Ca) (Sörensen et al., 1981). It was shown to be specific for nervous tissue (Kristjansson et al., 1982) and to have a synaptic localization throughout the brain (Oestreicher et al., 1981), presumably restricted to presynaptic membranes (Sörensen et al., 1981). Its phosphorylation is inhibited by ACTH but not by methionine-enkephaline (Zwiers et al., 1976, 1980).

The 43 K protein most likely is similar to the band F2 (Routtenberg et al., 1975), which is recently characterized as the $\alpha$ subunit of pyruvate dehydrogenase (see above). Indeed, in our bands this phosphoprotein was only found in fractions containing mitochondria.

After an osmotic shock of this crude fraction the light synaptic membranes were isolated by sucrose gradient centrifugation (Fig. 3, lane B) as described by Zwiers et al. (1976). The SPM shows a clear enrichment of phosphorylation of 48 K and 52 K. Thus, we concluded that the endogenous phosphorylation of the 50 K band takes place in material that sediments with the mitochondria whereas that of the 52 K band is associated with the SPM (Bär et al., 1982).

Subsequently, the proteins present in the P2 and SPM were separated two-dimensionally as described by Zwiers et al. (1979). Identification of the 50 K and 52 K proteins after autoradiography was possible using known properties of the two phosphoproteins: (1) the 50 K is not present in an SPM fraction; (2) the two different proteins show a different $Ca^{2+}$-dependency; (3) MW markers, as well as a phosphorylated SPM fraction were always applied to the same SDS gel on which the second dimension separation was run. The 50 K protein appears to be heterogenous after isoelectric focussing. The IEP of the components ranges from 3.5 to 4.3. The 52 K protein is present as a minor phosphoprotein, with an IEP of 5.3. It has been shown that the 50 K protein is strongly calcium-dependent in its phosphorylation and in the presence of calmodulin the calcium optimum is shifted towards lower concentrations of the divalent ion (Bär et al., 1982). In contrast, the endogenous phosphorylation of the 52 K protein is not sensitive to calcium. The IEP, $M_r$ and its insensitivity to calcium suggest that the 52 K protein is similar to p54p (Mahler et al., this volume). However, these authors report that in their system this protein is phosphorylated in a cAMP-dependent manner. When studied in a P2 fraction, in which this protein is a minor component, no effects of cAMP were found (Bär et al., 1981). Moreover, we have shown that the 50 K and 52 K proteins also differ with respect to their response to neuropeptide incubations of slices: only the 52 K protein shows an increased post-hoc phosphorylation after incubation with methionine-enkephalin, whereas the 50 K protein does not (compare Bär et al., 1980b). Furthermore, it is possible that the former protein corresponds to a band in the region of 50 K, sensitive to depolarizing conditions (Krueger et al., 1977) and a band sensitive to diphenylhydantoin, an anticonvulsant (DeLorenzo and Freedman, 1977).

As reported before, high frequent stimulation (15 pulses/sec) during 15 sec applied to the

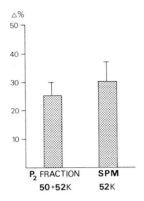

Fig. 4. Increase in phosphorylation of the 50–52 K proteins in different subcellular fractions in a post-hoc assay after high frequent stimulation of the hippocampal slice ($n = 6$) as compared to controls ($n = 6$).

perforant path fibres of the hippocampal slice, resulted primarily in an increased phosphorylation of a protein in a post-hoc assay using the P2 fraction (data given in Fig. 4). We demonstrated that 50 K and 52 K proteins behave differently after a tetanic stimulation. In the mitochondrial fraction, the 50 K protein did not show any change in phosphorylation after the tetanus, whereas the 52 K protein in the SPM showed a significant increase in $^{32}P$ incorporation of 30%. We therefore concluded that the increase of 24% after tetanus observed earlier (Bär et al., 1980a) in a P2 fraction is attributable to the 52 K component of the 50 K band (Bär et al., 1981, 1982).

## CONCLUDING REMARKS

In conclusion, these data confirm and extend our observations of the change in protein phosphorylation after tetanic stimulation of the perforant path. The data show that the effects are confined to a 52 K protein (IEP 5.3) whose phosphorylation occurs in a calcium-independent manner. It is worth mentioning that the change in phosphorylation brought about by the tetanic stimulation itself is absolutely dependent on the presence of calcium (Bär et al., 1980a). The localization studies carried out with various subcellular fractions point to a synaptic membrane rather than a mitochondrial origin of the 52 K phosphoprotein. Thus, in addition to the metabolic correlates discussed by Browning et al. (this volume) and Lynch and Schubert (1980) (energy metabolism and calcium in mitochondria), tetanic stimulation may indeed bring about changes in protein phosphorylation in synaptic membranes. Besides these phenomena we have found (Bär, 1982) that a tetanus provokes also a change in phosphoinositide metabolism, namely the hydrolysis of membrane-bound (poly) phosphoinositides (PI, DPI, TPI) yielding diacylglycerol (dAG) which may play a role in the fusion of synaptic vesicles and hence in transmitter release and may change membrane fluidity and thus membrane permeability. Also, dAG is phosphorylated to PA which may function as $Ca^{2+}$ ionophore (Harris et al., 1981; Salmon and Honeyman, 1980); in this way an influx of $Ca^{2+}$ can take place and cytosolic $Ca^{2+}$ may rise approximately 1000-fold. This increase would be maintained by a decreased activity of a mitochondrial enzyme pyruvate dehydrogenase which Browning et al. (this volume) showed to be affected by the tetanus. At the present moment we can only hypothesize that the change in phosphorylation of the 52 K protein may result also in an altered sensitivity of the postsynaptic membrane, towards the neurotransmitter. In order to determine the exact role of this protein in the process of LTP it is necessary to find its exact location and to characterize it in more detail. Such characterization will certainly give insight in the synaptic processes responsible for LTP.

## ACKNOWLEDGEMENTS

The authors wish to thank M. Boelen and W. Mollevanger for excellent experimental help. This research was in part supported by ZWO-FUNGO (The Hague) Grant No. 13-31-39.

## REFERENCES

Alger, B.E. and Teyler, T.J. (1976) Long-term and short-term plasticity in the CA, CA₂ and dentate regions of the hippocampal slice. *Brain Res.,* 110: 463–480.

Bär, P.R. (1982) *Membrane Phosphorylation and Nerve Cell Functions: Modulation and Nerve Cell Functions: Modulation by Neuropeptides.* Thesis, University Utrecht, The Netherlands.

Bär, P.R., Schotman, P., Gispen, W.H., Lopes da Silva, F.H. and Tielen, A.M. (1980a) Changes in synaptoc membrane phosphorylation after tetanic stimulation in the dentate area of the rat hippocampal slice. *Brain Res.,* 198: 478–484.

Bär, P.R., Schotman, P. and Gispen, W.H. (1980b) Enkephalins affect hippocampal membrane phosphorylation. *Eur. J. Pharmacol.,* 65: 165–174.

Bär, P.R., Boelen, M. and Gispen, W.H. (1981) Properties of two hippocampal phosphoproteins responsive to tetanic stimulation. In *Proc. of the 8th Meeting Int. Soc. Neurochem.,* (Abstr.), p. 326.

Bär, P.R., Tielen, A.M., Lopes da Silva, F.H., Zwiers, H. and Gispen, W.H. (1982) Membrane phosphoproteins of rat hippocampus: Sensitivity to tetanic stimulation and enkephalin. *Brain Res.,* in press.

Baudry, M. and Lynch, G. (1980) Hypothesis regarding the cellular mechanisms responsible for long-term synaptic potentiation in the hippocampus. *Exp. Neural.,* 68: 202–204.

Browning, M., Dunwiddie, T., Bennett, W., Gispen, W.H. and Lynch, G. (1979a) Synaptic phosphoproteins: Specific changes after repetitive stimulation of the hippocampal slice. *Science,* 203: 60–62.

Browning, M., Bennett, W. and Lynch, G. (1979b) Phosphoryl kinase phosphorylates a brain protein which is influenced by repetitive synaptic activation. *Nature (Lond.),* 278: 273–275.

Browning, M., Baudry, M., Bennett, W., Kelly, P. and Lynch, G. (1981) Evidence that high frequency stimulation influences the phosphorylation of pyruvate dehydrogenase and that the activity of this enzyme is linked to mitochondrial calcium sequestration. *Neurosci. Abstr.,* 71.

DeLorenzo, R.J. and Freedman, S.D. (1977) Possible role of calcium-dependent protein phosphorylation in mediating neurotransmitter release and anticonvulsant action. *Epilepsia,* 18: 357–365.

DiLauro, A., Schmid, R.W. and Meek, J.L. (1981) Is aspartic acid the neurotransmitter of the perforant path? *Brain Res.,* 207: 476–480.

Dudek, F.E., Deadwyler, S.A., Cotman, C.W. and Lynch, G. (1976) Intracellular responses from granula cell layer in slices of rat hippocampus: perforant path synapse. *J. Neurophysiol.,* 39: 383–393, 1976.

Dunn, A.J. (1976) The chemistry of learning and the formation of memory. In *Molecular and Functional Neurobiology,* W.H. Gispen (Ed.), Elsevier, Amsterdam, pp. 347–387.

Ehrlich, Y.H. and Routtenberg, A. (1974) Cyclic AMP regulates phosphorylation of three protein components of rat cerebral cortex membranes for thirty minutes. *FEBS Lett.,* 45: 237–243.

Forn, J. and Greengard, P. (1978) Depolarizing agents and cyclic nucleotides regulate the phosphorylation of specific neuronal proteins in rat cerebral cortex slices. *Proc. nat. Acad. Sci. (Wash.),* 75: 5195–5199.

Harris, R.A., Schmidt, J., Hitzemann, B.A. and Hitzemann, R.J. (1981) Phosphatidate as a molecular link between depolarization and neurotransmitter release in the brain. *Science,* 212: 1290–1291.

Heald, P.J. (1957) The incorporation of phosphate into cerebral phosphoprotein promoted by electrical impulses. *Biochem. J.,* 66: 659–663.

Heald, P.J. (1962) Phosphoprotein metabolism and ion transport in nervous tissue: a suggested connexion. *Nature (Lond.),* 193: 451–454.

Kristjansson, G.J., Zwiers, H., Oestreicher, A.B. and Gispen, W.H. (1982) Is the synaptic phosphoprotein B-50 specific for nervous tissue? *J. Neurochem.*, in press.

Krueger, B.K., Forn, J. and Greengard, P. (1977) Depolarization-induced phosphorylation of specific proteins, mediated by calcium ion influx, in rat brain synaptosomes. *J. biol. Chem.*, 252: 2764–2773.

Lopes da Silva, F.H. and Arnolds, D.E.A.T. (1978) Physiology of the hippocampus and related structures. *Annu. Rev. Physiol.*, 40: 185–216.

Lopes da Silva, F.H., Bär, P.R., Tielen, A.M. and Gispen, W.H. (1982) Plasticity in synaptic transmission and changes of membrane-bound protein phosphorylation. In *Chemical Transmission in the Brain*, R.M. Buys, P. Pévet and D.F. Swaab (Eds.), Progr. in Brain Res., Elsevier/North-Holland Biomedical Press, Amsterdam, in press.

Lynch, G. and Schubert, P. (1980) The use of in vitro brain slices for multidisciplinary studies of synaptic function. *Annu. Rev. Neurosci.*, 3: 1–22.

Morgan, D.G. and Routtenberg, A. (1980) Evidence that a 41,000 dalton brain phosphoprotein is pyruvate dehydrogenase. *Biochem. Biophys. Res. Commun.*, 95: 569–576.

Morgan, D.G. and Routtenberg, A. (1981) Brain pyruvate dehydrogenase: Phosphorylation and enzyme activity altered by a training experience. *Science*, in press.

Oestreicher, A.B., Zwiers, H., Gispen, W.H. and Roberts, S. (1981) Characterization of infant rat cerebral cortical membrane proteins phosphorylated in vivo. *J. Neurochem.*, in press.

Rodnight, R. (1979) Cyclic nucleotides as second messenger in synaptic transmission. *Int. Rev. Biochem.*, 26: 1–80.

Routtenberg, A., Ehrlich, Y.H. and Rabjohns, R.R. (1975) Effect of a training experience of phosphorylation of a specific protein in neurocortical and subcortical membrane preparations. *Fed. Prod.*, 34: 17.

Salmon, D.M. and Honeyman, T.W. (1980) Proposed mechanism of cholinergic action in smooth muscle. *Nature (Lond.)*, 284: 344–345.

Schwartz, J.H., Cezellucci, V.F. and Kandel, E.R. (1971) Functioning of identified neurons and synapses in abdominal ganglion of Aplysia in absence of protein synthesis. *J. Neurophysiol.*, 34: 939–953.

Schwartzkroin, P.A. and Wester, K. (1975) Long-lasting facilitation of a synaptic potential following tetanization on the in vivo hippocampal slice. *Brain Res.*, 89: 107–119.

Sörensen, R.G., Kleine, L.P. and Mahler, H.R. (1981) Presynaptic localization of phosphoprotein B-50. *Brain Res. Bull.*, 7: 57–61.

Spencer, W.A. and April, R.S. (1970) Plastic properties of monosynaptic pathways in mammals. In *Short-Term Changes in Neural Activity and Behaviour*, G. Horn and R.A. Hinde (Eds.), Cambridge University Press, Cambridge, pp. 433–474.

Storm-Mathisen, J. (1977) Localization of transmitter candidates in the brain: The hippocampal formation as a model. *Progr. Neurobiol.*, 8: 119–181.

Tielen, A.M., Lopes da Silva, F.H., Bär, P.R. and Gispen, W.H. (1982) Long-lasting post-tetanic stimulation in the dentate area of rat hippocampal slices and correlated changes in synaptic membrane phosphorylation. In *Mechanisms and Models of Neuroplasticity: The Role of Hippocampus Structures*, H. Matthies (Ed.), Raven Press, New York.

Weller, M. (1979) Protein Phosphorylation. Pion, London.

Zigmond, R.E. and Bowers, Ch. W. (1981) Influence of nerve activity on the macromolecule content of neurons and their effector organs. *Annu. Rev. Physiol.*, 43: 673–687.

Zwiers, H., Veldhuis, D., Schotman, P. and Gispen, W.H. (1976) ACTH, cyclic nucleotides and brain phosphorylation in vitro. *Neurochem. Res.*, 1: 669–677.

Zwiers, H., Tonnaer, J., Wiegant, V.M., Schotman, P. and Gispen, W.H. (1979) ACTH-sensitive protein kinase from rat brain membranes. *J. Neurochem.*, 33: 247–256.

Zwiers, H., Schotman, P. and Gispen, W.H. (1980) Purification and some characteristics of an ACTH-sensitive protein kinase and its protein in rat brain membranes. *J. Neurochem.*, 34: 1689–1700.

# Identification and Back-Titration
# of Brain Pyruvate Dehydrogenase:
# Functional Significance for Behavior

ARYEH ROUTTENBERG

*Cresap Neuroscience Laboratory, 2021 Sheridan Road,*
*Northwestern University, Evanston, IL 60201, U.S.A.*

## 1. INTRODUCTION: CAST OF CHARACTERS

The work on brain phosphoproteins in this laboratory has grown out of the demonstration, made first in 1975, that phosphate back-titration in vitro of electrophoretically separated brain phosphoproteins can be influenced by the in vivo state of the organism (Routtenberg, 1979b, for review). In the present chapter, I wish to review the evidence that indicates which of these substrate proteins are susceptible to alterations following in vivo functional manipulations and, as important, which proteins appear to be stable and uninfluenced by such manipulations.

It will be valuable to first present the cast of characters with which we will be dealing in this paper. To do so, then, Fig. 1 presents an autoradiographic profile of reaction products separated on a 10 % gel. The components in the gel that we will focus on are pointed out in the left hand side. We have used the nomenclature described in Mitrius et al. (1981), which divides the molecular weight ranges by letter, and then simply adds subscripts to that letter as the phosphoproteins are identified. The gels were divided into eight molecular weight ranges, designated A through H. A was greater than 160 000; B, 131 000–160 000; C, 91 000–130 000; D, 61 000–90 000; E, 51 000–60 000; F, 41 000–50 000; G, 21 000–40 000; and H, 20 000 or less. The bands that we shall be discussing in this paper are bands D-1, 86 000; D-2, 80 000; and D-3, 67 000. Bands D-1 and D-2 are proteins Ia and Ib of Ueda and Greengard (1977). E-1, 60 000; E-2, 54 000; and E-3, 51 000. As can be seen in this figure, bands E-1 and E-3 are reduced in their phosphorylation in the presence of EGTA and increased in the presence of calcium chloride, suggesting that these are calcium-dependent phosphoprotein bands. E-1 and E-3 are likely to be DPH-L and DPH-M, respectively, of DeLorenzo (1977) and E-3 is likely to be the 51 K protein described by Schulman and Greengard (1978). As demonstrated in Routtenberg et al. (1981), band E-2 demonstrates cyclic AMP (cAMP) stimulation, and is likely to be protein II of Ueda et al. (1973, 1979). Band F-1 is likely to be B-50 of Gispen and co-workers. Band F-2 is the α subunit of pyruvate dehydrogenase (PDH) as identified by Morgan and Routtenberg (1980).

Using 20 mM EDTA or 50 mM sodium fluoride, it can be readily observed that band F-2 is unique among phosphoproteins since it has a minimal magnesium requirement for phosphorylation. Thus, we can selectively phosphorylate band F-2 using 20 mM EDTA in a HEPES buffer.

Our initial functional studies, then, have focused on the bands just discussed, though this does not rule out other phosphoprotein substrates. Part of the reason for this focus of interest has been that, in the 30 000–90 000 mol. wt. range, we have observed larger changes than in

350

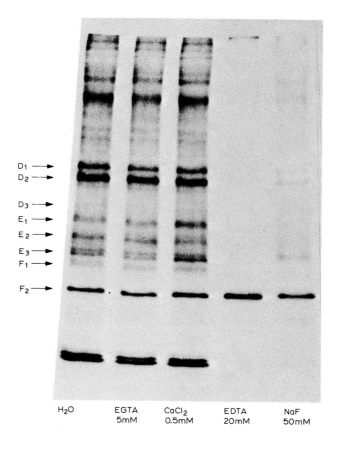

D₁ →
D₂ →

D₃ →
E₁ →
E₂ →
E₃ →
F₁ →

F₂ →

| H₂O | EGTA 5mM | CaCl₂ 0.5mM | EDTA 20mM | NaF 50mM |

Fig. 1. In vitro phosphorylation of hippocampal proteins: Selective preservation of band F-2 phosphorylation with 20 mM EDTA. Autoradiogram of the effects of various compounds on the activity of endogenous brain phosphorylation activity are presented in this figure. In order to assay phosphorylation activity, hippocampal P-2 fraction membranes were incubated in HEPES (pH 7.2) and MgCl₂ for 30 sec at 30°C. The modulatory compound was then added, followed 30 sec later by [³²P]ATP. The final reaction concentrations were 0.5 mg protein/ml, 5 μM ATP, 50 mM HEPES, 10 mM MgCl₂, plus the modulatory compound listed below the autoradiogram at the indicated concentration. Aliquots were removed to SDS-stop solution 0.5 min after ATP addition and slab gel electrophoresis was performed. EDTA is a potent inhibitor of protein kinase, apparently due to its chelation of the exogenous Mg²⁺, a required co-factor for many protein kinase enzymes. The failure of EDTA to inhibit band F-2 phosphorylation suggests that F-2 kinase has a reduced divalent cation requirement compared to other protein kinases. Like EDTA, fluoride ion, at high concentration, also inhibits most protein phosphorylation of band F-2. However, the inhibition of phosphorylation activity is less complete than with EDTA, and some inhibition of F-2 phosphorylation is apparent. At low concentrations, no inhibition of protein phosphorylation is observed with NaF. Thus, F-2 phosphorylation appears to be regulated differently from most intrinsic brain protein kinase enzymes. While stimulated by Ca²⁺, it is apparently not dependent upon this ion for activity since substantial phosphorylation occurs in the presence of EGTA. Magnesium ion requirement is low for the activity of F-2 kinase since EDTA blocks the phosphorylation of all bands except F-2. The NaF results confirm the independence of F-2 kinase from divalent cations (Morgan and Routtenberg, unpublished observations). These results are consistent with the identification of band F-2 as pyruvate dehydrogenase (Morgan and Routtenberg, 1980). While 5 mM EGTA, a specific calcium chelator, had a small inhibitory effect on endogenous brain membrane protein phosphorylation, CaCl₂ stimulated incorporation into several phosphoprotein bands. The most readily discernible stimulation occurred in bands F-1 and E-3, although some stimulation is also apparent in bands D-1, D-2 and F-2. This stimulation of these bands by Ca²⁺ ion corresponds well with the reports from several different laboratories (see Greengard, 1978, for review) on calcium-dependent phosphorylation in brain. (Autoradiograph prepared by David Morgan.)

other bands. We have also observed some rather dramatic changes, at times, in certain band H components in prior studies from our laboratory. These will be discussed briefly in a later section. We have focused, therefore, on those bands where the most dramatic changes have been observed.

In early studies where different gel systems were used, bands D-1 and D-2 were simply seen as one band referred to as band D, and bands F-1 and F-2 were observed as one band referred to as band F (Routtenberg and Ehrlich, 1975). Bands E-1, E-2 and E-3 were also observed as a single band, or a poorly differentiated multiple set of bands. With later modifications of the gel system we were able to observe the functional differentiation among certain of these bands, particularly band F-1 and band F-2.

## 2. BACK-TITRATION METHOD

I wish to introduce the term "back-titration" as employed by Sale and Randle (1981) to describe the phosphorylation of unoccupied sites in vitro which, by subtraction from partially phosphorylated forms, enables the determination of occupied sites in vivo. In our first back-titration study (Routtenberg et al., 1975) the estimation was a relative one, being a comparison among groups treated to different environmental conditions. Although of potential future value, we have not as yet attempted back-titration in comparison with fully dephosphorylated proteins.

It should be re-emphasized that we use an endogenous reaction that enables us to evaluate the net phosphorylation, based on substrate levels of kinase and phosphatase activities. Thus, no attempt is made in the basic endogenous assay to specify how these three factors contribute to the net substrate protein phosphorylation. As we identify certain brain phosphoproteins, such as the $\alpha$ subunit of pyruvate dehydrogenase (PDHa; Morgan and Routtenberg, 1980), where kinase and phosphatase inhibitors are known, then we can estimate the relative contribution of each factor. Moreover, these inhibitors can be used to preserve the in vivo state, and hence increase the accuracy of the back-titration method for evaluating the number of phosphorylatable sites present in vivo.

## 3. SEARCH FOR SUBSTRATE BRAIN PHOSPHOPROTEINS THAT MAY BE FUNCTIONALLY ALTERED

### 3.1. Duration of regulation of phosphorylation in vitro

Although potential linkages between synaptic transmission and molecular alterations had been earlier suggested (e.g., Kernell and Peterson, 1970), the demonstration of cAMP stimulation of phosphorylation of a band termed protein I by Johnson et al. (1972) offered considerable promise in providing a link between synaptic transmission and biochemical alterations in the cell (see, for review, Greengard and Kebabian, 1974). Although we had made several inquiries into the problem of functional/behavioral effects on protein metabolism (Routtenberg and Bondareff, 1971; Holian et al., 1971; Routtenberg et al., 1974), the substrate specificity of the effect of cAMP on a "specific protein (sic) in synaptic membrane fractions" (Johnson et al., 1972, p. 5650), made it attractive for study from the functional point of view.

In our first study, then, we sought to repeat the observations of Johnson et al. (1972) using a discontinuous gradient gel (7, 9 and 12 %) to improve separation of protein across a wider molecular weight spectra.

We found, indeed, that cAMP did stimulate the phosphorylation of protein I (termed band D) of 80 000 approximate mol. wt. (Ehrlich and Routtenberg, 1974). We also found to our initial surprise that another band (termed band E) of 53 000 approximate mol. wt. was also stimulated by cAMP. In a report that appeared while this first manuscript was in preparation, Ueda et al. (1973) did note the presence of another band (termed protein II) of molecular weight similar to band E, which was stimulated by cAMP.

Thus, we had obtained evidence in support of the view that two phosphoproteins were stimulated by cAMP.

In our initial study we noted, in contrast to Ueda et al. (1973), that band D was rapidly phosphorylated in the *absence* of cAMP at the first time point studied (20 sec). There was also a rapid dephosphorylation of band D, such that at 1 min little phosphorylation was observed in the absence of cAMP. Since in the presence of cAMP considerable phosphorylation of band D was observed, the result at 1,2,5 and 15 min was quite similar to that presented by Johnson et al. (1972) and Ueda et al. (1973). The argument has been advanced by Matus et al. (1979) that only with micromolar, but not millimolar, ATP concentrations, is cAMP stimulation observed. Possibly, at low ATP concentrations, cAMP stimulation is, in actuality, the retardation of ATP hydrolysis. The rapid phosphorylation and dephosphorylation of band D in the absence of cAMP may also be related to evidence indicating that this band is regulated by other factors, such as calcium (Sieghart et al., 1979).

Perhaps the most important new finding in out initial study was the discovery of a third major phosphoprotein band which we termed band F and which had an approximate molecular weight of 42–48 K (Ehrlich and Routtenberg, 1974). Band F had the highest phosphorylation in the absence of cAMP and the lowest percentage of stimulation by cAMP. In this and a subsequent full-length report (Routtenberg and Ehrlich, 1975), the differentiation of band F from other phosphoprotein bands, particularly bands D and E was emphasized. At that time, in fact, there was evidence to suggest that band F might in fact be a cAMP-independent phosphoprotein. This result was of importance since it contrasted with the emphasis by Greengard (1976) on the cAMP dependence of phosphorylation based on the hypothesis of Kuo and Greengard (1969) that all the effects of cAMP are mediated through the protein phosphorylation mechanism. The converse, however, did not appear to be true in the case of band F. There was evidence to suggest, nonetheless, that cAMP at micromolar ATP concentrations could stimulate phosphorylation of certain brain proteins.

In our initial report we also demonstrated that the cAMP stimulation of band D was most prominent in the synaptic fraction using the subcellular preparation of Davis and Bloom (1973). In reviewing Fig. 3 of Ehrlich and Routtenberg (1974) several features can now be understood. In the myelin fraction there is considerable amount of phosphate contained within a low molecular weight range, which we at that time referred to as band H. There is, moreover, evidence that certain myelin basic proteins are phosphorylated (see Sulakhe, this volume) and that their molecular weight is below 20 000. Thus, it is likely that it represents part of that component. There is also some evidence that the myosin light chain is present within band H (see Mahler, this volume).

Another interesting aspect of this subcellular preparation is the presence of a phosphorylated substrate, which is not stimulated by cAMP in its phosphorylation, immediately below what we termed band F. In all likelihood, since this has a lower molecular weight than pyruvate dehydrogenase (Morgan and Routtenberg, 1980), it may be band G (Routtenberg and Ehrlich, 1975), which may be of ribosomal origin (see Roberts, this volume; Ashby and Roberts, 1975).

These studies were based on the view that functional in vivo events would alter brain phosphorylation for a period of time. We were, therefore, interested initially (Ehrlich and Routtenberg, 1974; Routtenberg and Ehrlich, 1975) in the duration in which phosphorylation was detected and altered by cAMP. The main focus of interest in our studies was, therefore, the long duration of phosphorylation detected even 30 min after the initiation of a reaction. In the initial studies by Ueda et al. (1973) a 2 min reaction was used. Moreover, we emphasized the fact that certain bands, in the case of band D, were not phosphorylated when studied in the absence of cAMP, but remained phosphorylated 30 min after initiation of the reaction. We concluded that cAMP can maintain the state of phosphorylation for a period of 30 min. This result was considered important then for providing a potential change in a substrate protein consequent to a physiological stimulus.

An interesting feature of these results contrasts band D and band F phosphoproteins observed 15 min after the initiation of the reaction. In the absence of cAMP, band F has the highest level of phosphorylation of all phosphoproteins. Band D is barely detectable. In the presence of cAMP, band D is the most heavily phosphorylated at this same 15 min time point.

The exciting question which we next addressed was, which phosphoproteins, as studied in vitro, could be changed as a consequence of in vivo functional state? With respect to bands D and F, in particular, we were especially interested in their potential for being functionally altered, since both bands appeared to possess the ability to remain phosphorylated for a period of time, but appeared to do so using either a cyclic nucleotide-dependent or -independent mechanism.

It was our plan, then, to study the effects of behavioral manipulations on back-titration. We altered activity in brain functionally, using a physiologically meaningful, non-artificial, that is, environmental, method of stimulation.

## 3.2. *Effect of behavioral activation in a step-down apparatus on back-titration of electrophoretically separated brain phosphoproteins*

It seemed reasonable to suppose that phosphorylation of brain proteins in vitro would depend on the in vivo state of the animal. Moreover, the state of the animal's brain could be determined by the environmental conditions present prior to sacrifice. I based this view in part in analogy with the results of Horn et al. (1973), who demonstrated in vitro alterations in RNA polymerase in chick brain, following imprinting. The possibility existed then that alterations could be demonstrated in brain phosphoproteins in certain brain regions following behavioral activation. We, therefore, studied phosphoproteins in the neostriatal system, which our laboratory had indicated played a role in learning and memory (see Routtenberg and Kim, 1978, for review; Routtenberg and Holzman, 1973; Kim and Routtenberg, 1976, for experimental reports). We used the same behavioral situation which we had used to demonstrate that this system appeared to play a role, namely the step-down avoidance situation.

As has been pointed out elsewhere (Routtenberg, 1979b, 1982), it is necessary to be specific both from a behavioral point of view and from a neuroanatomical point of view in studying the effects of behavioral activation on molecular mechanisms. It is conceivable, given the differentiated function of the cerebrum, that locations in brain not participating in a particular behavioral function would be altered biochemically consequent to learning a particular situation. Were one to study phosphoproteins of whole brain, one would risk the loss of signal since a majority of brain phosphoproteins might in fact be unaltered in consequence to environmental stimulation.

We sought, therefore, to study particular brain locations, focusing our interest on the neostriatum. In the first report (Routtenberg et al., 1975), we demonstrated that the alterations observed in the neostriatum were present in band F but not in band D or band E. To my knowledge this is the first demonstration of the use of back-titration of brain proteins (later referred to as a "post-hoc" or "backwards" assay) to study functional manipulations. We emphasized these points: the effects of in vivo training on phosphate incorporation can be measured in vitro, that these effects were specific to particular phosphoproteins and they appeared to be long-lasting.

### 3.3. *Doubts about the role of phosphorylation in locus coeruleus and cerebellum and motor learning*

Consequent to our discovery that band F phosphorylation was altered after step-down training in the neostriatum (Routtenberg et al., 1975), it seemed possible that those animals that were trained in the apparatus to perform a particular mode of response may have demonstrated an altered phosphorylation in a motor-related structure such as neostriatum because they were required to perform a specialized motoric act. Moreover, the possibility was considered that the alteration detected could be related to the memory for this motor act.

A proposal similar to this was provided by Gilbert (1975), who suggested that the cerebellum, using the afferent input of the locus coeruleus, could be involved in the ability to remember movements. As briefly discussed elsewhere (Routtenberg, 1976), I found little support for the Gilbert position based on prior evidence reported from my laboratory. There was no apparent role of the locus coeruleus in memory (Santos-Anderson and Routtenberg, 1976), no involvement of the locus coeruleus in reinforcement mechanisms (Routtenberg, 1977) and no detectable alterations in the cerebellum membrane fractions in phosphorylation following training. While the specifics of the Gilbert proposal were not supported by our results, the view that a relation exists among reinforcement, learning and phosphorylation was indeed a reasonable one. A subsequent discussion of the triangulation of these relationships in another brain location, the frontal cortex, was provided a few years later (Routtenberg, 1979a).

An important point to emphasize with respect to evidence which is essentially negative, is that it differentiates brain locations with respect to the phosphorylation mechanism engaged. Thus, we demonstrated in the neostriatum that there were, in fact, training-related alterations in band F but not D and E indicating a molecular-specific response. At the anatomical level, one can note the absence of effects in the cerebellum, following step-down learning. In subsequent studies (Morgan and Routtenberg, in preparation) we did not observe alterations in band F phosphorylation in hippocampus following step-down learning. This differentiates the neostriatal system from brain locations, such as hippocampus, which appear not to participate or are not significantly altered by the behavioral activation.

In sum, we found little evidence in the spons, that the locus coeruleus and cerebellum were altered in phosphorylation following step-down avoidance learning. Moreover, telencephalic locations with a similar laminar organization to cerebellum, such as hippocampus, did not show alterations in phosphorylation following this type of training. These results illustrate a point to be made again later that the locus of molecular mechanism alteration in restricted brain locations depends on the behavioral situation to which the organism is exposed. Indeed, there may exist a functional metabolic impenetrability, so as to provide for the efficiency of an isolated mechanism.

In sum, with respect to the search for functionally altered substrate phosphoproteins, the evidence (Routtenberg et al., 1975) indicated that a cAMP-independent phosphoprotein band that we termed band F was, in fact, the major phosphoprotein band altered by a behavioral experience. This alteration was observed in neostriatum but not hippocampus or cerebellum.

# 4. DETAILED ANALYSIS OF THE IN VITRO PHOSPHORYLATION PROCEDURE: FUNCTIONAL MANIPULATIONS AND CROSS-LABORATORY REPLICABILITY

The past analyses of brain biochemistry in relation to learning (Glassman, 1969; Hyden and Lange, 1970; Shashoua, 1977) have provided an interesting and potentially important mechanisms for the molecular basis of memory. One major difficulty in understanding these results is the lack of replication by other laboratories. In some cases this is related to the difficulty of the procedures required to carry out the study. In others there have been problems with the analyses themselves.

It is important, then, that the phosphorylation changes that we have observed following functional manipulation can be replicated in other laboratories. Replication not only means that the same result is observed. It also provides a measure of difference between one laboratory and another, indicating, therefore, the robustness of the effect. Thus, replication not only provides support for the phenomenon but lends evidence to the generality of the biochemical and behavioral procedures which will not be precisely identical in two different laboratories. Moreover, should a replication attempt fail, one may be given insight into the potential variables that are important for determining the differences in observations.

In this regard, then, it is striking that several different laboratories have performed functional experiments subsequent to our initial demonstration of functional effects on band F phosphorylation, which have shown that a phosphoprotein band similar in molecular weight to band F, can be altered by electrical stimulation in isolated hippocampal slices (Browning et al., 1979a) by opiates (O'Callaghan et al., 1979; Davis and Ehrlich, 1979) and by peptides (Jolles et al., 1980). Moreover, peptide-related behavioral manipulations, such as neonatal handling, substantially reduce band F phosphorylation (Cain and Routtenberg, 1981). These various studies indicate that certain phosphoproteins in the 40 000–50 000 mol. wt. range can be altered following functional manipulations.

Understanding the significance of these functional manipulations depends upon the identification of the substrate protein. As will be discussed later, this identification has been made in the case of band F-2, which has been shown to be pyruvate dehydrogenase (Morgan and Routtenberg, 1980). The significance of alterations in the phosphorylation of this brain protein in relation to behavioral state will be considered in a later section.

It is important to emphasize replicated cases in which substrate proteins are *uninfluenced* by functional manipulations. Perhaps the most notable example is band D, protein I of Ueda et al (1973). In this case both in our laboratory and in other laboratories (e.g., Browning et al., 1979a; Bär et al., 1980) there have been minor or no effects of these functional manipulations on band D phosphorylation. Moreover, in our hands, we have observed little effect of such functional manipulations on the capacity of cAMP to stimulate phosphorylation of band D. One might have expected that while the basal levels of phosphorylation would be unaltered, perhaps the capacity of cAMP to stimulate would have been changed. Thus, there has been relatively good agreement among laboratories that few alterations occur in band D phosphorylation following functional treatment.

Under rather specialized circumstances, possible nonspecific effects on band D phosphorylation have been observed. Strombom et al., (1979) have reported alterations in this band following liquid nitrogen sacrifice. As there was no other band analyzed, the question of its specificity remains moot. In the Conway and Routtenberg (1978) study, no effects on band D were observed in cortical $P_2$ preparations. Bär et al. (1980) reported that band D phosphorylation was altered following synaptic activation only in the absence of calcium. Since synaptic transmission is blocked in such a case, the significance of this finding remains to be determined.

To increase the opportunity for replicability of functional manipulations among laboratories, as well as detailing some of the major determinants of the phosphorylation system, several key variables will now be considered. These are: (a) method of sacrifice; (b) buffer system used; (c) the subcellular fraction; (d) gel conditions; and (e) the data analysis.

One generality may be stated at the outset. The demonstration of functional effects using back-titration in the in vitro phosphorylation system is dependent upon the conditions used to arrive at the final product — the phosphorylated protein in the autoradiograph. As will be documented later, if the phosphorylation of the protein in vitro is unchanged, it could be due either to its true lack of functional responsivity or to the absence of the proper conditions for demonstrating its in vivo responsivity. A negative effect is, of course, difficult to establish, though such a "negative" demonstration using several different reaction conditions, would be of significant value.

### 4.1. *Method of sacrifice*

The transition from life to death critically influences back-titration of the brain protein phosphorylation in vitro. This rather provincial approach to existence is absolutely essential in defining the relation between environmental events and brain protein phosphorylation. In the simplest case, consider a functional in vivo manipulation, which could alter phosphorylation in vitro, but the method of sacrifice produces an effect that is equal and opposite to the functional effect. Thus, there would be no consequence detected in vitro to the functional manipulation even though it produced an effect in vivo.

Our initial reports which characterized the in vitro phosphorylation system made use of decapitation as the method of sacrifice (Ehrlich and Routtenberg, 1974; Routtenberg and Ehrlich, 1975). When sacrifice by decapitation was used, in functional studies, no effects of training were observed (Routtenberg, Conway and Ratliff, unpublished observations). Since rapid freezing did enable us to observe functional effects, we were led to consider the influence of method of sacrifice on phosphorylation of individual phosphoprotein substrates.

In experiments that measured cAMP in brain (Goldberg et al., 1970) decapitation produced a rapid rise in cAMP levels compared to rapid freezing in liquid nitrogen or microwave irradiation. The rise in phosphocreatinine levels and decrease in ATP levels was also prevented by rapid freezing or heating. It was concluded that liquid nitrogen or microwave irradiation sacrifice prevents enzymatic activity from substantially altering the in vivo levels. These findings have been confirmed and extended by Lust et al., (1980), in which detailed analysis of the cooling of the layers of the cortex have been provided. The evidence has indicated that rapid cooling of the cortex ($< 10$ sec) can be obtained with liquid nitrogen and that the use of a refrigerant, such as freon or isopropane to avoid the "oxygen skin", does not materially change the rate of freezing. Moreover, the deepest portions of rat or mouse brain are frozen within 30 sec.

It should be obvious that to study the endogenous phosphorylation after in vivo functional manipulations, the in vivo state must be preserved. In the study of back-titration using in vitro phosphorylation, the preferred method is clearly whole body immersion in liquid nitrogen, since the animal can be transferred from a wake, freely moving condition to death in less than 2 sec, and therefore relatively painlessly. Moreover, the frozen brain tissue leaves intact brain anatomy which can still be appreciated and hence dissected for regional analysis. Finally, enzymatic activity can be studied in vitro when the tissue is brought to the reaction temperature ($30°C$).

357

We initially reported our results concerning the effects of behavioral manipulation using liquid nitrogen sacrifice (Routtenberg et al., 1975; Ehrlich et al., 1977). We noted at that time that differences existed in the in vitro phosphorylation of animals sacrificed by decapitation as compared to those sacrificed by liquid nitrogen. It was essential, then, for us to compare the differences in these two methods. One method, decapitation, has been used extensively in the study of brain biochemistry, while the other method has been used infrequently.

We compared the phosphorylation of cerebral cortex of decapitated and liquid nitrogen sacrificed animals. (In the cerebral cortex and in the neostriatum the effects observed were similar. Since the neostriatum would undoubtedly reach freezing temperatures after cerebral cortex, it is unlikely that the functional differences that have been observed are related to the rate of freezing. Moreover, the pattern of phosphorylation in cerebral cortex and neostriatum is quite similar (Conway and Routtenberg, 1978, Fig. 1).)

The major difference observed as a consequence of sacrifice method was the increase in phosphorylation in band F of liquid nitrogen-treated tissue. This was observed in both the cerebral cortex and neostriatum. Also of interest was the absence of phosphorylation of a band now referred to as band D-3. There was a decrease in phosphorylation of band E following liquid nitrogen sacrifice.

As will be discussed shortly, the liquid nitrogen sacrifice-induced increase in phosphorylation of band F appears to be associated with band F-1 of 47 000 approximate mol. wt. Also of interest was the fact that another band, immediately below band F, was observed in decapitated preparations, but appeared not to be present in the liquid nitrogen preparation, or was decreased in phosphorylation following liquid nitrogen. If this band is F-2, the increase in phosphorylation of band F-2 following decapitation is consistent with its identification as the $\alpha$ subunit of pyruvate dehydrogenase (Morgan and Routtenberg, 1980, 1981a).

The interpretation of this result with band F-2 (PDH) is as follows: PDH dephosphorylation activates the PDH enzyme. In animals that are decapitated there is an increase in the activity of the enzyme (Jope and Blass, 1976). The increased enzyme activity would be accompanied by a phosphatase activation and dephosphorylation. Thus, phosphatase would cause a dephosphorylation in PDH in situ. When brought to the in vitro reaction for back-titration a net increase in phosphorylation would be observed. This logic can be similarly applied to the relative decrease in phosphorylation in PDH (band F-2) when rapid freezing is used since this would prevent the activation of PDH, thereby increasing its phosphorylation. When brought to the in vitro reaction, this PDH would be significantly less phosphorylated than its decapitated brother. Thus, the observed increase in PDH phosphorylation in decapitated vs. liquid nitrogen-sacrificed preparations can be ascribed to the greater back-titration of vacant sites, brought about by PDH phosphatase activation following decapitation sacrifice*.

Given our recent demonstration of behaviorally induced changes in PDH activity (Morgan and Routtenberg, 1981a), it is now rather clear why behaviorally induced alterations were not observed in PDH, using decapitated preparations. Decapitation would have a significantly greater effect than the alterations in PDH activation occurring as a consequence of training. More specifically, the vacant sites available for back-titration would be elevated in controls to the point where no differences among groups would be detected.

---

* The alterations in PDH brought about by training and those occurring consequently to decapitation are not necessarily related. For example, training-induced alterations in PDH may be related to the need for transmitter (the acetyl CoA moiety for acetylcholine synthesis; Benjamin and Quastel, 1981) while decapitation in all likelihood signals need for acetyl CoA for Kreb's cycle ATP production. In general, then, a widespread response of brain molecules to sacrifice conditions (e.g., cAMP, actylcholine or ATP) should not be taken to indicate that its function is not discrete and specific under physiological conditions.

It is interesting to note that band F-2 phosphorylation is decreased consequent to liquid nitrogen sacrifice, while F-1 phosphorylation is increased consequent to sacrifice. This calls attention to the fact, emphasized by Conway and Routtenberg (1979), that these two band F phosphoproteins are different proteins with different properties. It is important to indicate that these bands respond in an opposite manner to rapid freezing. The possibility suggested by Gispen and co-workers that band F-1 is a lipid kinase, a diphosphoinositide kinase, relates this band to the plasma membrane. The difference in phosphate incorporation of band F-1 between the liquid nitrogen sacrifice method and decapitation is the most dramatic of any of the bands in the cerebral cortex, showing a ratio of 3.39 (Conway and Routtenberg, 1978). A similar and parallel increase is noted in band H-4. Since this may be a phospholipid the parallel change in band F and in H-4 is not too surprising.

It is interesting that cAMP stimulation of band D was not significantly influenced by the method of sacrifice. Assuming that cAMP regulates band D phosphorylation in vivo (Strombom et al., 1979) one should assume that decapitation, by elevating cyclic nucleotide levels, would increase phosphorylation of band D in situ and hence lead to a decreased back-titration compared to liquid nitrogen-sacrificed animals. The absence of such a decrease remains an unsolved question.

In our first study of the transition states between life and death (Conway and Routtenberg, 1978), we used two methods of sacrifice to achieve the transition. In our follow-up study (Conway and Routtenberg, 1979), we effected the transition, in addition, by use of barbiturate anesthesia overdose. We also observed the effects of light and deep pentobarbital anesthesia on in vitro phosphorylation.

Of particular significance with respect to the discussion on sacrifice method is that the presence of anesthesia reversed the effects of liquid nitrogen sacrifice. Thus, the animal showed increased phosphorylation in band F-1 as a consequence of the rapid freezing but did not show a similar increase when that was preceded by barbiturate anesthesia. Thus, it can be concluded that tissue freezing per se and the consequences thereof are not sufficient to produce the elevation in band F-1 phosphorylation (Conway and Routtenberg, 1978). The elevation of band F-1 in liquid nitrogen sacrificed unanesthetized preparations likely involves the preservation of an increased number of available sites for back-titration in the awake brain. Pentobarbital anesthesia, then, causes an in vivo increment in band F-1 phosphorylation, depressing its phosphorylation in vitro. These results suggest that band F-1 phosphorylation may be related to the state of brain activation (Routtenberg, 1979b).

One drawback of the rapid freezing method is the inevitable alteration of membrane structure consequent to immersion in liquid nitrogen. This may be especially deleterious in studies which attempt to observe the effects of peptide hormone on phosphorylation, where interaction with the membrane is an important first step. Thus, for example, if one were interested in the effects of $ACTH_{1-24}$, such as has been shown by Jolles et al. (1980), on brain protein phosphorylation, it is not at all clear that the ACTH would have similar effects on rapidly frozen brain.

### 4.2. Buffer system

The effect of experience on band F phosphorylation (Routtenberg et al., 1975) was demonstrated using a Tris magnesium buffer. Ueda et al. (1973) used this buffer system to demonstrate the cAMP stimulation of protein I (band D). Moreover, our initial detailed characterization of the four phosphoproteins designated D, E, F and G (Routtenberg and Ehrlich, 1975) used this buffer system. Because of its hypotonicity, Conway and I determined whether any alterations would occur in the reaction if unbuffered 0.32 M sucrose was used in place of Tris, during subcellular preparation of the crude synaptosome and in the reaction mixture. As reported in Routtenberg (1979b, Fig. 6), there was in fact a considerable difference in the phosphorylation of all the phosphoprotein bands in iso-osmotic sucrose as compared to the hypo-osmotic buffer. This difference is especially evident in band F. No alterations were seen in the H bands, but bands D-1 and D-2 and band E were significantly increased in their phosphorylation in the sucrose buffer. The effects were particularly evident in the absence of cAMP.

Given the higher level of phosphorylation seen in sucrose, suggesting a more optimum set of conditions for phosphotransferase activity, we had planned on using this buffer system in functional experiments.

To our surprise the use of sucrose in a follow-up study on the effect of early neonatal handling on brain protein phosphorylation which used Tris buffer (Cain and Routtenberg, 1982) yielded a negative result. Since Holmes et al. (1977) indicated an alteration in phosphorylation as a consequence of handling in adult animals, we presumed that such an effect would be magnified if initiated at an earlier stage, namely from day 1 of birth, and then maintained for 25 days. The absence of an effect using sucrose was also disturbing since the first time we had performed this neonatal handling experiment, using Tris buffer, a significant decrease in phosphorylation of band F-1 was observed in handled animals relative to control animals. We were puzzled, then, that changing the buffer to optimize the reaction conditions (i.e., greater phosphotransferase activity) would vitiate the effect of handling on phosphorylation.

We took the set of samples that demonstrated no effect when sucrose was used as the "buffer", and resuspended them in a Tris buffer. To our surprise we found that alterations were now observed in the effects of handling on phosphorylation of band F-1. These results provide evidence, then, that samples which do not show a difference in phosphorylation as a consequence of functional stimulation, using one system (unbuffered 0.32 molar sucrose) do show a functionally significant difference when a Tris buffer system is used. This indicates then that the conditions which are optimal for demonstrating enzyme activity, may not be optimal for demonstrating functional differences. Potential mechanisms need to be determined, but it may be emphasized at this juncture that only certain buffers may permit accurate in vitro back-titration of functional in vivo differences.

The buffer system not only influences the outcome of an in vivo functional experience on in vitro phosphorylation, but also influences the effect of in vitro manipulations on in vitro phosphorylation.

A recent example from our laboratory comes from a series of studies (Morgan and Routtenberg, 1980) on the influence of modulators of pyruvate dehydrogenase phosphorylation. Thus, we have found that dichloroacetate, the substance which has been shown by Whitehouse et al. (1974) to inhibit PDH kinase, is only effective when used in phosphate buffer, but is explicitly ineffective when used in HEPES buffer (Morgan and Routtenberg, unpublished observations). It is to be emphasized that basal phosphorylation in vitro appears to be quite similar with the two buffers. It is not clear whether this effect is related to the increased permeability of mitochondrial membranes or the more ready access of ADP to the PDH complex (Pratt and Roche, 1979). Nonetheless, it is clear that the type of buffer chosen will determine whether inhibitors or facilitators of enzyme activity in an in vitro system will be effective.

The choice of buffer system used will be determined by or restricted to those buffers which are relevant to the enzyme under study. Thus, for example, in our experiments on training and PDH activity (Morgan and Routtenberg, 1981a), we were interested in studying both band F-2 phosphorylation and PDH activity from the same membrane preparation, of the same animal, from the same brain location. In order to study PDH activity, then, phosphate is the typical buffer system used. Thus, we looked at the effects of training as we had in the past (Routtenberg et al., 1975; Routtenberg and Benson, 1980), using this buffer system. We found, in fact, that we could replicate our earlier findings with regard to a training-induced increase in band F phosphorylation, using a phosphate buffer system. In fact, alterations in PDH activity were observed which were correlated with changes in band F-2 phosphorylation. We again did not observe alterations in band D or band E phosphorylation, suggesting that the negative results observed in prior experiments were not dependent solely on the use of Tris buffer. In the case, then, of training-related alterations of band F-2 phosphorylation, we have now observed significant changes using Tris and phosphate buffers. Thus, the functional effects related to band F-2 appear, in fact, not to be dependent on a particular buffer system.

In summary, while it is difficult to say that a particular buffer system should be used in back-titration studies which attempt to observe the effects of functional treatment on subsequent in vitro phosphorylation, it is clear that the buffer system selected will have an important if not a determining influence on the result obtained. It is also clear then that the selection of the buffer system can hardly be regarded as unimportant, and thus care must be given to its selection.

### 4.3. Subcellular system

In an effort to specify the subcellular location of the change in phosphorylation, it would seem advantageous to obtain reasonably pure subcellular components: synaptosomes, mitochondria, ribosomes, synaptic plasma membranes, myelin and so on. Thus, for example, considerable emphasis has been devoted to the possibility that functional alterations are likely to occur at the synaptic junction consequent to synaptic activation. One would wish to know, then, whether the alterations in phosphorylation that do occur are, in fact, located at such junctions.

This may appear to be a valuable approach to the study of phosphorylation changes in relation to function. However, alterations of the state of phosphorylation of a phosphoprotein could conceivably occur as the subcellular treatment (e.g., ultracentrifugation) becomes successively more harsh. Moreover, as pointed out by Matus et al. (1979), alterations can occur in subcellular fractions, so that components of the endogenous phosphorylation that are not normally associated, become so following subcellular fractionation. Thus, a "pure" synaptosome might demonstrate phosphorylation of a protein that normally does not occur at the synapse.

Another problem arises when considering the fact that the substrate, kinase and phosphatase should be present to study endogenous phosphorylation. The removal of the kinase or the substrate would of necessity eliminate phosphorylation of that protein, but it would not indicate whether it was the substrate or the kinase that was no longer present. Thus, the absence of phosphorylation would not necessarily mean that the substrate protein is not present in that subcellular fraction.

These considerations have led us to become more particular with respect to the gel conditions used to enable separation of phosphoprotein substrates, and to avoid the potential pitfaills of purified subcellular preparations. Thus, in our current studies (Morgan and Routtenberg, 1981a), we have used the homogenate preparation; while this loses the enrichment of synaptic material in the reaction mixture, it has the benefit of reducing the problems associated with subcellular fractionation. Moreover, we maintain our guarded interest in those phosphoproteins which we have observed in synaptic preparations (Ehrlich and Routtenberg, 1974) and have thus exploited, in some sense, the subcellular specificity by allowing the gel system to separate the proteins.

There are, in fact, other reasons why an approach which emphasizes subcellular purity may not be satisfactory. Consider, as an example, the role of PDH (band F-2). Assuming for the moment that the majority of PDH is located in the mitochondrial fraction, it is clear that in a purified mitochondrial preparation we are looking at PDH from several different subcellular sources: perinuclear, axon terminal and dendritic. Each of these locations is different with respect to function. Thus, it would be important to differentiate between the PDH activity from dendritic loci as opposed to that found in presynaptic terminals. There are several techniques for separating mitochondria along subcellular dimensions. All of them, however, provide essentially a relative degree of enrichment. Nonetheless, it would be instructive to study PDH from various subcellular locations in an effort to determine whether functional alterations in PDH are selective for a particular location. If this were so, clearly the percentage change in PDH would be much larger in certain subcellular compartments currently observed (Morgan and Routtenberg, 1981a).

Though the functional alterations observed on phosphorylation have been related to PDH, and hence mitochondrial systems, it is not to be concluded, therefore, that the effect is unrelated to the synaptic junction. As indicated in a representative dendritic spine synapse shown in Fig. 4 of Tarrant and Routtenberg (1979), mitochondria are present in presynaptic terminals and in postsynaptic dendrites in close proximity to the neck of the dendritic spine. Changes in presynaptic terminal mitochondrial PDH might be expected to influence synaptic activity at such an axon-dendritic synapse. Pysh and Khan (1970) have indicated that nearly 25 % of the total mean volume fraction of dendrites are mitochondrial, based on stereological analysis of electron micrographs of cerebellum and inferior colliculus. Alterations in PDH might alter postsynaptic, that is dendritic, responsivity. Because the mitochondria are found in heavy concentration in dendrites perhaps the alterations that we have observed in PDH activity following training (Morgan and Routtenberg, 1981) are derived from such postsynaptic sites.

In summary, this discussion serves to illustrate the complexity of issues surrounding attempts to use subcellular fractionation to specify the locale of functional changes in brain protein phosphorylation. No simple solution is apparent. The investigator need be cautious, then, in drawing conclusions that the site of activity is synaptic, when the phosphorylation changes observed are present in a synaptosomal preparation, however well purified. Similar caution is necessary when concluding that activity in "non-synaptic" preparations, such as the mitochondrial fraction is, therefore, unrelated to synaptic functions.

### 4.4. *Gel conditions*

In the past seven years we have used three different gel systems, a discontinuous three-layered (7, 9, 12 %) gel, a gradient (7–18 %) gel, and a single concentration 10 % gel (Laemmli, 1970). In the gradient and discontinuous gel systems, the attempt was to resolve proteins over a wide range of molecular weights, both below 20 000 and above 100 000. In our more recent experiments we have focused our analysis on proteins in the molecular weight range between 35 000 and 90 000. We have used the 10 % gel system, which more clearly resolves proteins in this molecular weight range, while providing less resolution in the higher and lower molecular weight ranges. Thus, as it became evident which range was of interest, we altered the gel system used.

The importance of enhancing gel resolution is illustrated in our studies on phosphorylation of proteins in the 40 000–50 000 mol. wt. range. Initially we observed alterations in the phosphorylation of a single band which we termed band F. Using the 10 % Laemmli (1970) gel, we have been able to separate band F into two components, band F-1 and band F-2. This system inter alia also enables a clear distinction between proteins D-1 and D-2 (Ia, Ib of Ueda and Greengard, 1977). It appears clear now that a part of the functional alterations in band F phosphorylation can be attributed to band F-2 (Routtenberg and Benson, 1980).

It is worth emphasizing the use of the term "band" rather than "protein" to refer to individual bands in the particular gel system. Even with the compelling evidence (see section 6) for identification of band F-2 as PDH, it is probable that there are other phosphoproteins in that location on the gel which are minor but present nonetheless. Thus, it is reasonable to refer to these separated components on the gel as "bands" rather than as individual "proteins" since they are potentially one of several at that location. A detailed analysis of brain phosphoproteins using two-dimensional gel electrophoresis can, at times, be valuable in this regard. It may be fruitful, as well, to cut out a particular band or spot, e.g., the $\alpha$ subunit of pyruvate dehydrogenase, and study the phosphate content of peptide fragments, using limited proteolysis (see Sale and Randle, 1981).

### 4.5. *Data analysis*

The approach to the study of brain phosphoproteins with respect to the evaluation of the data has taken several forms. The lack of consistency in the treatment of data may lead to several new problems.

With regard to densitometric analysis, Ueda et al. (1973) first suggested the densitometric quantification of the phosphorylated brain substrates, using a baseline, adjusted to background levels of density that surround each individual band. This analysis had been used by our laboratory, but required modification because of two significant problems. First, peak height was used as a measure of incorporation. The possibility exists that t phosphoprotein containing a considerable amount of phosphate would not be scored as such because it would be diffusely focused, and have a lower peak. It would be more accurate, then, to use the area of the curve rather than its peak height. This would conform more closely to the slicing and counting approach which takes into account adjacent gel slices in measuring the counts in the gel (e.g., Morgan and Routtenberg, 1979a).

A second problem involves the variations among samples in overall incorporation that are due either to the manipulation itself that precedes the reaction or due to some variability in tissue preparation or reaction conditions so that enzyme (kinase/phosphatase) activity is different. Assuming a linear relationship between the phosphorylated substrate and protein concentration, for example, it is reasonable to use a measure of incorporation that takes into account some overall level of incorporation. We have used, as an overall measure, the sum of densities of the individual bands on a particular gel sample (see Mitrius et al., 1981). Therefore, to demonstrate that the incorporation change in an individual band is not a function of some overall change, but is specific to that band, a percentage of total band density measure described by Mitrius et al. (1981) can be used. It should be emphasized that one does not confer specificity of a functional manipulation by analyzing or, indeed, isolating a single band. Since this practice is used, it is necessary to be cautious when evaluating an effect that is claimed to be band-specific.

At an early stage in the analysis of densitometric profiles it is important that a correlation be determined between the density of an individual band and its activity determined in a scintillation counter. Removing and counting individual bands and relating that to a density measure would be more accurate than simply taking individual gel slices at 1 mm intervals. Using the 1 mm slice technique, we have assessed the relation between densitometric values and counts/min found in individual slices. The correlation between the two was $+0.87$

(Ehrlich and Routtenberg, 1974). While demonstrating a significant high positive correlation, it is by no means perfect, and improvement in the densitometric analysis is still an important priority.

### 4.6. *Summary of methodological issues: Signs of health in resolving areas of conflict*

It is reasonable to conclude from consideration of methodological issues related to brain phosphoproteins and function, that this field has developed sufficiently so that specific, conflicting results can now be appreciated and perhaps resolved. One reason for this is the fact that several different laboratories are using similar in vitro phosphorylation techniques to study functional manipulations. This represents a significant advance over prior "brain macromolecules and behavior" experiments in which individual laboratories reported on alterations in a particular macromolecular species, but with neither replication nor explicit denial by others in the field. We are thus now approaching a time when a functional description of a set of identifiable brain phosphoproteins may be achieved. Moreover, from a nomenclature point of view we can identify these phosphoproteins and, in general, know that we are studying the same molecular species. Thus, it should be possible to identify phosphoproteins not solely on the basis of molecular weight, but on the basis of other features, i.e., cAMP stimulation (D-1, D-2, E-2), calcium sensitivity (E-1, E-3), post-mortem manipulation and response to anesthesia (F-1) and magnesium requirement (F-2), each of which may prove diagnostic for that substrate. The capacity to compare experimental results across laboratories, when the substrate protein is known to be the same, considerably increases the possibility of resolving conflicting results, facilitating the achievement of progress by replication.

Browning et al. (1979a) have reported that stimulation of the hippocampal slice produces a decrement in phosphorylation in a 40 K phosphoprotein, probably band F-2 or pyruvate dehydrogenase (Morgan and Routtenberg, 1980). Bär et al. (1980) have reported that stimulation in the same hippocampal slice preparation produces an increment in phosphorylation of a 50 K protein, which is immediately above their B-50 protein (probably E-3). Browning et al. (1979a) saw no change in this 50 K protein and Bär et al. (1980) saw no change in the 40 K protein. While there are several possible reasons why such differences were obtained, it is of interest to consider that the method of sacrifice might lead to differences in results observed. In both studies the animal is stunned by a blow to the head, the brain is quickly removed, and a hippocampal slice is incubated in a warm, moist, oxygenated medium. Perusal of the autoradiographs suggests that band F-1 may have been present in the preparation of Bär et al. (1980), but may have been absent in the preparation of Browning et al. (1979a). One thus needs to take into account the fact that as a consequence of this essentially post-mortem manipulation band F-1 may have been altered. Since the alteration in band F-1 was different in the two studies, the state of the slice may have been different. The response of other brain phosphoproteins, then, to repetitive stimulation may also have been different.

There is a paucity of evidence with respect to the relation between phosphorylation in the hippocampal slice and that found under other conditions, such as a freshly decapitated or quick frozen preparations. It would be valuable to compare the hippocampal slice and the liquid nitrogen-sacrificed preparation with respect to the basal levels of phosphorylation and the response to cAMP for example. Since the substrates studied by each group are known, it should be possible to resolve the conflict in results by determining the conditions which give rise to the particular results in the hippocampal slice preparation.

## 5. IN VIVO PHOSPHORYLATION

We have recently sought to determine whether, in fact, the electrophoretically separated phosphoproteins examined in vitro would be phosphorylated in vivo. It was conceivable, for example, given the Matus et al (1979) results, that in vitro phosphorylation of certain proteins might be related to a subcellular artefact. Moreover, band D-3 was only readily detected in its phosphorylation in post-mortem tissue (Conway and Routtenberg, 1979; Routtenberg et al., 1981), suggesting potential artefactual results such as protein denaturation exposing normally unphosphorylated sites for phosphate incorporation (Krebs, 1972). It was possible, then, that certain phosphoproteins would not necessarily be observed using in vivo methods. We also wished to observe differences in the pattern or rate of phosphorylation that might be different from those observed using the in vitro method. Finally, we had hoped to study the effects of functional manipulations on in vivo phosphorylation.

In a recent report, then, Mitrius et al. (1981) observed that those bands that are phosphorylated in vivo do, in fact, co-migrate with phosphoprotein bands observed in vitro. A similar finding, which however emphasized possible qualitative differences in phosphorylation, has been made by Berman et al. (1980). Of special interest in the report of Mitrius et al. (1981) was the fact that the highest levels of incorporation at the shortest time points were present in bands F-1 and F-2. Lesser degrees of phosphorylation were observed in bands D-1 and D-2 at these time points.

Even at the 2 min incorporation time phosphorylation of bands F-1 and F-2 could be detected with injection of as little as 25 $\mu$C [$^{32}$P] orthophosphate. Thus, bands F-1 and F-2 were highly phosphorylated at short incorporation times, but approached non-detectability at 24 h after incorporation. In contrast, band E increased its phosphorylation from the 20 min to the 24 h time point. Bands D-1 and D-2 showed no significant change in incorporation. Thus, the evidence gathered indicates that those phosphoprotein bands which are altered in their back-titration following functional manipulations are also the bands which in vivo are most rapidly turning over. This property makes them ideal substrates for the rapid alterations required to parallel rapid changes in electrical or synaptic activity following a functional manipulation.

In the one experiment which compared the effects of state of the animal on phosphorylation, we observed no band-specific effects of pentobarbital anesthesia when compared to awake preparations. The reasons for the lack of differences with respect to in vivo phosphorylation and method of sacrifice is probably related to the 60 min interval between the time of injection and the time of sacrifice and the use of tissue processing at 0–4°C which inhibits phosphatase activity (Mitrius, et al., 1981). There was some suggestion, although not consistent enough to be statistically significant, that a decrease in band F-2 phosphorylation in vivo occurred in decapitated preparations (Mitrius et al., 1981, Fig. 6) relative to animals decapitated while under barbiturate anesthesia. This difference would be expected on the basis of our identification of band F-2 as PDH (Morgan and Routtenberg, 1980), since under barbiturate, activity of the enzyme is lower than in the awake state. Following decapitation, there is a decreased dephosphorylation activation of PDH in the chronic or awake state (Jope and Blass, 1976). This could explain the decrease in band F-2 phosphorylation in vivo which we have, at times, observed.

Consistency is needed, therefore, in order to study the incorporation of orthophosphate in vivo as a function of an experimental manipulation. One would expect, for example, that since training causes an activation of PDH (Morgan and Routtenberg, 1981a) then a decrease in in vivo phosphorylation should be observed following training.

## 6. IDENTIFICATION OF BAND F-2 AS PDH

It is interesting that brain phosphoproteins have, in general, not been linked to particular non-neural phosphoproteins. It is perhaps most interesting that the well studied proteins Ia and Ib of Ueda and Greengard (1977), which have been characterized in detailed terms (see Ueda, this volume), have not yet been identified with a known protein. It may be that they are unique proteins, which are not found in other tissues. The evidence to date suggests that they may, indeed, be brain-specific proteins.

Considerable care must be made in making this judgement, however, since recent work in our laboratory, comparing rat and human bands D-1 and D-2 have shown differences in migration rate, indicating different characteristics of this protein pair in rat and human (Routtenberg et al., 1981). Thus, it is possible that bands D-1 and D-2 exist in non-neural tissue but that differences exist between neural and non-neural bands D-1 and D-2. It will be vital, then, to determine if there are such small differences in properties such that bands D-1 and D-2 in brain are, in fact, non-neural isozymes.

The strategy which our laboratory has undertaken from the outset in the study of brain proteins and function has been to survey the various proteins of a particular class, glycoproteins (e.g., Morgan and Routtenberg, 1979a) or phosphoproteins (Conway and Routtenberg, 1979) and to determine which members of the class are altered consequently to training. Thus, we have found that certain glycoproteins (Morgan and Routtenberg, 1979b) or phosphoproteins are altered consequently to functional manipulations, while others remain stable.

With respect to brain phosphoproteins, our strategy was to determine which phosphoproteins were altered using back-titration, and then describe the characteristics of such phosphoproteins in an effort to identify the particular molecule. We have made progress along these lines from studies initiated in 1970 to the recent identification of enzymatic changes following training (Morgan and Routtenberg, 1981).

In this section of the paper, then, I wish to discuss the steps that have been taken to identify band F-2 as PDH and to indicate also the considerable advantage in using specific kinase and phosphatase inhibitors that has been possible when identification is made. This should encourage the search for identification of other brain phosphoproteins with non-neural phosphoproteins.

It may be speculated that the lack of identification of brain phosphoproteins other than band F-2 stemmed from a view, now rapidly disappearing, that phosphoproteins that exist in brain must somehow be unique. Although this view is unlikely and not shared by many, the search for unique molecules which exist in brain and confer upon brain its uniqueness continues. It is entirely feasible that brain phosphoproteins, which are found in non-neural tissue, function in brain locations in the same fashion as in non-neural tissue. Conceivably, the uniqueness of brain resides less in its molecules and more in its structure, the organizational matrix in which the molecules are disposed.

Such a view emerges, in part, when considering the role of pyruvate dehydrogenase in brain function. The sequence of steps in identification of band F-2 as PDH are now considered. The work to be reviewed in the following section is based on the thesis of David Morgan (1981).

### 6.1. *Regulators of pyruvate dehydrogenase alter band F-2 phosphorylation*

The first work in our laboratory which indicated that band F-2 had certain unique properties was suggested by the effects of EDTA (shown in Fig. 1). We had observed that, in contrast to all other bands, band F-2 was readily phosphorylated in the virtual absence of magnesium. This suggested that band F-2 was a phosphoprotein whose kinase required no more than

366

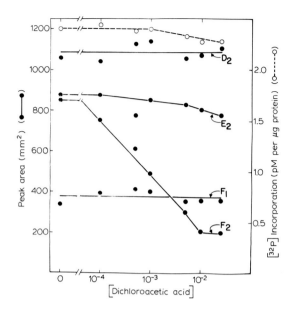

Fig. 2. The effects of increasing concentrations of dichloroacetic acid on brain protein phosphorylation. Brain homogenates at a protein concentration of 2.1 mg/ml were reacted with [$^{32}$P]ATP for 30 sec in the presence of several dichloroacetic acid concentrations. Aliquots were removed for polyacrylamide gel electrophoresis and TCA precipitation of protein. The effects of increasing concentrations of dichloroacetate on the total $^{32}$P incorporation into TCA precipitates and the incorporation of radioactivity into individual phosphoprotein bands (quantified densitometrically) are presented. The solid lines indicate the area of the individual peaks in mm$^2$. The TCA-precipitable $^{32}$P incorporation is indicated by the dashed line. The concentrations of dichloroacetate used were 0, 0.1, 0.5, 1.0, 5.0, 10.0 and 25.0 mM. (From Morgan and Routtenberg, 1980.)

micromolar quantities of magnesium. A phosphoprotein with such properties having a similar molecular weight was the $\alpha$ subunit of pyruvate dehydrogenase (PDH). Moreover, PDH phosphatase would be inhibited in the absence of magnesium. Thus, the phosphatase inhibition and presence of kinase activity leading to a substantial increase of band F-2 phosphorylation could be understood if band F-2 were PDH.

Because much had been known with regard to the control of PDH activity, Morgan and I (1980) set out to determine whether inhibitors of PDH kinase, such as dichloroacetate, would influence band F-2 phosphorylation. Fig. 2 shows that an increasing concentration of dichloroacetate selectively inhibits band F-2 phosphorylation. Other phosphoprotein bands were not influenced by dichloroacetate. We also demonstrated that the products (acetyl CoA, NADH) and substrates (CoA, NAD$^+$, pyruvate) of PDH would alter its phosphorylation in the expected direction. Thus, substrates of PDH would be expected to activate the enzyme by dephosphorylation, while products would be expected to inhibit the enzyme, by increased phosphorylation. Acetyl CoA, then, was found to increase phosphorylation. CoA, on the other hand, which would cause an activation, caused a decrease in phosphorylation. Pyruvate would be expected to cause an activation of the enzyme and hence cause a dephosphorylation.

Pyruvate at 5 mM decreased band F-2 phosphorylation by more than 50%. These results conformed precisely to those expected on the basis of our current understanding of the regulators of PDH activity (Reed et al., 1980), providing evidence that band F-2 was PDH.

### 6.2. *PDH activity correlates with band F-2 phosphorylation*

The evidence that we had gathered (Morgan and Routtenberg, 1980), then, indicated that manipulators of PDH kinase manipulate band F-2 phosphorylation in the expected direction, while manipulators of PDH phosphatase also manipulate band F-2. In all cases, the manipulation is selective for this phosphoprotein, i.e., other bands are not influenced at the same concentration levels that significantly alter band F-2 phosphorylation. Thus, there was no evidence that opposed the view that band F-2 was PDH. Indeed, as shown in Morgan and Routtenberg (1980, Fig. 2) the authentic $\alpha$ subunit of PDH, provided by L. Reed, co-migrated with our band F-2 from brain.

We wished to obtain more direct evidence for this association, determining whether pyruvate dehydrogenase activity would be inversely related to band F-2 phosphorylation as had been shown for non-neural PDH (Reed et al., 1980). That this would be the case in brain was suggested initially by the work of Siess et al. (1971). We, therefore, set up a parallel assay to study both PDH and band F-2 phosphorylation, the design of which is briefly described in Morgan and Routtenberg (1981). Thus, we hoped to discover in this parallel assay whether, for example, inhibition of PDH phosphatase would cause not only an increase of phosphorylation of band F-2, but a decrease in PDH enzyme activity. Also, we hoped to discover whether DCA would not only inhibit band F-2 phosphorylation as previously shown, but would elevate PDH activity by virtue of its capacity to inhibit PDH kinase. In Fig. 3 it can be seen, indeed, that alterations in phosphorylation are inversely related to the levels of enzyme activity. The time course of these changes are roughly parallel. The correlation of enzyme activity and PDH phosphorylation is $-0.91$. The inverse relation was most evident in the EDTA condition where the correlation between phosphorylation and PDH activity was $-0.99$. Thus, this inverse relation between PDH activity and band F-2 phosphorylation provides compelling evidence for the identification of band F-2 as PDH.

### 6.3. *The effect of avoidance training on PDH activity and back-titration of band F-2 and on PDH activity*

In prior reports we had shown that band F-2 phosphorylation is altered following an aversive experience using step-down training (Routtenberg and Benson, 1980). Because of the evidence just discussed, we would expect to observe alterations in PDH activity following training. We have recently shown that PDH activity is increased, in fact, at the same time that an increase in band F-2 phosphorylation is observed (Morgan and Routtenberg, 1981) following training.

Given the fact that PDH activity is inversely related to its phosphorylation, we can suggest a specific relation between back-titration of band F-2 and PDH enzyme activity. Moreover, the sequence of in vivo events and in vitro events can be considered. This is summarized in Fig. 4, which suggests that training leads to a speculated activation of PDH phosphatase (although it could also be an inhibition of kinase activity, for various reasons the regulation is likely to be on the phosphatase). This causes a net dephosphorylation in vivo. This activates the enzyme which is demonstrated in vitro using [$^{14}$C]pyruvate as substrate and a carbon trapping procedure to measure evolved $CO_2$. An increase in in vitro phosphorylation is also detected when the tissue is now brought to the in vitro back-titration assay since the available number of

368

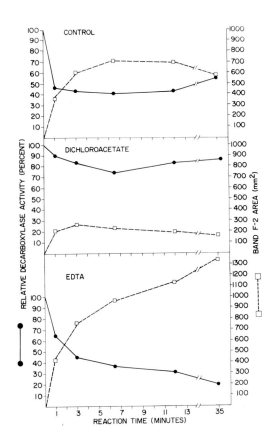

Fig. 3. The time course of pyruvate dehydrogenase activity and band F-2 phosphorylation under phosphorylating conditions. Brain homogenates were preincubated for 18 min at which time ATP alone (A), ATP plus 10 mM dichloroacetate (B), or ATP plus 9 mM EDTA (C) were added. Aliquots were removed immediately before and 1, 3, 6.5, 12 and 35 min after, the ATP addition. The pyruvate decarboxylase activity is expressed as the percentage of the value before the ATP addition. The 100 % values were 11.2 nmoles of carbon dioxide evolved per ng protein per min in condition A, 10.5 nmoles per ng per min in the presence of dichloroacetate, and 9.1 nmoles per ng per min in the excess EDTA condition. The values presented are the average of duplicate determinations. *Assay of pyruvate decarboxylase activity*. The release of [$^{14}$C]carbon dioxide from L-[$^{14}$C]pyruvate was measured using a vented center well reaction vessel within a liquid scintillation vial (Leiter et al., 1978). The fully activated homogenate material (see above) or material reacted with ATP were added to the center well through a serum bottle stopper. Following a 2 min incubation at 30°C, L-[$^{14}$C]pyruvate was added. The reaction was quenched after 3 min with 6 NaH$_2$SO$_4$ and the incubation was continued for 60 min to trap the evolved carbon dioxide in 0.3 ml of Nuclear Chicago Solubilizer. The center well was then removed and 12 ml of scintillation cocktail (Research Products) was added. The amount of carbon dioxide released during the assay was determined by liquid scintillation counting. The final concentrations in the assay vessel were 30 mM potassium phosphate (pH 7.7), 2 mM magnesium chloride, 2 mM dithiothreitol, 0.5 mM thiamine pyrophosphate, 6 mM NAD, 1.5 mM coenzyme A, 5 μg/ml phosphotransacetylase and 50 μg/ml lactate dehydrogenase. In the control and dichloroacetate conditions, the EDTA concentration was 4 mM and the magnesium concentration was increased to 5 mM. All determinations were made in duplicate. Preliminary experiments indicated that the decarboxylase activity was linear with respect to protein concentration and time up to 15 min. The phosphorylation of band F-2 using methods of Conway and Routtenberg (1979) was measured as the area minus baseline of the peak corresponding to band F-2 on the densitometric tracings. The decarboxylase activity and band F-2 phosphorylation were determined in separate ATP reactions run in parallel. The reaction for pyruvate decarboxylase activity was carried out with nonradioactive ATP. (Morgan and Routtenberg, 1982.)

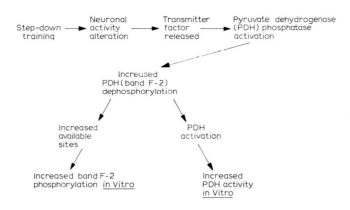

Fig. 4. Hypothesized sequence of events leading to PDH activation and its increased phosphorylation in vitro.

phosphate acceptor sites on the PDH molecule has been increased by the in vivo dephosphorylation occurring following training.

These results and the suggested sequence of events of Fig. 4 indicate certain predictions that can now be tested[*]. For example, in vivo phosphorylation of band F-2 should be decreased in animals following training. Another prediction is that PDH phosphatase, if activated by training, should produce a greater rate of dephosphorylation of band F-2, using methods in Mitrius et al. (1981).

This prediction serves to highlight one of the major strengths of back-titration in the in vitro phosphorylation procedure as applied to the study of functional effects on training. By observing a consequence of training on the in vitro system *and* by identification of the component substrate, one can then evaluate the kinase and phosphatase activity in an effort to specify what precise enzymatic alteration has taken place that has led to the observed result, in this case, an increase of in vitro phosphorylation of PDH. If PDH phosphatase can be shown to be activated then the next step in the process would be to specify the mechanism by which that activation takes place. This strategy illustrates the potential for describing the initiating and consequent metabolic events set into motion by training.

6.4. *Effects of appetitive training on back-titration of band F-2 phosphorylation*

Until recently we have focused our efforts on describing alterations in phosphorylation consequently to training motivated by painful or aversive stimuli. Recently we have begun to study the effects of training in a radial arm maze, an environment in which the animal is required to search for food in each of the eight arms which radiate like spokes from a central hub. By restricting arm entries to eight, the animal learns to enter all the arms without repeating an entry. We have studied the consequence of such learning on in vitro phosphorylation

[*] The point made in this figure that brain activity leads to alterations in PDH activity can be inferred on this basis: (1) Browning et al. (1979a) showed that repetitive stimulation altered a 40 000 mol. wt. phosphoprotein; (2) Browning et al. (1979b) indicated that a molecule of this molecular weight could be troponin; (3) Browning et al. (1981) indicate that a phosphoprotein of this molecular weight is pyruvate dehydrogenase. While suggestive, there is only indirect evidence that repetitive stimulation alters band F-2 phosphorylation or PDH activity (see Browning, this volume).

focusing interest on the hippocampus, since this structure's integrity is critical for the performance in this maze (Olton et al., 1978). Moreover, electrical stimulation which disorganizes specific hippocampal circuits (Collier et al., 1981) also confirms the involvement of the hippocampal formation in radial maze performance.

The question that we have asked is, presuming that hippocampal activity is altered during and perhaps consequent to performance (O'Keefe, 1979), what in vitro phosphorylation alterations might occur consequently to performing in the maze. We have found (Cain et al., 1981) that 24 h after performance in this maze, the levels of band F-2 phosphorylation are increased relative to control level of phosphorylation or 0 h after the last performance. Thus, in contrast to our results with an aversive task, alterations in phosphorylation following performance in an appetitive task cause no post-training alteration in in vitro phosphorylation of band F-2. Because the alteration is observed 24 h later, this result, if confirmed, is especially interesting since it calls attention to the possibility that PDH alterations are different in different tasks and in different brain locations. Thus, alterations in PDH phosphorylation are observed both at 0 and 24 h after step-down training in neostriatum and frontal cortex. In contrast, after radial maze training, to date differences have been observed 24 h, but not at 0 h. Interestingly, this effect is observed in dorsal hippocampus, but not in neostriatum.

## 6.5. *Implications of the response of brain PDH to changing environmental conditions*

Perhaps the search for an exotic molecule which would play a special role in memory functions, which we subjectively regard as critical for our intellectual life, may be inappropriate, and such functions are less mysterious than originally supposed. The possibility exists, then, that alterations in the intermediary metabolic states may, in fact, regulate those synaptic processes involving the release of transmitters, receptor activation and plasticity, for example. Thus, one view of our results might be that one now needs to search for a description of the cycle or sequence of intermediary metabolic events involved in the process of altering synaptic junction transmission following a training experience.

Another point of some importance is the possibility that we now have a foot-hold on a point in time in which a specifiable cell biological event occurs that, at the least, is active during the learning and memory process. It will be of special importance to determine, both those events which initiate and lead to alterations in PDH, as well as the consequences of changes in PDH activity. Such evaluation will also critically assess the precise role of PDH in learning and memory, since it may be the case that some as yet uncovered events that are linked to PDH activation are essential for the alterations related to learning and memory.

We appear to be at a level of study of phosphorylation that is specific with respect to mechanism. Knowledge of one specific protein potentially involved in the process permits us to be rather precise with respect to the tests that we can perform and the ability to either accept or reject with some degree of assurance the role of a particular metabolic process in the storage function of brain.

## SUMMARY

In 1975 we introduced an in vitro method for back-titration of brain phosphoproteins to determine the consequences of behavioral treatments on the available phosphorylatable sites of such proteins. This back-titration technique, in the endogenous phosphorylation system, measures the net phosphate incorporated as a consequence of both kinase and phosphatase activity.

We have found an alteration in available sites in a 41 K phosphoprotein following behavioral treatments involving training. The time and direction of alteration depends on the behavioral situation used. The task used also determines the regional location of this alteration. Several phosphoproteins including an 80 K protein, which is predominantly of synaptic vesicle origin, remain unchanged.

We have identified this 41 K phosphoprotein as pyruvate dehydrogenase (PDH). The evidence for thsi identification is based on the regulation of phosphorylation between band F-2 phosphorylation and PDH enzyme activity using parallel assays of the same tissue sample.

The back-titration method is influenced by procedural factors which alter, from the time before sacrifice to the time of assay, the amount of phosphate covalently bound to substrate proteins. The influence of method of sacrifice, buffer system, subcellular fraction and gel conditions on the accuracy of back-titration thus requires detailed consideration.

With the present use of conventional biochemical techniques, with the establishment of evidence that indicates that different laboratories are, in fact, working with the same phosphoproteins, with the use of back-titration to establish the consequences of functional/behavioral manipulations, and with the identification of a behaviorally responsive phosphoprotein as pyruvate dehydrogenase, the study of the macromolecular basis of behavior can be said to be established on a firm foundation. Understanding the function of brain phosphoproteins will require the identification of the sequence of cellular and molecular events set into motion by specific environmental conditions, particularly those involving learning and memory.

## ACKNOWLEDGEMENTS

Gratitude is expressed to Betty Wells for assistance in preparation of this manuscript. Support for the research was provided by N.I.M.H. research grant to A.R.

## REFERENCES

Ashby, C.D. and Roberts, S. (1975) Phosphorylation of ribosomal proteins in rat cerebral cortex in vitro. *J. biol. Chem.*, 250: 2546–2555.

Bär, P.R., Schotman, P., Gispen, W.H., Tielen, A.M. and Lopes Da Silva, F.H. (1980) Changes in synaptic membrane phosphorylation after tetanic stimulation in the dentate area of the rat hippocampal slice. *Brain Res.*, 198: 478–484.

Benjamin, A.M. and Quastel, J.H. (1981) Acetylcholine synthesis in synaptosomes: Mode of transfer of mitochondrial acetyl coenzyme A. *Science*, 213: 1495–1497.

Berman, R.F., Hullihan, J.P., Kinnier, W.J. and Wilson, J.E. (1980) Phosphorylation of synaptic membranes, *J. Neurochem.*, 34: 431–437.

Browning, M., Dunwiddie, T., Bennett, W., Gispen, W. and Lynch, G. (1979a) Synaptic phosphoproteins: Specific changes after repetitive stimulation of the hippocampal slice. *Science*, 203: 60–62.

Browning, M., Bennett, W. and Lynch, G. (1979b) Phosphorylase kinase phosphorylates a brain which is influenced by repetitive synaptic activation. *Nature (Lond.)*, 278: 273–275.

Browning, M., Bennett, W., Kelly, P. and Lynch, G. (1981) The 40,000 Mr phosphoprotein influenced by high frequency synaptic stimulation is the alpha subunit of pyruvate dehydrogenase. *Brain Res.*, 218: 255–264.

Cain, S.T. and Routtenberg, A. (1981) Endogenous phosphorylation in vitro: Effects of neonatal handling. *Fed. Proc.*, 40: 250.

Cain, S.T. and Routtenberg, A. (1982) Effects of handling on band F-1 phosphorylation. Submitted for publication.

Cain, S.T., Akers, R., Collier, T.J. and Routtenberg, A. (1981) Making memories of rewards in the environment metabolic: Radial maze learning alters pyruvate dehydrogenase in vitro phosphorylation. *Soc. Neurosci.*, 7: 457.

Collier, T.J., Miller, J.S., Quirk, G., Travis, J. and Routtenberg, A. (1981) Remembering rewards in the environ-

372

ment: Endogenous hippocampal opiates modulate reinforcement-memory associations. *Soc. Neurosci.,* Abstr. 1981.

Conway, R.G. and Routtenberg, A. (1978) Endogenous phosphorylation in vitro: Selective effects of sacrifice methods on specific brain proteins. *Brain Res.,* 139: 366–373.

Conway, R.G. and Routtenberg, A. (1979) Endogenous phosphorylation in vitro: Differential effects of brain state (anesthesia, post-mortem) on electrophoretically separated brain proteins. *Brain Res.,* 170: 313–324.

Davis, G.A. and Bloom, F.E. (1973) Isolation of synaptic junctional complexes from rat brain. *Brain Res.,* 62: 135–153.

Davis, L.G. and Ehrlich, Y.H. (1979) Opioid peptides and protein phosphorylation. *Adv. exp. med. Biol.,* 110: 233–244.

DeLorenzo, R.J. (1977) Antagonistic actions of diphenylhydantoin and calcium on the level of phosphorylation of particular rat and human brain proteins. *Brain Res.,* 134: 125–138.

Ehrlich, Y.H. and Routtenberg, A. (1974) Cyclic AMP regulates phosphorylation of three protein components of rat cerebral cortex mbranes for thirty minutes. *FEBS Lett.,* 45 (No. 1): 237–243.

Ehrlich, Y.H., Rabjohns, R.R. and Routtenberg, A. (1977) Experiential-input alters the phosphorylation of specific proteins in brain membranes. *Pharmacol. Biochem. Behav.,* 6: 169–174.

Gilbert, P. (1975) How the cerebellum memorizes movements. *Nature (Lond.),* 254: 688–689.

Glassman, E. (1969) The biochemistry of learning: An evaluation of the role of RNA and protein. *Annu. Ray. Biochem.,* 38: 605–646.

Goldberg, N.D., Lust, W.D., O'Dea, R.F., Wei, S. and O'Toole, A.G. (1970) A role of cyclic nucleotides in brain metabolism. In *Role of Cyclic AMP in Cell Function, Advances in Biochemical Psychopharmacology,* Vol. 3, P. Greengard and E. Costa (Eds.), Raven Press, New York, pp. 67–87.

Greengard, P. (1976) Possible role for cyclic nucleotides and phosphorylation of membrane proteins in the postsynaptic actions of neurotransmitters. *Nature (Lond.),* 260: 101–108.

Greengard, P. (1978) Phosphorylated proteins as physiological effectors. *Science,* 199: 146–152.

Greengard, P. and Kebabian, J.W. (1974) Role of cyclic AMP in synaptic transmission in the mammalian peripheral nervous system. *Fed. Proc.,* 33: 1059–1067.

Holian, O., Brunngraber, E.G. and Routtenberg, A. (1971) Memory consolidation and glycoprotein metabolism: A failure to find a relationship. *Life Sci.,* 10: 1029–1035.

Holmes, H., Rodnight, R. and Kapoor, R. (1977) Effect of electroshock and drugs administered in vivo on protein kinase activity in rat brain. *Pharmacol. Biochem. Behav.,* 6: 415–419.

Horn, G., Rose, S.P.R. and Bateson, P.P.G. (1973) Experience and plasticity in the central nervous system. *Science,* 181: 506–514.

Hyden , H. and Lange, P.W. (1970) Protein changes in nerve cells related to learning and conditioning. In *The Neurosciences, Second Study Program,* F. O. Schmitt (Ed.), The Rockefeller University Press, New York, pp. 278–289.

Johnson, E.M., Ueda, T., Maeno, H. and Greengard, P. (1972) Adenosine 3′,5′-monophosphate-dependent phosphorylation of a specific protein in synaptic membrane fractions from rat cerebrum. *J. biol. Chem.,* 247: 5650–5642.

Jolles, J., Zwiers, H., van Dongen, C.J., Schotman, P., Wirtz, K.W.A. and Gispen, W.H. (1980) Modulation of brain polyphosphoinositide metabolism by ACTH-sensitive protein phosphorylation. *Nature (Lond.),* 286: 623–625.

Jope, R. and Blass, J.P. (1976) The regulation of pyruvate dehydrogenase in brain in vivo. *J. Neurochem.,* 26: 709–714.

Kernell, D. and Peterson, R.P. (1970) The effect of spike activity versus synaptic activation on the metabolism of ribonucleic acid in a molluscan giant neurone. *J. Neurochem.,* 17: 1087–1094.

Kim, H.-J. and Routtenberg, A. (1976) Retention disruption following post-trial picrotoxin injection into the substantia nigra. *Brain Res.,* 113: 620–625.

Krebs, E.G. (1972) The mechanism of hormonal regulation by cyclic AMP. In *Endocrinology, Proc. Fourth Int. Congr. Endocrinology,* ICS 273, Excerpta Medica, Amsterdam, pp. 17–29.

Kuo, J.F. and Greengard, P. (1969) Cyclic nucleotide-dependent protein kinases. IV. Widespread occurrence of adenosine 3′,5′-monophosphate-dependent protein kinase in various tissues and phyla of the animal kingdom. *Proc. nat. Acad. Sci. (Wash.),* 64: 1349.

Laemmli, U.K. (1970) Cleavage of structural proteins during the assembly of the head of bacteriophage T4. *Nature (Lond.),* 227: 680–685.

Leiter, A.B., Weinberg, M., Isohashi, F., Utter, M.F. and Linn, T. (1978) Relationship between phosphorylation and activity of pyruvate dehydrogenase in rat liver mitochondria and the absence of such a relationship for pyruvate carboxylase. *J. biol. Chem.,* 253: 2716–2723.

Lust, W.D., Murakami, N., de Arzeredo, R. and Passonneau, J. (1980) A comparaison of methods for brain fixation. In *Cerebral Metabolism and Neural Function*, J. V. Passonneau, R.A. Hawkins, W.D. Lust and F.A. Welsh (Eds.), Williams and Wilkins, Baltimore, MD, pp. 10–19.

Matus, A.I., Ng, M.L. and Mazat, J.-P. (1979) Protein phosphorylation in synaptic membranes: Problems of interpretation. *Protein Phosphorylation and Bio-Regulation*, FMI-EMBO Workshop, Basel, pp. 25–35.

Mitrius, J.C., Morgan, D.G. and Routtenberg, A. (1981) In vivo phosphorylation following $^{32}$P-orthophosphate injection into neostriatum or hippocampus: Selective and rapid labeling of electrophoretically-separated brain proteins. *Brain Res.*, 212: 67–82.

Morgan, D.G. (1981) *The Phosphorylation of Brain Pyruvate Dehydrogenase and its Response to Behavioral Experience*. Dissertation, Northwestern University, Evanston, IL.

Morgan, D.G. and Routtenberg, A. (1979a) The incorporation of intrastriatally injected $^{3}$H-fucose into electrophoretically-separated synaptosomal glycoproteins. I. Time course of incorporation and molecular weight estimations. *Brain Res.*, 179: 329–341.

Morgan, D.G. and Routtenberg, A. (1979b) The incorporation of intracranially injected $^{3}$H-fucose into electrophoretically-separated glycoproteins of the neostriatal P-2 fraction. II. The influence of passive avoidance training. *Brain Res.*, 179: 343–354.

Morgan, D.G. and Routtenberg, A. (1980) Evidence that a 41,000 dalton brain phosphoprotein is pyruvate dehydrogenase. *Biochem. biophys. Res. Commun.*, 95 (No. 2): 569–576.

Morgan, D.G. and Routtenberg, A. (1981) Brain pyruvate dehydrogenase: Phosphorylation and enzyme activity altered by a training experience. *Science*, 214: 470–471.

Morgan, D.G. and Routtenberg, A. (1982) Regulation of brain PDH by the phosphorylation–dephosphorylation cycle. *Brain Res.*, in press.

O'Callaghan, J.P., Williams, N. and Clouet, D.H. (1979) The effect of morphine on the endogenous phosphorylation of synaptic plasma membrane proteins of rat striatum. *J. Pharmacol. exp. Ther.*, 208: 96.

O'Keefe, J. (1979) A review of the hippocampal place cells. *Progr. Neurobiol.*, 13: 419–439.

Olton, D.S., Walker, J.A. and Gage, F.H. (1978) Hippocampal connections and spatial discrimination. *Brain Res.*, 139: 295–308.

Pratt, M.L. and Roche, T.E. (1979) Mechanism of pyruvate inhibition of kidney pyruvate dehydrogenase kinase and synergistic inhibition by pyruvate and ADP. *J. biol. Chem.*, 254: 7191–7196.

Pysh, J.J. and Khan, T. (1970) Comparative electron microscopic variations in mitochondrial structure and content in rat brain. *J. Cell. Biol.*, 47: 163–164a.

Reed, L.J., Pettit, F.H., Yaaman, S.J., Teague, W.M. and Bielle, D.M. (1980) Structure, function and regulation of the mammalian pyruvate dehydrogenase complex. In *Enzyme Regulation and Mechanism of Action*, FEBS (Fed. of European Biochem. Soc.), P. Mildner and B. Ries (Eds.), Pergamon Press, New York, pp. 47–56.

Routtenberg, A. (1976) Self-stimulation pathways: Origins and terminations — a three stage technique. In: *Brain Stimulation Reward*, A. Wauquier and E. Rolls (Eds.), North-Holland Publ. Co., Amsterdam, pp. 31–39.

Routtenberg, A. (1977) Intracranial self-stimulation and memory processes — a common substrate. *Neurosci. Res. Progr. Bull.*, 15 (No. 2): 227–231.

Routtenberg, A. (1979a) The participation of brain stimulation reward substrates in memory: Anatomical and biochemical evidence. *Fed. Proc.*, 38: 2446–2453.

Routtenberg, A. (1979b) Anatomical localization of phosphoprotein and glycoprotein substrates of memory. *Progr. Neurobiol.*, 12: 85–113.

Routtenberg, A. (1982) Memory formation as a post-translational modification of brain proteins. In *Mechanisms and Models of Neural Plasticity, Proc. of the VIth International Neurobiological IBRO Symposium on Learning and Memory*, Vol. 9, C.A. Marsan and H. Matthies (Eds.), Raven Press, New York, pp. 17–24.

Routtenberg, A. and Benson, G. (1980) In vitro phosphorylation of a 41,000-MW protein band is selectively increased 24 h after footshock or learning. *Behav. neural Biol.*, 29 (2): 168–175.

Routtenberg, A. and Bondareff, W. (1971) Protein synthesis and memory consolidation: radioautographic study of intrahippocampal microinjections of (3)-leucine in awake freely moving rats. *Fed. Proc.*, 30: 215.

Routtenberg, A. and Ehrlich, Y.H. (1975) Endogenous phosphorylation of four cerebral cortical membrane proteins: Role of cyclic nucleotides, ATP and divalent cations. *Brain Res.*, 92: 415–430.

Routtenberg, A. and Holzman, N. (1973) Memory disruption by electrical stimulation of substantia nigra, pars compacta. *Science*, 181: 83–86.

Routtenberg, A. and Kim, H.-J. (1978) The substantia nigra and neostriatum: Substrates for memory consolidation. In *Cholinergic-Monoaminergic Interactions in the Brain*, L.L. Butcher (Ed.), Academic Press, New York, pp. 305–331.

Routtenberg, A., George, D., Davis, L. and Brunngraber, E. (1974) Memory consolidation and fucosylation of crude synaptosomal glycoproteins resolved by gel electrophoresis: A regional study. *Behav. Biol.*, 12: 461–475.

374

Routtenberg, A., Ehrlich, Y.H. and Rabjohns, R. (1975) Effect of a training experience on phosphorylation of a specific protein in neocortical and subcortical membrane preparations. *Fed. Proc.*, 34: 293.

Routtenberg, A., Morgan, D.G., Conway, R., Schmidt, M.J. and Ghetti, B. (1981) Human brain protein phosphorylation in vitro: Cyclic AMP stimulation of electrophoretically-separated substrates. *Brain Res.*, 222: 323–333.

Sale, G.J. and Randle, P.J. (1981) Occupancy of sites of phosphorylation in inactive rat heart pyruvate dehydrogenase phosphate in vivo. *Biochem. J.*, 193: 935–946.

Santos-Anderson, R. and Routtenberg, A. (1976) Stimulation of rat medial or sulcal prefrontal cortex during passive avoidance learning differentially influences retention performance. *Brain Res.*, 103: 243–259.

Schulman, H. and Greengard, P. (1978) Stimulation of brain membrane protein phosphorylation by calcium and an endogenous heat-stable protein. *Nature (Lond.)*, 271: 478–479.

Shashoua, V.E. (1977) Brain protein metabolism and the acquisition of new patterns of behavior. *Proc. nat. Acad. Sci. (Wash.)*, 74: 1743–1747.

Sieghart, W., Forn, J. and Greengard, P. (1979) $Ca^{2+}$ and cyclic AMP regulate phosphorylation of same two membrane-associated proteins specific to nerve tissue. *Proc. nat. Acad. Sci. (Wash.)*, 76: 2475–2479.

Siess, E., Wittmann, J. and Wieland, D. (1971) Interconversion and kinetic properties of pyruvate dehydrogenase from brain. *Hoppe-Seylers Z. physiol. Chem.*, 352: 447–452.

Strombom, U., Forn, J., Dolphin, A.C. and Greengard, P. (1979) Regulation of the state of phosphorylation of specific neuronal proteins in mouse brain by in vivo administration of anesthetic and convulsant agents. *Proc. nat. Acad. Sci. (Wash.)*, 76: 4687–4690.

Tarrant, S.B. and Routtenberg, A. (1979) The synaptic spinule in the dendritic spine: Electron microscopic study of the hippocampal dentate gyrus. *Tissue Cell*, 9: 461–473.

Ueda, T. and Greengard, P. (1977) Adenosine 3′,5′-monophosphate-regulated phosphoprotein system of neuronal membranes. I. Solubilization, purification and some properties of an endogenous phosphoprotein. *J. biol. Chem.*, 252: 5155–5163.

Ueda, T., Maeno, H. and Greengard, P. (1973) Regulation of endogenous phosphorylation of specific proteins in synaptic membrane fractions from rat brain by adenosine 3′,5′-monophosphate. *J. biol. Chem.*, 248: 8295–8305.

Ueda, T., Greengard, P., Berzins, K., Cohen, R.S., Blomberg, F., Grab, D.J. and Siekevitz, P. (1979) Subcellular distribution in cerebral cortex of two proteins phosphorylated by a cAMP-dependent protein kinase. *J. Cell Biol.*, 83: 308–319.

Whitehouse, S., Cooper, R.H. Randle, P.J. (1974) Mechanism of activation of pyruvate dehydrogenase by dichloroacetate and other halogenated carboxylic acids. *Biochem. J.*, 141: 761–774.

# Protein Phosphorylation in the Regulation and Adaptation of Receptor Function

YIGAL H. EHRLICH [1,2], SCOTT R. WHITTEMORE [1,3], MARK K. GARFIELD [1,4],
STEPHEN G. GRABER [1,2] and ROBERT H. LENOX [1]

[1]*Neuroscience Research Unit, Department of Psychiatry, Departments of* [2]*Biochemistry,* [3]*Physiology-Biophysics and* [4]*Pharmacology, University of Vermont College of Medicine, Burlington, VT 05405, U.S.A.*

## INTRODUCTION

During the last two decades, a large body of evidence has accumulated demonstrating that the phosphorylation and dephosphorylation of proteins play important and ubiquitous roles in the regulation of neural function (for reviews, see Greengard, 1976, 1978; Williams and Rodnight, 1977; Ehrlich, 1979, 1981). This evidence is based on two lines of investigation. First, the demonstration that various neurotransmitters, neurohormones and neurotropic factors, either directly or indirectly, regulate the phosphorylation of different proteins in neural tissue. The second line of investigation has demonstrated that various neuronal processes are regulated by phosphorylative activity. These include the metabolism and release of neurotransmitters, the induction and biosynthesis of neural-specific enzymes, axonal transport, chemically and electrically induced depolarization, receptor sensitivity, neuronal maturation and differentiation. Moreover, reports from several laboratories have implicated modifications in protein phosphorylation systems in processes whereby neurons respond with long-lasting alterations to persistent environmental, hormonal or pharmacological stimulations. These are just a few examples pertinent directly to neuronal function. In addition, several key cellular processes such as DNA and RNA synthesis, metabolism of carbohydrates, lipids, etc., membrane permeability, mitochondrial function, cell division and transitions in cell cycle have been shown to involve protein phosphorylation (for recent reviews, see Krebs and Rosen, 1981). This chapter is focused on studies of receptor function. We shall briefly review the evidence that activation of neural receptors results in altered protein phosphorylation, summarize studies demonstrating a role for this system in neuronal adaptation, and present some recent data from our laboratory indicating that endogenous phosphorylation systems of neural membranes may play a direct role in receptor-mediated transduction of signals across plasma membranes.

## ON THE SPECIFICITY IN PROTEIN PHOSPHORYLATION FUNCTION

In view of the great diversity of metabolic and physiological events regulated by protein phosphorylative activity, as outlined above, the first question that needs to be addressed in elucidating mechanisms of action is the element that provides specificity to this mode of regulation. The first clue to this question came from studies by P. Greengard and his colleagues (Johnson et al., 1972; Ueda et al., 1973), who demonstrated that synaptic membranes from rat

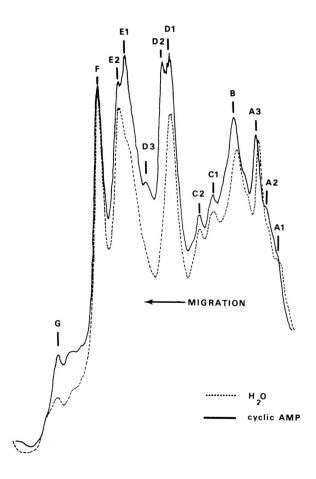

Fig. 1. Multiple endogenous protein phosphorylation systems in brain membranes. Membrane preparations were obtained form P2 fractions osmotically lysed in a buffer containing $50\mu$M CaCl$_2$ (Ehrlich and Routtenberg, 1974). Aliquots containing 40 $\mu$g protein were incubated for 1 min with $3\mu$M [$\gamma$-$^{32}$P]ATP and 10 mM MgCl$_2$, then subjected to SDS–slab gel electrophoresis as described previously (Ehrlich et al., 1977c). Autoradiographs of dried gels were scanned at 649 nm. Depicted are the scans of autoradiographs obtained from assays carried out in the presence (————) and absence (– – – –) of 5 $\mu$M cAMP. In addition to the phosphorylated protein bands A–G which are in the molecular weight range of 30 K–200 K, these membrane preparations contain seven phosphorylated protein components, designated H, in the molecular weight range of 10 K–20 K, whose phosphorylation is insensitive to exogenously added cAMP.

cerebrum contain two specific protein substrates whose phosphorylation is regulated by cyclic AMP (cAMP). Our initial reports (Ehrlich and Routtenberg, 1974; Routtenberg and Ehrlich, 1975) confirmed this finding and identified six additional proteins in synaptic membranes whose phosphorylation and dephosphorylation are carried out by protein kinase(s) and phosphatase(s) which constitute part of the structure of these membranes. We have designated these specific phosphoprotein bands by the letters A through H (see Fig. 1). The bands designated D and E were found to be identical to the cAMP-stimulated substrates designated as bands I and II by Ueda et al. (1973). The phosphorylation of a protein band designated G was virtually dependent on cAMP, while phosphorylation of bands A, B, C, F and H was only minimally affected by cyclic nucleotides. DeLorenzo (1976) and Schulman and Greengard (1978) have reported that synaptic membranes contain calcium-dependent protein kinase. The specific protein substrates phosphorylated by this activity produce the same phosphorylation pattern as our bands A, B, C, F and H. Indeed, we have found that the saturation of calcium-binding sites during our routine procedure of membrane preparation (Ehrlich and Routtenberg, 1974) is sufficient to fully support the activity of endogenous calcium-dependent protein phosphorylation in these membranes (Ehrlich et al., 1980b). Moreover, these recent studies have revealed that each of the protein components A trough H resolves into several distinct bands, for a total of 22 different phosphoproteins (Ehrlich, 1979). The endogenous phosphorylation of each of these protein bands exhibits differential sensitivity to various factors that affect protein phosphorylation in synaptic membranes. These include ATP to protein ratio, cyclic nucleotides, magnesium and calcium ion concentration, calmodulin, reaction time, etc. (Ehrlich and Routtenberg, 1974; Routtenberg and Ehrlich, 1975; Ehrlich et al., 1977c). An extensive investigation in the laboratory of H. Mahler (DeBlass et al., 1979; see also Mahler et al., this volume) has provided evidence that over 20 different endogenous phosphorylation systems of synaptic membrane preparations from rat brain are unequally distributed among various sub-synaptic organelles (synaptic plasma membranes, synaptic vesicles, postsynaptic densities, etc.). Thus, brain membranes, and in particular membranes of synaptic origin, contain a multiplicity of endogenous phosphorylation systems, each characterized by phosphorylating a different substrate. The differences in subcellular location and in phosphorylative properties among various phosphoproteins strongly suggest that each phosphorylation system may subserve a different role in the regulation of synaptic function. The specificity in this regulation is provided, in all likelihood, by the nature of the protein substrate.

The conclusion stated above implies that investigations which aim to assign a specific functional role for certain specific phosphoproteins could be aided by determining the properties that individual endogenous phosphorylation systems reveal in in vitro assays. Selective sensitivity to various agents in vitro may be indicative of the possible function that a given phosphoprotein plays in vivo. Our current studies, for example, investigate the possible role of endogenous protein phosphorylation systems in the regulation of adenylate cyclase activity. These studies will be discussed in greater detail later. Within the context of this section, it could be mentioned that adenylate cyclase activity is known to have different properties depending on whether the supporting cation for its activity is magnesium or manganese (Chech et al., 1980). Identification of endogenous protein phosphorylation systems with differential sensitivity to these two divalent cations may, therefore, be of value in such an investigation. This can be done by incubating membrane preparations that possess adenylate cyclase activity with $[\gamma\text{-}^{32}P]ATP$, in the presence of either $MgCl_2$ or $MnCl_2$. The results of such an experiment are depicted in Fig. 2. It can be seen that the phosphorylation of two closely migrating protein bands (in the molecular weight range of 40–60 kilodalton) responds reciprocally to the addition of $Mg^{2+}$ and $Mn^{2+}$ to the reaction medium. Whereas the phosphorylation of one band is stimulated by $Mn^{2+}$ and inhibited by $Mg^{2+}$, the other shows the opposite relationships. The same figure demonstrates that monovalent cations also affect endogenous phosphorylative activity, but in a manner less selective than that of divalent cations. For example, addition of 100 mM KCl to the reaction results in an overall decrease of $[^{32}P]$phosphate incorporation (Fig. 2). In addition to the theoretical value of the finding that physiological agents have selective effects on the phosphorylation of different protein substrates, the ability to conduct such manipulations in vitro also has some practical implications. Membranes can be incubated in vitro with ATP under various controlled conditions that produce a predetermined pattern of endogenously phosphorylated proteins (e.g. with $Mn^{2+}$ vs. $Mg^{2+}$, see Fig. 2). Washed and resuspended membranes can then be reincubated under identical conditions to measure another

378

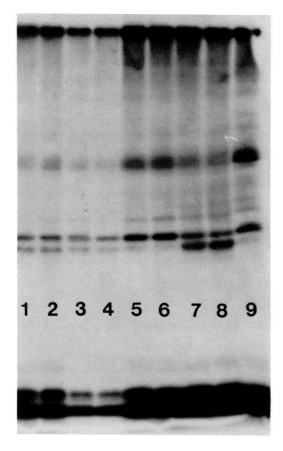

Fig. 2. Selective effects of divalent cations on endogenous phosphorylation of specific proteins. Membrane preparations (see Fig. 1) from rat neostriatum were assayed for endogenous phosphorylation during 1 min incubation with 3 $\mu$M [$\gamma$-$^{32}$P]ATP and either 10 mM MnCl$_2$ (lanes 1, 2, 7, 8) or 10 mM MgCl$_2$ (lanes 3, 4, 5, 6). The reaction medium in lanes 1–4 also included 100 mM KCl. Other reaction and electrophoresis conditions were as previously described (Ehrlich et al., 1980). Lane 9 contained reaction products from assay carried out with EGTA-washed membranes, incubated with 10 mM MgCl$_2$ and 5 $\mu$M cAMP. Bands I and II of Ueda et al. (1973) stand out under these conditions and serve as internal markers in the identification of other bands.

membrane-bound activity (e.g. adenylate cyclase, ATPase, etc.) — as a function of the phosphorylation state of a specific protein in these membranes. This investigative approach is used extensively in our current studies (see below).

The main conclusion of this section, that the specificity in the mode of regulation exerted by protein phosphorylation is determined by the nature of the substrate proteins, is based upon the multiplicity and differential sensitivity of endogenous phosphorylation systems acting simultaneously. Such a conclusion would be valid, however, only if the multiple systems are present in the same cell. The studies cited above investigated heterogeneous preparations from brain tissue which contain subcellular organelles from many different cells. It is, therefore, of importance to emphasize that membranes prepared from a homogeneous population of neuroblastoma cells grown in culture were found to have multiple endogenous phosphorylation systems which are as complex as those observed in brain membranes (Ehrlich et al., 1977d,

1978c). Furthermore, selective alterations in the phosphorylation of specific proteins have been detected when these cells were induced to differentiate in culture and to acquire many properties characteristic of mature neurons (Ehrlich et al., 1977c, 1978d). This indicates that different phosphoproteins of an individual neuronal cell may subserve different physiological functions, and that the relative activity of certain endogenous systems undergoes selective changes during the transition from multiplying neuroblasts to differentiated mature neurons.

## PHOSPHORYLATIVE RESPONSES TO NEURONAL STIMULATION

The suggestion that protein phosphorylation is intimately involved in synaptic function implies that it should be possible to detect changes in this system following neuronal stimulation. Indeed, such an observation was reported a quarter of a century ago by Heald (1957). He found that a brief depolarization of respiring slices from cerebral cortex by electrical pulses caused a significant increase in the amount of protein-bound phosphate in the tissue. These studies have been continued and expanded in the laboratory of R. Rodnight. The electrical stimulation-induced increase in protein-bound phosphate has been localized to membranes (Trevor and Rodnight, 1965) and within it, in neuron-enriched but not in glial-enriched fractions (Williams et al., 1974). Subsequent studies from the same laboratory have demonstrated that not only electrical, but also hormonal stimulation can induce an increase in protein-bound phosphate of cortical slices. Thus, the neurotransmitters norepinephrine, dopamine, GABA, histamine and serotonin are capable of increasing [$^{32}$P]phosphate incorporation into proteins of respiring slices (reviewed by Williams and Rodnight, 1977). The specific protein substrates whose phosphorylation is increased by either electrical or neurohormonal stimulation of brain slices have not been identified in these studies. Nonetheless, these reports were the first to indicate that activation of receptors by neurotransmitters results in altered membrane-bound protein phosphorylation activity.

The studies on effects of stimulation on protein phosphorylation in cortical slices cited above have used inorganic $^{32}$Pi to label intracellular ATP pools, and then determined phosphoprotein labeling by measuring $^{32}$P incorporation into alkali-labile phosphate of the slices. One of the reasons that the specific phosphoproteins involved had not been identified in these studies was the low specific activity obtained by this mode of labeling (M. Williams, personal communication). Some of these difficulties can be overcome by employing a paradigm of post-hoc analysis. In this experimental paradigm, the tissue is subjected to a stimulus, membranes or other subcellular fractions are prepared and then assayed in vitro for endogenous protein phosphorylation using high specific activity [$\gamma$-$^{32}$P]ATP as a phosphate donor. Proteins whose phosphorylation had been inhibited by the stimulus in vivo (or in situ) will have an increased number of available phosphorylation sites. This would be manifested by an apparent increase of [$^{32}$P]phosphate incorporation in vitro, and vice versa (Ehrlich et al., 1977a). Recent studies have used this experimental design in investigating the effects of electrical (Browning et al., 1979a,b) and hormonal (Bär et al., 1980) stimulation of hippocampal slices on the phosphorylation of specific protein bands. Earlier studies used this experimental paradigm in investigation of the responses of protein phosphorylation systems to neural stimulation in the brain of intact animals (Ehrlich et al., 1977a,e). However, special precautions are to be taken in using this paradigm, and these are discussed below.

In all studies of rapidly metabolized substances within the brain, the experimental animals are killed by methods enabling rapid fixation of the tissue, such as microwave irradiation or quick freezing in liquid nitrogen (for a recent review, see Lenox et al., 1981). Sacrifice

380

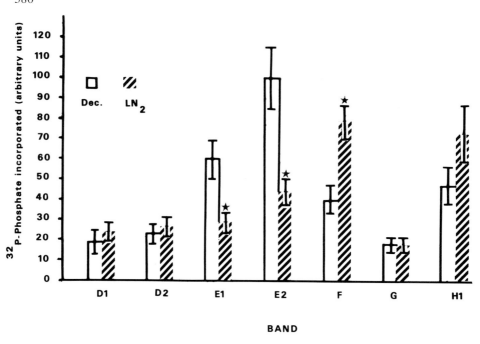

Fig. 3. Effects of decapitation on the in vitro phosphorylation of specific proteins in cortical membranes. Rats (100–140 g) were killed by head immersion in liquid $N_2$ ($LN_2$) or by decapitation (Dec.). The surface of the cerebral cortex was scraped off and used for preparing membrane fractions which were then assayed for endogenous phosphorylation. The amount of [$^{32}$P]phosphate incorporation into specific bands was quantitated by microdensitometry of autoradiographs and expressed in arbitrary density units. The histogram was reproduced from Ehrlich et al. (1978a) with permission. * Significantly different from Dec. $P < 0.05$.

methods that produce rapid post-mortem changes, such as decapitation, are avoided in these studies. The cycles of phosphorylation/dephosphorylation of membrane-bound proteins from brain are very rapid, particularly under conditions of limited ATP availability (Ueda et al., 1973; Ehrlich and Routtenberg, 1974; Zwiers et al., 1976). Decapitation is known to produce rapid ATP depletion in brain tissue (Duffy et al., 1972) and, therefore, may be expected to cause changes in protein phosphate metabolism. We have investigated this issue by examining the phosphorylation of specific proteins in cortical membranes prepared from rats sacrificed by decapitation as compared to corresponding preparations from rats sacrificed by head immersion in liquid nitrogen (Ehrlich et al., 1977e, 1978a). To control for the effects of freezing, the head of the decapitated animal was also immersed in liquid nitrogen prior to tissue processing. Crude synaptic membrane fractions from each group were incubated in vitro with $Mg \cdot AT^{32}P$ for 10 sec to pulse-label endogenous proteins, and $^{32}P$ incorporation into specific protein bands was determined by SDS–gel electrophoresis and autoradiography. The results, quantitated by densitometry of the autoradiographs, are depicted in Fig. 3. As compared to membranes from quick-frozen rats, decapitation caused selective and *bidirectional* changes in the in vitro phosphorylation of specific proteins. Phosphorylation of the protein bands designated E-1 and E-2 (apparent molecular weight of 56 K and 52 K) increased 2-fold after decapitation, while phosphorylation of band F (47 K) in these preparations showed a 50% decrease. In spite of the variety of manipulations and length of time required to prepare the membrane fragments used in these experiments, the consequences of decapitation were sufficiently stable to permit the detection of changes in protein phosphorylation by post-hoc analysis, utilizing an in vitro assay. Since changes in different bands occurred in opposing directions, the results cannot be explained merely on the basis of ATP depletion. Our interpretation of these findings (Ehrlich et al., 1977a, 1980b), which was also applied in other similar studies (Zwiers et al., 1977; Browning et al., 1979; Bär et al., 1980) has been that decreases and increases in the state of phosphorylation of specific proteins induced by a stimulus in vivo, results in respective increases and decreases of [$^{23}$P]phosphate incorporation into these bands in the post-hoc assay carried out in vitro.

The post-hoc analysis of membranes prepared from rats killed by quick freezing can be used to study transient changes in protein phosphorylation in vivo. Massive stimulation of central neurons is induced by electroconvulsive shock (ECS), and we have used this input to examine the rate and reversibility of phosphorylative changes induced by neuronal stimulation. Rats were administered ECS and then killed by head immersion in liquid nitrogen 10 sec (during tonic seizures), 30 sec (clonic seizures), 2 and 4 min (behavioral recovery) after the shock. Cortical membranes analyzed in vitro revealed that phosphorylation of the bands designated H (molecular weight 15–20 K) increased 100% over sham-shocked control during the tonic phase, reached maximum (400% increase) during the clonic phase, declined to 200% above control levels 2 min after shock, and returned to control level upon behavioral recovery of the animals from the effect of the electroshock (Ehrlich et al., 1980b). This study thus serves to demonstrate that neuronal stimulation produces rapid and REVERSIBLE changes in the phosphorylation of specific proteins of brain tissue. The mechanism underlying this phenomenon may involve selective activation of neural receptors.

## PROTEIN PHOSPHORYLATION AND RECEPTOR ACTIVATION

The massive stimulation of brain by ECS is known to involve increased synaptic activity due to enhanced release of neurotransmitters. One of its consequences is great elevation in the levels of cAMP in brain tissue (Lust et al., 1976). Activation of receptors by certain neurotransmitters results in increased intracellular cAMP levels, with consequent stimulation of cAMP-dependent protein kinase activity. Such a sequence of events has been shown recently by Nestler and Greengard (1980), using preparations of mammalian superior cervical sympathetic ganglion. The specific protein substrate involved is protein I, whose poperties are described in detail by T. Ueda in another chapter of this volume. These results strongly support the suggestion of Kuo and Greengard (1969), that protein phosphorylation plays a role in the mechanism of receptor activation as a third step, following the generation of cAMP. Interestingly, however, the protein substrates whose phosphorylation exhibited a marked response to ECS (Ehrlich et al., 1980b) do not constitute part of a cyclic nucleotide-sensitive system. It is possible, therefore, that receptor activation may affect protein phosphorylation via a mechanism that does not involve generation of cAMP or cyclic GMP (cGMP). In the case of surface receptors localized in plasma membranes and endogenous phosphorylation systems embedded within the same membranes, there may even be a direct interaction between the receptor and some elements of the protein phosphorylation system.

The best evidence available to date demonstrating that hormone–receptor interaction directly regulates membrane-bound protein phosphorylation comes from studies of non-neural systems. S. Cohen and his colleagues have shown that the binding of epidermal growth factor (EGF) to specific receptors in plasma membranes of the epidermoid cell line A-431 results in a

382

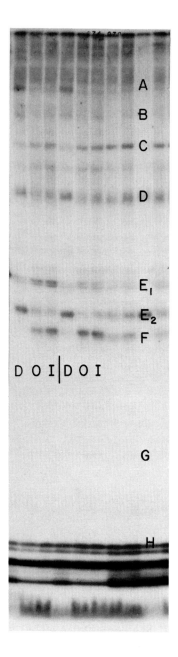

Fig. 4. Effects of dopamine on endogenous protein phosphorylation in neostriatal membranes. Synaptosomal preparations (P2) from rat neostriatum were osmotically shocked in the presence of 50 $\mu$M $CaCl_2$ and then washed in a buffer containing 50 mM KCl (Ehrlich, in preparation). Aliquots containing 60 $\mu$g protein were incubated (30 sec at 30°C) with 1 $\mu$M [$\gamma$-$^{32}$P]ATP and 10 mM $MgCl_2$ without additions (O), with 10 $\mu$M dopamine (D) or 10 $\mu$M (−)-isoproterenol (I). Stock solutions of dopamine (Sigma) in 1 mM HCl were stored at − 20°C, thawed and diluted before the assays. SDS-solubilized reaction products were separated in 30 cm long slab-polyacrylamide gel gradient (10–16%; exponential) and autoradiographed. In the autoradiograph, note the multiple effects of dopamine on different phosphoproteins, e.g. dopamine stimulated the phosphorylation of bands A, D and E-2, but inhibited bands C, E-1 and F.

marked stimulation of the in vitro phosphorylation of proteins in these membranes (Carpenter at al., 1978, 1979). Maximal stimulation of phosphorylation by EGF was obtained at a concentration ($3$–$4 \times 10^{-8}$ M) which is very similar to that required to saturate receptor binding sites ($1.6 \times 10^{-8}$ M). Detergent solubilization of the membranes extracted both $^{125}$I-EGF binding activity and EGF-stimulated endogenous phosphorylation activity. Affinity chromatography revealed that a protein band of molecular weight 150 K serves both as a binding site for EGF and as a substrate of EGF-enhanced phosphorylative activity. These studies not only demonstrate an inherent close relationship between receptor and protein phosphorylation, but also suggest that hormone–binding and kinase activities may be present in the same molecule (Cohen et al., 1980). An important property of the EGF receptor–protein kinase complex is that it phosphorylates tyrosine residues (rather than serine or threonine) of the protein substrate (Ushiro and Cohen, 1981). Undoubtedly, the importance of this refined difference will have to be investigated and clarified in all future studies of receptor–protein phosphorylation interactions.

The first studies to demonstrate direct effects of a neurohormone on protein phosphorylation in brain membranes were reported by Zwiers et al. (1976). They have demonstrated that the endogenous phosphorylation of proteins with molecular weights of 48 K and 15–20 K in synaptic membranes is selectively inhibited in vitro by $ACTH_{1-24}$. Continued investigation successfully isolated ACTH-sensitive kinase and its substrate protein and showed that this system is $Ca^{2+}$ dependent (for details, see Zwiers et al., this volume). Other studies by Gordon and Diamond (1979 review) have demonstrated that purified acetylcholine receptors isolated from Torpedo electroplax contain endogenous phosphorylative activity which is inhibited by cholinergic agonists. Our laboratory has reported interactions between opiate receptors and $Ca^{2+}$-sensitive endogenous phosphorylation systems of brain membranes (Ehrlich, 1979; Ehrlich et al., 1980a). Incubation of preparations containing synaptic membranes with nanomolar concentrations of etorphine or human $\beta$-endorphin resulted in over 2-fold stimulation of the phosphorylation of certain protein bands. This effect could be blocked by the specific narcotic antagonist, naloxone. In addition, nanomolar concentrations of $\beta$-endorphin or micromolar concentrations of methionine-enkephalin caused inhibition of phosphorylation of other protein bands, designated F (47 K) and H (15–20 K). This effect was naloxone-insensitive. Inhibition of calcium/calmodulin protein phosphorylation system in brain membranes mediated by benzodiazepine receptors was recently demonstrated by DeLorenzo et al. (1981). Ongoing studies in our laboratory have begun to provide evidence that classical neurotransmitters, the catecholamines, also exert direct effects on endogenous phosphorylative activity in brain membranes. The results of such an experiment are depicted in Fig. 4. Calcium-saturated membranes from rat neostriatum were assayed for endogenous phosphorylative activity in vitro in the presence of dopamine, or isoproterenol and for basal activity. In the autoradiograph, multiple and selective effects of dopamine on the phosphorylation of specific protein bands can be seen. Phosphorylation of band E-2, with estimated molecular weight of 50 K, was stimulated; confirming a previous report by Clement-Cormier (1980), using solubilized dopamine receptor preparations. In addition, dopamine caused increased phosphorylation of bands A and D and inhibition in bands C, E-1 and F. Addition of (−)-isoproterenol, a noradrenergic ligand, had minimal effects on neostriatal membranes, but was inhibitory in phosphorylation assays carried out with cortical membranes (Whittemore et al., 1981).

The common denominator to all the reports cited above is that a receptor ligand, interacting with neural membranes, produced selective changes in the phosphorylation of specific protein components present in these membranes. These effects did not require prior changes in intracellular concentrations of ATP, cAMP or cGMP and, in some cases, could be blocked by the presence of specific antagonists to the receptor under investigation. These findings strongly indicate that neurohormone interaction with membrane receptors has direct effects on protein phosphorylation. Studies of a non-neural system have shown that a molecule serving as a binding site of the receptor also possesses protein kinase activity. Future studies should determine whether such a close relationship also exists in neural receptors.

## PHOSPHORYLATIVE MODIFICATIONS IN RECEPTOR ADAPTATION

Numerous studies have demonstrated that long-term exposure of experimental animals to psychotropic drugs results in altered receptor function. In general, chronic exposure to agonists can produce receptor subsensitivity, whereas chronic treatment with antagonists may result in receptor supersensitivity. Current opinion holds that the need for a long-term exposure reflects the occurrence of adaptive changes involving yet unidentified enzymatic machinery of the neuron (for review, see Bonnet, 1979). The demonstration that endogenous protein phosphorylation systems in synaptic membranes are tightly linked to certain neuroreceptors (see preceding section) has suggested to us the possibility that a modification in endogenous protein phosphorylative activity may constitute a site of molecular adaptation in processes whereby persistent hormonal, pharmacological or environmental stimulations induce long–lasting alterations in receptor function (Ehrlich, 1979). Indirect evidence in support of this suggestion comes from studies which have demonstrated that treatments which induce receptor adaptation also cause alterations in the phosphorylation of specific proteins in synaptic membranes. Thus, chronic neuroleptic exposure caused increased protein phosphorylation in neostriatal membranes (Ehrlich and Brunngraber, 1976); whereas long-term narcotic exposure produced a decrease in phosphorylation of specific proteins in such preparations (Bonnet et al., 1978; Ehrlich et al., 1978b). Interestingly, the specific proteins whose phosphorylation was affected by chronic treatments with incremental doses of morphine (the bands designated F and H) were the same as those inhibited by endorphins in vitro (Ehrlich et al., 1980a). The neuronal adaptation occurring during the development of narcotic dependence does not involve changes in opiate binding and is thought to take place at another action site of this receptor complex (Bonnet et al., 1978). Long-lasting alterations in a phosphorylation system sensitive to opiates may be involved in the mechanisms underlying this phenomenon (Brann and Ehrlich, in preparation).

A more direct evidence for the role of protein phosphorylation in receptor adaptation has been provided by studies on the process of desensitization. Chuang and Costa (1979) have shown temporal correlation between down-regulation of $\beta$-adrenergic receptors in turkey erythrocytes and increased phosphorylation of membrane-bound proteins. Birnbaumer and his colleagues reported that luteinizing hormone-induced desensitization of hormone-sensitive adenylate cyclase in a cell-free preparation exhibits critical dependence on $Mg^{2+}$ and ATP. This desensitization could be reversed by addition of a phosphoprotein phosphatase, partially purified from the cytosol of the cells under investigation (Hunzicker-Dunn et al., 1979). Studies on the role of protein phosphorylation in processes determining receptor sensitivity in neural tissue were carried out by Gnegy et al. (1976, 1977; Gnegy and Treisman, 1981). These reports demonstrated that dopamine sensitivity of striatal adenylate cyclase depends on the amount of membrane-bound calmodulin; the latter decreases with increased phosphorylation state of membrane-bound proteins. Thus, studies of several receptor systems indicate that decreased sensitivity of hormine-coupled adenylate cyclase is associated with increased

385

phosphorylation of membrane proteins, and vice versa. Modifications in protein phosphorylation systems may, therefore, be responsible for neural adaptations that involve altered receptor sensitivity.

## PROTEIN PHOSPHORYLATION IN THE REGULATION OF
## ADENYLATE CYCLASE

The involvement of phosphoproteins in processes underlying the desensitization of receptor-coupled adenylate cyclase activity raises the possibility that adenylate cyclase activity itself is regulated by protein phosphorylation. Since adenylate cyclase utilizes Mg·ATP as a substrate, it is obvious that endogenous phosphorylation systems are also in operation whenever adenylate cyclase activity is being measured in preparations containing synaptic membranes. To solve a methodological problem in experimental testing of such a possibility, we have developed a two-phase assay (Whittemore et al., 1981). In these assays, lysed synaptosomal preparations from rat cerebral cortex are first preincubated under various phosphorylating conditions; this phase is terminated by rapid chilling of the reaction mixture to 0°C and centrifugation. The sedimented membranes are washed in a cold buffer containing EGTA and devoided of $Mg^{2+}$. The final pellet is resuspended in a buffer used for assaying adenylate cyclase activity, and formation of $[^{32}P]cAMP$ from $[\alpha-^{32}P]ATP$ is then measured during very short reaction times (10–120 sec). In the first series of experiments in this line of investigation, we measured adenylate cyclase activity in the reincubation under conditions permitting estimation of both the initial rate and extent of cAMP formation during such short reaction periods (for details, see legend to Fig. 5, and Whittemore et al., 1981). Using these assay conditions, we have compared adenylate cyclase activity in phosphorylated versus dephosphorylated membranes. Phosphorylated membranes were prepared by preincubating lysed synaptosomal fractions with 2 mM ATP in the presence of 10 mM $MgCl_2$. Preliminary

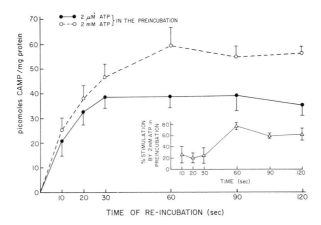

Fig. 5. Effects of PREincubation under phosphorylating conditions on adenylate cyclase activity in cortical membranes. The P2 fraction from rat cerebral cortex was osmotically lysed in a buffer containing 1 mM Tris–HCl (pH 7.4) and 2 mM EGTA. $MgCl_2$ was added to make 10 mM and the preparation then incubated for 5 min at 30°C with either 2 $\mu$M or 2 mM ATP. The membranes were sedimented and washed twice (at 0°C) with the same buffer. Resuspended pellets were assayed for adenylate cyclase activity at 5.0 mg protein/ml in a buffer containing 50 mM Tris–maleate (pH 7.4), 10 mM $MgCl_2$, 0.2 mM EGTA and 1 mM IBMX (a phosphodiesterase inhibitor). $[\alpha-^{32}P]ATP$ (100 $\mu$M) served as substrate and $[^{32}P]cAMP$ formation was monitored as described by Whittemore et al. (1981).

386

experiments confirmed previous reports that after 5 min incubation under these conditions membrane-bound proteins are at peak phosphorylation state. Dephosphorylated membranes were prepared using the same preincubation conditions, but with 2 *micro*molar (instead of 2 mM) ATP. As reported by several laboratories (Ueda et al., 1973; Ehrlich and Routtenberg, 1974; Zwiers et al., 1976), at this low ATP concentration, most all of the phosphate incorporated initially into membrane proteins is hydrolysed by phosphatase action during 5 min incubation. After these preincubations, sedimented and washed membranes were assayed for adenylate cyclase activity. As can be seen in Fig. 5, the extent of cAMP formation in the *re*incubation was 60–80% greater in membranes *pre*incubated with 2mM ATP than in those preincubated with 2 $\mu$M ATP. This effect was highly reproducible and significant at all time points in which cAMP formation is at steady-state levels (60–120 sec). It should be pointed out here that we have previously reported (Whittemore et al., 1981) that the steady state achieved at these time points is due to ATP depletion as well as effective phosphodiesterase inhibition.

The effects of preincubation with ATP on the extent of cAMP formation in the reincubation is not seen when preincubations are extended beyond 5 min (see inset in Fig. 6), suggesting that this effect may be reversed by *de*phosphorylation. To test this possibility we have utilized [$\gamma$-S]ATP in the preincubation. This analog of ATP is used by protein kinase to thiophosphorylate proteins. The thiophosphoester bond formed, which resists phosphatase action, has been successfully utilized in studies of smooth muscle to demonstrate the role of protein phosphorylation in excitation–contraction cycles (Cassidy et al., 1979). When cortical membranes were preincubated with [$\gamma$-S]ATP for 5 min and then washed and reincubated under conditions described in the legend to Fig. 5, cAMP formation was elevated 400% above that of control preparations (zero preincubation time or no [$\gamma$-S]ATP, see Fig. 6). 2 mM ATP under the same preincubation conditions produced only 70% activation, which was reversed at longer preincubation times. Prolonging preincubation with [$\gamma$-S]ATP, on the other hand, resulted in further activation, up to 700% increase following 40 min preincubation (Fig. 6).

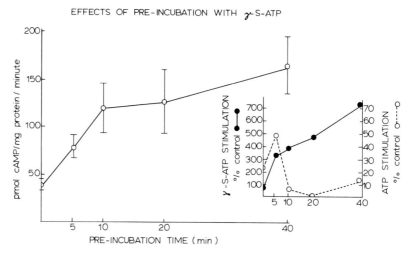

Fig. 6. Reversible and irreversible activation of adenylate cyclase. Osmotically lysed P2 preparation (see Fig. 5) was preincubated with 2$\mu$M ATP (control) or 2 mM ATP (– – – –) or 2 mM [$\gamma$-S]ATP (————) for various periods as indicated in the abcissa. cAMP formation in washed and resuspended membranes was carried out as described in the legend to Fig. 5. Note that maximal stimulation of adenylate cyclase activity with ATP (about 50%), is reached after preincubation for 5 min, and then declines rapidly. With [$\gamma$-S]ATP, however, increasing preincubation time results in further activation.

To enable better assessment of the effects of irreversible thiophosphorylation on cAMP formation by cortical membranes, we have modified the reincubation conditions and included an ATP regeneration system in the second phase of the assay. With this system, linear kinetics of adenylate cyclase activity can be assessed in the reincubation (see Fig. 7). Using this assay, we have measured various parameters of the activation. As depicted in Fig. 7, the rate of adenylate cyclase activity in the reincubation is dependent on the concentration of [$\gamma$-S]ATP included in the preincubation. A concentration of 250 $\mu$M [$\gamma$-S]ATP was saturating. As determined by regression line analysis (see table inset in Fig. 7), half-maximal increase in the

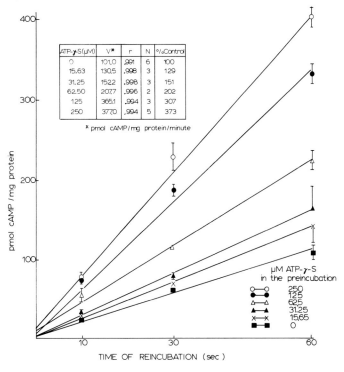

Fig. 7. Effects of [$\gamma$-S]ATP concentration on activation of adenylate cyclase in cortical membranes. The kinetics of adenylate cyclase activity were evaluated by using assay conditions permitting constant ATP concentration. This was achieved by including 3 IU of creatine kinase and 5 mM of creatine phosphate in the REincubation phase of the reaction. In the assay depicted above, preincubation time was kept constant (40 min) and the concentration of [$\gamma$-S]ATP was varied from 0 to 250 $\mu$M. For details, see text.

velocity *(V)* of cAMP formation in the reincubation is produced by preincubation with 40 $\mu$M [$\gamma$-S]ATP. Using the same experimental design, we have tested the effects of preincubation time with [$\gamma$-S]ATP (Fig. 8), and of $Mg^{2+}$ concentration (not shown). It was found that the activation is $Mg^{2+}$ and time-dependent. Most (60%) of the activation occurs during 10 min preincubation and this effect requires free $Mg^{2+}$ ions (buffered with EDTA) at a concentration at least 10 $\mu$M above that needed to saturate the ATP present in the reaction medium.

Incubation of thiophosphorylated membranes with 0.75 M NaCl and two washes at this high salt concentration had only minimal effects on the activation of adenylate cyclase, by [$\gamma$-S]ATP, thus establishing its irreversibility and suggesting that formation of a covalent bond

388

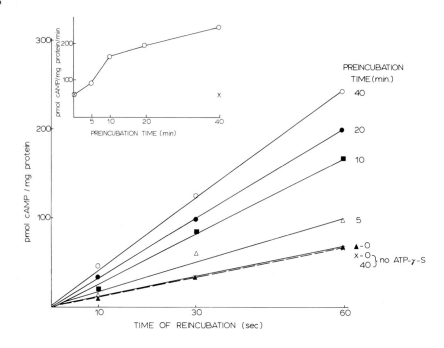

Fig. 8. Effect of preincubation time on activation of cortical adenylate cyclase by [γ-S]ATP. Assays were carried out as described in the legend to Fig. 7, except that preincubation time was varied and [γ-S]ATP concentration (250 μM) was kept constant. Note that preincubation of membranes without [γ-S]ATP (×––×) had no effects on adenylate cyclase activity.

underlies this process. To test this possibility in a more direct fashion, we have carried out the preincubation phase of several assays with $^{35}$S-labeled [γ-S]ATP. Aliquots of membranes entering the reincubation phase of the assay were solubilized in SDS and subjected to slab-gel electrophoresis. An autofluorograph of such a gel is depicted in Fig. 9. Seven minor and two major thiophosphorylated protein bands could be identified, the latter two migrated in the molecular weight range of 40–60 K. Further studies, to be reported in detail elsewhere, found a correlation coefficient of 0.96 between adenylate cyclase activation and $^{35}$S incorporation into the slower of these two major bands (M.W., 54 K).

A recent report from the laboratory of A. Gilman has demonstrated charge differences between the guanine-nucleotide regulatory protein (the G/F factor) of adenylate cyclase from the uncoupled (UNC) mutant and wild-type S49 lymphoma cells. It has been pointed out that "phosphorylation of the substrates for cholera toxin in UNC is an attractive but (yet) unsubstantiated possibility" (Schleifer et al., 1980, p. 2643). Previous studies demonstrated influences of G/F factor on basal adenylate cyclase activity in a $Mg^{2+}$-dependent fashion (Cech et al., 1980). Our results on the effects of [γ-S]ATP on adenylate cyclase are not yet conclusive, and perhaps mechanisms other than protein phosphorylation play a role in bringing about the observed activation. Nonetheless, we now have the data base essential for continued investigation on the role of membrane-bound protein phosphorylation in the regulation of cyclase activity and its relationship to the function of the G/F factor.

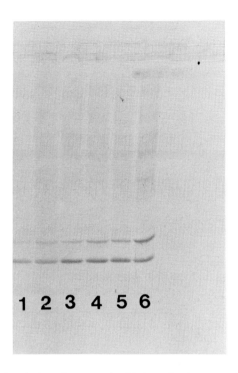

Fig. 9. Thiophosphorylation of cortical membrane proteins. To determine the pattern of thiophosphorylated proteins in our preparation, the preincubation phase of the assay (see legend to Fig. 7) was carried out with 10 $\mu$M [$\gamma$-S]ATP (Boehringer-Mannheim) containing 2 $\mu$Ci [$\gamma$-$^{35}$S]ATP (from New England Nuclear) per reaction tube. Reaction products were subjected to SDS–gel electrophoresis in 7–16 % exponential polyacrylamide gradient. Stained gels were treated for 45 min with 1 M sodium salicylate, dried, and exposed to X-ray film for 3 days. In the autofluorograph depicted here, the incubation time was varied as follows: lane (1) 0, (2) 10 min, (3) 20 min, (4) 50 min, (5) 90 min and (6) 120 min.

## PROTEIN PHOSPHORYLATION AND SIGNAL TRANSDUCTION ACROSS PLASMA MEMBRANES

The previous section presented data demonstrating temporal and quantitative correlation between thiophosphorylation of specific proteins and adenylate cyclase activation in membranes from rat cerebral cortex. However, direct evidence for the existence of cause–effect relationships between these two enzymatic systems is still lacking. Achievement of this goal, and particularly demonstrating conclusively that such processes play a role in receptor-mediated events, requires the solution of several experimental difficulties. The mammalian nervous system contains heterogeneous cell populations, multiple receptor types and subtypes, and the concentration of specific receptors is rather low. Considering the complexity and multiplicity of neuronal protein phosphorylation systems, the task of elucidating mechanisms of activation or inhibition of such molecular events by neurotransmitters in brain preparations is formidable. Some of these difficulties can be overcome by studying model systems. Somatic hybridization of the mouse neuroblastoma clone NB 18-TG2 with the rat glioma clone C6B7-1 yielded a hybrid clone that had been extensively investigated in recent years since it was found to possess a large number of neuronal properties. Briefly, neuroblastoma × glioma (NG)

390

clones have: action potential-$Na^+$ channels (Catteral and Nirenberg, 1973); electrical excitability (Nelson et al., 1976); muscarinic-cholinergic, $\alpha_2$-adrenergic and opiate receptors (Sharma et al., 1977; Sabol and Nirenberg, 1979; Nathanson et al., 1978) as well as adenylate and guanylate cyclase activities coupled to these receptors (ibid.); a choline uptake system (McGee, 1980); $Na^+$ GTP-regulated adenylate cyclase and receptor-binding sites (Blume et al., 1979) and cholera toxin-sensitive, receptor-coupled adenylate cyclase system (Propst and Hamprecht, 1981). Numerous laboratories now utilize NG cells as a model system for the investigation of neural function. The advantage of using hybrid NG cells over neuroblastoma (NB) cell lines derives from the great sensitivity to alterations in $Ca^{2+}$ ion concentration (a characteristic of excitable cells) which is displayed by NG cells but not by their parental NB clone (Brandt et al., 1980; Kurzinger et al., 1980). Finally, following cAMP-induced differentiation in culture, NG cells demonstrate the ultimate property of mature neurons: the ability to form functional synapses (Nelson et al., 1976; Christian et al., 1977).

We have recently begun utilizing NG cells in studies on the role of protein phosphorylation in receptor function (Ehrlich et al., 1981). The availability of intact, viable cells provided the

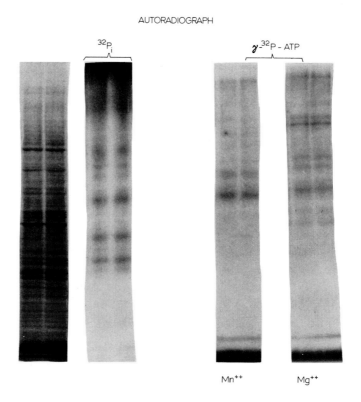

Fig. 10. Protein phosphorylation in intact neuroblastoma × glioma hybrid cells. Cells of the clone NG108-15 were grown in culture, harvested at 50% confluency and resuspended in a modified Krebs–Ringer solution (Brandt et al., 1980). To test for endogenous phosphorylative activity utilizing extracellular ATP, intact, viable cells (50 000 cells/100 $\mu$l) were incubated for 30 sec with 1 $\mu$M [$\gamma$-$^{32}$P]ATP added to the incubation medium which had been supplemented with either 4 mM $MgCl_2$ ($Mg^{++}$) or 4 mM $MnCl_2$ ($Mn^{++}$). SDS-solubilized cells were subjected to gel electrophoresis and autoradiography as described in the legend to Fig. 2. The pattern of proteins phosphorylated by intracellular ATP was examined in cells incubated for 1 h with inorganic $^{32}$Pi then washed twice and subjected to SDS electrophoresis on the same gel gradient.

opportunity to examine whether protein phosphorylation activity occurs on the outer surface of plasma membranes. It is well known that ATP is co-released with neurotransmitters upon neuronal stimulation. Such extracellular ATP may be utilized by protein kinases localized pericellularly to phosphorylate endogenous proteins in plasma membranes. Indication that such activity indeed operates in neural tissue was provided by comparing phosphorylation patterns obtained with intact synaptosomes and lysed synaptic plasma membranes (Ehrlich, unpublished observations). However, as even the most purified synaptosomal preparations contain a large amount of membrane fragments, clear-cut conclusions could not be drawn from these observations. In the present studies, intact NG cells were incubated for 30 sec with $[\gamma\text{-}^{32}P]ATP$ added to the extracellular medium, and then solubilized in SDS. Autoradiography of electrophoresed reaction products revealed $[^{32}P]$phosphate incorporation into specific protein bands. Pulsing for the same period with inorganic $^{32}Pi$ did not yield any detectable bands. Moreover, after incubation with $^{32}Pi$ for 1 h, when intracellular pools of ATP are labeled and used by phosphorylation systems inside the cells, the autoradiographic pattern obtained was different from that obtained by labeling with extracellular $AT^{32}P$ (Fig. 10). This indicates that ectokinase in NG cells can utilize extracellular ATP to phosphorylate endogenous proteins localized in the plasma membranes. This phosphorylation system also demonstrates selectivity in the phosphorylation of specific proteins. Fig. 10, for example, demonstrates differential effects of $Mg^{2+}$ and $Mn^{2+}$ on different bands. We have also established that this activity is linearly proportional to the concentration of ATP added to the extracellular medium.

Intracellular adenylate cyclase activity in intact cells can be conveniently measured by prelabeling with tritiated adenine. We have used this assay to investigate the possible invol-

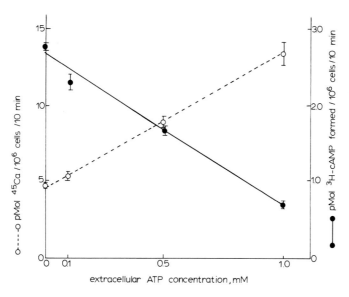

Fig. 11. Effects of extracellular ATP on adenylate cyclase activity and calcium uptake of NG108-15 cells. To measure adenylate cyclase activity in intact cells, intracellular ATP pools were labeled by preincubation with [³H]adenine (2 $\mu$Ci/10⁶ cells for 1 h). The amount of [³H]cAMP formed was measured after 10 min incubation of washed cells at 37°C; with 0.5 $\mu$M prostaglandin E$_1$, 1 mM RO 20-1724 (a phosphodiesterase inhibitor) and various ATP concentrations added to the standard incubation medium (see legend to Fig. 10). Uptake of Ca²⁺ was measured by incubating the cells for 10 min at 37°C in the same medium supplemented with 2 $\mu$Ci of ⁴⁵CaCl$_2$/10⁶ cells, and terminated by rapid filtration over GFC filters.

vement of ectokinase activity in the regulation of intracellular adenylate cyclase. As seen in Fig. 11, increasing extracellular ATP concentration resulted in decreased cAMP formation from intracellular [³H]ATP, indicating a transmembrane phenomenon. It has been reported that PGE₁-stimulated cAMP formation in intact NG cells is inhibited by increase of Ca²⁺ flux into the cells (Brandt et al., 1980). Indeed, we have found that under conditions that extracellular ATP inhibits the cyclase, there is a parallel increase in calcium uptake by NG cells (Fig. 11). Future studies should attempt to provide further evidence to the possibility that phosphorylation of membrane-bound proteins by ectokinase(s) regulate receptor-coupled adenylate cyclase in a mechanism that involves control of calcium ion movements across the plasma membrane.

## CONCLUSIONS AND FUTURE DIRECTIONS

The discovery and identification of specific receptors for neurohormones was accompanied by the admonition (Goldstein, 1973) that binding alone cannot account for receptor function. It

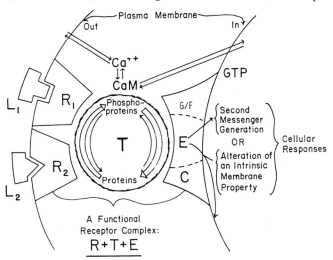

Fig. 12. Hypothetical role for protein phosphorylation in the transducing mechanism of receptor complexes. R, recognition site. Confers *specificity* to the binding of ligands (L). $R_1$, $R_2$, recognition sites for two different hormones. T, transducing mechanism. Confers *a conformational change,* which is necessary for the activation or inhibition of E, depending on the properties of $R_1$ and $R_2$. This process MUST BE REVERSIBLE. E, effector site. Initiates the chain of events which lead to cellular responses to L. E may be a system that generates a second messenger such as cAMP (then E contains guanine nucleotide-regulatory protein(s): G/F; and catalytic subunit-C of adenylate cyclase), or an intrinsic membrane activity, e.g. ion channels.

*Hypothesis:* "T" may be an endogenous phosphorylation system regulated by $L_1$ or $L_2$. By regulating the cycles of endogenous phosphorylation, $L_1$ may activate E and perhaps also alter some properties of $R_2$. A cyclic alteration in the phosphorylation state of membrane-bound proteins is catalyzed by enzymes (protein kinase and phosphoprotein phosphatase) that constitute part of the structure of these membranes. This mechanism can provide a means to carry out reversible conformational changes, which may be necessary for activation and inactivation of the effector (e.g. adenylate cyclase). In the event that it can be shown that such an endogenous phosphorylation system is under the control of L·R and that agonist-induced changes in phosphorylative activity stimulate and/or inhibit adenylate cyclase, it would be demonstrated that protein phosphorylation can fulfill a role in the transducing mechanism. In such case, the specificity of receptor function would be determined by properties inherent to the "recognition site". The expression of receptor function would be determined by the identity of the "effector site", but the "transducing mechanism" could be general in nature.

has been postulated that the interaction of agonists with their recognition sites produces a conformational change which triggers the chain of events leading to cellular responses. The phosphorylation and dephosphorylation of proteins provide the means to carry out reversible conformational changes that can mediate functional alterations. Studies using homogeneous membrane preparations have implicated phosphorylation and dephosphorylation of proteins in the re-arrangement of membrane components (Gazzit et al., 1976). This chapter has summarized studies demonstrating that membrane-bound protein phosphorylation systems are controlled by neurotransmitters on the one hand, and could play a role in the regulation of receptor-coupled effector sites, such as adenylate cyclase, on the other hand. The hypothetical relationships that may be presumed to exist on the basis of these findings are illustrated in Fig. 12 and detailed in its legend. We offer this working hypothesis as a guideline whose value should be judged primarily on the basis of the experimental tests that it will generate in future studies.

## ACKNOWLEDGEMENTS

We wish to thank Mr. Roger A. Lambert for expert technical assistance and Mrs. Ginger McDowell for excellent secretarial help in preparing the manuscript.

The studies described herein were supported in part by a USPHS grant DA02747 from the National Institute on Drug Abuse.

## REFERENCES

Bär, P.R., Schotman, P. and Gispen, W.H. (1980) Enkephalins affect hippocampal membrane phosphorylation. *Eur. J. Pharmacol.*, 65: 165–174.

Blume, A.J., Boone, G. and Lichtshtein, D. (1979) Regulation of the neuroblastoma × glioma hybrid opiate receptors by $Na^+$ and guanine nucleotides. In *Advances in Experimental Medicine and Biology*, Vol. 116, Y.H. Ehrlich, J. Volavka, L.G. Davis and E.G. Brunngraber (Eds.), Plenum Press, New York–London, pp. 163–174.

Bonnet, K.A. (1979) Adaptive alterations in receptor mediated processes and their implications for some mental disorders. In *Advances in Experimental Medicine and Biology*, Vol. 116, Y.H. Ehrlich, J. Volavka, L.G. Davis and E.G. Brunngraber (Eds.), Plenum Press, New York–London, pp. 247–260.

Bonnet, K.A., Branchey, L.B., Friedhoff, A.J. and Ehrlich, Y.H. (1978) Long-term narcotic exposure reduces caudate cyclic nucleotide levels, protein kinase and tyrosine hydroxylase activities. *Life Sci.*, 22: 2003–2008.

Brandt, M., Buchen, C. and Hamprecht, B. (1980) Relationship between the actions of calcium ions, opioids, and prostaglandin $E_1$ on the level of cyclic AMP in neuroblastoma × glioma hybrid cells. *J. Neurochem.*, 34: 643–651.

Browning, M., Dunwiddie, T., Bennet, W., Gispen, W. and Lynch, G. (1979a) Synaptic phosphoproteins: Specific changes after repetitive stimulation of the hippocampal slice. *Science*, 203: 60–62.

Browning, M., Bennet, W. and Lynch, G. (1979b) Phosphorylase kinase phosphorylates a brain protein which is influenced by repetitive synaptic activation. *Nature (Lond.)*, 278: 273–275.

Carpenter, G., King, L. and Cohen, S. (1978) Epidermal growth factor stimulates phosphorylation in membrane preparations in vitro. *Nature (Lond.)*, 276: 409–410.

Carpenter, G., King Jr., L. and Cohen, S. (1979) Rapid enhancement of protein phosphorylation in A-431 cell membrane preparations by epidermal growth factor. *J. biol. Chem.*, 254: 4884–4891.

Cassidy, P., Hoar, P.E. and Kerrick, W.G.L. (1979) Irreversible thiophosphorylation and activation of tension in functionally skinned rabbit ileum strips by $^{35}S$-ATPγS. *J. biol. Chem.*, 254: 11148–11153.

Catterall, W.A. and Nirenberg, M. (1973) Sodium uptake associated with activation of action potential ionophores of cultured neuroblastoma and muscle cells. *Proc. nat. Acad. Sci. (Wash.)*, 70: 3769–3763.

Cech, S.Y., Broaddus, W.C. and Maguire, M.E. (1980) Adenylate cyclase: The role of magnesium and other divalent cations. *Mol. cell. Biochem.*, 33: 67–92.

Christian, C., Nelson, P.G., Peacock, J. and Nirenberg, M. (1977) Synapse formation between two clonal cell lines. *Science*, 196: 995–998.

394

Chuang, D.M. and Costa, E. (1979)β-Adrenergic receptors of frog erythrocytes. *Neurochem. Res.,* 4: 777–793.

Clement-Cormier, Y.C. (1980) Dopamine receptor: Isolation, purification and regulation. In *Receptors for Neuro-transmitters and Peptide Hormones,* G. Pepeu, M.J. Kuhar and S.J. Enna (Eds.), Raven Press, New York, pp. 159–167.

Cohen, S., Carpenter, G. and King, L. (1980) Epidermal growth factor–receptor protein kinase interactions. *J. biol. Chem.,* 255: 4834–4842.

DeBlas, A.L., Wang, Y.J., Sorensen, R. and Mahler, H.R. (1979) Protein phosphorylation in synaptic membranes regulated by adenosine 3′:5′-monophosphate: Regional and subcellular distribution of the endogenous substrates. *J. Neurochem.,* 33: 647–659.

DeLorenzo, R.J. (1976) Calcium-dependent phosphorylation of specific synaptosomal fraction proteins: possible role of phosphoproteins in mediating neurotransmitter release. *Biochem. biophys. Res. Commun.,* 71: 590–597.

DeLorenzo, R.J., Burdette, S. and Holderness, J. (1981) Benzodiazepine inhibition of the calcium-calmodulin protein kinase system in brain membrane. *Science,* 213: 546–549.

Duffy, T.E., Nelson, S.R. and Lowry, O.H. (1972) Carbohydrate metabolism during acute hypoxia and recovery. *J. Neurochem.,* 19: 959–977.

Ehrlich, Y.H. (1979) Phosphoproteins as specifiers for mediators and modulators in neuronal function. In *Advances in Experimental Medicine and Biology,* Vol. 116, Y.H. Ehrlich, J. Volavka, L.G. Davis and E.G. Brunngraber (Eds.), Plenum Press, New York–London, pp. 75–101.

Ehrlich, Y.H. (1981) Protein phosphorylation, neuronal receptors and seizures in the CNS. In *Status Epilepticus,* C. Wasterlain, A.V. Delgado-Escueta and R. Porter (Eds.), Raven Press, New York, in press.

Ehrlich, Y.H. and Brunngraber, E.G. (1976) cAMP-stimulated phosphorylation of proteins after chronic chlorproma-zine. *Trans. Am. Soc. Neurochem.,* 7: 109 (abstr.).

Ehrlich, Y.H. and Routtenberg, A. (1974) Cyclic AMP regulates the phosphorylation of three proteins of rat cerebral cortex membranes for thirty minutes. *FEBS Lett.,* 45: 237–243.

Ehrlich, Y.H., Rabjohns, R. and Routtenberg, A. (1977a) Experiential-input alters the phosphorylation of specific proteins in brain membranes. *Pharmacol. Biochem. Behav.,* 6: 169–174.

Ehrlich, Y.H., Bonnet, K.A., Davis, L.G., and Brunngraber, E.G. (1977b) Protein phosphorylation in neostriatal membranes: Involvement of specific phosphoproteins in narcotic addiction. In *Developments in Neuro-science,* Vol. 2, S. Roberts, A. Lajtha and W. Gispen (Eds.), Elsevier, Amsterdam, pp. 273–278.

Ehrlich, Y.H., Davis, L.G., Gilfoil, T. and Brunngraber, E.G. (1977c) Distribution of endogenously phosphorylated proteins in subcellular fractions of rat cerebral cortex. *Neurochem. Res.,* 2: 533–548.

Ehrlich, Y.H., Brunngraber, E.G., Sinah, P.K. and Prasad, K.N. (1977d) Specific alterations in phosphorylation of cytosol proteins from differentiating neuroblastoma cells grown in culture. *Nature (Lond.),* 265: 238–240.

Ehrlich, Y.H., Davis, L.G. and Brunngraber, E.G. (1977e) Effects of seizure-producing stimulation on protein phosphorylation in cortical membranes. *Soc. Neurosci. Abstr.,* 3: 139.

Ehrlich, Y.H., Davis, L.G. and Brunngraber, E.G. (1978a) Effects of decapitation stress on protein phosphorylation in cortical membranes. *Brain Res. Bull.,* 3: 251–256.

Ehrlich, Y.H., Bonnet, K.A., Davis, L.G. and Brunngraber, E.G. (1978b) Decreased phosphorylation of specific proteins in neostriatal membranes from rats after long-term narcotic exposure. *Life Sci.,* 23: 137–146.

Ehrlich, Y.H., Prasad, K.N., Davis, L.G., Sinah, P.K. and Brunngraber, E.G. (1978c) Endogenous phosphorylation of specific proteins in subcellular fractions from malignant and cAMP-induced differentiated neuroblastoma cells in culture. *Neurochem. Res.,* 3: 803–813.

Ehrlich, Y.H., Davis, L.G., Keen, P. and Brunngraber, E.G. (1980a) Endorphin-regulation of protein phosphoryla-tion in brain membranes. *Life Sci.,* 26: 1765–1772.

Ehrlich, Y.H., Reddy, M.N., Keen, P. and Davis, L.G. (1980b) Transient changes in the phosphorylation of cortical membrane proteins after electroconvulsive shock. *J. Neurochem.,* 34: 1327–1330.

Ehrlich, Y.H., Garfield, M.K. and Lenox, R.H. (1981) Protein phosphorylation on the surface of neuroblastoma cells. *Trans. Am. Soc. Neurochem.,* 12: 229 (abstr.).

Gazitt, Y., Ohad, I. and Loyter, A. (1976) Phosphorylation and dephosphorylation of membrane proteins as a possible mechanism for structural rearrangement of membrane components. *Biochim. biophys. Acta,* 436: 1–14.

Gnegy, M. and Treisman, G. 1981) Effect of calmodulin on dopamine-sensitive adenylate cyclase activity in rat striatal membranes. *Mol. Pharmacol.,* 19: 256–263.

Gnegy, M.E., Uzunov, P. and Costa, E. (1976) Regulation of dopamine stimulation of striatal adenylate cyclase by an endogenous $Ca^{++}$-binding protein. *Proc. nat. Acad. Sci. (Wash.),* 73: 3887–3890.

Gnegy, M., Uzunov, P. and Costa, E. (1977) Participation of an endogenous $Ca^{++}$-binding protein activator in the development of drug-induced supersensitivity of striatal dopamine receptors. *J. Pharmacol. exp. Ther.,* 202: 558–564.

Goldstein, A. (1973) In *Pharmacology and the Future of Man,* Karger, Basel, pp. 140–150.

Gordon, A.S. and Diamond, I. (1979) Phosphorylation of the acetylcholine receptor. In *Advances in Experimental Medicine and Biology*, Vol. 116, Y.H. Ehrlich, J. Volavka, L.G. Davis and E.G. Brunngraber (Eds.) Plenum Press, New York–London, pp. 175–198.

Greengard, P. (1976) Possible role of cyclic nucleotides and phosphorylated membrane proteins in post-synaptic actions of neurotransmitters. *Nature (Lond.)*, 260, 101–105.

Greengard, P. (1978) *Cyclic Nucleotides, Phosphorylated Proteins and Neuronal Function*, Raven Press, New York.

Heald, P.J. (1957) The incorporation of phosphate into cerebral phosphoprotein promoted by electrical impulses. *Biochem. J.*, 66: 659–663.

Hunzicker-Dunn, M., Derda, D., Jungmann, R.A. and Birnbaumer, L. (1979) Resensitization of the desensitized follicular adenylyl cyclase system to luteinizing hormone. *Endocrinology*, 104: 1785–1793.

Johnson, E.M., Ueda, T., Maeno, H. and Greengard, P. (1972) Cyclic AMP-dependent phosphorylation of a specific protein in synaptic membranes. *J. biol. Chem.*, 247: 5650–5652.

Krebs, E.G. and Rosen, O.M. (Eds.) (1981) *Protein Phosphorylation: Proceedings of Eighth Cold Spring Harbor Conference on Cell Proliferation*, CSH Press, New York.

Kuo, J.E. and Greengard, P. (1969) Cyclic nucleotide-dependent protein kinase. IV. Wide-spread occurrence of adenosine 3′,5′-monophosphate-dependent protein kinase in various tissues and phyla of the animal kingdom. *Proc. nat. Acad. Sci. (Wash.)*, 64: 1349–1355.

Kurzinger, K., Stadtkus, C. and Hamprecht, B. (1980) Uptake and energy-dependent extrusion of calcium in neural cells in culture. *Eur. J. Biochem.*, 103: 597–611.

Lenox, R.H., Kant, G.J. and Meyerhoff, J.L. (1981) Rapid enzyme inactivation. In *Handbook of Neurochemistry*, Vol. II, 2nd edn., A. Lajtha (Ed.), Plenum Press, New York, in press.

Lust, E.D., Goldberg, N.D. and Passonneau, J.V. (1976) Cyclic nucleotides in murine brain: the temporal relationship of changes induced in adenosine 3′,5′-monophosphate and guanosine 3′,5′-monophosphate following maximal electroshock or decapitation. *J. Neurochem.*, 26: 5–10.

McGee, R. (1980) Choline uptake by the neuroblastoma × glioma hybrid, NG108-15. *J. Neurochem.*, 35: 829–837.

Nathanson, N.M., Klein, W.L. and Nirenberg, M. (1978) Regulation of adenylate cyclase activity mediated by muscarinic acetylcholine receptors. *Proc. nat. Acad. Sci. (Wash.)*, 73: 123–127.

Nelson, P., Christian, C. and Nirenberg, M. (1976) Synapse formation between clonal neuroblastoma glioma hybrid cells and striated muscle cells. *Proc. nat. Acad. Sci. (Wash.)*, 73: 123–127.

Nestler, E.J. and Greengard, P. (1980) Dopamine and depolarizing agents regulate the state of phosphorylation of protein I in the mammalian superior cervical sympathetic ganglion. *Proc. nat. Acad. Sci. (Wash.)*, 77: 7479–7483.

Propst, F. and Hamprecht, B. (1981) Opioids, noradrenaline and GTP analogs inhibit cholera toxin activated adenylate cyclase in neuroblastom × glioma hybrid cells. *J. Neurochem.*, 36: 580–588.

Routtenberg, A. and Ehrlich, Y.H. (1975) Endogenous phosphorylation of four proteins in cerebral cortex membranes. Role of cyclic nucleotides, ATP and divalent cations. *Brain Res.*, 92: 415–430.

Sabol, S. and Nirenberg, M. (1979) Regulation of adenylate cyclase of neuroblastoma × glioma hybrid cells by alpha-adrenergic receptors. *J. biol. Chem.*, 254: 1913–1920.

Schleifer, L.S., Garrison, J.C., Sternweis, P.C., Northup, J.K. and Gilman, A.G. (1980) The regulatory component of adenylate cyclase from uncoupled S49 lymphoma cells differs in charge from the wild type protein. *J. biol. Chem.*, 255: 2641–2644.

Schulman, M. and Greengard, P. (1978) Stimulation of brain membrane protein phosphorylation by calcium and an endogenous heat-stable protein. *Nature (Lond.)*, 271: 478–479.

Sharma, S., Klee, W. and Nirenberg, M. (1977) Opiate-dependent modulation of adenylate cyclase. *Proc. nat. Acad. Sci. (Wash.)*, 74: 3365–3369.

Trevor, A.J. and Rodnight, R. (1965) The subcellular localization of cerebral phosphoproteins sensitive to electrical stimulation. *Biochem. J.*, 95: 889–896.

Ueda, T., Maeno, H. and Greengard, P. (1973) Regulation of endogenous phosphorylation of specific proteins in synaptic membrane fractions from rat brain by adenosine 3′:5′-monophosphate. *J. biol. Chem.*, 248: 8295–8305.

Ushiro, H. and Cohen, S. (1981) Identification of phosphotyrosine as a product of epidermal growth factor-activated protein kinase in A-431 cell membranes. *J. biol. Chem.*, 255: 8363–8365.

Whittemore, S.R., Lenox, R.H., Hendley, E.D. and Ehrlich, Y.H. (1981) Protein phosphorylation mediates effects of isoproterenol on adenylate cyclase activity in rat cortical membranes. *Neurochem. Res.*, 6: 777–787.

Williams, M. and Rodnight, R. (1977) Protein phosphorylation in nervous tissue: possible involvement in nervous tissue function and relationship to cyclic nucleotide metabolism. *Progr. Neurobiol.*, 8: 183–250.

Williams, M., Pavlik, A. and Rodnight, R. (1974) Turnover of protein phosphorus in respiring slices of guinea pig cerebral cortex: cellular localization of phosphoprotein sensitive to electrical stimulation. *J. Neurochem., 22*: 373–376.

Zwiers, H., Veldhuis, H.D., Schotman, P. and Gispen, W.H. (1976) ACTH, cyclic nucleotides and brain protein phosphorylation in vitro. *Neurochem. Res., 1*: 669–677.

Zwiers, H. Weigant, V.M., Schotman, P. and Gispen, W.H. (1977) Intraventricular administered ACTH and changes in rat brain protein phosphorylation: A preliminary report. In *Developments in Neuroscience,* Vol. 2, S. Roberts, A. Lajtha and W. Gispen (Eds.), Elsevier, Amsterdam, pp. 267–272.

# Modulation of Adenylate Cyclase by Protein Phosphorylation: Effects of ACTH

V.M. WIEGANT, J.M.H.M. REUL and W.H. GISPEN

*Division of Molecular Neurobiology, Rudolf Magnus Institute for Pharmacology, and Institute of Molecular Biology, University of Utrecht, Urecht, The Netherlands*

## INTRODUCTION

Previous studies from our laboratory have demonstrated that neuropeptides related to ACTH may function as regulators of brain adenylate cyclase activity (Wiegant et al., 1979). In $\mu$M and higher concentrations $ACTH_{1-24}$ inhibits the activity of adenylate cyclase in brain synaptic plasma membranes in vitro. The presence of calcium ions is essential for this effect (Wiegant et al., 1979; Wiegant, Reul and Gispen, unpublished), indicating that the inhibition of adenylate cyclase by $ACTH_{1-24}$ involves a calcium-dependent process.

From other investigations it became clear that ACTH and congeners specifically inhibit the endogenous phosphorylation of a number of proteins in brain synaptic plasma membranes in vitro (Zwiers et al., 1976, 1978). The peptide concentration at which this effect occurs, is identical to that needed for the inhibition of adenylate cyclase. Zwiers et al. (1978, 1979, 1980) have shown that the inhibition by ACTH of the phosphorylation of at least one specific membrane protein, B-50, is the result of a direct interaction of the peptide with a calcium-dependent, cyclic AMP (cAMP)-insensitive, protein kinase.

Structure–activity relationships for this effect appeared to be very similar to those found for the inhibition of adenylate cyclase (Wiegant et al., 1981). In general, the determination of adenylate cyclase is performed using ATP as a substrate, under conditions where phosphorylation of proteins can also take place. Interestingly, the inhibitory effect of the peptide on adenylate cyclase and on B-50 protein kinase turned out to be dependent on the concentration of ATP in the incubation mixture (Wiegant et al., 1979; Zwiers et al., 1978). These similarities between the interactions of ACTH with adenylate cyclase and endogenous protein phosphorylation in brain synaptic plasma membranes (dose range, structure–activity relationships, calcium dependence and ATP dependence) led us to consider that ACTH influences adenylate cyclase activity through a mechanism involving peptide-sensitive phosphorylation. This consideration is in line with recent observations by Richards et al. (1981) and Ehrlich et al. (this volume) that membrane phosphoproteins are involved in the regulation of basal and receptor-coupled adenylate cyclase activity.

In the present report we present experimental data supporting this idea. It is suggested that phosphate turnover in the membrane may function as an important pathway for neuromodulators to change the efficacy of transmitter adenylate cyclase interactions, thereby modulating nerve impulse flow.

## EXPERIMENTAL DESIGN

Light synaptic plasma membranes (SPM) were prepared according to Terenius et al. (1973) from rat cerebral cortex, septum, basal ganglia and hippocampi. To control the state of phosphorylation of the membrane proteins prior to the determination of adenylate cyclase activity, a two-phase incubation system was used. First, membranes were incubated at 30° C in buffer (20 mM Tris–HCl, pH 7.5), containing 5 mM $Mg^{2+}$ for 30 min, in the presence or absence of $10^{-4}$ M $ACTH_{1-24}$ and of varying amounts of ATPγS. This analog of ATP is used by protein kinases as a phosphate donor. As the thiophosphate-ester bond is not hydrolysed by phosphatases as a substrate, thiophosphorylation in essence is an irreversible process (Gratecos and Fischer, 1974; Cassidy et al., 1979). Immediately after the incubation, the membranes were rapidly spun down, washed twice with ice-cold buffer and resuspended. Aliquots of the suspension were then reincubated to determine the adenylate cyclase activity. Adenylate cyclase assays were carried out at 30° C for 5 min, using 0.5 mM [ $\alpha$-$^{32}$P]ATP as substrate in the presence of 5 mM $Mg^{2+}$, an ATP-regenerating system, and caffeine to inhibit phosphodiesterase activity. Samples were processed and cAMP accumulation was determined as previously described (Wiegant et al., 1979). In parallel reincubations the amount of free phosphorylatable sites in the membrane suspension was estimated. Aliquots were reincubated for 10 sec at 30° C in the presence of 7.5 $\mu$M [γ-$^{32}$P]ATP, 10 mM $Mg^{2+}$ and 1 mM $Ca^{2+}$. Phosphoproteins were solubilized with SDS, separated by SDS–polyacrylamide gel electrophoresis (SDS–PAGE) and visualized by autoradiography according to Zwiers et al. (1976). Incorporation of [$^{32}$P]phosphate into specific protein bands was determined by liquid scintillation counting.

## RESULTS

Rat brain SPM were incubated for 30 min in the presence of various concentrations of ATPγS, then washed twice at 4° C and resuspended in buffer. Reincubation of aliquots of this suspension for 10 sec in the presence of [γ-$^{32}$P]ATP resulted in the incorporation of [$^{32}$P]phosphate into proteins. Subsequently, these proteins were solubilized and then separated on SDS–PAGE. As is illustrated by the autoradiograph (Fig. 1), the incorporation of phosphate was inversily related to the concentration of ATPγS employed in the incubation. Radiolabelling of all phosphoprotein bands present was decreased by incubation with ATPγS. Maximal inhibition of incorporation of phosphate into proteins was observed at 1 mM ATPγS. The absolute amount of phosphate incorporated during reincubation into the two most prominent phosphoprotein bands (apparent molecular weights 48 K and 56 K) was determined by liquid scintillation counting. Phosphate labelling of these proteins showed an inverse linear relationship with the log concentration of ATPγS present in the incubation (Fig. 2). From the data depicted in Fig. 2, the $EC_{50}$ of ATPγS on phospholabelling of these bands was computed, being 60 and 20 $\mu$M, respectively.

As expected, ATPγS did not abolish the protein kinase activity of the membranes. For histone added to the reincubation mixture became highly phosphorylated by endogenous SPM protein kinases, irrespective of the ATPγS concentration during the incubation (data not shown). These data suggest that ATPγS does not affect the process of phosphorylation in SPM, but indeed serves as a (thio)phosphate donor resulting in irreversible thiophosphorylation of membrane proteins.

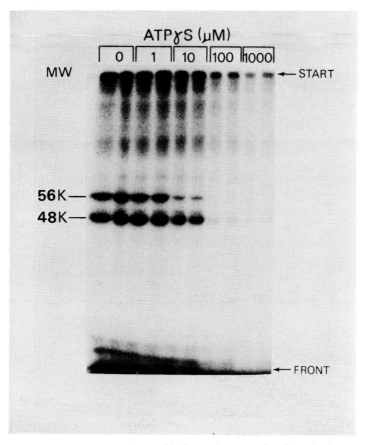

Fig. 1. Effect of ATPγS on the phosphorylation of brain membrane proteins. Synaptic plasma membranes were incubated with 5 mM $Mg^{2+}$ and various concentrations of ATPγS, washed and resuspended in buffer. Aliquots were reincubated with [$\gamma^{32}$P]ATP (7.5 $\mu$M) in the presence of $Mg^{2+}$ (10 mM) and $Ca^{2+}$ (1 mM). Proteins were solubilized with SDS and separated by SDS–polyacrylamide slab gel electrophoresis. The radiolabelled protein bands were visualized by autoradiography. The autoradiograph depicted here shows the inverse relationship between incorporation of [$^{32}$P]phosphate and the concentration of ATPγS during the incubation. Incubation in the presence of 1000 $\mu$M ATPγS completely prevented incorporation of phosphate into proteins during reincubation. The major phosphoprotein bands in this preparation had apparent molecular weights of 48 K and 56 K.

Also, following incubation with ATPγS, aliquots of the membrane suspension were reincubated for 5 min in a system containing 0.5 mM [$\alpha$-$^{32}$P]ATP to assess the effect of thiophosphorylation on the activity of adenylate cyclase. Fig. 3 shows that incubation of SPM in the presence of ATPγS markedly stimulated the basal activity of adenylate cyclase in a concentration-dependent manner. A linear relationship existed between the activity of the enzyme and the log concentration of ATPγS used in the incubation. Half-maximal stimulation was observed at a concentration of 60 $\mu$M, whereas maximal stimulation occurred at 0.5 mM ATPγS. By comparing Figs. 1, 2 and 3, a strong correlation between the degree of phosphate incorporation into proteins and the activity of adenylate cyclase in the same membrane preparation becomes apparent.

400

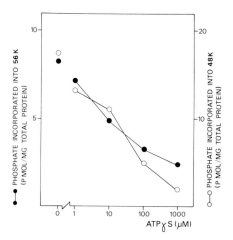

Fig. 2. Effect of ATPγS on phosphate incorporation into distinct brain membrane phosphoproteins. Synaptic plasma membranes were incubated with various concentrations of ATPγS, washed, reincubated in the presence of [γ-$^{32}$P]ATP and separated by SDS–polyacrylamide gel electrophoresis as described in the legend to Fig. 1. The 48 K and 56 K phosphorprotein bands were excised from the gel. Radioactivity in these bands was determined by liquid scintillation counting and the incorporation into both bands showed inverse correlation with the concentration of ATPγS during the incubation.

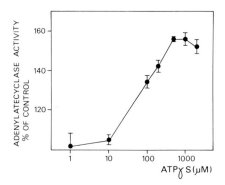

Fig. 3. Activation of brain membrane adenylate cyclase by ATPγS. Synaptic plasma membranes were incubated with various concentrations of ATPγS under phosphorylation conditions (5 mM Mg$^{2+}$), washed, resuspended and reincubated to assay adenylate cyclase activity. ATPγS dose dependently activated adenylate cyclase. Values are expressed as mean ± S.E.M. of triplicate determinations. Basal adenylate cyclase activity in this experiment: 720.3 ± 2.3 pmoles/mg protein/min.

Incubation of SPM in the presence of $10^{-4}$ M ACTH$_{1-24}$ under non-phosphorylating conditions (i.e., in absence of ATP or ATPγS), resulted in a strong inhibition (32%) of adenylate cyclase activity detected by reincubation in the presence of [α-$^{32}$P]ATP (Fig. 4). In a parallel reincubation with [γ-$^{32}$P]ATP a large decrease in the incorporation of phosphate was observed in the 48 K protein band, but also the labelling of the 56 K band was affected (Fig. 5).

When membrane phosphoproteins are saturated with phosphate, as is the case after incubation with 1000 μM ATPγS (Fig. 2), a change in the activity of protein kinase cannot be expressed in an altered degree of phosphate incorporation in the reincubation. Indeed, $10^{-4}$ M

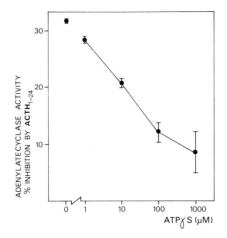

Fig. 4. Effect of ATP$\gamma$S on ACTH$_{1-24}$-induced inhibition of adenylate cyclase. Synaptic plasma membranes were incubated with various concentrations of ATP$\gamma$S in the presence or absence of $10^{-4}$ M ACTH$_{1-24}$ under phosphorylating conditions (5 mM Mg$^{2+}$). Membranes were washed, resuspended and adenylated cyclase activity was determined. The expression of the inhibitory effect of the peptide on adenylate cyclase activity depended on the concentration of ATP$\gamma$S during the incubation. Incubation with 1000 $\mu$M ATP$\gamma$S abolished the effect of the peptide. The values are expressed as mean $\pm$ S.E.M. of triplicate incubations. Basal adenylate cyclase activity in this experiment: $836.6 \pm 19.4$ pmoles/mg protein/min.

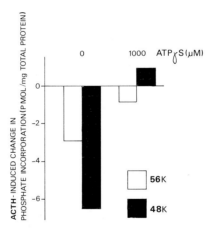

Fig. 5. Effect of ATP$\gamma$S on the ACTH$_{1-24}$-induced inhibition of phosphate incorporation into SPM proteins. Synaptic plasma membranes were incubated with or without 1000 $\mu$M ATP$\gamma$S in the presence or absence of $10^{-4}$ M ACTH$_{1-24}$. The membranes were washed, resuspended, reincubated with 7.5 $\mu$M [$\gamma$-$^{32}$P]ATP and separated by SDS–polyacrylamide gel electrophoresis. The 48 K and 56 K protein bands were excised from the gel. Radioactivity in these bands was determined by liquid scintillation counting. ACTH$_{1-24}$ inhibited phosphate incorporation into both protein bands. Incubation with 1000 $\mu$M ATP$\gamma$S abolished this effect of the peptide.

ACTH$_{1-24}$ did not affect phospholabelling of the 48 K and 56 K proteins in membranes incubated with 1000 $\mu$M ATP$\gamma$S (Fig. 5). Interestingly, in the same membranes thiophosphorylation also antagonized the expression of the effect of ACTH$_{1-24}$ on adenylate cyclase activity. No inhibition by the peptide was found after incubation with 1000 $\mu$M ATP$\gamma$S (Fig. 4).

## DISCUSSION

In the presence of ATP$\gamma$S, protein kinase substrate proteins are irreversibly (thio)phosphorylated (Gratecos and Fischer, 1974; Cassidy et al., 1979). In this study we have used this feature to predetermine the degree of phosphorylation of synaptic plasma membranes by incubation with varying concentrations of ATP$\gamma$S. Subsequently, the degree of (thio)phosphorylation was monitored by short reincubation of the membranes in the presence of [$\gamma$-$^{32}$P]ATP. Under these conditions, $^{32}$P-labelled phosphate is only bound to free un(thio)phosphorylated sites. Previously, it was determined that the phosphorylation conditions used (7.5 $\mu$M ATP) did not result in complete saturation of the acceptor proteins (Wiegant et al., 1978). Yet, by employing this method, a good reflection of the degree of (thio)phosphorylation of membrane proteins at the start of the reincubation could be obtained (Figs. 1 and 2). Our data show that the process of thiophosphorylation is proportional to the concentration of ATP$\gamma$S used in the incubation medium, and that thiophosphorylation was maximal at 1 mM ATP$\gamma$S (Figs. 1 and 2).

The basal activity of adenylate cyclase was directly related to the concentration of ATP$\gamma$S used in the incubation (Fig. 3) and therefore to the state of (thio)phosphorylation of the membranes. These results corroborate those of Ehrlich et al. (this volume), and they indicate that brain basal adenylate cyclase activity is stimulated by phosphorylation of membrane proteins. Quantitative analysis of the two major phosphoprotein bands with apparent molecular weights of 56 K and 48 K (Fig. 2) revealed a close correlation between thiophosphorylation of these bands and the activity of adenylate cyclase. However, as we did not analyse the kinetics of thiophosphorylation of these and other proteins in more detail, no conclusion can be drawn with respect to the role individual phosphoproteins may play in the regulation of the multicomponent adenylate cyclase system, Ehrlich et al. (this volume) studied the incorporation of thiophosphate into membrane proteins using $^{35}$S-labelled ATP$\gamma$S in a comparable experimental system. Interestingly, they reported on (thio)phosphorylation of two protein bands in SPM with molecular weights between 40 and 60 K and also described a correlation of the phosphorylation of these proteins with the activation of adenylate cyclase. It remains to be shown whether both studies indeed deal with the same phosphoproteins.

ACTH$_{1-24}$ inhibits the phosphorylation of a number of SPM proteins via interaction with endogenous protein kinase(s) (Zwiers et al., 1976). Notably, the peptide was shown not to influence brain membrane phosphoprotein phosphatase activity (Zwiers et al., 1978). It should be kept in mind that the experimental set up of our previous studies on the effect of neuropeptides on brain protein phosphorylation greatly differ from those employed here (Zwiers et al., 1976, 1978). The differences in incubation conditions (time of exposure to ACTH$_{1-24}$, incubation/reincubation, etc.) may be cause of the different phosphorylation pattern and sensitivity of the kinases to ACTH. For instance, recently we reported that exposure of membranes to a number of fragments of ACTH resulted in the release of a protein (molecular weight 41 K) from these membranes (Aloyo et al., 1982). Albeit that the meaning of this observation is not yet totally understood, it certainly may have resulted in differences between previous and present endogenous membrane phosphorylation. Although no proper immunochemical or two-dimensional identification of the 48 K protein band was performed, it is almost certain that this protein is identical to the B-50 protein first described by Zwiers et al. (this volume).

The inhibitory effect of ACTH$_{1-24}$ on SPM protein kinase(s) could be detected by reincubation in the presence of [$\gamma$$^{32}$P]ATP, even after the membranes had been washed extensively (cf. Fig. 5). The adenylate cyclase assay was performed under phosphorylating conditions

(0.5 mM ATP, 5 mM Mg$^{2+}$). Hence, it could be that the inhibition of adenylate cyclase activity by ACTH$_{1-24}$ in fact is the result of a lower degree of phosphorylation of a number of proteins essential in adenylate cyclase regulation.

Inhibition of protein kinase by ACTH$_{1-24}$ will only result in a lower degree of phosphorylation of substrate proteins, if these are present in a relatively dephosphorylated from as is the case after incubation of SPM in the absence of ATPγS. Indeed, no inhibition of phosphorylation by the peptide was observed when complete and irreversible (thio)phosphorylation had taken place (Fig. 5). Also, under these conditions, the adenylate cyclase activity was not inhibited by the peptide.

In conclusion, the present results strongly support the idea that phosphoproteins in the membrane are intimately involved in the regulation of adenylate cyclase activity (Richards et al., 1981; Whittemore et al., 1981; Ehrlich et al., this volume). Moreover, they indicate neuropeptides like ACTH can alter adenylate cyclase activity by changing the state of phosphorylation of one or more relevant phosphoproteins. At present, no information on the exact nature and role of the phosphoprotein(s) is available. However, there seems to be a strong parallel to the observed regulation of membrane DPI kinase by the degree of phosphorylation of B-50 (Jolles et al., 1980, 1981). With respect to adenylate cyclase, it has been suggested (Schleifer et al., 1980) that phosphorylation of the guanine nucleotide regulatory protein may be involved in the regulation of the activity of the receptor adenylate cyclase complex. Such a mechanism would allow putative neuromodulators like ACTH and other neuropeptides to change the efficacy of neurotransmission by affecting membrane processes involved in the generation of second messengers (cAMP, calcium).

REFERENCES

Aloyo, V.J., Zwiers, H. and Gispen, W.H. (1982) ACTH$_{1-24}$ releases a protein from synaptosomal plasma membranes. *J. Neurochem.,* in press.

Cassidy, P., Hoar, P.E. and Kerrick, W.G.L. (1979) Irreversible thiophosphorylation and activation of tension in functionally skinned rabbit ileum strips by $^{35}$S-ATPγS. *J. biol. Chem.,* 254: 11148–1153.

Gratecos, D. and Fischer, E.H. (1974) Adenosine 5'-*O* (3-thiotriphosphate) in the control of phosphorylase activity. *Biochem. biophys. Res. Commun.,* 58: 960–967.

Jolles, J., Zwiers, H., van Dongen, C., Schotman, P., Wirtz, K.W.A. and Gispen, W.H. (1980) Modulation of brain polyphosphoinositide metabolism by ACTH-sensitive protein phosphorylation. *Nature (Lond.),* 286: 623–625.

Jolles, J., Zwiers, H., Dekker, A., Wirtz, K.W.A. and Gispen, W.H. (1981) Corticotropin (1–24)-tetracosapeptide affects protein phosphorylation and polyphosphoinositide metabolism in rat brain. *Biochem. J.,* 194: 283–291.

Richards, J.M., Tierney, J.H. and Swislocki, N.I. (1981) ATP-dependent activation of adenylate cyclase. *J. biol. Chem.,* 256: 8889–8891.

Schleifer, L.S., Garrison, J.C., Sternweis, P.C., Northup, J.K. and Gilman, A.G. (1980) The regulatory component of adenylate cyclase from uncoupled S49 lymphoma cells differs in charge from the wild type protein. *J. biol. Chem.,* 255: 2641–2644.

Terenius, L. (1973) Stereospecific interaction between narcotic analgesics and a synaptic plasma fraction of rat cerebral cortex. *Acta pharmacol. Toxicol.,* 32: 317–320.

Whittemore, S.R., Lenox, R.H., Hendley, E.D. and Ehrlich, Y.H. (1981) Protein phosphorylation mediated effects of isoproterenol on adenylate cyclase activity in rat cortical membranes. *Neurochem. Res.,* 6: 775–785.

Wiegant, V.M., Zwiers, H., Schotman, P. and Gispen, W.H. (1978) Endogenous phosphorylation of rat brain synaptosomal plasma membranes in vitro: Some methodological aspects. *Neurochem. Res.,* 3: 443–453.

Wiegant, V.M., Dunn, A.J., Schotman, P. and Gispen, W.H. (1979) ACTH-like neurotropic peptides: possible regulators of rat brain cyclic AMP. *Brain Res.,* 168: 565–584.

Wiegant, V.M., Zwiers, H. and Gispen, W.H. (1981) Neuropeptides and brain cAMP and phosphoproteins. *Pharmacol. Ther.,* 12: 463–490.

404

Zwiers, H., Veldhuis, H.D., Schotman, P. and Gispen, W.H. (1976) ACTH, cyclic nucleotides, and brain protein phosphorylation in vitro. *Neurochem. Res.,* 1: 669–677.

Zwiers, H., Wiegant, V.M., Schotman, P. and Gispen, W.H. (1978) ACTH-induced inhibition of endogenous rat brain protein phosphorylation in vitro: structure–activity. *Neurochem. Res.,* 3: 455–463.

Zwiers, H., Tonnaer, J., Wiegant, V.M., Schotman, P. and Gispen, W.H. (1979) ACTH-sensitive protein kinase from rat brain membranes. *J. Neurochem.,* 33: 247–256.

Zwiers, H., Schotman, P. and Gispen, W.H. (1980) Purification and some characteristics of an ACTH-sensitive protein kinase and its substrate protein in rat brain membranes. *J. Neurochem.,* 34: 1689–1700.

# ACTH and Synaptic Membrane Phosphorylation in Rat Brain

H. ZWIERS, J. JOLLES, V.J. ALOYO, A.B. OESTREICHER and W.H. GISPEN

*Division of Molecular Neurobiology, Rudolf Magnus Institute for Pharmacology and Institute of Molecular Biology, State University of Utrecht, 8 Padualaan, 3508 TB Utrecht, The Netherlands*

## ACTH AND BRAIN FUNCTION

In the last decades it has become increasingly clear that adrenocorticotropic hormone (ACTH) influences the behavior of both animal and man by a direct action on the nervous system. De Wied and his co-workers demonstrated that the N-terminus of the polypeptide hormone is responsible for the behavioral activity. Fragments of that region possess full behavioral and neurophysiological activity but lack the classical endocrine effects of ACTH. The term "neuropeptides" was chosen to designate those peptides that act directly on the nervous system. In an attempt to formulate a unifying theory for the behavioral action of ACTH, Bohus and De Wied suggested that the peptide influences motivation or attention, resulting in improved performance in a variety of behavioral tests (Bohus and De Wied, 1980).

In view of the possible clinical relevance of ACTH and congeners, more knowledge is required on the neurochemical mechanism of action. It is possible that the peptide is a neurotransmitter in a peptidergic synapse. Firing of the presynaptic nerve cell would result in the release of ACTH in the synaptic cleft. However, at present there is insufficient experimental support for the hypothesis that ACTH acts as a classical neurotransmitter in the CNS. Currently, the influence of ACTH-like neuropeptides on brain neuronal activity is best formulated as neurohormonal or neuromodulatory (Gispen et al., 1979). When ACTH acts as a neurohormone it reaches its target in the brain via the liquor or blood circulation. An example of such a mode of action may be trophic influence of the peptide on nervous tissue. This influence is evidenced by an enhanced protein synthesis (Dunn and Schotman, 1981) and cell repair (Bijlsma et al., 1981). The neuromodulatory action of the peptide involves its release in the vicinity of the synaptic cleft, and the modulation of synaptic efficacy.

Recent research into the mechanism of action of ACTH-like neuropeptides has therefore focussed on the molecular events that are known to be crucial for membrane function.

## ACTH AND THE PHOSPHORYLATION OF SYNAPTIC MEMBRANE PROTEINS

Fragments of the synaptic plasma membrane are the richest known source of protein phosphorylating systems in mammalian tissues. This suggests that they may be involved in synaptic transmission. The hypothesis that a change in the state of phosphorylation of membrane protein may govern the ion permeability of the neural membrane, and thus may play a key role in determining the functional activity of the neuron has stimulated a great amount of

406

research. Originally, attention was focussed on the cyclic AMP (cAMP)-dependent phosphorylation. The cAMP-dependent phosphorylating system in synaptic membranes have been investigated in several laboratories and are discussed in great detail in several other chapters in this volume.

Other protein phosphorylating systems have been described in brain which are sensitive to $Ca^{2+}$ but not to cAMP (Rodnight, 1980). Synaptic plasma membranes contain the so-called B-50 protein (Fig. 1), which is an acceptor protein that is phosphorylated in a $Ca^{2+}$-sensitive and cAMP-insensitive way. The phosphorylation of this protein is sensitive to ACTH and some of its behaviorally active fragments. Extensive studies have been performed on the extraction of this protein and of its protein kinase from the synaptic membrane and its purification and characterization.

Treatment of SPM with 0.5% Triton X-100 in 75 mM KCl solubilized 15% of the total B-50 protein kinase activity and preserved the sensitivity of the enzyme to $ACTH_{1-24}$. Column chromatography of the solubilized material over DEAE-cellulose pointed to the presence of multiple protein kinase activities, one of which was the ACTH-sensitive B-50 protein kinase (Zwiers et al., 1979). The column fractions containing the B-50 protein kinase were subjected to ammonium sulfate precipitation and a protein fraction (57–82% ammonium sulfate)

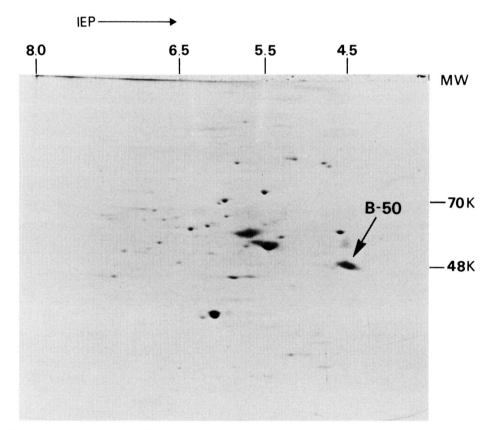

Fig. 1. Two-dimensional separation of synaptosomal plasma membrane proteins from rat brain cortex. Separation in the first dimension was performed with isoelectric focusing (pH 3–9) in polyacrylamide. The second dimension was a separation based on molecular weight in a SDS–polyacrylamide slab gel. B-50 appeared to be one of the most acidic proteins of SPM (IEP 4.5).

enriched in endogenous B-50 phosphorylation activity was obtained. The time course of the endogenous phosphorylation of B-50 in this fraction showed a linear incorporation with time for at least 10 min and a maximal incorporation of 0.65 mole P/mole B-50 was reached after 60 min. The inhibition of ACTH$_{1-24}$ of the protein kinase was dose-dependent; the half-maximal effective concentration $5 \times 10^{-6}$ M, being 10–20 times lower as compared to intact SPM. The B-50 protein kinase required both magnesium and calcium for optimal activity (Gispen et al., 1979; Zwiers et al., 1980a). After two-dimensional electrophoresis on polyacrylamide slab gels, the B-50 protein kinase and the B-50 protein could be further identified, purified and characterized. The isoelectric point (IEP) of the kinase in 5.5 and the apparent molecular weight 70 K, whereas the IEP of the substrate protein B-50 is 4.5 and the apparent molecular weight 48 K. Amino acid analysis on $\mu$g quantities of purified kinase and B-50 protein revealed basic/acid amino acid ratios in agreement with the respective IEPs (Zwiers et al., 1980a).

Although the B-50 protein band as separated on SDS–polyacrylamide gels consists of more than one protein as was seen after two-dimensional separation, the major component is the phosphoprotein B-50 (Fig. 1) (Zwiers et al., 1980a). Therefore, it was decided to try to raise antibodies to the protein B-50 using B-50 material isolated from rat brain SPM and separated in one dimension on SDS–polyacrylamide slab gels (Oestreicher et al., 1979, 1981). The presence of specific antibodies to B-50 in rabbit antiserum was demonstrated by an immuno-peroxide staining method. By use of this peroxidase–antiperoxidase (PAP) method, the immunohistochemical localization of B-50 was studied in sections of rat brain cerebellum and hippocampus. In agreement with the presumed synaptic origin of B-50, the antiserum reacted with tissue components in brain regions rich in synaptic contacts. In contrast, white matter and cell perikarya were virtually without immuno staining. The staining pattern was markedly similar to that found by others using synaptic antigens (Matus et al., 1976) and suggests that at the cellular level there is a restricted localization of the B-50 protein (i.e., synaptic region) but at the brain regional level the protein seems ubiquitous. In order to obtain insight in the question of whether the B-50 protein was specific for nervous tissue, we monitored the endogenous phosphorylation of proteins in three subcellular fractions ($1000 \times g$ and $150000 \times g$ supernatants; $150000 \times g$ pellet) obtained from seven different organs of the rat (brain, liver, lung, skeletal muscle, heart, spleen and adrenal cortex; Kristjansson et al., 1982). In agreement with Carstens and Weller (1979) the particulate fractions of brain displayed the highest phosphorylating activity. Furthermore, a relative enrichment of endogenous B-50 protein phosphorylation was observed when purified SPM was used. This observation is in line with previous studies indicating that in brain tissue the B-50 protein was mainly found in regions rich in synaptic projections (Oestreicher et al., 1981) and in the synaptic region predominantly in the presynaptic membranes (Sörensen et al., 1981). Endogenous phosphorylation of a 48 K protein, which could be inhibited by ACTH$_{1-24}$ was only observed in the $1000 \times g$ supernatant and the $150000 \times g$ particulate fraction from brain. The absence of a phosphorlated protein band with $M_r$ 48 K (B-50) in the other organs studied per se is not convincing evidence that indeed the phosphate acceptor protein was not present. For, in the absence of the corresponding protein kinase, no phosphorylation of B-50 would be measured despite the fact that B-50 itself was present in the fractions studied. Therefore, we focussed on two-dimensional separation and immunochemical identification of the B-50 protein itself. A two-dimensional separation technique consisting of IEF followed by SDS–PAGE rendered data suggesting that B-50 is only present in those fractions where endogenous phosphorylation of this protein was observed, e.g., subcellular fractions from brain containing particulate material ($1000 \times g$ supernatant, $150000 \times g$ pellet; Kristjansson et al., 1982).

408

To further substantiate this tentative conclusion that B-50 is exclusively localized in brain particulate material, gel sections containing SDS–PAGE separated proteins obtained from the various subcellular fractions were incubated with the antiserum to B-50. In agreement with our two-dimensional PAGE results, the immunochemical procedure did not demonstrate the presence of B-50 in cell fractions of organs other than the particulate fraction of brain tissue (Kristjansson et al., 1982).

We studied the regional distribution of endogenous B-50 phosphorylating activity in brain tissue under conditions that measured the initial reaction velocity (Wiegant et al., 1978). The data suggest that there are indeed differences in endogenous phosphorylation reaction velocity in different brain regions. The highest value was found in SPM from septal origin, the lowest in SPM from medulla spinalis. It is of interest that in SPM of septal origin $ACTH_{1-24}$ is more effective in inhibiting B-50 protein kinase as compared to SPM from total brain (Fig. 2). The

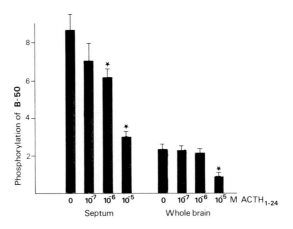

Fig. 2. Effect of $ACTH_{1-24}$ on phosphorylation of B-50 in SPM obtained from septum or from whole rat brain. Aliquots of 20 $\mu$g of SPM protein were phosphorylated in the presence of various concentrations of $ACTH_{1-24}$. Proteins were separated bt SDS–PAGE and the amount of $^{32}P$ incorporated into B-50 was determined by liquid scintillation counting. Incorporation is expressed as fmoles phosphate incorporated into B-50 per $\mu$g total SPM protein ($\pm$ S.E.M., $n = 4$). * Significantly different from control values.

septal area has previously been reported to be essential for the expression of some of the behavioral effects of ACTH-like peptides (Van Wimersma Greidanus et al., 1975). Also other studies point to a special relationship between ACTH and the septum: stereospecific uptake mechanism (Verhoef et al., 1977a,b); specific transport of pituitary ACTH into the septal complex (Mezey et al., 1978), ACTH containing nerve fiber projections (Krieger et al., 1980) and ACTH-induced increase in septal cAMP in vivo (Wiegant et al., 1979).

Thus, it may well be that the modulation of the degree of membrane phosphoprotein underlies some of the behavioral activities of ACTH. The specificity of the ACTH/B-50 protein kinase interaction being provided for by local delivery of peptidergic synapses in the brain.

SPECIFIC PROTEOLYTIC BREAKDOWN OF PROTEIN B-50

In the procedure to isolate and purifiy the ACTH-sensitive membrane B-50 substrate protein/protein kinase complex, dialysis of the protein fraction was one of the tools used. Davis and Ehrlich (1979) reported that after dialysis of SPM a general enhancement of endogenous protein phosphorylation could be observed. They suggested the presence of a dialysable phosphorylation inhibiting factor. Also, in our hands dialysis of the $ASP_{57-82}$ protein fraction led to a marked enhancement of — in this case — only the phosphorylation of the B-50 protein. As the effect of prior dialysis was evident at 3 different purification stages we could rule out that the enhancement was caused by the removal of certain ions such as NaCl or ammonium sulfate. Next, the dialysate of $ASP_{57-82}$ proteins obtained from 150 g rat brain tissue was lyophilized, resuspended in water and subjected to HPLC in a system developed to separate small molecular weight peptides (MW < 4000; Loeber et al., 1979). When tested in the endogenous phosphorylation assay only one peak displayed the inhibiting activity. Based on its sensitivity to pronase or acid hydrolysis and the nature of the separation system used, the factor was thought to be a small peptide. Indeed, amino acid analysis of the inhibiting fraction revealed the presence of a basic peptide of approximately 15 amino acids with a molecular weight in the order of 1650 (phosphorylation inhibiting peptide, PIP; Zwiers et al., 1980b). Furthermore, we reported preliminary evidence that during dialysis PIP occurred in the dialysate as the result of a specific proteolytic cleavage of the B-50 protein. In collaboration with the laboratory of Dr. Henry Mahler, we substantiated this working hypothesis that B-50 is subject to proteolysis yielding a small fragment PIP and a larger breakdown product B-60 (MW 46 K) (Zwiers et al., 1982). The ammonium sulfate precipitate containing the highest endogenous B-50 phosphorylating activity, also contains protease activity. When incubated in the absence of calcium a time-dependent decrease of the protein B-50 is observed with a concomi-

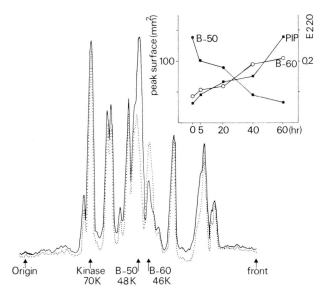

Fig. 3. Densitometric scans of Fast Green-stained protein profiles of $ASP_{57-82}$ proteins after SDS–polyacrylamide slab gel electrophoresis before (————) and after ( . . . . .) dialysis for 20 h at 4° C. Insert: Surface area of the peaks of B-50 and B-60 as a function of the dialysis time. The amount of PIP in the dialysate is indicated by the extinction at 220 nm of the PIP-containing fraction obtained by high pressure liquid chromatography.

tant appearance of phosphoprotein B-60 and PIP (Fig. 3). Addition of calcium and/or calmodulin enhances the protease activity whereas the substrate specificity is lost. Results of both isoelectric focussing and peptide mapping indicate that B-50 and B-60 are related proteins (Zwiers et al., 1982).

If this proteolysis is also taking place in vivo, this mechanism opens the possibility for specific proteolysis of B-50 in synaptic membranes, releasing a peptide (PIP) inhibiting the B-50 protein kinase and thus modulating the degree of B-50 phosphorylation.

## HOW DOES ACTH INHIBIT THE PHOSPHORYLATION OF B-50?

As is discussed elsewhere (Aloyo et al., this volume), there is good reason to suppose that the B-50 kinase first isolated by Zwiers et al. (1980a) is identical to the protein kinase C isolated by Nishizuka and co-workers (this volume). The apparent ubiquitous localization of the C kinase, the restricted localization of B-50 and the fact that the B-50 protein kinase co-purified with the B-50 protein, suggest that in brain part of the B-50 kinase forms a complex with its membrane substrate protein B-50. By what mechanisms is this membrane complex affected by ACTH? As reviewed by Witter (1980) there is little evidence so far pointing to classical binding sites as assessed by radioligand assays. In relatively high concentrations ACTH and related peptides may interfere with the specific binding of dihydromorphin and naloxone to opiate receptors in SPM obtained from rat brain (Terenius, 1975; Terenius et al., 1975; Gispen et al., 1976). As preincubation with naloxone did not counteract the effect of ACTH on B-50 kinase (Zwiers et al., 1981) but did so of that of met-enkephalin on the phosphorylation of a 50 K protein in subcellular fractions of hippocampal tissue (Bär et al., 1980), it was concluded that occupation of opiate receptors was not involved in B-50 kinase inhibition.

At present, not having brain ACTH receptors in hand, we are left with the working hypothesis that ACTH directly affects membrane properties (fluidity, see Herskowitz, this volume) and/or the B-50 protein kinase.

In a first attempt to approach this hypothesis experimentally, we noted that incubation of SPM with ACTH-like peptides, as performed when studying the effect of the peptide on the endogenous phosphorylation, results, in addition to the inhibition of the protein kinase, also in a release of a 41 K protein (Aloyo et al., 1982). Although the dose–response relationship for the release of the 41 K protein and the inhibition of the B-50 protein kinase by $ACTH_{1-24}$ (Zwiers et al., 1976) are in the same order of magnitude, the discrepancy between the structure–activity relationships for extraction of 41 K protein and inhibition of B-50 phosphorylation suggests that the two peptide effects are only remotely related. Thus, although removal of the 41 K band results in the reduction of endogenous B-50 phosphorylation, there are sequences of ACTH such as $(1–16)-NH_2$ which do not release the 41 K band but do inhibit the phosphorylation of B-50. Even more disconcerting is the lack of effect of the sequence (11–24) on the B-50 phosphorylation yet it strongly releases the 41 K band (Aloyo et al., 1982).

Preliminary evidence shows that the $ACTH_{1-24}$ cannot be removed from the 41 K protein indicating an interaction between the two polypeptides. Although we are not certain about the biological significance of the release of 41 K, it is of sufficient interest for further research in view of the lack of success of finding binding of labeled ACTH to brain membranes (Witter, 1980). Thus, although in the $ACTH_{1-24}$ extract the presence of the 41 K protein was observed, at present it would appear that the release of this band is not the sole explanation for the

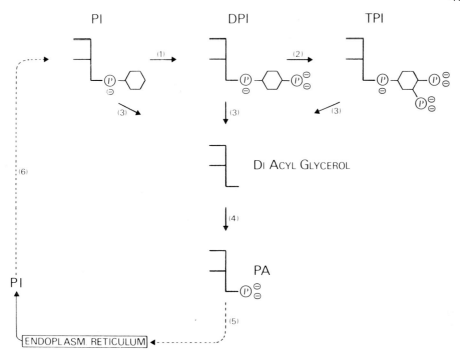

Fig. 4. Metabolism of polyphosphoinositides. Phosphatidyl-*myo*-inositol (PI) and its phosphorylated derivates phosphatidyl-*myo*-inositol 4-phosphate (DPI) and phosphatidyl-*myo*-inositol 4,5-diphosphate (TPI) are rapidly inter-converted by lipid kinases and/or phosphomonoesterases (1 and 2). A polyPI-specific phosphodiesterase can hydrolyse the phosphodiester linkage in a phospholipase C-type manner, thereby yielding 1,2-diacylglycerol (3). This substance is rapidly phosphorylated to phosphatidic acid (PA) (4). All these reactions take place at the plasma membrane. Resynthesis of PI from PA takes place in the endoplasmic reticulum, and the transport of the lipid between plasma membrane and intracellular membrane is performed by phospholipid-exchanging proteins.

inhibition of B-50 protein kinase. It is entirely possible that the interaction with the 41 K protein relates to other known chemical effects of ACTH in the brain.

## INOSITOL PHOSPHOLIPIDS AND THE METABOLISM OF $Ca^{2+}$ AT THE CELL MEMBRANE

Not only phosphoproteins, but also phospholipids are involved in processes that are crucial for synaptic membrane function. The inositol phospholipids (Fig. 4) are implicated in receptor activation, $Ca^{2+}$ entry through the membrane and membrane (de)polarization. The original interest in phosphatidylinositol (PI) arose from the observation that acetylcholine-treated pancreas showed a large increase in the incorporation of radioactive phosphate into phosphatidic acid (PA) and PI (Michell, 1975). It is now clear that the initial event in the so-called "PI response" is the breakdown of PI. The 1,2-diacylglycerol which is formed, is rapidly phosphorylated to PA. Because this structure is again the precursor of PI, the increase in [$^{32}$P]PA and [$^{32}$P]PI manifests a prior breakdown of PI. It has since been found that PI has a special role in the responses of cells to external stimuli such as hormones and neurotransmitters. It appears that the response can be elicited in virtually any type of cell.

By 1974 it was realized that the PI response is not evoked by stimuli that induce the intracellular production of cAMP. Instead, the stimuli that enhance the metabolism of PI have a mode of action on their target cells which involves $Ca^{2+}$ in some essential way. The hypothesis put forward by Michell (1975) states that PI breakdown precedes the influx of $Ca^{2+}$ into the cell, and that this PI response is the mechanism whereby receptor activation at the plasma membrane controls the influx of $Ca^{2+}$ into the cell.

Although at present it is not totally clear whether $Ca^{2+}$ influx is the cause or the consequence of the PI response, some link between both processes must exist (Michell and Kirk, 1981). Furthermore, $Ca^{2+}$ is involved in the metabolism of the so-called polyphosphoinositides (polyPI). Both phosphatidylinositol 4-phosphate (DPI) and phosphatidylinositol 4,5-diphosphate (TPI) bind $Ca^{2+}$ very avidly, and it has been proposed that they have an important role in the de- or hyperpolarization of the neuronal membrane (Torda, 1974). However, the experimental data on the involvement of DPI and TPI in cell membrane function have been ambiguous in view of the exceedingly rapid metabolism of these substances. It has only recently been found that the breakdown of DPI and TPI at the cytoplasmic side of the plasma membrane is accelerated by agents that induce an influx of $Ca^{2+}$ into the cell (e.g., muscarinic cholinergic or $\alpha$-adrenergic in rabbit iris muscle; the $Ca^{2+}$ ionophore A23187 in synaptosomes and in erythrocytes). It has been concluded from these studies that the breakdown of DPI and TPI is a consequence of the $Ca^{2+}$ influx.

These recent studies are interesting in yet another aspect: they reveal that a decrease in DPI/TPI is accompanied by an increase in PA. This may reflect the fact that breakdown of DPI and TPI results in the formation of diacylglycerol which is rapidly phosphorylated to PA. So the formation and the disappearance of the polyphosphoinositides may be different manifestations of the same phenomenon.


## ACTH AND THE METABOLISM OF THE INOSITOL PHOSPHOLIPIDS

There were several reasons why we have started to investigate the possible relationship between protein phosphorylation and polyPI metabolism. In the first place, as described above, both processes were thought to serve a similar physiological function; secondly, because the B-50 protein phosphorylation was critically dependent on the presence of $Ca^{2+}$, whereas this ion is also critically involved in the interconversion of the polyPI.

The first demonstration that ACTH affects brain polyPI metabolism was in prelabeled synaptosomes (Jolles et al., 1979). However, the experimental approach used prevented conclusions as to the molecular mechanism involved. We have therefore turned to the approach that has been used for many years in the study of protein phosphorylation: ATP was used as the phosphate precursor, and brain subcellular fractions were incubated under hypotonic conditions for very short incubation times (seconds). It was found that indeed the phosphorylation of proteins and lipids could be measured at the same moment (Jolles et al., 1981a). Moreover, very specific effects of ACTH were monitored: the peptide inhibited the formation of phosphoprotein and PA and stimulated the formation of TPI (Fig. 5). (Note this inverse relationship between PA and TPI which is also described in the preceding paragraph.)

With regard to the molecular mechanisms involved it appeared that ACTH acted on the kinases for both protein (Zwiers et al., 1978) and lipid (Jolles et al., 1981a), but not on the respective phosphatases. Furthermore, the ion $Ca^{2+}$ was of critical importance for both B-50 protein phosphorylation and TPI formation. These two processes were inversely related as B-50 phosphorylation was maximal in the presence of $Ca^{2+}$ whereas TPI formation was

413

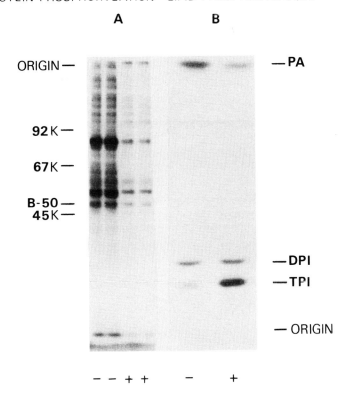

PROTEIN PHOSPHORYLATION   LIPID PHOSPHORYLATION

Fig. 5. Autoradiogram (A) after protein separation by polyacrylamide gel electrophoresis, showing the endogenous phosphorylation profile of the lysed P2 fraction obtained from the subcortical part of the rat brain tissue. The position of molecular weight marker proteins and of B-50 protein is indicated. Autoradiogram (B) after lipid extraction and thin layer chromatography. The position of the separated lipids is shown on the right. The absence (−) and presence (+) of 100 μM ACTH$_{1-24}$ in the incubations is indicated.

maximal in the absence of this ion. There were also other correlations between both processes. The dose–response relationship of ACTH was identical for the phosphorylation of the different membrane components. Furthermore, the same regions in the ACTH molecule were found to contain the site(s) that were important for B-50 phosphorylation, for TPI/PA formation and for behavioral activity in vivo (Zwiers et al., 1978; Gispen et al., 1979; Jolles et al., 1981b).

Taken together, the evidence provided in this paragraph suggested that a correlation might exist between B-50 protein phosphorylation and PA/TPI formation, and that in fact such a relationship might underly the mechanism of action of ACTH.

## WHAT IS THE RELATIONSHIP BETWEEN PROTEIN AND LIPID PHOSPHORYLATION?

The hypothesis that lipid and protein phosphorylation might have to do with each other was advanced by selectively extracting the protein kinase complex from the membrane and testing its ability to use exogenously added DPI as lipid substrate. Indeed, this purified enzyme

414

fraction containing the substrate protein (B-50) and its kinase was able to phosphorylate DPI to TPI (Jolles et al., 1980). The sensitivity to ACTH appeared similar to that obtained in intact membranes, and the degree of B-50 phosphorylation was a determining factor for TPI production (i.e., DPI kinase activity). This latter conclusion emerged from experiments in which the B-50 protein was prephosphorylated before the measurement of its DPI kinase activity. The amount of TPI formation decreased with the increasing amount of prephosphorylated B-50. We concluded that there may be one peptide-sensitive kinase complex that can act both as a lipid kinase and as a protein kinase (Jolles et al., 1980).

In view of the literature data that phosphorylation is a process which can regulate enzyme activity in general and protein kinase activity in particular (Krebs and Beavo, 1979), we have proposed the following working hypothesis: B-50 may be a regulating factor to or the regulatory subunit of the DPI kinase, the autophosphorylation of which determines the lipid kinase activity. ACTH interferes with the B-50 autophosphorylation and thereby activates the DPI kinase (Fig. 6). This explains why inhibited B-50 phosphorylation is always accompanied by stimulated TPI formation. The enzyme activation is possibly performed by dissociation of the holoenzyme.

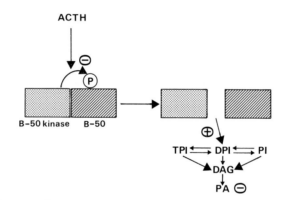

Fig. 6. Relationschip between ACTH-sensitive phosphorylation of protein and of lipid. In this working model B-50 in its phosphorylated form is bound to the B-50 kinase. By inhibiting the phosphorylation of B-50 ACTH induces the dissociation of the complex. The free B-50 acts as a modulator of the system that controls the phosphorylation state of the phosphoinositides.

It is of interest to note that the characteristics of the protein kinase used in our studies resemble those of the protein kinase which has been studied extensively at the Kobe University in Japan. These investigators described a multifunctional protein kinase in brain that was independent of cyclic nucleotides. Using histone as exogenous protein substrate they found that the kinase activity was absolutely dependent on the presence of $Ca^{2+}$ and 1,2-diacylglycerol (Kishimoto et al., 1980). Because diglyceride is the breakdown product of PI, this suggests that this kinase may have another importance function in the PI response (see also Nishizuka and Aloyo et al., both this volume).

Taken together, these and our own studies support the notion that protein phosphorylation and polyphosphoinositide metablism are related. Now what does this tell us about cell membrane functioning and about the response of the membrane to extracellular agents such as neuropeptides?

## PROTEIN PHOSPHORYLATION AND MEMBRANE FUNCTION

Protein phosphorylation was thought to be the final common pathway that mediates the effects of all intracellular second messengers. Upon phosphorylation, the protein conformation would alter, thereby opening or closing an ion pore and thus changing the membrane permeability (Greengard, 1978). Although the hypothesis that ion permeability is caused by protein phosphorylation is an attractive one, there is no conclusive evidence. It has been shown that isoproterenol (which causes an intracellular increase in cAMP) increases the influx of sodium ions into turkey erythrocytes, and also increases the phosphorylation of globin, a 230 K intrinsic protein of the plasma membrane (Alper et al., 1980). However, it is by no means clear whether protein phosphorylation is the result or the cause of the influx, or possibly only a correlate.

Therefore, another hypothesis was formulated that is in line with the experimental data discussed: protein phosphorylation, although a very important process, is not the final pathway. It is a link in a chain of events, and the metabolism of the phosphoinositides is another link. The phosphate acceptor protein may be (part of) a membrane enzyme which by reversible phosphorylation and dephosphorylation is converted from an active into an inactive state and vice versa (Fig. 6). Therefore, and in view of the data presented in the last paragraph, this hypothesis suggests that phosphorylation of a quantitatively minor membrane protein (e.g., B-50 protein) can bring about profound changes in membranes characteristics by changing the content of the phosphoinositides. The demonstration that ACTH influences this process provides experimental evidence for a modulatory role of this peptide in ongoing neurotransmission.

## ACKNOWLEDGEMENTS

The authors thank Jan Brakkee, Lia Claessens, Greet Hoekstra and Ed Kluis for their contributions to the content and for the prepration of this manuscript.

### REFERENCES

Aloyo, V.J., Zwiers, H. and Gispen, W.H. (1982) $ACTH_{1-24}$ releases a protein from synaptosomal plasma membranes. *J. Neurochem.*, 38: 871–875.

Alper, S.L., Beam, K.G. and Greengard, P. (1980) Hormonal control of $Na^+/K^+$ contransport in turkey erythrocytes. *J. biol. Chem.*, 255: 4864–4871.

Bär, P.R., Schotman, P. and Gispen, W.H. (1980) Enkephalins affect hippocampal membrane phosphorylation. *Eur. J. Pharmacol.*, 65: 165–174.

Bohus, B. and De Wied, D. (1980) Pituitary-adrenal system hormones and adaptive behavior. In *General, Comparative and Clinical Endocrinology of the Adrenal Cortex,* Vol. 3, I. Chester Jones and I.W. Henderson, (Eds.), Academic Press, New York, pp. 265–347.

Bijlsma, W.A., Jennekens, F.G.I., Schotman, P. and Gispen, W.H. (1981) Effects of corticotrophin (ACTH) on recovery of sensori-motor function in the rat: structure–activity study. *Eur. J. Pharmacol.*, 76, 73–79.

Carstens, M. and Weller, M. (1979) A comparison of the intrinsic protein kinase activities of membrane preparations from various tissues. *Biochem. biophys. Acta,* 551: 420–431.

Davis, L.G. and Ehrlich, Y.H. (1979) Opioid peptides and protein phosphorylation. *Adv. exp. Med. Biol.,* 116: 233–244.

Dunn, A.J. and Schotman, P. (1981) Effects of ACTH and related peptides on cerebral RNA and protein synthesis. *Pharmacol. Ther.,* 12: 353–372.

Gispen, W.H., Buitelaar, J., Wiegant, V.M., Terenius, L. and De Wied, D. (1976) Interaction between ACTH fragments, brain opiate receptors and morphine-induced analgesia. *Eur. J. Pharmacol.*, 39: 393–397.

Gispen, W.H., Zwiers, H., Wiegant, V.M., Schotman, P. and Wilson, J.E. (1979) The behaviorally active neuropeptide ACTH as neurohormone and neuromodulator: the role of cyclic nucleotides and membrane phosphoproteins. *Adv. exp. Med. Biol.*, 116: 199–224.

Greengard, P. (1978) Phosphorylated proteins as physiological effectors. Protein phosphorylation may be a final common pathway for many biological regulatory agents. *Science*, 199: 146–152.

Jolles, J., Wirtz, K.W.A., Schotman, P. and Gispen, W.H. (1979) Pituitary hormones influence polyphosphoinositide metabolism in rat brain. *FEBS Lett.*, 105: 110–114.

Jolles, J., Zwiers, H., Van Dongen, C., Schotman, P., Wirtz, K.W.A. and Gispen, W.H. (1980) Modulation of brain polyphosphoinositide metabolism by ACTH-sensitive protein phosphorylation. *Nature (Lond.)*, 286: 623–625.

Jolles, J., Zwiers, H., Dekker, A., Wirtz, K.W.A. and Gispen, W.H. (1981a) Corticotropin-(1–24)-tetracosapeptide affects protein phosphorylation and polyphosphoinositide metabolism in rat brain. *Biochem. J.*, 194: 283–291.

Jolles, J., Bär, P.R., Gispen, W.H. (1981b) Modulation of brain polyphosphoinositide metabolism of ACTH and $\beta$-endorphin: structure–activity studies. *Brain Res.*, in press.

Kishimoto, A., Takai, Y., Mori, T., Kikkawa, U. and Nishizuka, V. (1980) Activation of calcium and phospholipid-dependent protein kinase by diacylglycerol, its possible relation to phosphatidylinositol turnover. *J. biol. Chem.*, 255: 2273–2276.

Krebs, E.G. and Beavo, J.E. (1979) Phosphorylation–dephosphorylation of enzymes. *Annu. Rev. Biochem.*, 48: 923–961.

Krieger, D.T., Liotta, A.S., Browstein, M.J. and Zimmerman, E.A. (1980) ACTH, $\beta$-lipotropin and related peptides in brain, pituitary and blood. *Recent Progr. Horm. Res.*, 36: 272–344.

Kristjansson, G.I., Zwiers, H., Oestreicher, A.B. and Gispen, W.H. (1982) Evidence that the synaptic phosphoprotein B-50 is localized exclusively in nerve tissue. *J. Neurochem.*, in press.

Loeber, J.G., Verhoef, J., Burbach, J.P.H. and Witter, A. (1979) Combination of high pressure liquid chromatography and radioimmunoassay is a powerful tool for the specific and quantitative determination of endorphins and related peptides. *Biochem. biophys. Res. Commun.*, 86: 1288–1295.

Matus, A.I., Jones, D.H. and Mughal, S. (1976) Restricted distribution of synaptic antigens in the neuronal membrane. *Brain Res.*, 103: 171–175.

Mezey, E., Palkovits, M., De Kloet, E.R., Verhoef, J. and De Wied, D. (1978) Evidence for pituitary-brain transport of a behaviorally potent ACTH analog. *Life Sci.*, 22: 831–838.

Michell, R.H. (1975) Inositol phospholipids and cell surface receptor function. *Biochem. biophys. Acta*, 415: 81–148.

Michell, R.H. and Kirk, C.J. (1981) Why is phosphatidylinositol degraded in response to stimulation of certain receptors? *Trends phys. Sci.*, 2: 86–89.

Oestreicher, A.B., Zwiers, H., Schotman, P. and Gispen, W.H. (1979) Immunohistochemical studies of a phosphoprotein band (B-50) modulated in rat brain membranes by ACTH. In *Abstr. 7th Int. Meeting of the ISN*, p. 509.

Oestreicher, A.B., Zwiers, H., Schotman, P. and Gispen, W.H. (1981) Immunohistochemical localization of a phosphoprotein (B-50) isolated from rat brain synaptosomal plasma membranes. *Brain Res. Bull.*, 6: 145–153.

Rodnight, R. (1980) Cyclic nucleotides, calcium ions and protein phosphorylation in neurotransmission. In *Synaptic Constituents in Health and Disease*, M. Brzin, D. Sket and H. Bachelard (Eds.), Pergamon Press, London, pp. 81–96.

Sörensen, R.G., Kleine, L.P. and Mahler, H.R. (1981) Presynaptic localization of phosphoprotein B-50. *Brain Res. Bull.*, 7: 57–61.

Terenius, L. (1975) Effect of peptides and amino acids on dihydromorphine binding to the opiate receptor. *J. Pharm. Pharmacol.*, 27: 450–452.

Terenius, L., Gispen, W.H. and De Wied, D. (1975) ACTH-like peptides and opiate receptors in the rat brain: structure–activity studies. *Eur. J. Pharmacol.*, 33: 395–399.

Torda, C. (1974) Model of molecular mechanism able to generate a depolarization–hyperpolarization cycle. *Int. Rev. Neurobiol.*, 16: 1–66.

Van Wimersma Greidanus, Tj.B., Bohus, B. and De Wied, D. (1975) CNS sites of action of ACTH, MSH and vasopressin in relation to avoidance behavior. In *Anatomical Endocrinology*, W.E. Stumph and L.D. Grant (Eds.), Karger, Basel, pp. 284–289.

Verhoef, J., Palkovits, M. and Witter, A. (1977a) Distribution of behaviorally highly potent $ACTH_{4-9}$ analog in rat brain after intraventricular administration. *Brain Res.*, 126: 89–104.

Verhoef, J., Witter, A. and De Wied, D. (1977b) Specific uptake of a behaviorally potent $^3$H-ACTH$_{4-9}$ analog in the septal area after intraventricular injection in rats. *Brain Res.*, 131: 117–128.

Wiegant, V.M., Zwiers, H., Schotman, P. and Gispen, W.H. (1978) Endogenous phosphorylation of rat brain synaptosomal plasma membranes in vitro: Methodological aspects. *Neurochem. Res.*, 3: 443–453.

Wiegant, V.M., Dunn, A.J., Schotman, P. and Gispen, W.H. (1979) ACTH-like neurotropic peptides: possible regulators of rat brain cyclic AMP. *Brain Res.*, 168: 565–584.

Witter, A. (1980) On the presence of receptors for ACTH-neuropeptides in the brain. In *Receptors for Neurotransmitters and Peptide Hormones*, G.C. Pepeu, M. Kuhar and L. Enna (Eds.), Raven Press, New York, pp. 407–414.

Zwiers, H., Veldhuis, D., Schotman, P. and Gispen, (1976) ACTH, cyclic nucleotides and brain protein phosphorylation in vitro. *Neurochem. Res.*, 1: 669–677.

Zwiers, H., Wiegant, V.M. Schotman, P. and Gispen, W.H. (1978) ACTH-induced inhibition of endogenous rat brain protein phosphorylation in vitro: structure–activity. *Neurochem. Res.*, 3: 455–463.

Zwiers, H., Tonnaer, J., Wiegant, V.M., Schotman, P. and Gispen, W.H. (1979) ACTH-sensitive protein kinase from rat brain membranes. *J. Neurochem.*, 33: 247–256.

Zwiers, H., Schotman, P. and Gispen, W.H. (1980a) Purification and some characteristics of an ACTH-sensitive protein kinase and its substrate protein in rat brain membranes. *J. Neurochem.*, 34: 1689–1700.

Zwiers, H., Verhoef, J., Schotman, P. and Gispen, W.H. (1980b) A new phosphorylation-inhibiting peptide (PIP) with behavioral activity from rat brain membranes. *FEBS Lett.*, 112: 168–172.

Zwiers, H., Aloyo, V.J. and Gispen, W.H. (1981) Behavioral and neurochemical effects of the new opioid peptide dynorphin (1–13): comparison with other neuropeptides. *Life Sci.*, 28: 2545–2551.

Zwiers, H., Gispen, W.H., Kleine, L. and Mahler, H.R. (1982) Specific proteolysis of a brain membrane phosphoprotein (B-50): effects of calcium and calmodulin. *Neurochem. Res.*, 7: 127–137.

# The Modulation of Protein Phosphorylation and Receptor Binding in Synaptic Membranes by Changes in Lipid Fluidity: Implications for Ageing

MOSHE HERSHKOWITZ[1], DAVID HERON[1], DAVID SAMUEL[1] and MEIR SHINITZKY[2]

*Departments of [1]Isotope Research and [2]Membrane Research, The Weizmann Institute of Science, Rehovot 76100, Israel*

## 1. INTRODUCTION

Phosphorylation and dephosphorylation of membrane proteins are intermediate steps in signal transduction by hormones and neurotransmitters (Williams and Rodnight, 1977; Greengard, 1978; Zwiers et al., 1978). These processes are regulated by cyclic nucleotides (Routtenberg and Ehrlich, 1975; Greengard, 1976) and by ions (DeLorenzo, 1976; Hershkowitz, 1978; Schulman and Greengard, 1978), and are probably dependent on membrane dynamics.

Complex, sequential membranal events can be classified into two categories: active, metabolically driven, and passive. Active processes are characterized by energy consumption (e.g. ATP-linked) which can be blocked by metabolic poisons and low temperatures. These processes are long-term in nature and require a specific compartmental strucutre. Most of these processes are associated with the cytoskeletal network (Edelman, 1976; Nicolson, 1976). Passive processes, on the other hand, are directly related to diffusion (lateral, rotational or vertical) and are therefore largely determined by membrane lipid fluidity (Shinitzky and Henkart, 1979). These processes do not require metabolic energy and can proceed in isolated membranes. Alteration of membrane lipid fluidity can therefore passively and instantaneously modulate (Shinitzky, 1979) receptors (Heron et al., 1980a,b), antigens (Shinitzky and Souroujon, 1979) and enzymes (Sandermann, 1978). The following study describes the passive modulation of protein phosphorylation and receptor binding by in vitro or in vivo lipid manipulations.

## 2. MODULATION OF LIPID FLUIDITY IN CRUDE SYNAPTOSOMAL MEMBRANES ($P_2m$)

The main physiological determinant of membrane lipid fluidity is the cholesterol to phospholipid (C/PL) mole ratio (Cooper, 1978; Shinitzky and Henkart, 1979). This parameter can be modulated by membrane rigidification either in vivo or in vitro, with either cholesterol (Cooper et al., 1975), or hydrophilic cholesterol esters such as cholesteryl hemisuccinate (CHS) (Shinitzky et al., 1979), or fluidization with egg lecithin (Cooper et al., 1975; Heron et

420

al., 1980a). In this study we have used CHS and egg lecithin for membrane lipid manipulation.

The media for the lipid modulation were prepared as described (Heron et al., 1980a): cholesteryl hemisuccinate (CHS) was dissolved in hot glacial acetic acid (40 mg/ml). One volume of the hot solution was added with a preheated pipette into 100 vol. of a medium containing 3.5% polivinylpyrolidone, MW 40 000 (PVP), 50 mM Tris–HCl, pH 7.4, with vigorous stirring. The pH was then immediately readjusted to 7.4 with solid Tris free base. The resulting translucent syspension of CHS in 170 mM Tris–acetate buffer was then used for increasing the membrane lipid microviscosity ($\bar{\eta}$). Solution of crude egg lecithin (80 mg/ml) was prepared in a similar manner to form the corresponding medium, used for membrane fluidization. The PVP–lipid complexes are fine dispersions of small particles which act similarly to lipoproteins (Pal et al., 1981).

Membrane lipid microviscosity ($\bar{\eta}$, the reciprocal of fluidity), was determined by fluorescence depolarization of a lipid probe, 1,6-diphenyl-1,3,5-hexatriene (DPH), according to the method of Shinitzky and Barenholz (1978), as described by Heron et al. (1980a). Forebrains of male Wistar rats (2–3 months old) were used for $P_2m$ preparations according to Hofstein et al. (1980).

Lipid manipulation was carried out by incubation of 1 vol. of $P_2m$ suspension (2–4 mg protein/ml) with 1–10 vol. of the PVP–lipid dispersions (CHS or egg lecithin) for up to 2 h, with constant shaking at room temperature. The membranes were then washed twice with 50 mM Tris–HCl buffer pH 7.4. Measurements of $\bar{\eta}$ were carried out with samples containing about 40 $\mu$g protein suspended in 2 ml DPH dispersion in phosphate-buffered saline (PBS). In parallel, samples from the same membrane suspensions were used for protein phosphorylation and receptor-binding experiments (see below). A typical profile of the apparent $\bar{\eta}$ in the treated membranes as a function of the lipid concentrations is shown in Fig. 1. A wide range of $\bar{\eta}$ values could thus be obtained (between approximately 3 and 7 poise), in a reversible manner.

## 3. PROTEIN PHOSPHORYLATION AS A FUNCTION OF MEMBRANE LIPID FLUIDITY MANIPULATED IN VITRO

The apparent endogenous phosphorylation of membrane proteins is the net result of a series of processes: the hydrolysis of ATP by protein kinase, the effective encounters between the

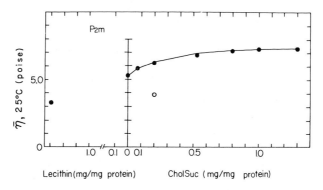

Fig. 1. The microviscosity ($\bar{\eta}$, 25°C, poise) of $P_2m$ after treatment with lipids at various concentrations ( ●——● ). Incubation of $P_2m$ with the lipids was carried out for 30 min at room temperature as described in the text. The open circle represents $\bar{\eta}$ of $P_2m$ treated initially with CHS (0.2 mg/mg protein), followed by a treatment with egg lecithin (1.3 mg/mg protein). Each experiment was repeated three times with similar results.

phosphorylated kinase and the target protein, the rate of phosphate transfer from the kinase to its target protein and the dephosphorylation by phosphatases (Rubin and Rosen, 1975). These processes can, in principle, be affected by the membrane lipid fluidity.

$P_2m$ samples of different membrane fluidity (see section 2) were phosphorylated for 30 sec with $[\gamma\text{-}^{32}P]ATP$ as described by Hershkowitz (1978) and Hofstein et al. (1980). The phosphorylated proteins were then analyzed by polyacrylamide gel electrophoresis, followed by autoradiography (Hofstein et al., 1980). The phosphorylation was quantitized by densitometry of the autoradiograms.

Fig. 2 presents the phosphorylation pattern of the $P_2m$ proteins at increasing $\bar\eta$ values. Several proteins seem to undergo phosphorylation, but are differently affected by the changes in lipid fluidity. This autoradiogram was further analyzed by densitometry as shown in Fig. 3. Good resolution was obtained for proteins A, B, C and 47 K (see Fig. 2) and the quantitative level of phosphorylation is shown separately for each protein in Fig. 4. The phosphorylation of proteins A and 47 K is changed to a lesser extent than the phosphorylation of proteins B and C which are markedly affected by the increase in $\bar\eta$ though the profiles of the changes are different. The phosphorylation of protein B is triphasic, namely a sharp increase upon a very small increase in $\bar\eta$, followed by a plateau and then another sharp increase. Band B, however, consists of at least two proteins (DeLorenzo, personal communication). On the other hand, the phosphorylation of protein C is a typical optimum curve, with an activity peak (when $\bar\eta$ is increased by about 15 %) which is about 5-fold compared to control (vehicle treated). This is

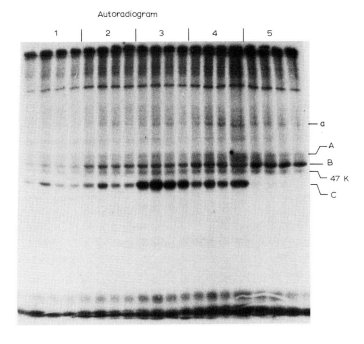

Fig. 2. Autoradiogram of $^{32}P$ incorporated into $P_2m$ proteins after various lipid treatments: 1, vehicle-treated (170 mM Tris–acetate buffer containing 3.5 % PVP, pH 7.4); 2, CHS (0.1 mg/mg protein); 3, CHS (0.2 mg/mg protein); 4, CHS (0.5 mg/mg protein); 5, CHS (0.8 mg/mg protein). The second column for each treatment represents phosphorylation in the presence of papaverin ($5 \cdot 10^{-4}$ M). The other columns represent triplicates of basal phosphorylation. Incubation of $P_2m$ with the lipid was carried out for 30 min at room temperature. Phosphorylation of $P_2m$ proteins was carried out for 30 sec at room temperature. For more details, see text. These experiments were repeated five times, with similar results.

422

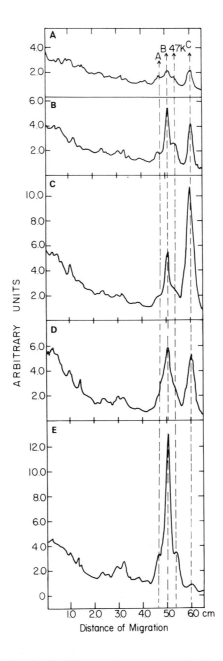

Fig. 3. Densitograms of the phosphorylated P₂m proteins presented in Fig. 2. Densitometry was performed with a Joyce–Loebel microdensitometer. A, B, C, D, E correspond to 1, 2, 3, 4, 5 in Fig. 2.

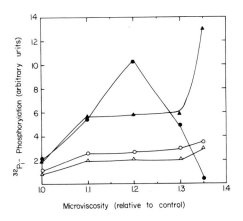

Fig. 4. The phosphorylation of $P_2m$ proteins as a function of the increased membrane microviscosity. The values were calculated from the areas under the appropriate peaks of the densitograms presented in Fig. 3. △--- -△ , protein A; ○——○, 47 K; ●——● , C; ▲——▲, B.

followed by a sharp decrease, down to zero phosphorylation, when $\eta$ is further increased (by about 40 %) by CHS treatment.

The changes in protein phosphorylation induced by an increase in $\eta$, can be reversed by membrane fluidization (i.e. decrease in $\eta$) with egg lecithin, as shown in Fig. 5. The increase in the phosphorylation of proteins B, C and 47 K (Fig. 5, lane 2) as a result of CHS treatment (about 15 % increase in $\eta$, which corresponds to the peak value in Fig. 4) is reversed by subsequent treatment with egg-lecithin (Fig. 5, lane 3) to a level similar to that of control (Fig. 5, lane 1). However, when membrane rigidification exceeds the peak value, subsequent treatment with egg lecithin causes further reduction in the phosphorylation of protein C (Fig. 6), indicating that an irreversible loss of activity had occurred.

In the presence of papaverin and cyclic AMP (cAMP), the phosphorylation of the various proteins was augmented (see Figs. 2 and 6) as expected (Hershkowitz, 1978). It is of interest that the level of augmentation by cAMP and papaverin was not affected by the various lipid treatments (see Fig. 2). This suggests that these phosphorylation stimulants affect a step in the process of phosphorylation which is independent of lipid fluidity.

The positional features of proteins a, B, C and 47 K in the membrane were tested by phosphorylation after treatment with high salt (0.6 M KCl), or with non-ionic detergent (0.5 % Triton X-100). Neither of these treatments affected the basal or the cAMP-stimulated phosphorylation. Protein A, on the other hand, could be eliminated from the membrane with 0.5 % Triton X-100. These results indicate that all five heavily phosphorylated proteins are integral membrane proteins and that protein A has a weaker association with the membrane.

The phosphorylation of proteins a and A, which are designated by others as I and II, is cAMP-dependent (Ueda et al., 1973). Protein 47 K is probably identical to protein 48 K, and its phosphorylation can be inhibited by ACTH (Zwiers et al., 1978). The phosphorylation of protein C is implicated in a series of physiological functions, such as release of neurotransmitters (Hershkowitz, 1978), electrical stimulation (Browning et al., 1979), cell energetics (Magilen et al., 1981) and calcium transport (Browning et al., 1981).

In general two main kinetic parameters may be affected by changes in membrane lipid fluidity. The degree of exposure of integral membrane proteins may be increased upon an increase in $\eta$, due to vertical displacement (Bochorov and Shinitzky, 1976; Shinitzky, 1979).

424

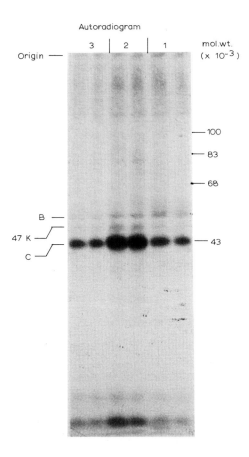

Fig. 5. Autoradiogram of $^{32}$P incorporated into the $P_2$m proteins preincubated as follows: 1, with the PVP medium only; 2, with CHS (0.24 mg/mg protein) for 30 min; 3, with CHS (0.24 mg/mg protein) followed by lecithin (1.3 mg/mg protein), 30 min for each treatment. Markers for molecular weights are phosphorylase A, lactoperoxidase, bovine serum albumin and ovalbumin.

Therefore, the available fraction of protein kinase to the ATP, as well as the availability of the target proteins to transphosphorylation are expected to increase with $\bar{\eta}$. On the other hand, the increase in $\bar{\eta}$ will concomitantly reduce the turnover of enzymatic processes (Gavish and Werber, 1979), as well as the rates of lateral encounters (Hanski et al., 1979) which determine the rate constant for transphosphorylation. Therefore, the net effect of membrane lipid fluidity on complex processes such as protein phosphorylation may adopt a bell-shaped curve with a specific optimal fluidity, typical for each system (Yuli et al., 1981; Shinitzky, 1979). In case of irreversible loss of activity at high $\bar{\eta}$ values (e.g. due to protein shedding, see Heron et al., 1980b, 1981; Muller and Shinitzky, 1981), the descending phase of the bell-shaped curve will become apparently steeper. The data presented for the phosphorylation of protein C fit this model (see Fig. 4). The phosphorylation profiles of the other proteins presented in Fig. 4, are presumably the result of even more complicated processes, yet all of the proteins exhibit an appreciable increase in the phosphorylation, with the slight initial increase in $\bar{\eta}$.

Transient changes in membrane fluidity similar in magnitude to those applied in this study (about $\pm 10\%$) are physiologically relevant. Such changes in membrane fluidity were ob-

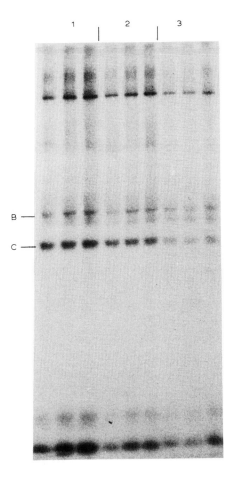

Fig. 6. Autoradiogram of $^{32}$P incorporated into the P$_2$m proteins preincubated as follows: 1, with the PVP medium only; 2, with CHS (0.5 mg/mg protein) for 60 min; 3, with CHS (0.5 mg/mg protein) followed by lecithin (1.3 mg/mg protein), 60 min for each treatment.

served upon the creation of transmembrane electrical potential (Corda et al., 1981; George-scauld and Duclohier, 1978), small changes in pH (Schachter and Shinitzky, 1977), calcium binding (Jacobson and Papahadjopoulos, 1975), specific binding of hormones (Luly and Shinitzky, 1979) and neurotransmitters (Schneeweiss et al., 1979; Rosenberg, 1977) and transmethylation of phospholipids (Hirata and Axelrod, 1978). The temporal change in lipid fluidity can thus regulate synaptic transmission processes.

Longer term changes in lipid fluidity are generally cumulative and progressive, and, beyond a certain threshold, are irreversible. Such changes may take place during cell growth (Muller et al., 1980) cellular differentiation (Arndt-Jovin et al., 1976; DeLaat et al., 1978; Ip and Cooper, 1980), and certain clinical disorders such as hypertension (Montenay-Garestier et al., 1981), cirrhosis (Cooper et al., 1975), chronic alcoholism (Johnson et al., 1979; Chin et al., 1978), morphine addiction (Heron et al., 1982) and ageing (Heron et al., 1980a; Rivnay et al., 1979; Rouser et al., 1972).

Protein phosphorylation is the terminal step in cyclic nucleotide-mediated processes

(Greengard, 1978; Williams and Rodnight, 1977). It is also involved in ion transport (Rudolf and Greengard, 1974), calcium uptake (Weller and Morgan, 1977), neurotransmitter release (DeLorenzo, 1976 Hershkowitz, 1978; Sieghart et al., 1979; Michaelson and Avissar, 1979), acetylcholine receptor modulation (Teichberg et al., 1977; Gordon et al., 1977), signal transduction by peptides (Zwiers et al., 1978; Bär et al., 1980), enzyme regulation (Magilen et al., 1981), and bioelectrical activity (Browning et al., 1979). The phosphorylation of protein C in particular has been shown to be involved in most of these processes (Hershkowitz, 1978; (Browning et al., 1979, 1981; Magilen et al., 1981). The sensitivity of the phosphorylation of protein C to small changes in lipid fluidity could thus be expressed in these physiological processes. It is of interest that the modulation of protein C phosphorylation by calcium and papaverin (Hershkowitz, 1978) is smaller than that induced by changes in lipid fluidity.

## 4. RECEPTOR BINDING AND LIPID FLUIDITY

Receptors, like other membrane-bound proteins, can be freely diffusible entities or anchored to the cytoskeletal network. Again, it is to be expected that lipid fluidity will affect the freely diffusible receptors selectively. The formation of ligand–receptor complexes depends on the affinity between the two and the accessibility of the receptor-binding sites. Both of these parameters can be affected by lipid fluidity in freely diffusible receptors (Heron et al., 1980a,b, 1981; Shinitzky, 1979). The constraints imposed on the receptor by the surrounding lipids can induce subtle conformational changes in the binding sites which, in turn, can effect its affinity. The accessibility of receptors to their ligands can be modulated by changes in lipid fluidity due to vertical displacement (Heron et al., 1980a,b; Borochov and Shinitzky, 1976; Shinitzky, 1979). This parameter can be resolved under saturation conditions.

The binding capacity of various receptors were tested as a function of lipid fluidity, in crude membrane preparation obtained from the mouse forebrain. $\beta$-Adrenergic receptor binding was assayed essentially according to Uprichard et al. (1978), using [$^3$H]dihydroalprenolol (DHA). Serotonin and opiate receptor binding were assayed as previously described (Heron et al., 1980a,b) using [$^3$H]serotonin and [$^3$H]naloxone, respectively. Diazepam receptor was assayed with [$^3$H]flunitrazepam as previously described (Grimm and Hershkowitz, 1981) and the muscarinic receptor was assayed using [$^3$H]quinoclidinyl-benzilate (QNB), essentially as described by Yamamura and Snyder (1974). Lipid manipulations and measurements of membrane lipid microviscosity ($\bar{\eta}$), were carried out as described in section 2. Ligand-binding assays were carried out at saturation concentrations.

Fig. 7 summarizes the specific binding profiles as a function of $\bar{\eta}$, for all five receptors. It can be clearly seen that while the ligand binding to the muscarinic and diazepam receptors remains practically unaffected, the ligand binding to the $\beta$-adrenergic, serotonin and opiate receptors is markedly affected by changes in lipid fluidity. The binding to this latter group of receptors decreases upon membrane fluidization, presumably due to the masking of their binding sites by membrane lipids. Increase in $\bar{\eta}$, on the other hand, augments the binding to all the three receptors, but to different extents. Thus an increase of about 30 % in $\bar{\eta}$ causes a 2-fold increase in opiate binding, a 3-fold increase in serotonin binding and a 15-fold increase in $\beta$-adrenergic binding. At higher $\bar{\eta}$ values the opiate and serotonin binding reach a maximum at $\bar{\eta} = 135$ % and $\bar{\eta} = 175$ %, respectively. The apparent decrease in the binding beyond these peaks, is attributed to shedding of the receptors from the membrane (Heron et al., 1980a,b, 1981). This is supported by the fact that only up to the peaks, the changes in binding by lipid manipulations could be reversed (Heron et al., 1980a,b, 1981). Preliminary data also indicate

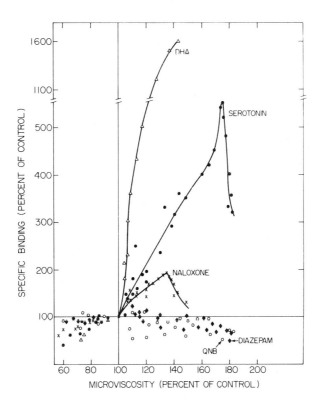

Fig. 7. The specific binding at saturation of [³H]DHA (8 nM), [³H]serotonin (4 nM), [³H]naloxone (2 nM), [³H]QNB (1 nM) and [³H]flunitrazepam (1 nM) to crude mouse forebrain membrane at varying microviscosity ($\bar{\eta}$). The values of the control samples were: $\bar{\eta} = 5.3 \pm 0.2$ (poise, 25°C) and specific binding of [³H]DHA = 11.5 ± 2.0 pmoles/g wet weight tissue, [³H]serotonin = 2.5 ± 0.5 pmoles/g, [³H]naloxone = 4.5 ± 1.0 pmoles/g, [³H]QNB = 15.0 ± 3.0 pmoles/g, [³H]flunitrazepam = 30 ± 5 pmoles/g. Measurements of $\bar{\eta}$ were carried out in duplicate. Binding assays were carried out in triplicate with the labeled ligand only and in triplicate with the unlabeled ligands, $10^{-4}$ M propranolol, $10^{-5}$ M serotonin, $10^{-5}$ M morphine, $10^{-4}$ M atropine, or $10^{-5}$ M diazepam. At least three experiments were carried out with each ligand. Displacement with other ligands was carried out in order to confirm specificity.

that the missing specific binding beyond the peak value could be quantitatively detected in the supernatant.

These results indicate that under normal physiological conditions, only a fraction of the opiate, serotonin and $\beta$-adrenergic receptors are available for ligand binding, while the rest are burried and therefore may function as a reservoir. This reservoir may be available for immediate recruitment, during fluctuating physiological or environmental conditions, such as in supersensitivity. It is suggested that the muscarinic and diazepam receptors are less diffusible than the other three receptors, and are presumably associated with the cytoskeletal network.

Under adverse hyperlipidemic conditions where membrane microviscosity is increased, overexposure of membrane proteins can result in an irreversible loss of function due to shedding or enzymatic degradation (Heron et al., 1980a,b, 1981). Such processes are pertinent to ageing in its advanced stages.

428

## 5. PROTEIN PHOSPHORYLATION AND RECEPTOR BINDING IN BRAINS OF SENESCENT MICE

It is well documented that during ageing, there is a marked increase in C/PL mole ratio, in the sphingomyelin content in various tissues and in particular, in the brain (Rouser et al., 1972). These changes in lipid composition render the membranes more viscous (Heron et al., 1980a,b; Rivnay et al., 1979). In line with the results obtained after in vitro lipid manipulation presented in the previous sections, it was to be expected that the changes in receptor binding and protein phosphorylation in the brain of old mice would correspond to the changes predicted by the in vitro studies.

Young adult (2–3 months) and old (24–27 months) male Eb/Bl mice were used in all experiments. The membrane preparation used in this study was synaptic plasma membranes (SPM), obtained from the forebrain, according to Jones ánd Matus (1974). All other procedures were carried out as described in the previous sections.

The microviscosities (at 25°C) of SPM which were used in the phosphorylation and receptor-binding experiment were $5.4 \pm 0.2$ and $7.2 \pm 0.5$ poise for the young and old mice, respectively.

Fig. 8 presents the basal endogenous phosphorylation patterns of the phosphoroproteins in SPM of young (Y) and old (OC) mice. Except for protein 47 K, no appreciable difference in the phosphorylation patterns could be observed. The phosphorylation of the 47 K protein is significantly higher (about 2-fold) in old as compared to young. In the presence of 8-bromo-cAMP (Fig. 9), the protein phosphorylation was markedly augmented (up to 2-fold) only in young animals, with no significant effect in old ones.

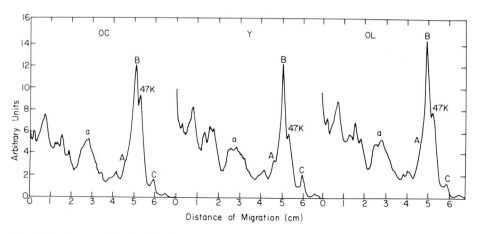

Fig. 8. Densitograms of the phosphorylated proteins in SPM from forebrain of 3-month- (Y) and 26-month-old mice (OC), as well as 26-month-old mice treated with the active lipids AL (OL). For details, see text.

The lack of response to cAMP stimulation in old mice could not originate from an increase in the activity of phosphodiesterase, since in our assays we used the analog 8-bromo-cAMP which freely permeates the lipid bilayer and is resistant to hydrolysis by phosphodiesterase. Thus, the failure of cAMP stimulation in old mice could stem from a reduction in the affinity between cAMP and the kinase regulatory subunit. It is more likely, however, that it is due to increased restriction by membrane lipids of the dissociation between the bound regulatory and

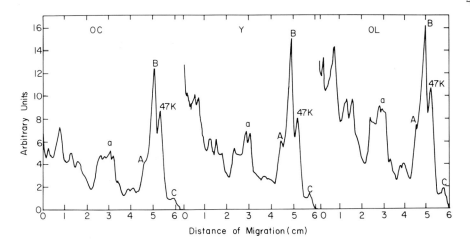

Fig. 9. Densitograms of the phosphorylated proteins in SPM in the presence of $10^{-6}$ M 8-bromo-cAMP. Details are given in the legend to Fig. 8 and in the text.

the catalytic subunits which is a prerequisite for further transphosphorylation. In the cascade of membranal events, which are triggered by hormones and neurotransmitters, phosphorylation step plays a prominent role. When phosphorylation is impaired, as in ageing, its rate constant may be reduced to a level which is rate-limiting.

The serotonin receptor was selected as a representative example of receptor modulation in ageing. The basal binding of serotonin to SPM from old mice was about 50 % higher than that to SPM from young ones in agreement with values for human brain by Shih and Young (1978). However, when the membranes were rigidified in vitro with CHS, the binding of serotonin

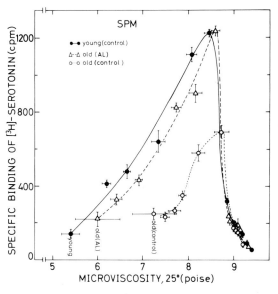

Fig. 10. The specific binding of [³H]serotonin to SPM from forebrains of 3-month-old mice, 26-month-old untreated mice, and 26-month-old mice fed with the active lipids (AL), as a function of increasing concentrations of CHS. See legend to Fig. 7.

increased to a peak of about 7-fold in young mice with only a 3-fold increase in old ones. The profiles of serotonin binding vs. $\eta$ were similar to those obtained for $P_2m$ (see Fig. 7). These results indicate that the total binding capacity stored in the membrane in young mice is about double that in old animals.

Scatchard analyses of serotonin binding in SPM from young mice indicate the presence of high- and low-affinity sites (data not shown), as has been previously reported (Heron et al., 1980a,b). In SPM from old mice only low-affinity sites could be detected, similar to the trend observed upon in vitro rigidification (Heron et al., 1980a).

Ageing is characterized by the loss of ability to maintain homeostasis, especially under stress (Adelman, 1975; Finch et al., 1969; Gregerman and Bierman, 1974). For example, it has been shown that in aged rats, the density of $\beta$-adrenergic receptors could not be increased in response to various stimuli (Greenberg and Weiss, 1978, 1979). This could be accounted for by the decrease in the number of hidden receptors in the membrane, as demonstrated here for serotonin receptors (Fig. 10). Consequently, in aged tissue, the plasticity based on the capacity for adaptive receptor modulation in response to fluctuating physiological or environmental conditions is suppressed. Under resting conditions, the differences between young and old are not so obvious. However, on imposing a challenge which perturbs the system, the differences in plasticity become apparent. It has been shown, for example, that in aged rats there is impaired synaptic potentiation upon repetitive electrical stimulation (Landfiels and Lynch, 1977; Landfield et al., 1978). Thus, cAMP-stimulated protein phosphorylation is much more in the young mice as compared to old. Similarly, CHS could unmask many more receptors in the SPM from young as compared to old mice.

We suggest that changes of this sort may occur in vivo during ageing, and stem from an impaired "homeoviscous adaptation" mechanism (Sinensky, 1974, 1980; Cossins et al., 1978). This fundamental mechanism, which is responsible for maintaining a constant membrane lipid fluidity, has been shown to operate under various conditions of stress such as in alcoholism (Johnson et al., 1979; Chin et al., 1978), through adjustments of membrane lipid composition (Hazel and Prosser, 1974). In ageing, where the membrane is rigidified by an increase in cholesterol and sphingomyelin, the rate of lipid adjustment is presumably too slow to cope fully with the rate of accumulation of cholesterol and sphingomyelin. Up to a certain stage, external intervention with potent membrane-fluidizing lipids could restore the proper membrane fluidity, and consequently functional plasticity will be regained. Such an approach is described in the next section.

## 6. REVERSAL OF MEMBRANE PROPERTIES IN SENESCENT MICE BY DIETARY "ACTIVE LIPIDS"

As outlined above, membrane hyperviscosity is implicated in the etiology of many disorders which are relevant to ageing. Based on this assumption, membrane fluidization both *in vitro* and *in vivo* was attempted with various preparations of egg-lecithin (phosphatidylcholine, PC). Three sources were tested: (1) Grade I (+ 99%) egg PC from "Lipid-Products", Nutfield, England. (2) Crude egg-lecithin grade II, type IX ($\sim$ 60% PC) from Sigma (St. Louis, MO). (3) "Active-lipid" (AL), a special lipid mixture from egg-yolk where the active ingredients are phospholipids, mainly PC, from "AL Laboratories", P.O. Box 1215, Ojai, 93023, California. Substantial membrane fluidization of various tissues in both *in vitro* and *in vivo* experiments was achieved only with AL. It can operate by several mechanisms, such as extraction of excess cholesterol by passive translocation (Cooper, 1978), by direct incorporation (Bakaradjieva et al., 1979) or by exchange with membrane lipids of higher microviscosity (Wirtz and Zilversmith, 1968). When AL was tested for membrane fluidization in vitro, with erythrocytes or lymphocytes, it was found to be much more effective than pure egg lecithin (to be published).

Young and old mice (see section 5) were fed with a 5 % mixture of AL in rat purina chow for 10–20 days. The food was freshly prepared each day by mixing an alcoholic solution of AL with ground purina chow, followed by thorough drying. Each animal received on the average 250 mg AL per day per os. Control groups were fed in a similar manner, but without the AL supplement. The animals were then sacrificed and SPM were isolated and assayed as described in the previous sections.

The lipid microviscosity of the SPM from the old mice treated with AL was $\bar{\eta}_{25°C} = 6.0 \pm 0.5$ poise, which is considerably lower than that of the untreated (control) old mice ($\bar{\eta}_{25°C} = 7.2 \pm 0.5$ poise) and only slightly above that of young mice ($\bar{\eta}_{25°C} = 5.4 \pm 0.2$ poise). At the same time fluidization of the hyperviscous SPM by AL restored the phosphorylation patterns under cAMP stimulation completely (see Fig. 9). In addition, the profile of serotonin binding was almost completely restored to the level for young mice (see Fig. 10) and the high-affinity binding sites reappeared (data not shown). It is interesting to note that treatment of young mice with AL has no apparent effect on either membrane fluidity, protein phosphorylation or serotonin binding. Presumably, restoration of membrane lipid fluidity in old mice shifts the equilibrium position of the receptors to their original state, where they are less vulnerable to degradation or shedding (Heron et al., 1980a,b, 1981). Restored membrane dynamics may also be responsible for the recovery of cAMP-stimulated phosphorylation. It is hoped that these results may afford a new approach for the treatment of impaired brain functions associated with ageing. Further experiments along this line are now in progress.

## SUMMARY

In this study protein phosphorylation and receptor binding were markedly modulated by lipid manipulations in vitro, which alter brain membrane fluidity in a reversible manner. In the ageing brain, where membrane lipid composition is altered, synaptic plasma membranes become hyperviscous, which modulates both protein phosphorylation and receptor binding. These changes were reversed by a diet supplemented with "active lipid" (AL), which is highly effective in membrane fluidization, both in vitro and in vivo. A new approach for the treatment of various behavioral symptoms of senescence in suggested.

## ACKNOWLEDGEMENT

The skilful technical assistance of Mali Israeli and Rachel Haimovich is gratefully acknowledged.

### REFERENCES

Adelman, R.C. (1975) Impaired hormonal regulation of enzyme activity during ageing. Fed. Proc., 34(2): 179.
Arndt-Jovin, D.J., Ostertag, W., Eisen, H., Klimek, F. and Jovin, T. (1976) Studies of cellular differentiation by automated cell separation: Two model systems — Friend virus-transformed cells and hydra attenuata. J. Histochem. Cytochem., 24: 332–350.
Bakardjieva, A., Galla, H.J. and Helmreich, E.J.M. (1979) Modulation of $\beta$-receptor adenylate cyclase interactions in cultured Chang liver cells by phospholipid enrichment. Biochemistry, 18: 3016–3023.

432

Bär, H.P., Schotman, P. and Gispen, W.H. (1980) Enkephalins affect hippocampal membrane phosphorylation. *Eur. J. Pharmacol.*, 65: 165–174.

Borochov, H. and Shinitzky, M. (1976) Vertical displacement of membrane proteins mediated by changes in microviscosity. *Proc. nat. Acad. Sci. (Wash.)*, 73: 4526–4530.

Browning, M., Bennett, W. and Lynch, G. (1979) Phosphorylase kinase phosphorylates a brain protein which is influenced by repetitive synaptic activation. *Nature (Lond.)*, 278: 273–275.

Browning, M., Baudry, M., Bennett, W.F. and Lynch, G. (1981) Phosphorylation-mediated changes in pyruvate dehydrogenase activity influence pyruvate-supported calcium accumulation by brain mitochondria. *J. Neurochem.*, 36: 1932–1940.

Chin, J.H., Parsons, L.M. and Goldstein, D.B. (1978) Increased cholesterol content of erythrocyte and brain membranes in ethanol-tolerant mice. *Biochim. biophys. Acta*, 513: 358–363.

Cooper, R.A. (1978) Influence of increased membrane cholesterol on membrane fluidity and cell function in human red blood cells. *J. supramol. Struct.*, 8: 413–430.

Cooper, R.A., Arner, C.E., Wiley, J.S. and Shattil, S.J. (1975) Modification of red cell membrane structure by cholesterol-rich lipid dispersions. *J. clin. Invest.*, 55: 115–126.

Corda, D., Pasternak, C. and Shinitzky, M. (1981) Increase in lipid microviscosity of unilamellar vesicles upon the creation of transmembrane potential. *J. Membrane Biol.*, 65: 235–242.

Cossins, A.R., Christiansen, J. and Prosser, C.L. (1978) Adaptation of biological membranes to temperature. *Biochim. biophys. Acta*, 511: 442–454.

DeLaat, S.W., van der Saag, P.T., Neleman, S.A. and Shinitzky, M. (1978) Microviscosity changes during differentiation of neuroblastoma cells. *Biochim. biophys. Acta*, 509: 188–193.

DeLorenzo, R.J. (1976) Calcium-dependent phosphorylation of specific synaptosomal fraction proteins: Possible role of phosphoproteins in mediating neurotransmitter release. *Biochem. biophys. Res. Commun.*, 71: 590–597.

Edelman, G.M. (1976) Surface modulation in cell recognition and cell growth. *Science*, 192: 218–226.

Finch, C.E., Foster, J.R. and Mirsky, A.E. (1969) Ageing and the regulation of cell activities during exposure to cold. *J. gen. Physiol.*, 54: 690–712.

Gavish, B. and Werber, M.M. (1979) Viscosity-dependent structural fluctuations in enzyme catalysis. *Biochemistry*, 18: 1269–1275.

Georgescauld, D. and Duclohier, A. (1978) Transient fluorescence signals from pyrene labelled pike nerves during action potential: Possible implication for membrane fluidity changes. *Biochem. biophys. Res. Commun.*, 85: 1186–1191.

Gordon, A.S., Davis, C.G. and Diamond, I. (1977) Phosphorylation of membrane proteins at a cholinergic synapse. *Proc. nat. Acad. Sci. (Wash.)*, 74: 263–267.

Greenberg, L.H. and Weiss, B. (1978) β-Adrenergic receptors in aged rat brain: Reduced number and capacity of pineal gland to develop supersensitivity. *Science*, 201: 61–63.

Greenberg, L.H. and Weiss, B. (1979) Ability of aged rats to alter beta-adrenergic receptors of brain in response to repeated administration of reserpine and desmethylimipramine. *J. Pharmacol. exp. Ther.*, 211: 309–316.

Greengard, P. (1976) Possible role for cyclic nucleotides and phosphorylated membrane proteins in post-synaptic actions of neurotransmitters. *Nature (Lond.)*, 260: 101–108.

Greengard, P. (1978) Phosphorylated proteins as physiological effectors. *Science*, 199: 146–152.

Gregerman, R.I. and Bierman, E.L. (1974) Ageing and hormones. In *Textbook of Endocrinology*, R.H. Williams (Ed.), W.B. Saunders, Philadelphia, PA, pp. 1059–1070.

Grimm, V.E. and Hershkowitz, M. (1981) The effect of chronic diazepam treatment on discrimination performance and $^3$H-flunitrazepam binding in the brains of shocked and non-shocked rats. *Psychopharmacology*, 74: 132–136.

Hanski, E., Rimon, G. and Levitzki, A. (1979) Adenylate cyclase activation by the β-adrenergic receptors as a diffusion-controlled process. *Biochemistry*, 18: 846–853.

Hazel, J.R. and Prosser, C.L. (1974) Molecular mechanisms of temperature compensation in poikilotherms. *Physiol. Rev.*, 54: 620–677.

Heron, D., Shinitzky, M., Hershkowitz, M. and Samuel, D. (1980a) Lipid fluidity markedly modulates the binding of serotonin to mouse brain membrane. *Proc. nat. Acad. Sci. (Wash.)*, 77: 7463–7467.

Heron, D., Hershkowitz, M., Shinitzky, M. and Samuel, D. (1980b) The lipid fluidity of synaptic membranes and the binding of serotonin and opiate ligands. In *Neurotransmitters and their Receptors*, U.Z. Littauer, Y. Dudai, I. Silman, V.I. Teichberg and Z. Vogel (Eds.), John Wiley, New York, pp. 125–138.

Heron, D., Israeli, M., Hershkowitz, M., Shinitzky, M. and Samuel, D. (1981) Lipid-induced modulation of opiate receptors in mouse brain membranes. *Eur. J. Pharmacol.*, 72: 361–364.

Heron, D., Shinitzky, M., Zamir, N. and Samuel, D. (1982) Adaptive modulation of brain membrane lipid fluidity in drug addiction and denervation supersensitivity, *Biochem. Pharmacol.*, in press.

Hershkowitz, M. (1978) Influence of calcium on phosphorylation of a synaptosomal protein. *Biochim. biophys. Acta*, 542: 274–283.

Hirata, F. and Axelrod, J. (1978) Enzymatic methylation of phosphatidylethanolamine increases erythrocyte membrane fluidity. *Nature (Lond.)*, 275: 219–220.

Hofstein, R., Hershkowitz, M., Gozes, I. and Samuel, D. (1980) The characterization and phosphorylation of an actin-like protein in synaptosomal membranes. *Biochim. biophys. Acta*, 624: 153–162.

Ip, S.H.C. and Cooper, R.A. (1980) Decreased membrane fluidity during differentiation of human promyelocytic leukemia cells in culture. *Blood*, 56: 227–252.

Jacobson, K. and Papahadjopoulos, D. (1975) Phase transitions and phase separations in phospholipid membranes induced by changes in temperature, pH and concentration of bivalent cations. *Biochemistry*, 14: 152–170.

Johnson, D.A., Lee, N.M., Cooke, R. and Loh, H. (1979) Adaptation to ethanol-induced fluidization of lipid bilayers: Cross tolerance and reversibility. *Mol. Pharmacol.*, 17: 52–55.

Jones, D.G. and Matus, A.I. (1974) Isolation of synaptic plasma membrane from brain by combined floatation-sedimentation density gradient centrifugation. *Biochim. biophys. Acta*, 356: 276–287.

Landfield, P.W. and Lynch, G. (1977) Impaired monosynaptic potentiation in vitro hippocampal slices from aged, memory-deficient rats. *J. Gerontol.*, 32: 523–533.

Landfield, P.W., McGaugh, J.L. and Lynch, G. (1978) Impaired synaptic potentiation processes in the hippocampus of aged, memory-deficient rats. *Brain Res.*, 150: 85–101.

Luly, P. and Shinitzky, M. (1979) Gross structural changes in isolated liver cell plasma membrane upon binding of insulin. *Biochemistry*, 18: 445–450.

Magilen, G., Gordon, A., Au, A. and Diamond, I. (1981) Identification of a mitochondrial phosphoprotein in brain synaptic membrane preparations. *J. Neurochem.*, 36: 1861–1864.

Michaelson, D.M. and Avissar, S. (1979) $Ca^{2+}$-dependent protein phosphorylation induced by $K^+$ depolarization of the purely cholinergic Torpedo synaptosomes. *Proc. nat. Acad. Sci. (Wash.)*, 76: 6336–6340.

Montenay-Garestier, T., Aragon, I., Devynck, M.A., Meyer, P. and Helene, C. (1981) Evidence for structural changes in erythrocyte membranes of spontaneously hypertensive rats: A fluorescence polarization study. *Biochem. biophys. Res. Commun.*, 100: 660–665.

Muller, C.P. and Shinitzky, M. (1981) Passive shedding of erythrocyte antigens induced by membrane rigidification. *Exp. Cell Res.*, 136: 53–62.

Muller, C.P., Volloch, Z. and Shinitzky, M. (1980) Correlation between cell density, membrane fluidity and the availability of transferrin receptors in Friend erythroleukemia cells. *Cell Biophys.*, 2: 233–240.

Nicolson, G.L. (1976) Transmembrane control of the receptors on normal and tumor cells: I. Cytoplasmic influence over cell surface components. *Biochim. biophys. Acta*, 457: 57–108.

Pal, R., Barenholz, Y. and Wagner, R.R. (1981) Depletion and exchange of cholesterol from the membrane of vesicular stomatitis virus by interaction with serum lipoproteins or polyvinylpyrrolidone complexed with bovine serum albumin. *Biochemistry*, 20: 530–539.

Rivnay, B., Globerson, A. and Shinitzky, M. (1979) Viscosity of lymphocyte plasma membrane in old mice and its possible relation to serum cholesterol. *Mech. Age Dev.*, 10: 71–79.

Rosenberg, P.H. (1979) Effects of halothane, lidocaine and 5-hydroxytryptamine on fluidity of synaptic plasma membranes, myelin membranes and synaptic mitochondrial membranes. *Arch. Pharmacol.*, 307: 199–206.

Rouser, G., Kitchensky, G., Yamamoto, A. and Baxter, C.F. (1972) Lipids in the nervous system of different species as a function of age: Brain, spinal cord peripheral nerves, purified whole cell preparations and subcellular particulates: Regulatory mechanisms and membrane structure. *Adv. Lipid Res.*, 10: 261–360.

Routtenberg, A. and Ehrlich, H.Y. (1975) Endogenous phosphorylation of four cerebral cortical membrane proteins: Role of cyclic nucleotides, ATP and divalent cations. *Brain Res.*, 92: 415–430.

Rubin, C.S. and Rosen, O.M. (1975) Protein phosphorylation. *Annu. Rev. Biochem.*, 44: 831–887.

Rudolph, S.A. and Greengard, P. (1974) Regulation of protein phosphorylation and membrane permeability by $\beta$-adrenergic agents and cyclic adenosine $3':5'$-monophosphate in the ovian erythrocyte. *J. biol. Chem.*, 249: 5684–5687.

Sandermann Jr., J. (1978) Regulation of membrane enzymes by lipids. *Biochim. biophys. Acta*, 515: 209–237.

Schachter, D. and Shinitzky, M. (1977) Fluorescence polarization studies of rat intestinal microvillus membranes. *J. clin. Invest.*, 59: 536–542.

Schneeweiss, F., Naquira, D., Rosenheck, K. and Schneider, A.S. (1979) Cholinergic stimulants and excess potassium ion increase the fluidity of plasma membrane isolated from adrenal chromaffin cells. *Biochim. biophys. Acta*, 555: 460–471.

Schulman, H. and Greengard, P. (1978) $Ca^{2+}$-dependent protein phosphorylation system in membranes from various tissues and its activation by "calcium-dependent regulator". *Proc. nat. Acad. Sci. (Wash.)*, 75: 5432–5436.

434

Shih, J.C. and Young, H. (1978) The alteration of serotonin binding sites in aged human brain. *Life Sci.*, 23: 1441–1448.

Shinitzky, M. (1979) The concept of passive modulation of membrane responses. *Dev. Cell Biol.*, 4: 173–181.

Shinitzky, M. and Barenholz, Y. (1978) Fluidity parameters of lipid regions determined by fluorescence polarization. *Biochim. biophys. Acta*, 515: 367–394.

Shinitzky, M. and Henkart, P. (1979) Fluidity of cell membranes: Current concepts and trends. *Int. Rev. Cytol.*, 60: 121–147.

Shinitzky, M. and Souroujon, M. (1979) Passive modulation of blood group antigens. *Proc. nat. Acad. Sci. (Wash.)*, 76: 4438–4440.

Shinitzky, M., Skornick, Y. and Haran-Ghera, N. (1979) Effective tumor immunization induced by cells of elevated membrane lipid microviscosity. *Proc. nat. Acad. Sci. (Wash.)*, 76: 5313–5316.

Sieghart, W., Forn, J. and Greengard, P. (1979) $Ca^{2+}$ and cyclic AMP regulate phosphorylation of same two membrane-associated proteins specific to nerve tissue. *Proc. nat. Acad. Sci. (Wash.)*, 76: 2475–2479.

Sinensky, M. (1974) Homeoviscous adaptation: A homeostatic process that regulates the viscosity of membrane lipids in *Escherichia coli*. *Proc. nat. Acad. Sci. (Wash.)*, 71: 522–525.

Sinensky, M. (1980) Adaptive alteration in phospholipid composition of plasma membranes from a somatic cell mutant defective in the regulation of cholesterol biosynthesis. *J. Cell Biol.*, 166–169.

Strittmatter, W.J., Hirata, F., Axelrod, J., Mallorga, P., Tallman, J.F. and Hennelberry, R.C. (1979a) Benzodiazepine and $\beta$-adrenergic receptor ligands independently stimulate phospholipid methylation. *Nature (Lond.)*, 282: 857–859.

Strittmatter, W.J., Hirata, F. and Axelrod, J. (1979b) Phospholipid methylation unmasks cryptic $\beta$-adrenergic receptors in rat reticulocytes. *Science*, 204: 1205–1207.

Teichberg, V.I., Sobel, A. and Changeux, J.P. (1977) In vitro phosphorylation of the acetylcholine receptor. *Nature (Lond.)*, 267: 540–541.

Ueda, T., Maeno, H. and Greengard, P. (1973) Regulation of endogenous phosphorylation of specific proteins in synaptic membrane fractions from rat brain by adenosine $3':5'$-monophosphate. *J. biol. Chem.*, 248: 8295–8305.

Uprichard, D.C., Bylund, D.B. and Snyder, S.H. (1978) $(+)$-[$^3$H]Epinephrine and $(-)$-[$^3$H]dihydroalprenolol binding to $\beta_1$- and $\beta_2$-noradrenergic receptors in brain, heart, and lung membranes. *J. biol. Chem.*, 253: 5090–5101.

Weller, M. and Morgan, I.G. (1977) A possible role of the phosphorylation of synaptic membrane proteins in the control of $Ca^{2+}$ permeability. *Biochim. biophys. Acta*, 465: 527–534.

Williams, M. and Rodnight, R. (1977) Protein phosphorylation in nervous tissue: Possible involvement in nervous tissue function and relationship to cyclic nucleotide metabolism. In *Progress in Neurobiology*, Vol. 8, G.A. Kerku and J.W. Phillis (Eds.), Pergamon Press, Oxford, pp. 183–250.

Wirtz, K.W.A. and Zilversmit, D.B. (1968) Exchange of phospholipids between liver mitochondria and microsomes in vitro. *J. biol. Chem.*, 243: 3596–3602.

Yamamura, H.I. and Snyder, S.H. (1974) Muscarinic cholinergic binding in rat brain. *Proc. nat. Acad. Sci. (Wash.)*, 71: 1725–1729.

Yuli, I., Wilbrandt, W. and Shinitzky, M. (1981) Glucose transport through cell membrane of modified lipid fluidity. *Biochemistry*, 20: 4250–4256.

Zwiers, H., Wiegant, V.M., Schotman, P. and Gispen, W.H. (1978) ACTH-induced inhibition of endogenous rat brain protein phosphorylation in vitro: Structure activity. *Neurochem. Res.*, 3: 455–463.

# Proposed Role of Phosphoproteins
# in Visual Function

DEBORA B. FARBER

*Jules Stein Eye Institute, U.C.L.A. School of Medicine, Los Angeles, CA 90024, U.S.A.*

## INTRODUCTION

Studies attempting to unravel the mechanism of the visual process have multiplied in the last decade. However, the question of how retinal photoreceptor cells function is still not completely resolved. This brief review will summarize some biochemical aspects of the present knowledge on this topic and point out the possible involvement of phosphoproteins in the pathways that regulate transduction and adaptation. We will restrict our attention to vertebrate rod photoreceptors since the biochemistry and physiology of these cells are being studied most actively.

## THE ROD PHOTORECEPTOR AND THE VISUAL PROCESS

The rod photoreceptor has distinct morphological regions (Fig. 1). The outer segment contains tightly packed membranous discs which are encased by, but not attached to, the plasmalemma of the cell. Most of the visual pigment rhodopsin is located in the disc membranes but the plasmalemma also has rhodopsin (Jan and Revel, 1974; Dewey et al., 1969). The outer segment is the site of visual transduction, where light is detected and absorbed.The rod inner segment is rich in mitochondria; here the metabolic and synthetic machinery of the cell produce the energy-rich nucleoside triphosphates, ATP and GTP, which are sent to the outer segments. Thus, although outer segments are unable to generate these compounds by themselves via oxidative metabolism, they have millimolar concentrations of both ATP and GTP that are extensively used in many reactions. The rest of the photoreceptor cell is constituted by a nucleus, located in the cell soma and a synaptic ending joined to the cell soma by a short axon.

The initial step of the visual process is the absorption of a photon by the 11-*cis* retinal chromophore of rhodopsin. This causes the photochemical isomerization of the chromophore to the *all-trans* configuration, which is followed by a sequence of dark reactions producing metastable intermediates. The final products of the "bleaching" of rhodopsin are, at least in vitro, free *all-trans* retinal and opsin (Wald, 1968). The absorption of light by the visual pigment causes a transient suppression of the sodium permeability of the photoreceptor plasmalemma and, as a consequence of this, the cell hyperpolarizes (Werblin, 1974).

The link between photon capture in the disc membrane and the change in potential of the plasma membrane would be easy to visualize if one supposed that light causes the discs to

436

release a "second messenger" which diffuses to the plasmalemma and reduces its conductance for $Na^+$ (Baylor and Fuortes, 1970; Hagins, 1972; Cone, 1973). In addition, an extraordinary amplification of the light signal is needed, that is, many molecules of this substance would have to be released since a single absorbed photon can transiently reduce a rod's $Na^+$ current by about 3% (Cone and Pak, 1971). Furthermore, the effect of the second messenger should be fast, in the order of milliseconds, since this is the time frame in which the change in conductance occurs.

## THE CALCIUM HYPOTHESIS

Studies by Hagins and Yoshikami (1974) led them to propose a model in which $Ca^{2+}$ sequestered within the discs in the dark-adapted state is released into the cytoplasm when light is absorbed by rhodopsin and then it binds to the $Na^+$ channels of the plasmalemma, inhibiting the sodium entrance across the outer segment membrane. Thus, this model suggests that the amplification of the initial light signal is brought about by the intracellular transmitter $Ca^{2+}$. Although several laboratories have reported experiments designed to prove the release from rod outer segments of many $Ca^{2+}$ within milliseconds of light exposure (Hendricks et al., 1974; Liebman, 1974; Hemminki, 1975; Weller et al., 1975b; Sorbi and Cavaggioni, 1975; Szuts and Cone, 1977; Smith et al., 1977; Kaupp and Junge, 1977), there is no conclusive evidence as yet that validates Hagins and Yoshikami's hypothesis.

## THE CYCLIC GMP HYPOTHESIS

Another possible intermediate in the visual process is cyclic GMP (cGMP). The metabolism and content of this cyclic nucleotide are regulated by light. Rod outer segments of dark-adapted retinas from several species possess high levels of cGMP (Krishna et al., 1976; Orr et al., 1976) and high levels of the enzymes required for cGMP synthesis and degradation (Krishna et al., 1976; Pannbacker, 1973a; Pannbacker et al., 1972; Goridis and Virmaux, 1974; Miki et al., 1973). Upon bleaching of rhodopsin, cGMP phosphodiesterase activity is increased (Miki et al., 1973) and this occurs within milliseconds of light absorption (Yee and Liebman, 1978). Correspondingly, there is a rapid decrease in the levels of cGMP of isolated rod outer segments. Woodruff et al. (1977) reported that the bleaching of one rhodopsin molecule leads to the hydrolysis of $5 \times 10^4$ molecules of cGMP and that this occurs with a half-time of 125 msec. The speed and amplification of the phosphodiesterase reaction suggest that the light-activated hydrolysis of cGMP could be a stage in visual transduction. The decrease in cGMP concentration is reversible and is a function of light intensity, as is the recovery of membrane potential after illumination (Woodruff and Bownds, 1979; Kilbride and Ebrey, 1979; Lolley et al., 1979).

Several factors contribute to the large amplification of the light signal. A light-activated GTPase appears to be obligatory for phosphodiesterase activation (Wheeler and Bitensky, 1977; Robinson and Hagins, 1977; Kühn, 1978, 1980; Bignetti et al., 1978; Godchaux and Zimmerman, 1979). Moreover, Shinozawa et al. (1980) reported that a "helper" protein is required for expression of the GTPase activity. Fung et al. (1981) named "transducin" (T) the protein with GTPase activity that forms a complex with GTP in an exchange reaction ($T \cdot GDP + GTP \rightarrow T \cdot GTP + GDP$) catalyzed by bleached rhodopsin. Transducin is composed of three polypeptide chains, $\alpha$, $\beta$ and $\gamma$ and, upon illumination, GTP binds to the $\alpha$ subunit.

These authors showed that T·GTP can be formed with a high degree of amplification (approximately 500 molecules of T·GTP are produced for each molecule of bleached rhodopsin) in the absence of cGMP phosphodiesterase and that cGMP phosphodiesterase on unilluminated disc membranes can be fully activated by T·GTP. Thus, they proposed that transducin is the first amplified intermediate in cGMP hydrolysis. The transducin of Fung et al. (1981) and the GTPase with the "helper" protein of Shinozawa et al., (1980) may correspond to the same molecular complexes.

Other possible controls of cGMP phosphodiesterase which seem to be involved in the regulation of the visual process have been described, including a protein inhibitor (Dumler and Etingof, 1976; Sitaramayya et al., 1977; Berman and Usova, 1978; Hurley and Ebrey, 1979; Baehr et al., 1979). Liebman and Pugh (1979, 1980) showed that ATP concentration can control the activation–inactivation sequence of phosphodiesterase, and Kawamura and Bownds (1981) indicated that the ATP effect depends on the $Ca^{2+}$ concentration of the incubation medium. Furthermore, Robinson et al. (1980) reported the presence of a $Ca^{2+}$-dependent regulator. Calcium ions seem to regulate the levels of cGMP not only by control of phosphodiesterase but also of guanylate cyclase activity (Lolley and Racz, 1981). Removal of $Ca^{2+}$ increases cGMP concentration (Cohen et al., 1978) whereas addition of $Ca^{2+}$ suppresses the dark permeability of rod outer segments and decreases their cGMP levels (Woodruff and Bownds, 1979).

Electrophysiological studies also support the hypothesis that cGMP is involved in the visual process (Lipton et al., 1977a,b). Intracellular injection of cGMP depolarizes the plasma membrane of rod outer segments within milliseconds and increases both the latency and amplitude of the response to illumination (Nicol and Miller, 1978; Miller and Nicol, 1979).

## CYCLIC NUCLEOTIDE-DEPENDENT PHOSPHORYLATIONS

How is the light-induced change in cGMP concentration translated into a physiologically significant message? It is possible that the levels of cGMP regulate the phosphorylation of specific proteins which, in turn, could be involved in the control of functions that are fundamental for the cell (Farber et al., 1978). This seems to be the case for neurons, where phosphoproteins have been implicated in the control of membrane permeability to certain ions (Nathanson, 1977).

With the exception of a brief communication by Pannbacker (1973b) about a cyclic nucleotide-dependent kinase in rod outer segments, most of the work done until 1977 on the phosphorylating systems of the photoreceptors concentrated on the protein kinase that uses bleached rhodopsin as substrate. This enzyme acts independent of cyclic nucleotides. The significance of the phosphorylation of the visual pigment will be considered later in this review.

Cyclic nucleotide-dependent protein kinase of bovine rod outer segments has been studied by Farber et al. (1979). The enzyme can be extracted with Tris buffer and, after high speed centrifugation, is obtained in soluble form. This kinase is unaffected by light and is half-maximally stimulated by $1 \times 10^{-7}$M cyclic AMP (cAMP) and $4$–$5 \times 10^{-6}$M cGMP. In addition to its in vitro activation by lower concentrations of cAMP than cGMP, DEAE-cellulose chromatography demonstrates that most of the soluble kinase activity corresponds to the type II of cAMP-dependent protein kinases, with lesser amounts of type I. The presence of a cAMP-dependent protein kinase in rod outer segments appears to be paradoxical since their levels of cGMP are higher by severalfold than those of cAMP (Krishna et al., 1976; Orr et al.,

1976), and the concentration of cGMP but not of cAMP is regulated by light (Woodruff et al., 1977). Thus, Farber et al. (1979) have suggested that although the cyclic nucleotide-dependent protein kinase of rod outer segments has the characteristics of a cAMP-dependent enzyme, it is modulated directly in vivo by light-induced changes in cGMP levels.

Only one protein of the soluble fraction of rod outer segments is phosphorylated in a cyclic nucleotide-dependent manner. This protein has a molecular weight of 30 000 as estimated by SDS–polyacrylamide gel electrophoresis and, in the native state, it may exist as a dimer or, possibly, as a large aggregate (Farber et al., 1979). The 30 000 dalton protein has been found in the rod outer segment extracts of bovine, mouse and rat (Lolley et al., 1977). Pannbacker (1974) also observed a similar protein in human rod outer segments with an estimated molecular weight of 25 000. In rod outer segments of frog (Polans et al., 1979) and toad (Farber and Lolley, unpublished observations), the 30 000 dalton protein is not detected but, instead, two proteins of molecular weight 12 000 and 13 000 are phosphorylated in the dark by a cyclic nucleotide-dependent mechanism and are dephosphorylated by illumination. Polans et al. (1979) showed that rephosphorylation is achieved after illumination ceases; moreover, addition to the incubation medium of cGMP or of drugs that increase cGMP concentration increases the phosphorylation of the two proteins and, conversely, a decrease in the levels of cGMP caused by $Ca^{2+}$ decreases the level of phosphorylation of the 12 000 and 13 000 dalton proteins. Thus, light-induced changes in cGMP concentration may control the amount of bovine 30 000 or frog 12 000 and 13 000 dalton proteins present in the rod outer segment cytosol.

Based on the above observations, Farber et al. (1978) proposed a model which assumes a link between the absorption of light by rhodopsin in the rod outer segment disc membranes and the changes in ion permeability of the plasmalemma through the cGMP modulation of protein kinase activity and the effect of the resulting phosphoproteins. An updated version of the model will be discussed at the end of this review.


## PHOSPHORYLATION OF RHODOPSIN

The phosphorylation of rhodopsin, the main protein of the rod outer segment disc membranes, may also be an important event for vision. Rhodopsin spans the disc membrane thickness (Hubbell et al., 1977; Hubbell and Fung, 1978) crossing the membrane interface a minimum of three times. The C terminus is located at the cytoplasmic surface of the disc (Hargrave and Fong, 1977; Hubbell and Fung, 1978) and the N terminus at the intradiscal surface (Röhlich, 1976; Hargrave, 1977; Hubbell and Fung, 1978; Adams et al., 1979). Light causes conformational changes at both ends of the protein (Corless, 1972; Chen and Hubbell, 1973, 1978; Chabre, 1975; Saibil et al., 1976) which may originate the activation of cGMP phosphodiesterase. Moreover, rhodopsin is phosphorylated only after being bleached; thus, light-induced conformational changes may transform rhodopsin into the acceptable substrate for protein kinase (Weller et al., 1975a; Frank and Buzney, 1975). The membrane protein kinase of rod outer segments that phosphorylates rhodopsin is not activated by light and the reaction is a slow, dark process which has been reported to take from only a few minutes to more than 1 h (Kühn and Dreyer, 1972; Bownds et al., 1972; Frank et al., 1973; Kühn and Bader, 1976). The action spectrum of the light effect coincides with the absorption spectrum of rhodopsin (Bownds et al., 1972). Either ATP or GTP can act as phosphate donors, but it remains to be settled which of the two nucleotides is the one preferred (Chader et al., 1976, 1980; Miller and Paulsen, 1975; Weller et al., 1976; Shichi and Somers, 1978). The substrate specificity of the enzyme is also an open question. Some authors have reported that bleached rhodopsin is the only substrate (Weller et al., 1975a; Shichi and Somers, 1978) while others have been able to phosphorylate in addition proteins such as histone, protamine or phosvitin (Pannbacker, 1973b; Kühn et al., 1973; Frank and Bensinger, 1974; Frank and Buzney, 1975; Chader et al., 1976). The discrepancy in these observations may be related to the purity of the enzyme preparation. However, the only kinase that seems to phosphorylate bleached rhodopsin is that of the rod outer segments; protein kinases from other tissues are ineffective (Frank and Buzney, 1975).

Rhodopsin kinase is a cyclic nucleotide-independent enzyme (Kühn and Dryer, 1972; Frank et al., 1973; Weller et al., 1975a). It can be extracted with aqueous buffers from dark-adapted but not from illuminated rod outer segments (Kühn, 1978) because it binds to the freshly bleached membranes. The enzyme is released again after dark adaptation. This reversible binding was used by Kühn (1978) to partially purify rhodopsin kinase, which he reports has a molecular weight of 67 000–69 000 in contrast to the apparent molecular weight of 50 000–53 000 found by Shichi and Somers (1978).

Earlier work using bovine rod outer segments had shown that the stoichiometry of phosphorylation at saturating light levels varied between 0.3 and 2 moles of phosphate per mole of rhodopsin (Kühn and Dryer, 1972; Frank et al., 1973). However, Shichi and Somers (1978) determined that only a small fraction of bovine rhodopsin is phosphorylated in rod membranes, about 16% total pigment, and that these rhodopsin molecules contained 5 moles of phosphate/mole of pigment. Sale et al. (1978) reported similar results; in addition, they digested the phosphorylated rhodopsin with papain and found that one of the three fragments obtained (molecular weight 6000) contained all the phosphorylation sites. This suggests that one specific domain of rhodopsin is susceptible to multiple phosphorylation. Adams et al. (1979) demonstrated that these phosphorylation sites are on the interdiscal surface, where the C terminus is located. Shichi and Somers (1978) also showed that newly formed discs present in the basal region of the rod outer segment, and the plasma membrane that is continuous with them, are phosphorylated preferentially to older discs. This provides evidence of biochemical heterogeneity in different regions of the outer segments.

In contrast to the results obtained when the phosphorylation of rhodopsin is studied using bovine tissue, fully bleached frog rod outer segments bind 4 moles of phosphate per mole of rhodopsin (Miller and Paulsen, 1975; Kühn et al., 1977) but, at lower levels of illumination (less than 1% rhodopsin bleached), they incorporate up to 40–50 phosphates per mole of rhodopsin (Bownds et al., 1972; Miller et al., 1977). These authors suggest that since it is unlikely that each rhodopsin molecule binds more than 4–5 phosphates (Kühn and McDowell, 1977), unbleached rhodopsin must be phosphorylated. The possiblity of such an amplification in the phosphorylation of rhodopsin is as yet an unsettled issue.

Several laboratories have measured the activity of the phosphoprotein phosphatase that removes the phosphate groups from phosphorylated rhodopsin (Kühn, 1974; Weller et al., 1975a; Kühn and Bader, 1976). There is agreement that the reaction is very slow and that it is not affected by cyclic nucleotides (Goridis and Weller, 1976). Thus, the slow rate of both processes, phosphorylation and dephosphorylation of rhodopsin, indicate that these reactions could not be involved in visual excitation. On the other hand, Kühn et al. (1977) have found that the time required for dephosphorylation in the dark of intact frog retinas is similar to the time required for dark adaptation after a strong illumination. This could suggest that the state of phosphorylation of rhodopsin may be involved in controlling the light sensitivity of the rods, perhaps by regulating some properties of the photoreceptor membranes such as their $Ca^{2+}$ permeability. Weller et al. (1975b) observed that light increases the $Ca^{2+}$ permeability of rod outer segment discs, whereas phosphorylation of the bleached rhodopsin lowers the $Ca^{2+}$ permeability. On the basis of these data, Weller et al. (1975c) proposed a model in which the phosphorylation of rhodopsin would turn the rod outer segments "off" by preventing the light-induced $Ca^{2+}$ release. Return of the light-exposed phosphorylated discs to the dark would promote rhodopsin dephosphorylation and the discs would be switched "on" again. Such a process, in which the sensitivity of photoreceptors to light is modulated by the phosphorylation/dephosphorylation of rhodopsin, could have an important role in light and dark adaptation. This hypothesis remains to be proven.

Another possibility suggested by Liebman and Pugh (1979, 1980) and by Hubbell and Bownds (1979) is that the phosphorylation of rhodopsin may be a means to turn-off the light-activated phosphodiesterase. Light adaptation could then result from the accumulation of inactive phosphodiesterase which would be unable to link photon absorption to the decrease in cGMP concentration. Recent data by Aton and Litman (1981) show that the level of phosphodiesterase activity in rod outer segments decreases when the extracts are incubated with phosphorylated discs membranes; furthermore, it seems that the higher the degree of rhodopsin phosphorylation in the membranes, the lower the phosphodiesterase activity that is observed in the incubated mixture. However, Kawamura and Bownds (1981) refer in their paper to some experiments by Hermolin and Bownds, not published as yet, which show that ATP inactivates phosphodiesterase under conditions that suppress rhodopsin phosphorylation.

The proteins of rod outer segments are phosphorylated selectively in response to biological signals which might correspond to those that act in vivo. This was demonstrated by Farber et al. (1979) in an experiment in which they combined the Tris-extracted soluble fraction of rod outer segments with "purified rhodopsin" membranes, that is, rod outer segment membranes that had been depleted of protein kinase activity and that had rhodopsin as the major protein, as revealed by SDS gel electrophoresis. Aliquots of the mixture were phosphorylated under different conditions, with or without cyclic nucleotides, in the dark or in the light. As expected, the authors found that in the dark, the 30 000 dalton soluble protein was phosphorylated and that this reaction was stimulated by cyclic nucleotides; no phosphorylation of rhodopsin was observed. Upon bleaching the membranes however, rhodopsin and the 30 000 dalton protein both incorporated phosphate, but only the soluble protein showed higher incorporation in the presence of cyclic nucleotides. Thus, the signal "light" promotes the phosphorylation of the membrane protein rhodopsin, independent of cyclic nucleotides, and the signal "high levels of cGMP" stimulates the phosphorylation of a 30 000 dalton soluble protein, independent of light.

## CONCLUDING REMARKS

Fig. 1 summarizes all of the observations that have been described in this review. It shows that the photoreceptor cell produces its ATP and GTP in the mitochondria of the inner segment. Guanylate cyclase, which is localized in the connecting cilium primarily (Fleischman and Denisevich, 1979) synthesizes cGMP from GTP. In the dark, the levels of cGMP are high because of minimal phosphodiesterase activity and they stimulate a soluble cyclic nucleotide-dependent protein kinase. This enzyme, in the presence of ATP, phosphorylates a soluble protein (molecular weight 30 000 in bovine rod outer segments). As proposed by Farber et al. (1978) this phosphoprotein is in high concentration in the dark-adapted state and it interacts with the plasmalemma of the rod outer segments. The 30 000 dalton phosphoprotein facilitates the free movement of ions across the open channels of the membrane either by direct interaction or by binding $Ca^{2+}$. This sequence of events provides a mechanism for the

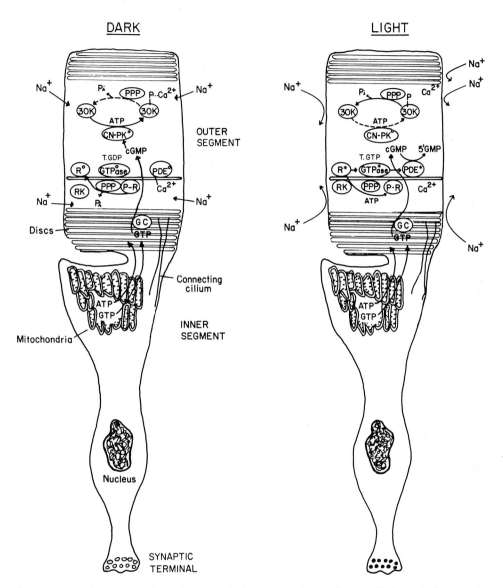

Fig. 1. Proposed involvement of phosphoproteins in the pathways that regulate transduction and adaptation. For explanation of the model, see text. GC, guanylate cyclase; $R^o$ and $R^*$, unbleached and bleached rhodopsin, respectively; GTPase$^o$ and GTPase$^*$, inactive and light-activated GTPase, respectively; PDE$^o$ and PDE$^*$, inactive or showing minimal activity and light-activated phosphodiesterase, respectively; T·GDP, inactive complex of transducin with GDP; T·GTP, activated complex of transducin with GTP; CN-PK$^o$ and CN-PK$^*$, inactive and activated cyclic nucleotide-dependent protein kinase, respectively; 30 K, soluble protein, molecular weight 30 000; 30 K-P, soluble phosphorylated protein, molecular weight 30 000; PPP, phosphoprotein phosphatase; RK, rhodopsin kinase; P-R, phosphorylated rhodopsin.

442

sustained state of depolarization that characterizes dark-adapted rod outer segments.

Fig. 1 also shows that in the dark, transducin is bound to GDP which keeps its GTPase activity inhibited and rhodopsin kinase is free in the cytosol. In addition, phosphoprotein phosphatase removes phosphate from phosphorylated rhodopsin, a process that could be related to dark adaptation.

In the light, bleached rhodopsin catalyzes the exchange of GDP for GTP on transducin, and this activated GTPase activates in turn the phosphodiesterase which hydrolyzes cGMP to 5′-GMP in a matter of milliseconds. The reduction in cGMP concentration does not allow for the activation of the soluble cyclic nucleotide-dependent protein kinase. This, together with the continued activity of phosphoprotein phosphatase, decreases the concentration of the 30 000 dalton phosphoprotein. The net result is a reverse of the dark condition, e.g., closure of the ion channels and hyperpolarization of the photoreceptor cell.

Also depicted in Fig. 1 (in the light) is the phosphorylation of bleached rhodopsin by the membrane-bound rhodopsin kinase. As mentioned above, this could be a means for reducing the sensitivity of the photoreceptor cell to light. Thus, the phosphorylation–dephosphorylation reactions of rhodopsin may be involved in dark/light adaptation.

In summary, we can state that specific phosphoproteins of rod photoreceptor cells may be involved in the modulation or perhaps regulation of visual function.


## ACKNOWLEDGEMENTS

The author wishes to thank Dr. Rehwa Lee for helpful criticism of the manuscript and Mrs. Inga Anderson for her expert assistance in its preparation.

This work was supported by RCDA EY 144 and grants EY 2651 and EY 331 of the National Eye Institute and by the Medical Research Service of the Veterans Administration.

## REFERENCES

Adams, A.J., Somers, R.L. and Shichi, H. (1979) Spatial arrangement of rhodopsin in the disk membrane as studied by enzymatic labeling. *Photochem. Photobiol.*, 29: 687–692.

Aton, G.B. and Litman, B.J. (1981) The ability of rhodopsin to light activate ROS phosphodiesterase is reduced by phosphorylation. *Invest. Ophthalmol. visual Sci.*, 20, Suppl.: 208.

Baehr, W., Devlin, M.J. and Applebury, M. (1979) Isolation and characterization of cGMP phosphodiesterase from bovine rod outer segments. *J. biol. Chem.*, 254: 11669–11677.

Baylor, D.A. and Fuortes, M.G.F. (1970) Electrical responses of single cones in the retina of the turtle. *J. Physiol. (Lond.)*, 207: 77–92.

Berman, A.L. and Usova, A.A. (1978) Protein inhibitor of the retinal cyclic nucleotide phosphodiesterase: Its localization in the outer segment of a photoreceptor. *Biokeimiia*, 43: 486–490.

Bignetti, E., Cavaggioni, A. and Sorbi, R.T. (1978) Light-activated hydrolysis of GTP and cyclic GMP in the rod outer segments. *J. Physiol. (Lond.)*, 279: 55–69.

Bownds, D., Dawes, J., Miller, J. and Stahlman, M. (1972) Phosphorylation of frog photoreceptor membranes induced by light. *Nature new Biol.*, 237: 125–127.

Chabre, M. (1975) X-Ray diffraction of retinal rods. I. Structure of disc membrane, effect of illumination. *Biochim. biophys. Acta*, 382: 322–335.

Chader, G.J., Fletcher, R.T., O'Brien, P.J. and Krishna, G. (1976) Differential phosphorylation by GTP and ATP in isolated rod outer segments of the retina. *Biochemistry*, 15: 1615–1620.

Chader, G.J., Fletcher, R.T., Russell, P. and Krishna, G. (1980) Differential control of protein kinase activities of the retinal photoreceptor. Cation effects on phosphorylation by adenosine and guanosine 5′-triphosphates. *Biochemistry*, 19: 2634–2638.

Chen, Y.S. and Hubbell, W.L. (1973) Temperature and light dependent structural changes in rhodopsin-lipid membranes. *Exp. Eye Res.*, 17: 517–532.

Chen, Y.S. and Hubbell, W.L. (1978) Reactions of the sulfhydryl groups of membrane-bound bovine rhodopsin. *Mem. Biochem.*, 1: 107–130.

Cohen, A.I., Hall, I.A. and Ferrendelli, J.A. (1978) Calcium and cyclic nucleotide regulation in incubated mouse retinas. *J. gen. Physiol.*, 71: 595–612.

Cone, R.A. (1973) The internal transmitter model for visual excitation: some quantitative implications. In *Biochemistry and Physiology of Visual Pigments*, H. Langer (Ed.), Springer, New York, pp. 275–282.

Cone, R.A. and Pak, W.L. (1971) The early receptor potential. In *Handbook of Sensory Physiology*, Vol. 1, W.R. Loewenstein (Ed.), Springer, Berlin, pp. 345–365.

Corless, J.M. (1972) Lamellar structure of bleached and unbleached rod photoreceptor membranes. *Nature (Lond.)*, 237: 229–231.

Dewey, M.M., Davis, P.K., Blasie, J.K. and Barr, L. (1969) Localization of rhodopsin antibody in the retina of the frog. *J. mol. Biol.*, 39: 395–405.

Dumler, I.L. and Etingof, R.N. (1976) Protein inhibitor of cyclic adenosine 3′:5′-monophosphate phosphodiesterase in retina. *Biochem. biophys. Acta*, 429: 474–478.

Farber, D.B., Brown, B.M. and Lolley, R.N. (1978) Cyclic GMP: Proposed role in visual cell function. *Vision Res.*, 18: 497–499.

Farber, D.B., Brown, B.M. and Lolley, R.N. (1979) Cyclic nucleotide dependent protein kinase and the phosphorylation of endogenous protein of retinal rod outer segments. *Biochemistry*, 18: 370–378.

Fleischman, D. and Denisevich, M. (1979) Guanylate cyclase of isolated bovine retinal rod axonemes. *Biochemistry*, 18: 5060–5066.

Frank, R.N. and Bensinger, R.E. (1974) Rhodopsin and light-sensitive kinase activity of retinal rod outer segments. *Exp. Eye Res.*, 18: 271–280.

Frank, R.N. and Buzney, S.M. (1975) Mechanism and specificity of rhodopsin phosphorylation. *Biochemistry*, 14: 5110–5117.

Frank, R.N., Cavanagh, H.D. and Kenyon, K.R. (1973) Light stimulated phosphorylation of bovine visual pigments by ATP. *J. biol. Chem.*, 218: 596–609.

Fung, B.K.-K., Hurley, J.B. ans Stryer, L. (1981) Flow of information in the light-triggered cyclic nucleotide cascade of vision. *Proc. nat. Acad. Sci. (Wash.)*, 78: 152–156.

Godchaux III, W. and Zimmerman, W.F. (1979) Membrane-dependent guanine nucleotide binding and GTPase activities of soluble protein from bovine rod cell outer segments. *J. biol. Chem.*, 254: 7874–7884.

Goridis, C. and Virmaux, N. (1974) Light-regulated guanosine 3′,5′-monophosphate phosphodiesterase of bovine retina. *Nature (Lond.)*, 248: 57–58.

Goridis, C. and Weller, M. (1976) A role for cyclic nucleotides and protein kinase in vertebrate photoreception. *Adv. Biochem. Psychopharmacol.*, 15: 391–412.

Hagins, W.A. (1972) The visual process: excitatory mechanisms in the primary photoreceptor cells. *Annu. Rev. Biophys. Bioeng.*, 1: 131–158.

Hagins, W.A. and Yoshikami, S. (1974) A role for calcium in excitation of retinal rods and cones. *Exp. Eye Res.*, 18: 299–305.

Hargrave, P.A. (1977) The amino-terminal tryptic peptide of bovine rhodopsin. A glycopeptide containing two sites of oligosaccharide attachment. *Biochem. Biophys. Acta*, 492: 83–94.

Hargrave, P.A. and Fong, S. (1977) The amino and carboxyl-terminal sequence of bovine rhodopsin. *J. supramol. Struct.*, 6: 559–570.

Hemminki, K. (1975) Light-induced decrease in calcium binding to isolated bovine photoreceptors. *Vision Res.*, 15: 69–72.

Hendricks, T., Daeman, F.J.M. and Bonting, S.L. (1974) Biochemical aspects of the visual process XXV. Light-induced movements in isolated frog rod outer segments. *Biochim. biophys. Acta*, 345: 468–473.

Hubbell, W.L. and Bownds, M.D. (1979) Visual transduction in vertebrate photoreceptors. *Annu. Rev. Neurosci.*, 2: 17–34.

Hubbell, W.L. and Fung, B.K.-K. (1978) The structure and chemistry of rhodopsin: relationship to models of function. In *Membrane Transduction Mechanisms*, R.A. Cone and J. Dowling (Eds.), Raven Press, New York, pp. 17–25.

Hubbell, W.L., Fung, B., Chen, Y. and Hong, K. (1977) Molecular anatomy and light-dependent processes in photoreceptor membranes. In *Vertebrate Photoreception*, H.B. Barlow and P. Fatt (Eds.), Academic Press, London, pp. 41–59.

Hurley, J.B. and Ebrey, T.G. (1979) Regulation of rod outer segment phosphodiesterase. *Biophysics*, 25: 314a.

Jan, L.Y. and Revel, J.-P. (1974) Ultrastructural localization of rhodopsin in the vertebrate retina. *J. Cell Biol.*, 62: 257–273.

Kaupp, U.B. and Jung, W. (1977) Rapid calcium release by passively loaded retinal discs on photoexcitation. *FEBS Lett.*, 81: 229–232.

444

Kawamura, S. and Bownds, M.D. (1981) Light adaptation of the cyclic GMP phosphodiesterase of frog photoreceptor membranes mediated by ATP and calcium ions. *J. gen. Physiol.*, 77: 571–591.

Kilbride, P. and Ebrey, T.G. (1979) Light initiated changes of cyclic GMP levels in the frog retina measured with quick freezing techniques. *J. gen. Physiol.*, 74: 415–426.

Krishna, G., Krishnan, N., Fletcher, R.T. and Chader, G. (1976) Effects of light on cyclic GMP metabolism in retinal photoreceptors. *J. Neurochem.*, 27: 717–722.

Kühn, H. (1974) Light dependent phosphorylation of rhodopsin in living frogs. *Nature (Lond.)*, 250: 588–592.

Kühn, H. (1978) Light-regulated binding of rhodopsin kinase and other proteins to cattle photoreceptor membranes. *Biochemistry*, 17: 4389–4395.

Kühn, H. (1980) Light- and GTP-regulated interaction of GTPase and other proteins with bovine photoreceptor membranes. *Nature (Lond.)*, 283: 587–589.

Kühn, H. and Bader, S. (1976) The rate of rhodopsin phosphorylation in isolated retinas of frog and cattle. *Biochim. biophys. Acta*, 428: 13–18.

Kühn, H. and Dreyer, W.J. (1972) Light-dependent phosphorylation of rhodopsin by ATP. *FEBS Lett.*, 20: 1–6.

Kühn, H. and McDowell, J.H. (1977) Isoelectric focusing of phosphorylated cattle rhodopsin. *Biophys. Struct. Mech.*, 3: 199–203.

Kühn, H., Cook, J.H. and Dreyer, W.J. (1973) Phosphorylation of rhodopsin in bovine photoreceptor membranes: a dark reaction after illumination. *Biochemistry*, 12: 2495–2502.

Kühn, H., McDowell, J.H., Leser, K.H. and Bader, S. (1977) Phosphorylation of rhodopsin as a possible mechanism of adaptation. *Biophys. Struct. Mech.*, 3: 175–180.

Liebman, P.A. (1974) Light-dependent $Ca^{++}$ content of rod outer segment disk membranes. *Invest. Ophthalmol.*, 13: 700–701.

Liebman, P.A. and Pugh Jr., E.N. (1979) The control of phosphodiesterase in rod disk membranes — kinetics, possible mechanisms and significance for vision. *Vision Res.*, 19: 375–380.

Liebman, P.A. and Pugh Jr., E.N. (1980) ATP mediates rapid reversal of cyclic GMP phosphodiesterase activation in visual receptor membranes. *Nature (Lond.)*, 287: 734–736.

Lipton, S.A., Ostroy, S.E. and Dowling, J.E. (1977a) Electrical and adaptive properties of rod photoreceptors in *Bufo marinus*. I. Effects of altered extracellular $Ca^{2+}$ levels. *J. gen. Physiol.*, 70: 747–770.

Lipton, S.A., Rasmussen, H. and Dowling, J.E. (1977b) Electrical and adaptive properties of rod photoreceptors in *Bufo marinus*. II. Effects of cyclic nucleotides and prostaglandins. *J. gen. Physiol.*, 70: 771–791.

Lolley, R.N. and Racz, E. (1981) Calcium regulation of receptor guanylate cyclase activity. *Invest. Ophthalmol. visual Sci.*, 20, Suppl.: 210.

Lolley, R.N., Brown, B.M. and Farber, D.B. (1977) Protein phosphorylation in rod outer segments from bovine retina: cyclic nucleotide-activated protein kinase and its endogenous substrate. *Biochem. biophys. Res. Commun.*, 78: 572–578.

Lolley, R.N., Racz, E. and Farber, D.B. (1979) Recovery of retinal cyclic GMP content after light or drug treatment. *Invest. Ophthalmol. visual Sci.*, 18, Suppl.: 21.

Miki, N., Keirns, J.J., Marcus, F.R., Freeman, J. and Bitensky, M.W. (1973) Regulation of cyclic nucleotide concentrations in photoreceptors: An ATP-dependent stimulation of cyclic nucleotide phosphodiesterase by light. *Proc. nat. Acad. Sci. (Wash.)*, 70: 3820–3824.

Miller, W.H. and Nicol, G.D. (1979) Evidence that cyclic GMP regulates membrane potential in rod photoreceptors. *Nature (Lond.)*, 280: 64–66.

Miller, J.A. and Paulsen, R. (1975) Phosphorylation and dephosphorylation of frog rod outer segment membranes as part of the visual process. *J. biol. Chem.*, 250: 4427–4432.

Miller, J.A., Paulsen, R. and Bownds, M.D. (1977) Control of light-activated phosphorylation in frog photoreceptor membranes. *Biochemistry*, 16: 2633–2639.

Nathanson, J.A. (1977) Cyclic nucleotides and nervous system function. *Physiol. Rev.*, 57: 157–256.

Nicol, G.D. and Miller, W.H. (1978) Cyclic GMP injected into retinal rod outer segments increases latency and amplitude of response to illumination. *Proc. nat. Acad. Sci. (Wash.)*, 75: 5217–5220.

Orr, H.T., Lowry, O.H., Cohen, A.I. and Ferrendelli, J.A. (1976) Distribution of 3′:5′-cyclic AMP and 3′:5′-cyclic GMP in rabbit retina in vivo: Selective effects of dark and light adaptation and ischemia. *Proc. nat. Acad. Sci. (Wash.)*, 73: 4442–4445.

Pannbacker, R.G. (1973a) Control of guanylate cyclase activity in the rod outer segment. *Science*, 182: 1138–1140.

Pannbacker, R.G. (1973b) Protein kinases and protein phosphorylation in the rod outer segment. In *Prostaglandins and Cyclic AMP*, R.H. Kahn and W.E. Lands (Eds.), Academic Press, New York, pp. 251–252.

Pannbacker, R.G. (1974) Cyclic nucleotide metabolism in human photoreceptors. *Invest. Ophthalmol.*, 13: 535–538.

Pannbacker, R.G., Fleischman, D.E. and Reed, D.W. (1972) Cyclic nucleotide phosphodiesterase: High activity in a mammalian photoreceptor. *Science*, 175: 757–758.

Polans, A.S., Hermolin, J. and Bownds, M.D. (1979) Light-induced dephosphorylation of two proteins in frog rod outer segments. Influence of cyclic nucleotides and calcium. *J. gen. Physiol.*, 74: 595–613.

Robinson, P.R., Kawamura, S., Abramson, D. and Bownds, M.D. (1980) Control of the cyclic GMP phosphodiesterase of frog photoreceptor membranes. *J. gen. Physiol.*, 76: 631–645.

Robinson, W.E. and Hagins, W.A. (1977) A light-activated GTPase in retinal rod outer segments. *Biophys. J.*, 17: 196a.

Rölich, P. (1976) Photoreceptor membrane carbohydrate on the intradiscal surface of retinal rod disks. *Nature (Lond.)*, 263: 789–791.

Saibil, H., Chabre, M. and Worcester, D. (1976) Neutron diffraction studies of retinal rod outer segment membranes. *Nature (Lond.)*, 262: 266–270.

Sale, G.J., Towner, P. and Akhtar, M. (1978) Topography of the rhodopsin molecule. Identification of the domain phosphorylated. *Biochem. J.*, 175: 421–430.

Shichi, H. and Somers, R.L. (1978) Light-dependent phosphorylation of rhodopsin. Purification and properties of rhodopsin kinase. *J. biol. Chem.*, 253: 7040–7046.

Shinozawa, T., Uchida, S., Martin, E., Cafiso, D., Hubbell, H. and Bitensky, M. (1980) Additional component required for activity and reconstitution of light-activated vertebrate photoreceptor GTPase. *Proc. nat. Acad. Sci. (Wash.)*, 77: 1408–1411.

Sitaramayya, A., Virmaux, N. and Mandel, P. (1977) On a soluble system for studying light activation of rod outer segment cyclic GMP phosphodiesterase. *Neurochem. Res.*, 2: 1–10.

Smith, H.G., Fager, R.S. and Litman, B. (1977) Light-activated calcium release from sonicated bovine retinal rod outer segment disks. *Biochemistry*, 16: 1399–1405.

Sorbi, R.T. and Cavaggioni, A. (1975) Effect of strong illumination on the ion efflux from the isolated discs of frog photoreceptors. *Biochim. biophys. Acta*, 394: 577–585.

Szuts, E.Z. and Cone, R.A. (1977) Calcium content of frog rod outer segments and discs. *Biochim. biophys. Acta*, 468: 194–208.

Wald, G. (1968) Molecular basis of visual excitation. *Science*, 162: 230–239.

Weller, M., Virmaux, N. and Mandel, P. (1975a) Light-stimulated phosphorylation of rhodopsin in the retina: The presence of a protein kinase that is specific for photobleached rhodopsin. *Proc. nat. Acad. Sci. (Wash.)*, 72: 381–385.

Weller, M., Virmaux, N. and Mandel, P. (1975b) Role of light and rhodopsin phosphorylation in control of permeability of retinal rod outer segment discs to $Ca^{++}$. *Nature (Lond.)*, 256: 68–70.

Weller, M., Goridis, C., Virmaux, N. and Mandel, P. (1975c) Hypothetical model for possible involvement of rhodopsin phosphorylation in light and dark adaptation in retina. *Exp. Eye Res.*, 21: 405–408.

Weller, M., Virmaux, N. and Mandel, P. (1976) The relative specificity of opsin kinase towards ATP and GTP and the lack of effect of cyclic nucleotides on the activity of the enzyme. *Exp. Eye Res.*, 23: 65–67.

Werblin, F.S. (1974) Organization of the vertebrate retina: Receptive fields and sensitivity control. In *The Eye*, Vol. 6, H. Davson and L.T. Graham Jr. (Eds.), Academic Press, New York, pp. 257–281.

Wheeler, G.L. and Bitensky, M.W. (1977) A light-activated GTPase in vertebrate photoreceptors: Regulation of light-activated cyclic GMP phosphodiesterase. *Proc. nat. Acad. Sci. (Wash.)*, 74: 4238–4242.

Woodruff, M.L. and Bownds, M.D. (1979) Amplitude, kinetics, and reversibility of a light-induced decrease in guanosine 3',5'-cyclic monophosphate in frog photoreceptor membranes. *J. gen. Physiol.*, 73: 629–653.

Woodruff, M.L., Bownds, D., Green, S.H., Morrisey, J.L. and Shedlovsky, A. (1977) Guanosine 3',5'-cyclic monophosphate and the in vitro physiology of frog photoreceptor membranes. *J. gen. Physiol.*, 69: 667–679.

Yee, R. and Liebman, P.A. (1978) Light-activated phosphodiesterase of the rod outer segment. Kinetics and parameters of activation and deactivation. *J. biol. Chem.*, 253: 8902–8909.

# Author Index

# Subject Index

454